Derby Hospitals NHS Foundation
Trust
Library and Knowledge Service

D1766224

Derby Hospitals NHS Foundation
Trust
Library and Knowledge Service

Pulmonary Rehabilitation

Pulmonary Rehabilitation

Edited by

Claudio F. Donner MD
Head, Division of Pulmonary Disease, Fondazione Salvatore
Maugeri, IRCCS, Veruno, Italy

Nicolino Ambrosino MD
Head, Pulmonary Division, Cardio-Thoracic Department,
Azienda Ospedaliera-Universitaria Pisana, Cisanello, Pisa, Italy

Roger Goldstein FRCP(c)
Professor of Medicine and Physical Therapy,
University of Toronto, West Park Hospital, Toronto,
Ontario, Canada

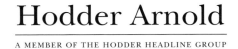

Hodder Arnold

A MEMBER OF THE HODDER HEADLINE GROUP

First published in Great Britain in 2005 by
Hodder Education, a member of the Hodder Headline Group,
338 Euston Road, London NW1 3BH

http://www.hoddereducation.com

Distributed in the United States of America by
Oxford University Press Inc.,
198 Madison Avenue, New York, NY10016
Oxford is a registered trademark of Oxford University Press

© 2005 Edward Arnold

All rights reserved. Apart from any use permitted under UK copyright law,
this publication may only be reproduced, stored or transmitted, in any form,
or by any means with prior permission in writing of the publishers or in the
case of reprographic production in accordance with the terms of licences
issued by the Copyright Licensing Agency. In the United Kingdom such
licences are issued by the Copyright Licensing Agency: 90 Tottenham
Court Road, London W1T 4LP.

Whilst the advice and information in this book are believed to be true and
accurate at the date of going to press, neither the author[s] nor the publisher
can accept any legal responsibility or liability for any errors or omissions
that may be made. In particular, (but without limiting the generality of the
preceding disclaimer) every effort has been made to check drug dosages;
however it is still possible that errors have been missed. Furthermore,
dosage schedules are constantly being revised and new side-effects
recognized. For these reasons the reader is strongly urged to consult the
drug companies' printed instructions before administering any of the drugs
recommended in this book.

British Library Cataloguing in Publication Data
A catalogue record for this book is available from the British Library

Library of Congress Cataloging-in-Publication Data
A catalog record for this book is available from the Library of Congress

ISBN-10:   0 340 810173
ISBN-13:   978 0 340 81017 0

1 2 3 4 5 6 7 8 9 10

Commissioning Editor: Joanna Koster
Development Editor: Sarah Burrows
Project Editor: Naomi Wilkinson
Production Controller: Lindsay Smith
Cover Design: Sarah Rees
Cover Photographs: Elderly woman receiving lung function test (Henny Allis/Science Photo Library);
Measuring maximum oxygen uptake during exercise (St Bartholomew's Hospital/Science Photo Library)

Typeset in 10/12 pt Minion by Charon Tec Pvt. Ltd, Chennai, India
Printed and bound in Great Britain by CPI Bath

What do you think about this book? Or any other Hodder Arnold title?
Please visit our website at www.hoddereducation.com

Contents

Contributors

Nicolino Ambrosino
Head, Pulmonary Division
Cardio-Thoracic Department
Azienda Ospedaliera-Universitaria Pisana
Pisa, Italy

Lorenzo Appendini MD
Division of Pulmonary Disease
Fondazione Salvatore Maugeri, IRCCS
Istituto Scientifico di Veruno
Veruno, Italy

Monica Avendaño MD
West Park Hospital
University of Toronto
Toronto, Canada

John R. Bach MD
Department of Physical Medicine and Rehabilitation
UMDNJ – New Jersey Medical School
Newark, NY, USA

Luca Bianchi MD
Department of Respiratory Medicine and Rehabilitation
Fondazione Salvatore Maugeri, IRCCS
Istituto Scientifico di Gussago
Gussago, Italy

Jean Bourbeau MD MSc FRCPC
Respiratory Division, Department of Medicine
McGill University Health Centre
Montreal, Quebec, Canada

Alberto Braghiroli MD
Division of Pulmonary Disease
Fondazione Salvatore Maugeri, IRCCS
Istituto Scientifico di Veruno
Veruno, Italy

Rachel A. Brown PhD
The Sackler Institute of Pulmonary Pharmacology
GKT School of Biomedical Science and Medicine
King's College London
London, UK

Kai-Håkon Carlsen MD PhD
Professor of Paediatric Allergology and Respiratory Medicine
University of Oslo; and
Professor of Sport Medicine
Norwegian University of Sport and Physical Education
Norway

Mauro Carone MD
Division of Pulmonary Disease
Fondazione Salvatore Maugeri, IRCCS
Istituto Scientifico di Veruno
Veruno, Italy

Richard Casaburi PhD MD
Chief, Division of Respiratory and Critical Care Physiology and Medicine
Harbor-UCLA Research and Education Institute
Torrance, CA, USA

Bartolome R. Celli MD
Tufts University School of Medicine
Boston, USA

Gerard J. Criner MD
Professor of Medicine
Director, Pulmonary and Critical Care Medicine
Temple University School of Medicine
Temple Lung Center
Philadelphia, PA, USA

Marc Decramer MD PhD
Pulmonary Rehabilitation (Respiratory Division)
UZ Gasthuisberg
Leuven, Belgium

Claudio F. Donner MD
Division of Pulmonary Disease
Fondazione Salvatore Maugeri, IRCCS
Istituto Scientifico di Veruno
Veruno, Italy

Sarah L. Elkin
Consultant Respiratory Physician
Department of Cystic Fibrosis
Royal Brompton & Harefield NHS Trust
London, UK

Karl Olov Fagerström
Fagerström Consulting and
Smokers Information Center
Helsingborg, Sweden

Bonnie F. Fahy RN MN
Pulmonary Clinical Nurse Specialist
Pulmonary Rehabilitation Coordinator
St. Joseph's Hospital and Medical Center
Phoenix, AZ, USA

Katia Foglio MD
Department of Respiratory Medicine and Rehabilitation
Fondazione Salvatore Maugeri, IRCCS
Istituto Scientifico di Gussago
Gussago, Italy

Steven E. Gay MD MS
Division of Pulmonary and Critical Care Medicine
University of Michigan Health System
Ann Arbor, MI, USA

Allen I. Goldberg MD MBA Master FCCP
Past President,
American College of Chest Physicians

Roger S. Goldstein FRCP(C)
Professor of Medicine and Physical Therapy
University of Toronto
West Park Hospital
Toronto, Ontario, Canada

Rik Gosselink PT PhD
Respiratory Division
Universitaire Zeikenhuizen Leuven
Department of Rehabilitation Services
Katholieke Universitat Leuven, Belgium

Timothy L. Griffiths PhD FRCP
Senior Lecturer in Respiratory Medicine
University of Wales College of Medicine
Llandough Hospital
Penarth, Vale of Glamorgan, UK

Marta Gudjónsdóttir PhD
Reykjalundur Rehabilitation Centre
Mosfellsbaer, Iceland

Gordon H. Guyatt MD MSc
Department of Clinical Epidemiology and Biostatistics
McMaster University and Health Sciences Center
Hamilton, Ontario, Canada

Khin M. Gyi MRCP
Consultant Physician
Royal Brompton Hospital & Harefield NHS Trust
London, UK

Paul Hernandez MDCM FRCPC
Medical Director and Respirologist
Pulmonary Rehabilitation Program
QEII Health Sciences Centre
Associate Professor of Medicine
Dalhousie University
Halifax, NS, Canada

Rick V. Hodder MD FRCPC
Professor of Medicine
University of Ottawa
Respirologist and Chief, Department of Critical Care
The Ottawa Hospital
Ottawa, Canada

Margaret E. Hodson MD MSc FRCP DA
Professor of Respiratory Medicine
Department of Cystic Fibrosis
Royal Brompton & Harefield NHS Trust
London, UK

Paul W. Jones MD
Professor, Division of Physiological Medicine
St George's Hospital Medical School
London, UK

Ulrick Keil
Department of Cardiology
University of Münster
Münster, Germany

Yves Lacasse MD
Centre de Recherche, Hôpital Laval
Institut Universitaire de Cardiologie et de Pneumologie
Université Laval
Québec, Canada

Suzanne C. Lareau RN MS
Clinical Educator, Instructor of Nursing
University of New Mexico
College of Nursing
USA

Mirco Lusuardi MD
Director, Cardio-Pulmonary Rehabilitation Programme
San Sebastiano Hospital
Correggio, Italy

Donald A. Mahler MD
Section of Pulmonary and Critical Care Medicine
Dartmouth-Hitchcock Medical Center
Lebanon, USA

Barry J. Make MD
Director, Emphysema & Pulmonary Rehabilitation
National Jewish Center for Immunology & Respiratory Medicine
Denver, CO, USA

François Maltais MD
Respirologist
Centre de Pneumologie
Hôpital Laval
Professor
Department of Medicine
Université Laval
Quèbec, Canada

Ubaldo Martin MD
Pulmonary and Critical Care Medicine
Temple University School of Medicine
Temple Lung Center
Philadelphia, PA, USA

F. J. Martinez MD
Division of Pulmonary and Critical Care Medicine
University of Michigan Medical Center
Ann Arbor, MI, USA

Walter T. McNicholas MD FRCP
Newman Professor
Department of Respiratory Medicine
University College Dublin
Dublin, Ireland

Michael D. L. Morgan MD
Consultant Physician
Department of Respiratory Medicine and Thoracic Surgery
Glenfield Hospital
University Hospitals of Leicester
Leicester, UK

Stefano Nardini
Chief, Pulmonary Division
Ospedale di Vittorio Veneto
Vittorio Veneto, Italy

Matthew T. Naughton MBBS MD FRACP
Associate Professor
Medical Faculty
Monash Univerity
Australia

Stefano Nava MD
Professor of Medicine
Clinica Del Lavoro e della Riabilitazione
Fondazione Salvatore Maugeri, IRCCS
Istituto Scientifico di Pavia
Pavia, Italy

Denis E. O'Donnell MD FRCPI FRCPC
Division of Respiratory & Critical Care Medicine
Department of Medicine
Queen's University
Kingston, Ontario, Canada

C. P. Page
The Sackler Institute of Pulmonary Pharmacology
GKT School of Biomedical Science and Medicine
King's College London
London, UK

Antonio Patessio MD
Division of Pulmonary Diseases
Fondazione Salvatore Maugeri, IRCCS
Istituto Scientifico di Veruno
Veruno, Italy

Victor Pinto-Plata MD
Tufts University School of Medicine
Boston, MA, USA

Fabio Pitta PT MSc
Department of Rehabilitation Sciences
Katholieke Universiteit Leuven
Belgium

Stephen I. Rennard MD
University of Nebraska Medical Center
Omaha, NE, USA

Andrew L. Ries MD MPH
Professor of Medicine and Family & Preventive Medicine
University of California
San Diego, CA, USA

Dominique Robert MD
Professor of Medicine, University Claude Bernard; Chief of the
Department of Intensive Care and Emergency Medicine; and
President of the Association Lyonnaise de Logistique Post
Hospitalière
Lyon, France

Josep Roca
Servei di Pneumologia
Hospital Clínic
Villarroel 170
Barcelona, Spain

Graham Rocker MA MHSc DM FRCP FRcPc
Respirologist
QEII Health Sciences Centre
Professor of Medicine
Dalhousie University
Halifax, NS, Canada

Andrea Rossi MD
Responsabile, UO Pneumologia
"Ospedali Riuniti di Bergamo"
Azienda Oispedaliera
Bergamo, Italy

Didier Saey PhT MSc
Hopital Laval
Québec, Canada

Andrew Sandford PhD
Assistant Professor
University of British Columbia
McDonald Research Wing/iCAPTURE Center
St Paul's Hospital
Vancouver, Canada

Annemie M. W. J. Schols MD
Department of Pulmonology
Maastricht University
Maastricht, The Netherlands

Holger Schünemann MD PhD
State University of New York at Buffalo, NY; and
McMaster University, Hamilton, Canada

John M. Shneerson MA DM FRCP
Consultant Physician
Director, Respiratory Support and Sleep Centre
Papworth Hospital NHS Trust
Cambridge, UK

Sally J. Singh PhD
Consultant Clinical Scientist
Department of Respiratory Medicine and Thoracic Surgery
Glenfield Hospital
University Hospitals of Leicester
Leicester, UK

Judith Soicher MSc
Respiratory Epidemiology and Clinical Research Unit
Montreal Chest Institute of the Royal Victoria Hospital
McGill University Health Centre
Toronto, Canada

Brian L. Tiep MD
Medical Director
Respiratory Disease Management Institute
Irwindale, CA, USA

Thierry Troosters PT PhD
Postdoctoral Fellow FWO-Vlaanderen
Pulmonary Rehabilitation (Respiratory Division)
UZ Gasthuisberg
Leuven, Belgium

Michele Vitacca MD
Division of Pulmonary Diseases
Fondazione Salvatore Maugeri, IRCCS
Istituto Scientifico di Gussago
Gussago, Italy

Nha Voduc MD FRCPC
Division of Respiratory & Critical Care Medicine
Department of Medicine
Queen's University
Kingston, Ontario, Canada

Katherine Webb MSc
Division of Respiratory & Critical Care Medicine
Department of Medicine
Queen's University
Kingston, Ontario, Canada

Peter J. Wijkstra MD
Department of Pulmonary Diseases
University Hospital Groningen
Groningen, The Netherlands

Emiel Wouters
Department of Pulmonology
University Hospital Maastricht
Maastricht, The Netherlands

N. Zamel MD
Department of Medicine
University of Toronto
Toronto, Canada

Richard ZuWallack MD
St Francis Hospital
Hartford, CT, USA

Foreword

The art and practice of pulmonary rehabilitation finds its roots in the tuberculosis era, beginning in the late 1800s. Following imposed bed rest, those who recovered with various stages of pulmonary insufficiency, and in a state of poor physical condition, learned that daily walks relieved dyspnoea, stimulated appetite and enhanced sleep and a feeling of well being. Early leaders including Albert Haas and Alvan Barach became champions of pulmonary rehabilitation in the mid 1900s. They had little scientific evidence of benefit, but as astute observers, became convinced that PR had a lot to offer.

The advent of ambulatory oxygen stimulated the Denver group to start a pilot pulmonary rehabilitation programme in the mid 1960s. This was the first organized programme that offered physiologic evidence of improvement and global functioning such as walk tolerance. Many more formal studies proving the scientific value of PR followed as pioneered by Andrew Ries, Roger Goldstein and Mary Burns, amongst many others. PR was the standard of care comparison for lung volume reduction therapy as conducted in the NETT. Thus, today, PR is established as the standard of care for many patients with chronic respiratory insufficiency, often due to COPD, interstitial fibrosis, cystic fibrosis, kyphoscoliosis and fibrotic residuals of tuberculosis and other infectious diseases of the lungs. The techniques of exercise training, the use of ambulatory oxygen, breathing training, nutritional support, and spiritual encouragement are principles that will aid many in their goals of living longer and better lives with chronic respiratory insufficiency. The authors of this new book are to be congratulated on taking a fresh approach to transferring knowledge about PR, but wisely adhere to the sound foundations, for PR, that were well established by our predecessors.

Thomas L. Petty
Denver, CO, USA

Preface

Chronic obstructive pulmonary disease (COPD) is the most widespread non-communicable respiratory disease in the world. It is also one of the major causes of morbidity worldwide and the only cause of mortality whose incidence continues to rise. Although COPD has been recognized by the World Health Organization as a major public health problem, governments and health authorities are only just beginning to acknowledge its impact on society. By 2020, COPD will rank fifth, globally, as a cause of disability, and third as cause of mortality.

In the last decade, important advances in our understanding of the primary and secondary impairments associated with chronic respiratory diseases have led to a better appreciation of the role of pulmonary rehabilitation as an integral part of disease management. Randomized controlled trials, using valid, reproducible and interpretable outcome measures, have provided sufficient evidence of effectiveness for pulmonary rehabilitation to be endorsed by professional societies around the world. This recognition appears increasingly in the form of international statements, such as the joint European Respiratory Society and American Thoracic Society 2005 "Statement on Pulmonary Rehabilitation".

Pulmonary rehabilitation programmes are included, as the prevailing standard of care, in the clinical management of patients with chronic respiratory diseases. Ongoing advances in basic and clinical research are helping to better define the components and likely outcomes associated with this treatment modality.

This textbook provides a detailed review of the major aspects of pulmonary rehabilitation, taken from recent, peer-reviewed reports, which have contributed to its establishment as a scientific discipline. The major goal of the book is to provide those interested in this area with useful tools that will help them to establish and evaluate a programme of pulmonary rehabilitation. Contributing authors have been asked to include specific outcome measures, whenever possible, and to identify key articles in support of their conclusions.

Pulmonary rehabilitation involves integrating health care habits into the lifelong management of patients with chronic respiratory disease. Systemic manifestations (secondary impairments) are often more amenable to treatment than the damaged airways and lung parenchyma (primary impairment). To be successful, rehabilitation requires a dynamic collaboration between the patient, the family and the health care providers.

Each chapter addresses a different aspect of what becomes a comprehensive strategy for pulmonary rehabilitation, aimed at improving functional exercise capacity and health-related quality of life as well as reducing the health care resources required per patient. The authors have condensed an enormous amount of literature, drawn mainly from the last decade, to provide the best possible support to clinical practice for health care providers working in the challenging field of pulmonary rehabilitation. We hope that readers will find this area of health care as rewarding to their patients and themselves as we, the editors, have.

Claudio F. Donner
Nicolino Ambrosino
Roger Goldstein

The foundations of pulmonary rehabilitation

Definition and rationale for pulmonary rehabilitation

M. LUSUARDI, N. AMBROSINO, C. F. DONNER

SUMMARY

Pulmonary rehabilitation can be traced back to medical textbooks of a century ago, when the prevalence of respiratory disorders was very different from today. Pneumonia and tuberculosis were the main lung disorders. Rehabilitation was confined to kinesiotherapy, but the concepts of improving oxygenation and functional exercise capacity were clearly expressed (1). It was 50 years ago that pulmonary rehabilitation (PR) began to be systematically applied, by Dr Alvin Barach, who was the first person to apply positive pressure mechanical ventilation in the 1940s and the first to administer oxygen during exercise in the 1950s, using an ambulatory small cylinder (2). At around the same time, oxygen-supported exercise began to be applied in England by Cotes and Gilson (3).

In 1948 the World Health Organization (WHO) adopted a definition of health as 'a state of complete physical, mental and social well-being rather than the absence of disease or infirmity' (4).

We searched PubMed (5) for review papers and clinical trials with the terms 'respiratory or pulmonary rehabilitation' among key words (without language limitation) from 1940 to 2003 (Table 1.1). We noted a progressive increase in the number of articles from six reviews and two clinical trials in the 1960s, to 271 reviews and 285 clinical trials in the 1990s, demonstrating the recent interest in PR. Since the International Year of Disabled Persons (1981) there have been significant changes in the concepts of disability and rehabilitation that have undoubtedly spurred the development of PR. Since then, the traditional medical model of disability has incorporated social aspects such as limited participation in school, work and social activities. These limitations are now viewed as resulting from societal barriers to their participation. The rights of individuals with disabilities to enjoy the same opportunities as others in their communities and society are now well recognized, but there are still many disabled people who do not have equal opportunities to health care or rehabilitation services (6).

The steep increase in clinical trials in the 1990s (Table 1.1) reflects both the large increase in patients with chronic respiratory conditions being referred for rehabilitation and the establishment of a more scientific basis for PR, especially well designed trials with valid, responsive and interpretable outcome measures. This is in keeping with the movement towards testing the efficacy and the effectiveness of multidisciplinary medical and surgical management in the clinical setting (7, 8).

Other factors that have promoted the growth of PR include the accessibility of simple instruments, such as spirometers, to assist physicians in diagnosing and stratifying

Table 1.1   *Number of review and clinical trial papers with the terms respiratory or pulmonary rehabilitation among key words in the PubMed in the decades 1940–1999 and in the period 2000–2003*

	1940–49	1950–59	1960–69	1970–79	1980–89	1990–99	2000–03
Reviews	0	0	6	34	80	271	153
Clinical trials	0	0	2	15	57	285	155

Box 1.1   Definitions of pulmonary rehabilitation

Pulmonary Rehabilitation Committee of the American College of Chest Physicians (ACCP), 1974; American Thoracic Society (ATS), 1981 (10)

Pulmonary rehabilitation is an art of medical practice wherein an individually tailored, multidisciplinary program is formulated which, through accurate diagnosis, therapy, emotional support and education, stabilizes or reverses both the physio- and psychopathology of pulmonary diseases and attempts to return the patient to the highest possible capacity allowed by his pulmonary handicap and overall life situation.

European Respiratory Society (ERS) Rehabilitation and Chronic Care Scientific Group, 1992 (11)

Pulmonary rehabilitation aims to restore patients to an independent, productive and satisfying life and prevent further clinical deterioration to the maximum extent compatible with the stage of the disease.

National Institutes of Health (NIH), 1994 (14)

Pulmonary rehabilitation is a multidimensional continuum of services directed to persons with pulmonary disease and their families, usually by an interdisciplinary team of specialists, with the goal of achieving and maintaining the individual's maximum level of independence and functioning in the community.

European Respiratory Society, 1997 (15)

Pulmonary rehabilitation is a process which systematically uses scientifically based diagnostic management and evaluation options to achieve the optimal daily functioning and health-related quality of life of individual patients suffering from impairment and disability due to chronic respiratory disease, as measured by clinically and/or physiologically relevant outcome measures.

Joint ACCP/AACVPR (American Association of Cardiovascular and Pulmonary Rehabilitation) Evidence-Based Guidelines, 1997 (16)

- Pulmonary rehabilitation is a well established and widely accepted therapeutic tool that improves the quality of life and functional capacity of chronic lung disease patients.
- Used in conjunction with standard medical therapy for chronic lung disease, pulmonary rehabilitation can alleviate symptoms and optimize a patient's physical and psychological functioning.
- Pulmonary rehabilitation is appropriate for any patient with stable chronic respiratory disease and severe or disabling dyspnoea on exertion.
- The primary goal of pulmonary rehabilitation is to restore the chronic lung disease patient to the highest possible level of independent function.

British Thoracic Society (BTS) guidelines for the management of COPD 1997 (17)

The restoration of the individual to the fullest medical, mental, emotional, social and vocational potential of which he/she is capable.

American Thoracic Society, 1999 (18)

Pulmonary rehabilitation is a multidisciplinary program of care for patients with chronic respiratory impairment that is individually tailored and designed to optimize physical and social performance and autonomy.

Italian Association of Hospital Pneumologists (AIPO), 2001 (20)

Long-term assessment and management of patients with chronic respiratory failure.

American Association for Respiratory Care (AARC) Clinical Practice Guideline on Pulmonary Rehabilitation, 2002 (19)

Pulmonary rehabilitation is a restorative and preventive process for patients with chronic respiratory disease.

Description/definition
Pulmonary rehabilitation (PR) has been defined as a 'multidisciplinary program of care for patients with chronic respiratory impairment that is individually tailored and designed to optimize physical and social performance and autonomy'.

chronic respiratory disease as well as simple measures (6-min walking test, shuttle walk test), to assess disability in the PR setting (9). For some patients, technical enhancements with devices for long-term oxygen therapy or non-invasive ventilation have improved health-related quality of life and, in some instances, survival. We have therefore included such devices as integral components of PR.

DEFINITIONS

The first authoritative statement on PR from the American College of Chest Physicians (ACCP) and the American Thoracic Society (ATS) in 1974 introduced PR as an art, according to a definition published a few years later in the *American Review of Respiratory Diseases* (Box 1.1) (10). Although in this definition a scientific foundation for PR was not explicitly stated, three important features of PR were highlighted: individualization, multidisciplinarity and attention to the different components of the disease and their impact on daily life. Since the 1981 ACCP/ATS statement, the clinical effectiveness and scientific foundation of PR have been firmly established.

In 1992, the European Respiratory Society (ERS) integrated in the definition the concept that aspects of PR can influence disease progression. Smoking cessation and long-term oxygen therapy are the only two components of PR that influence the natural history of chronic obstructive pulmonary disease (COPD) (11–13).

The definition adopted in the US (National Institutes of Health) in 1994 provided a comprehensive view of PR as a multidimensional continuum of services for the patient and the family supplied by an integrated team of specialists in complementary disciplines, having as a goal the independent living and functioning of the patient within society (14).

In 1997 the definitions of both the European Respiratory Society (ERS) and the ACCP/American Association of Cardiovascular and Pulmonary Rehabilitation (AACVPR) stressed the need for an evidence-based understanding of the components of PR as well as the need for functional as well as health status outcomes (15, 16). In the same year the British Thoracic Society (BTS), in its guidelines for the management of COPD, defined PR as a restoration of the best possible physiological, psychological and social potentials for the individual, quoting the ATS definition of 1981 (17).

In 1999, the ATS emphasized the three traditional attributes of PR (patient individuality, the use of a multidisciplinary approach and the optimization of physical and social autonomy) (18). In 2002 the American Association for Respiratory Care (AARC) added that PR should be both restorative and preventive (19).

In 2001, the Italian Association of Hospital Pneumologists (AIPO) adopted (20) a much simplified definition of rehabilitation, which included patients with chronic respiratory failure (CRF) in need of lifelong management. It reflected the rationale for PR expressed by the ERS in 1997 as 'a process of patient management required to systematically apply all existing treatment options available for the widest possible range of patients with chronic lung disease' (15) and also softened the distinction between traditional routine clinical care and pulmonary rehabilitation. The chest physician in charge of the patient would perform both activities, but what could change would be the organization and the location of the intervention.

In the AIPO definition, management of end-stage lung disease is implicit. Hence the field of rehabilitation extends to palliative care of the very severe respiratory patient. One reason for this is that, with the resurgence of surgical treatments such as lung transplantation and lung volume reduction, the role of pre- and postoperative rehabilitation has become crucial.

In summary, the main points in common among the various definitions of pulmonary rehabilitation include:

- focus on chronic respiratory patients and their care-givers
- individualization of the programme
- an ongoing multidisciplinary intervention
- outcomes based on physiological, psychological and social measures that consider a global dimension to the individual's health.

GOALS OF PULMONARY REHABILITATION

In view of the irreversible nature of the underlying damage to the respiratory system, the primary goals of PR are to control symptoms, especially dyspnoea, improve functional capacity (mainly exercise performance) and enhance health status.

Rationale

The rationale for pulmonary rehabilitation may be 'patient-centred', based on the respiratory condition as it affects the individual, or 'society-centred', based on disease epidemiology and the societal costs.

PATIENT–CENTRED RATIONALE

Do chronic respiratory patients need rehabilitation?

Stable or intermittent impairment of respiratory function of moderate to severe degree leads to significant disability, i.e. inability to cope with the usual tasks of daily life. Dyspnoea is the main factor, but cough, muscle weakness and fatigue also play a role. Handicap is a consequence to the individual as a result of a combination of physiological, psychological and social factors. The three 'historical' disease dimensions of impairment, disability and handicap, as defined by the WHO in 1980, are given in Box 1.2.

The International Classification of Impairments, Disabilities and Handicaps (ICIDH) was first published by the WHO in 1980. The revised ICIDH-2 has been available in its final form since May 2001. The revision process resulted in a change of name to 'The International Classification of Functioning, Disability and Health'. This new name is accompanied by a change of emphasis from negative descriptions of impairments, disabilities and handicaps to neutral descriptions of body

---

Box 1.2   Definitions of disease dimensions according to the WHO, 1980[a]

- Impairment – any loss or abnormality of psychological, physiological or anatomical structure or function resulting from disease
- Disability – restriction or lack, resulting from an impairment of ability to perform an activity within the range considered normal
- Handicap – disadvantage resulting from the disability preventing fulfilment of a role that is considered normal depending on age, sex, social and cultural factors for that individual

---

[a]From the preamble to the Constitution of the World Health Organization as adopted by the International Health Conference, New York, 19–22 June, 1946; signed on 22 July 1946 by the representatives of 61 States (Official Records of the World Health Organization, no. 2, p. 100) and entered into force on 7 April 1948.

---

structure and function, activities and participation. A further change is the recognition of the importance of the role of environmental factors that interact with a health condition either to facilitate functioning or to create barriers for people with disabilities.

Since most of the publications on PR have used the original terms of impairment, disability and handicap, we have continued to use them in this chapter.

Is pulmonary rehabilitation effective for the individual patient?

The positive scientific evidence for PR has consolidated since the 1980s. A meta-analysis by Lacasse *et al.* (21) demonstrated that PR is effective in the management of patients with COPD, improving dyspnoea and mastery over the disease. An update published by the same group in 2002 (22) confirmed the moderately large and clinically significant improvements in dyspnoea, fatigue and the patients' sense of control over their condition, together with a modest improvement in exercise capacity (22).

A recent meta-analysis by Salman *et al.* (23) noted that PR improved exercise capacity and reduced shortness of breath provided that the rehabilitation programmes include at least lower-extremity training. The study also reported that patients with mild-to-moderate COPD benefited from short- and long-term rehabilitation, whereas rehabilitation programmes of at least 6 months are indicated for patients with severe COPD (23).

The scientific evidence is mostly in reference to COPD, since this disease represents the largest application of PR both for epidemiological reasons and due to the chronic, slowly progressive nature of the condition. Patients with other chronic respiratory disorders, such as asthma or bronchiectasis, thoracic wall deformities and neuromuscular conditions, may also benefit from PR as well as respiratory patients who undergo major thoracic or abdominal surgery. Evidence of effectiveness in these other conditions is limited by the lack of

clinical trials. For example, removal of lung secretions is generally considered a key intervention in the rehabilitation of patients with bronchiectasis. A systematic review (24) by the Cochrane Airways Group found only seven trials with an acceptable design, but these were small and not generally of high quality. The authors concluded that 'there was not enough evidence to support or refute the use of bronchial hygiene physical therapy in people with chronic obstructive pulmonary disease and bronchiectasis' (24).

Many items in COPD guidelines are still based on expert opinion rather than on systematic reviews. Randomized controlled trials with adequate sample sizes are needed to correctly define the rationale for PR in disorders other than COPD. Furthermore, as noted in a review by Lacasse and Goldstein (25), most overviews on PR in COPD published from 1985 to 1995 did not use a scientific methodology similar to those used for many of the primary studies that they summarize. As a consequence, the conclusions of such overviews are only partially supported by the results extracted from the primary studies. Lacasse and Goldstein's review highlights the need for evidence-based overviews of the literature as a basis for implementing new rehabilitation programmes, although it obviously does not negate the validity of the content of many of the overviews analysed (25).

SOCIETY–CENTRED RATIONALE

Epidemiology and social costs

Chronic lung disease globally is associated with considerable mortality and morbidity and imposes a huge burden on the utilization of health care resources in both Western and developing countries throughout the world. COPD, in particular, is the fourth leading cause of death in the USA after heart disease, cancer and cerebrovascular disease. In 1990 COPD was ranked 12th as a burden of disease, but by 2020 it is projected to rank fifth. Despite the obvious burden, there is a lack of recognition of COPD as a disease among the general public, and also among health-care professionals, as shown by its under-diagnosis and inadequate management (26).

According to the large-scale international survey 'Confronting COPD in North America and Europe' conducted in seven countries (Canada, France, Italy, The Netherlands, Spain, UK and USA) to investigate the burden of COPD, a high economic impact of COPD on the health care system and society was determined in each country. The mean annual direct costs of the disease spanned from particularly high levels in the USA (US$4119 per patient) and Spain ($3196 per patient) to relatively low levels in The Netherlands ($606) and France ($522) with intermediate levels for Italy (1261.25 euros [~$1600] per patient) and the UK (£819.42 [~$1500] per patient).

Lost productivity due to COPD had a particularly high impact on the economy in France, The Netherlands and the UK, accounting for 67, 50 and 41 per cent of overall costs, respectively, ranging from over $5646 in the USA to $1023 in The Netherlands. The majority (52–84 per cent) of direct costs associated with COPD were due to in-patient hospitalizations in five out of seven countries (27, 28). In all of the participating countries, COPD was under-diagnosed (9–30 per cent of patients), despite symptoms consistent with COPD, and under-treated (up to 65 per cent of patients did not receive regularly prescribed medication). Patients reported poor symptom control and considerable use of health care resources. The survey also demonstrated that the societal costs of COPD were four to 17 times higher in patients with severe COPD than in patients with mild COPD. Patients with co-morbid conditions (30–57 per cent of patients in each country) were also particularly costly to society (27).

These results suggest that to alleviate the burden of COPD on the health care system and society, improvements in its management are required, with earlier diagnosis, interventions aimed at preventing exacerbations and delaying the progression of disease (smoking cessation and oxygen therapy in particular) and rehabilitation of those who are moderately to severely disabled.

The chances that we will be affected by a disability have increased due to advances in medical technology that have extended our life expectancies. In the USA, general disability ranks among the nation's biggest public health concerns, encompassing an estimated 52 million Americans. Disability due to a definite disorder can be expressed by the index 'disability-adjusted life-year' (DALY), i.e. the sum of years lost because of premature mortality and years of life lived with disability, adjusted for the severity of disability. COPD is one of the leading causes of DALYs lost worldwide, increasing from 2.1 per cent of total DALYs in 1990 (12th cause) to 4.1 per cent in 2020 projections (fifth cause) (29).

Socioeconomic outcomes of PR

The costs of PR programmes are not trivial, largely because many professionals with great expertise in different fields are involved. Highly sophisticated technical instrumentation is often utilized, but these costs are more easily paid off. Goldstein *et al.* (30) calculated that the numbers of subjects needed to be treated (by in-patient rehabilitation) to improve one subject were as follows: 4.1 for dyspnoea, 4.4 for fatigue, 3.3 for emotion, and 2.5 for mastery, with an incremental cost of achieving improvements beyond the minimal clinically important difference in three of the above domains (dyspnoea, emotional function and mastery) of Canadian $11 597 (~US$9500) per patient. Ninety per cent of these costs were attributable to the in-patient phase of the programme (30). Are these costs justified by the outcomes of PR? Rigorous studies on PR are needed in which cost-effectiveness is a major outcome measure. Some authors believe that 'hospital days' are not an appropriate outcome measure since hospitalization of chronic respiratory patients, COPD in particular, is generally caused by acute exacerbations, an event that rehabilitation is not expected to prevent (31). However, this point of view cannot be fully accepted, since several components of PR are potentially useful in preventing exacerbations in general (i.e. not only those due to infectious agents), such as smoking cessation, chest physiotherapy, nutritional support, long-term oxygen therapy (LTOT) and non-invasive ventilation (NIV). Griffiths *et al.* (32) demonstrated that an outpatient pulmonary rehabilitation programme for 200 patients, mainly with COPD, produced a cost per quality-adjusted life-years (QALY) ratio within bounds considered to be cost-effective and likely to result in financial benefits to the health service.

The Griffiths *et al.* study concluded that PR reduced the days of hospitalization for patients with COPD (32). As health care systems differ from country to country, rigorous studies should verify the socioeconomic outcomes of PR in each geographic context.

In conclusion, there is a significant body of evidence, at least for COPD, that pulmonary rehabilitation programmes improve an individual's functional capability and health status. The socioeconomic impact of PR should be established for each jurisdiction. Answers regarding the best approach to service delivery, programme duration and components should be promoted by those who specialize in PR programmes (20).

Key points

- The modern, global approach to patients with chronic respiratory disorders has gained ground progressively in the face of the significant increase in COPD.
- Pulmonary rehabilitation has developed in the last few years as a field of respiratory medicine with the specific task of applying evidence-based knowledge and methods to intervene in all the disease dimensions, so as to enable the individual to achieve the best health status possible.
- Documentary evidence exists on the clinical effectiveness of pulmonary rehabilitation, particularly in COPD patients.
- Reduction of both health care resource utilization and social costs is also a desirable outcome, and a definite demonstration of this in the most appropriate health care setting is the object of current research.

REFERENCES

1. Mariani F. La kinesiterapia nelle malattie dell'apparato respiratorio. In: *La terapia moderna*. Milan: Vallardi Editore, 1911; 270–5.
2. Barach A, Bickerman H, Beck G. Advances in the treatment of non-tuberculous pulmonary disease. *Bull NY Acad Med* 1952; 28: 353–84.
3. Cotes JE, Gilson JC. Effect of oxygen in exercise ability in chronic respiratory insufficiency: use of a portable apparatus. *Lancet* 1956; 1: 822–6.
4. World Health Organization. Preamble to the Constitution of the World Health Organization as adopted by the International Health Conference, New York, 19–22 June, 1946; signed on 22 July 1946 by the representatives of 61 States (Official Records of the World Health Organization, no. 2, p. 100) and entered into force on 7 April 1948. Geneva: WHO.
5. National Library of Medicine. Online. http://www4.ncbi.nlm.nih.gov/entrez/query.fcgi.

6. Krishnan JA, Diette GB, Rand CS. Disparities in outcomes from chronic disease. *Br Med J* 2001; **323**: 950.

7. Kollef MH. Outcomes research: starting to make its mark in defining optimal respiratory care practices. *Respir Care* 1998; **43**: 629–31.

8. Morgan MDL, Singh SJ. The practical implementation of multidisciplinary pulmonary rehabilitation. *Monaldi Arch Chest Dis* 1998; **4**: 391–3.

9. Dyer CA, Singh SJ, Stockley RA *et al*. The incremental shuttle walking test in elderly people with chronic airflow limitation. *Thorax* 2002; **57**: 34–8.

◆10. Hodgkin JE, Farrell MJ, Gibson SR *et al*. American Thoracic Society. Medical Section of the American Lung Association. Pulmonary rehabilitation. *Am Rev Respir Dis* 1981; **124**: 663–6.

◆11. Donner CF, Howard P. Pulmonary rehabilitation in chronic obstructive pulmonary disease (COPD) with recommendations for its use. *Eur Respir J* 1992; **5**: 266–75.

●12. Anthonisen NR, Connett JE, Kiley JP *et al*. Effects of smoking intervention and the use of an inhaled anticholinergic bronchodilator on the rate of decline of FEV1. *J Am Med Assoc* 1994; **272**: 1497–505.

●13. British Research Medical Council Working Party. Long-term domiciliary oxygen therapy in chronic hypoxic cor pulmonale complication in chronic bronchitis and emphysema. *Lancet* 1981; **1**: 681–6.

14. NIH Workshop Summary. Pulmonary rehabilitation research. *Am J Respir Crit Care Med* 1994; **149**: 825–33.

◆15. Donner CF, Muir JF. Selection criteria and programmes for pulmonary rehabilitation in COPD patients. ERS task force position paper. *Eur Respir J* 1997; **10**: 744–57.

◆16. ACCP/AACVPR Pulmonary Rehabilitation Guidelines Panel. Pulmonary rehabilitation: joint ACCP/AACVPR evidence-based guidelines. American College of Chest Physicians/American Association of Cardiovascular and Pulmonary Rehabilitation. *Chest* 1997; **112**: 1363–96.

◆17. The COPD Guidelines Group of the Standards of Care Committee of the BTS. BTS guidelines for the management of chronic obstructive pulmonary disease. *Thorax* 1997; **52**(Suppl. 5): S1–28.

◆18. Official statement of the American Thoracic Society. Pulmonary rehabilitation-1999. *Am J Respir Crit Care Med* 1999; **159**: 1666–82.

19. American Association for Respiratory Care (AARC). Clinical practice guideline on pulmonary rehabilitation. *Respir Care* 2002; **47**: 617–25.

20. Ambrosino NA, Bellone AF, Gigliotti FA *et al*. Raccomandazioni sulla riabilitazione respiratoria. *Rassegna di Patologia dell'Apparato Respiratorio* 2001; **3**: 164–80.

●21. Lacasse Y, Wong E, Guyatt GH *et al*. Meta-analysis of respiratory rehabilitation in chronic obstructive pulmonary disease. *Lancet* 1996; **348**: 1115–19.

22. Lacasse Y, Brosseau L, Milne S *et al*. Pulmonary rehabilitation for chronic obstructive pulmonary disease. *Cochrane Database Syst Rev* 2002; **3**: CD003793.

23. Salman GF, Mosier MC, Beasley BW, Calkins DR. Rehabilitation for patients with chronic obstructive pulmonary disease: meta-analysis of randomized controlled trials. *J Gen Intern Med* 2003; **18**: 213–21.

24. Jones AP, Rowe BH. Bronchopulmonary hygiene physical therapy for chronic obstructive pulmonary disease and bronchiectasis. *Cochrane Database Syst Rev* 2000; **2**: CD000045.

25. Lacasse Y, Goldstein RS. Overviews of respiratory rehabilitation in chronic obstructive pulmonary disease. *Monaldi Arch Chest Dis* 1999; **54**: 163–7.

◆26. Pauwels RA, Buist AS, Calverley PM, Jenkins CR, Hurd SS; GOLD Scientific Committee. Global strategy for the diagnosis, management, and prevention of chronic obstructive pulmonary disease. NHLBI/WHO Global Initiative for Chronic Obstructive Lung Disease (GOLD) Workshop summary. *Am J Respir Crit Care Med* 2001; **163**: 1256–76.

27. Wouters EF. Economic analysis of the Confronting COPD survey: an overview of results. *Respir Med* 2003; **97**(Suppl. C): S3–14.

28. Dal Negro R, Rossi A, Cerveri I. The burden of COPD in Italy: results from the Confronting COPD survey. *Respir Med* 2003; **97**(Suppl. C): S43–50.

●29. Murray CJ, Lopez AD. Evidence-based health policy – lessons from the Global Burden of Disease Study. *Science* 1996; **274**: 740–3.

30. Goldstein RS, Gort EH, Guyatt GH, Feeny D. Economic analysis of respiratory rehabilitation. *Chest* 1997; **112**: 370–9.

31. Clark CJ, Decramer M. The definition and rationale for pulmonary rehabilitation. *Eur Respir Mon* 2000; **13**: 1–6.

32. Griffiths TL, Phillips CJ, Davies S *et al*. Cost effectiveness of an outpatient multidisciplinary pulmonary rehabilitation programme. *Thorax* 2001; **56**: 779–84.

2

International trends in the epidemiology of chronic obstructive pulmonary disease

YVES LACASSE, ROGER S. GOLDSTEIN

INTRODUCTION

Cigarette smoking is the most important cause of chronic obstructive lung diseases (1, 2). Most surveys suggest that tobacco-related conditions, particularly chronic obstructive pulmonary disease (COPD), remain important problems in both the developed and developing worlds, and will probably be so for many years to come. COPD is currently the fourth leading cause of death in the world (3). Strategies aimed at reducing the burden of COPD include continuing anti-smoking campaigns (primary prevention), early detection and intervention among those individuals at risk for the late consequences of COPD (secondary prevention) (4), and the widespread application of effective therapeutic modalities in reducing the complications of the disease (tertiary prevention). Respiratory rehabilitation clearly falls into the latter category.

National and international statistics often provide the rationale for implementing new programmes aimed at reducing the disease burden. The primary objective of this chapter is to review the literature surrounding the epidemiology of COPD and emphasize the difficulties in defining COPD for clinical, research or epidemiological purposes. We hope to provide the basis for rehabilitation from an epidemiological perspective.

DEFINITIONS OF COPD

Definition of COPD in clinical practice

The Global Initiative for Chronic Obstructive Lung Disease (GOLD) defined COPD as 'a disease state characterized by airflow limitation that is not fully reversible. The airflow limitation is usually progressive and associated with an abnormal inflammatory response of the lung to noxious particles or gases' (5). Other professional organizations have adopted similar definitions, some of which include smoking as the leading cause of COPD (6–10). The definitions reflect the heterogeneity of the disease. Figure 2.1 illustrates the difficulty in differentiating, in both clinical practice and clinical trials, COPD (subsets 3, 4 and 5 in Fig. 2.1) from asthma with incompletely remitting airflow obstruction (subsets 6, 7 and 8). Both conditions (COPD and asthma) may also coexist (6).

Spirometry has become the gold standard for detecting airflow obstruction. It is reproducible, standardized and objective (8). There are often differences in the spirometric definitions of COPD among the various professional organizations (Box 2.1). Therefore, estimates of the prevalence of COPD might be substantially different, depending on the criteria used to diagnose the disease (11). The threshold between 'normal' and 'abnormal' is still ill-defined. A vivid illustration of this issue comes from a German study examining the distribution of the COPD stages as classified according to the GOLD guidelines (12). In this study, files from 1434 consecutive patients, visiting a lung specialist for the first time in 1995, were assessed retrospectively. Patients were classified (stages 0–3) according to the clinical and physiological parameters proposed by the guidelines; 37 per cent were classified stage 0 ('at risk'). The initial GOLD stages were correlated with age, duration of symptoms and pack-years of smoking. The authors correctly pointed out that patients now fulfilling the criteria of stage 0 COPD would have previously been labelled as having chronic bronchitis.

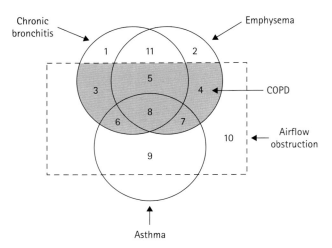

Figure 2.1 *Schema of chronic obstructive pulmonary disease (COPD). This non-proportional Venn diagram shows subsets of patients with chronic bronchitis, emphysema and asthma. The subsets comprising COPD are shaded. Patients with asthma whose airflow obstruction is fully reversible (subset 9) are not considered to have COPD. Because in many cases it is virtually impossible to differentiate patients with asthma whose airflow obstruction does not remit completely from persons with chronic bronchitis or emphysema who have partially reversible airflow obstruction with airway hyperreactivity, patients with unremitting asthma are classified as having COPD (subsets 6, 7 and 8). Non-obstructive chronic bronchitis and emphysema recognized on radiological assessment without airflow limitation (subsets 1, 2 and 11) are not classified as having COPD. COPD does not encompass airflow obstruction associated with other lung diseases (such as cystic fibrosis of diffuse bronchiectases – subset 10). In such circumstances, the patients should be classified as having 'secondary airflow obstruction'. Reproduced with permission from American Thoracic Society (6).*

Box 2.1 Spirometric definitions of COPD according to published practice guidelines

- GOLD (Global Initiative for Chronic Obstructive Lung Disease) (5)
  - mild COPD: FEV_1/FVC <70%
- American Thoracic Society (10)
  - obstructive abnormality is interpreted when the FEV_1/FVC ratio is below normal range
  - mild COPD: % pred FEV_1 <100 and ⩾70
- European Respiratory Society (7)
  - FEV_1 <80% predicted, FEV_1/FVC and other indices of expiratory flow reduced
- British Thoracic Society (8)
  - FEV_1 <80% predicted, FEV_1/FVC <70%
- Canadian Thoracic Society (9)
  - FEV_1 <80% predicted, FEV_1/FVC <70%

Another study illustrated the extent to which COPD may be over-diagnosed, when the GOLD criteria were applied to healthy, never having smoked, asymptomatic, elderly individuals (age ⩾70 years) (13). In a random, well defined subgroup of 208 never-smoker respondents with no current respiratory disease or significant dyspnoea, 71 were able to perform an acceptable spirometry; 35 per cent of them had a forced expiratory volume in 1 second/forced vital capacity (FEV_1/FVC) <70 per cent and would be classified by the GOLD guidelines as having stage 1 COPD. The authors concluded that the criteria used to define the various stages of COPD needed to be age-specific.

We support the notion that the diagnosis of COPD should include spirometric indices that are associated with the risk of significant morbidity or mortality. Individuals free of symptoms and presenting with a normal FEV_1, even with an FEV_1/FVC <70 per cent, should not be classified as having COPD. Clues as to what really defines COPD, in terms of spirometry, were provided by the Renfrew and Paisley (Scotland) survey (14). This longitudinal study of 15 411 adults aged 45–64 years when first examined (1972–1976) provided 15-year follow-up data on all-cause mortality, ischaemic heart disease, lung and other cancers, stroke and respiratory diseases. Almost 80 per cent of the eligible individuals took part in the survey and more than 99 per cent of them had measures of FEV_1 available for analysis. Significant trends of increasing risks with diminishing FEV_1 were apparent for both sexes for all causes of death examined after adjustment for age, cigarette smoking, diastolic blood pressure, cholesterol level, body mass index (BMI) and social class. For mortality from respiratory causes, the relative hazard ratio became significant for those in the second quintile of FEV_1 (73–86 per cent predicted for men; 75–89 per cent predicted for women).

Definition of COPD in clinical research

In some trials, the term 'COPD' encompasses any pulmonary disease with symptoms of respiratory obstruction or secretion. Using this definition, almost 90 per cent of the patients enrolled in an evaluation of an educational intervention for COPD had asthma (15). Most often, investigators conducting clinical trials in COPD have required patients to have a clinical diagnosis of COPD, a history of smoking and objective evidence of airway obstruction. This operational definition of COPD remains imperfect. For instance, in their comparison of the bronchodilator effects of aerosolized albuterol and ipratropium bromide, Easton *et al.* (16) noted changes in FEV_1 of up to 40 per cent among COPD patients receiving albuterol and ipratropium bromide successively. Although the study excluded patients with a history suggestive of asthma, the average response to bronchodilators was appreciably greater than that typically observed in clinical practice.

Unfortunately, there are no simple and reliable indices that differentiate 'pure' COPD from asthma with incompletely reversible airflow obstruction. A preserved carbon monoxide diffusing capacity and a higher ratio of airway to parenchymal abnormalities on high-resolution computed tomograms is found more frequently in asthma with incomplete reversibility than in COPD (17). However, the substantial overlap in results between populations makes these features of little help in classifying individual patients. Induced sputum eosinophilia may provide a simple way to predict the beneficial effect of steroid treatment in smokers with airflow obstruction by identifying patients with an asthmatic type of airway inflammation (18). However, this innovative strategy requires further study.

Despite the difficulty in correctly classifying patients with chronic airflow limitation, the strict exclusion of patients with an asthmatic component is of limited relevance for most components of the management of COPD. For instance, although the underlying pathology defining both COPD and asthma with incomplete reversibility is initially confined to the lungs, the associated physical deconditioning and the emotional responses contribute greatly to the resulting morbidity. Respiratory rehabilitation is likely to address the consequences of chronic airflow obstruction irrespective of the underlying mechanisms of both diseases. Hence, the authors of a recent research synthesis of respiratory rehabilitation did not find any difference in the effects of rehabilitation on exercise capacity or quality of life in controlled clinical trials which compared COPD patients with or without reversibility (19).

However, in studying other aspects of the disease, such as airway inflammation and the role of inhaled steroids in COPD, exclusion (or, at least, subgroup analysis) of patients with asthma with incomplete reversibility of airway obstruction (or COPD accompanied by significant airway hyperreactivity) becomes crucial. It is possible that much of the controversy surrounding the effectiveness of inhaled steroids in COPD may result from the heterogeneity of the study populations. One might expect that, at best, inhaled steroids would reduce the accelerated annual decline of FEV_1 over time in patients with COPD (20). A meta-analysis of inhaled steroids in COPD (21) found a small increase in prebronchodilator FEV_1 over a 2-year period in patients with moderate to severe COPD treated with relatively high doses of inhaled corticosteroids, raising the question as to how many of those included had underlying asthma.

In a trial of inhaled corticosteroids in patients with COPD, Bourbeau et al. (22) attempted to confine the intervention to the large subgroup of patients with COPD who did not benefit from oral steroids. Therefore, during phase I of their study, the investigators submitted their initial cohort of patients to a 2-week course of oral prednisone (40 mg daily). Only those patients whose FEV_1 had not improved by at least 15 per cent and 200 mL compared with their baseline values after the 2-week course of oral prednisone (the 'non-responders') were then eligible for the second phase of the study, a 6-month randomized placebo-controlled trial of inhaled corticosteroids. This design differs from that used in the ISOLDE study (23) in which COPD patients were given a short course of oral corticosteroids immediately after being randomized to receive either long-term inhaled steroids or placebo. This strategy did not exclude patients with airway hyperreactivity.

Definition of COPD in epidemiological research

Halbert et al. (24) recently published a critical evaluation of the literature addressing the epidemiology of COPD. Thirty-two sources of COPD prevalence rates were identified and broadly grouped into one of four categories according to the methods used to classify patients: (i) spirometry with or without clinical examination; (ii) presence of respiratory symptoms; (iii) patient-reported disease; and (iv) expert opinions. Overall, COPD prevalence rates ranged from <1 to >18 per cent depending on the methods used to estimate prevalence. Another useful review of the prevalence of COPD is found in Coultas and Mapel (25).

SPIROMETRY

Spirometry is likely to provide the most reliable data regarding the prevalence of COPD. When spirometry was rigorously measured, the prevalence of COPD ranged from 4 to 10 per cent (24). An important report on the prevalence of COPD, based on spirometric measurement, came from the National Health and Nutrition Examination Survey (NHANES III) (1980–1994) of 20 050 US adults (26); 6.8 per cent of this population had reduced lung function (an FEV_1 <80 per cent predicted and a FEV_1/FVC <0.7). Of these individuals, 63.3 per cent had not been diagnosed with obstructive lung disease. Of those with an FEV_1 <50 per cent predicted, 44.0 per cent did not have such a diagnosis. Undiagnosed airflow obstruction was associated with a health impact. The prevalence of respiratory symptoms increased even among those with mild impairment, and the presence of symptoms increased consistently with increasing severity of the FEV_1 impairment (27). NHANES III also emphasized that spirometry was not used widely in clinical practice.

RESPIRATORY SYMPTOMS

In Halbert's review, the symptom-based diagnosis of COPD yielded higher rates than spirometry alone, although the diagnosis was limited to chronic bronchitis defined by Medical Research Council criteria (28). A recent study raised concerns regarding the accuracy of the COPD prevalence derived from self-reported symptoms or diagnosis (29). The primary objective of this study was to determine the degree to which new, self-reported, diagnosis of chronic bronchitis and a physician-confirmed diagnosis of chronic bronchitis satisfied the symptom criteria of cough and sputum production for at least 3 months per year for at least two consecutive years. Data were drawn from the Tucson Epidemiologic Study of Obstructive Lung Disease, a longitudinal population study that enrolled a stratified sample of 1655 households in Tucson, Arizona, in the mid-1970s. Participants were administered standardized questionnaires during 12 different surveys 1–1.5 years apart. The study population included 4034

Table 2.1 *Concordance of the diagnosis of chronic bronchitis with symptom criteria. Reproduced with permission from Bobadila et al. (29)*

	Self-reported diagnosis of chronic bronchitis	
	Met the Ciba Guest Symposium criteria of chronic bronchitis	Did not meet the Ciba Guest Symposium criteria of chronic bronchitis
Physician confirmation status		
Yes	52	363
No	4	62
Total	56	425

individuals, of whom 481 (11.9 per cent) were given the diagnosis of chronic bronchitis, either on the basis of self-reported diagnosis (i.e. a positive answer to the following question: 'Since the last questionnaire, have you had chronic bronchitis?') or a physician-confirmed diagnosis. Concordance of the diagnosis with symptom criteria for chronic bronchitis (Table 2.1) proved to be poor. The authors concluded that responses to respiratory questionnaires did not provide an accurate clinical diagnosis.

PATIENT–REPORTED DISEASES

The 1994–95 Canadian National Population Health Survey reflected several limitations in data collection, including the computation of prevalence rates from self-report surveys (30). Estimates of the prevalence of COPD were derived from the individual's response to the following question: 'Do you have chronic bronchitis or emphysema diagnosed by a health professional?'. The respondents' answers were not validated by further investigation. We emphasized that the information reported should be thought of as the perceived prevalence. If individuals with non-obstructive bronchitis were included, then the survey might have overestimated the true prevalence of COPD in the community. However, as the survey could not capture undiagnosed individuals or those unaware of their diagnosis, the true prevalence might have been underestimated. The direction of the bias, if any, is uncertain. We concur with Halbert's view that the burden of COPD is underestimated (24).

INTERNATIONAL TRENDS IN COPD-SPECIFIC MORTALITY

Several factors limit the comparison of international data related to COPD mortality, including (31, 32):

- the lack of standardization of death certification and coding practices
- international differences in diagnostic practices
- availability and quality of medical care
- differences in the completeness and coverage of death data
- incorrect or systematic biases in diagnosis

- misinterpretation of International Classification of Diseases (ICD) rules for selection of the underlying cause of death.

We accessed the WHO mortality database and computed the COPD-specific mortality rates for the population aged ≥55 years. The mortality rates for men and women are shown in Figs 2.2(a) and (b), respectively. These illustrations show much heterogeneity in the death rates across the selected countries. The 30-fold difference between the highest and lowest reported mortality rates is considerably greater than that normally expected, illustrating the limitations of the data.

Mortality from COPD is related to the severity of the disease (33). The recent follow-up of the first National Health and Nutrition Examination Survey (NHANES I) reported on 5542 individuals who had their pulmonary function measured in 1971–75 (34). Follow-up surveys were conducted until 1992, at which time 96 per cent of the original cohort had been successfully traced. The Kaplan–Meier curve for death among the participants stratified by degree of lung function impairment is presented in Fig. 2.3. Whether the same death rates can be applied worldwide is doubtful given the widespread disparity in care around the world. Given that mortality may also be affected by health-related quality of life, independently of spirometry, this aspect of the epidemiology of COPD immediately becomes more complicated. An interesting report (35) noted that the categorization of patients with COPD by dyspnoea was useful in predicting health-related quality of life as well as improvements following rehabilitation. The authors wondered whether it might also predict mortality. After following 183 patients over 5 years, they concluded that categorization of COPD based on dyspnoea was more discriminating than staging disease severity based on flow rates, for predicting their 5 year survival. Therefore, outcome measures for future epidemiological studies that aim to predict survival will likely be expanded to include categorization based on dyspnoea as well as measures of FEV_1.

SOCIOECONOMIC IMPLICATIONS OF COPD AROUND THE WORLD

The burden of COPD may be examined from the perspective of society as well as from the points of view of patients, physicians and health care payers (36).

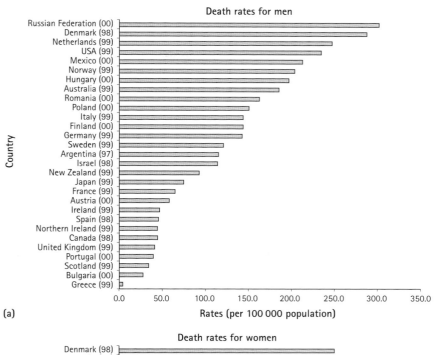

(a)

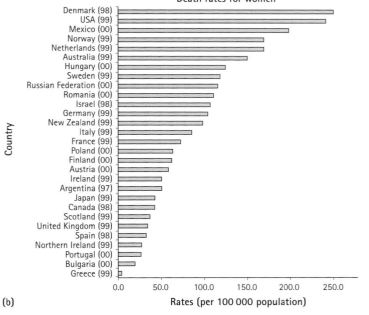

(b)

Figure 2.2 *Age-adjusted death rates for chronic obstructive pulmonary disease (COPD) by country and sex (a, men; b, women) in individuals aged ≥ 55 years. Year for which data are given is in parentheses.*

Quality of life

Multiple studies have demonstrated the negative impact of COPD on health-related quality of life. Their review is beyond the scope of this chapter. The impairment is only loosely related to the severity of airflow limitation. Even patients with mild disease show substantially compromised quality of life (37). Co-morbidities only partly influence the observed pattern of deterioration of quality of life with worsening stage of the disease.

Data collected as part of the Inhaled Steroids in Obstructive Lung Disease (ISOLDE) trial in COPD provided useful information regarding the decline in quality-of-life scores over an extended period of time (23). In this study, 751 patients were randomized to receive either fluticasone propionate or placebo. Patients completed the St George's Respiratory questionnaire and the Short-Form 36 (SF-36) at baseline and every 6 months for 3 years. Health status declined progressively in all components of both questionnaires. The rate of deterioration in health status was linear. Although smokers had worse baseline quality-of-life scores than ex-smokers, smoking had no influence on decline in health status over time (Fig. 2.4) (38). Of note, reduced generic and disease-specific qualities of life are independent risk factors for mortality, even after adjustment for age, FEV_1 and BMI (Fig. 2.5) (39).

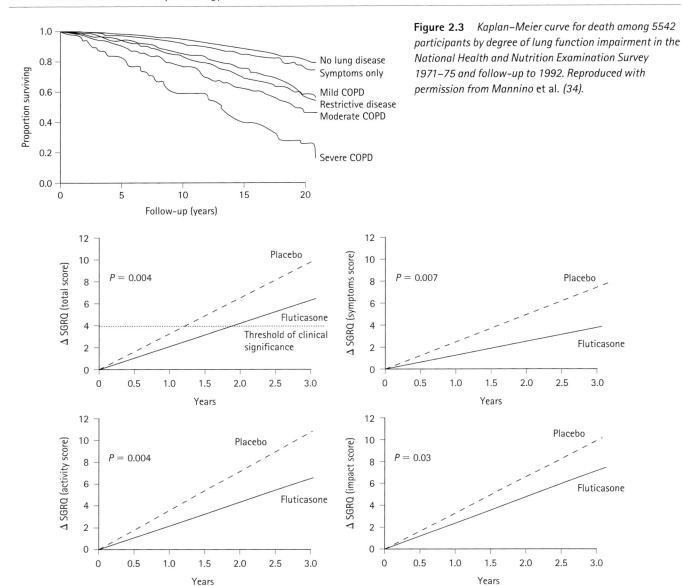

Figure 2.3 *Kaplan–Meier curve for death among 5542 participants by degree of lung function impairment in the National Health and Nutrition Examination Survey 1971–75 and follow-up to 1992. Reproduced with permission from Mannino et al. (34).*

Figure 2.4 *Slope of deterioration in health status measured by the St George's Respiratory Questionnaire (SGRQ) in the ISOLDE Study. Reproduced with permission from Spencer et al. (38).*

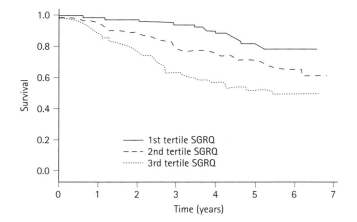

Figure 2.5 *Kaplan-Meier survival curves according to tertiles of the St George's Respiratory Questionnaire in 312 male patients with COPD. Reproduced with permission from Domingo-Salvany et al. (39).*

Social implications

Until recently, little was known about work loss attributable to COPD. This may have been because COPD was often considered to be a disease of the elderly, who are usually retired. Nevertheless, data from the Confronting COPD International Survey confirmed the great burden to society and high individual morbidity associated with COPD in North America and Europe (40). In this survey, more than 200 000 households were screened by random-digit dialling in the United States, Canada, France, Italy, Germany, the Netherlands, Spain and the United Kingdom; 3265 individuals (mean age, 63 years; 44 per cent female) with COPD (or symptoms of chronic bronchitis) were identified. Forty-five per cent of those <65 years reported work loss in the past year because of COPD. In the Canadian cohort of the Confronting COPD Survey, on average, 10 days of work had been lost during the

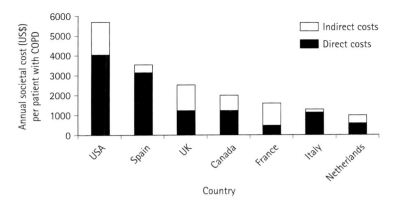

Figure 2.6 *Annual societal cost per patient with COPD in seven countries participating in the Confronting COPD Survey. All costs are in US dollars (2000). Reproduced with permission from Wouters (48).*

12-month period prior to the survey (41). In addition, 3 per cent of the sample reported that a care-giver had lost work because of the disease.

Secondary analyses of the NHANES III revealed that individuals with COPD were less likely to be in the labour force than those without COPD. Mild, moderate and severe COPD were associated with, respectively, a 3.4, 3.9 and 14.4 per cent reduction in the labour force participation rate relative to those without COPD (42). The Survey of Income and Program Participation (43) indicated that in 1991, adults with chronic respiratory disorders had an average annual earning loss of US$3143 compared with individuals without chronic respiratory conditions (44).

Economic implications

Because of the heterogeneity in methodology, the literature on the economic burden of COPD is difficult to review (45). Such an attempt was made in 2000 by Sullivan *et al.* (46). The authors reported that, according to estimates from the NHLBI, the annual cost of COPD to the United States was $23.9 billion in 1993. This included $14.7 billion in direct expenditures for medical care services, $4.7 billion in indirect morbidity costs, and $4.5 billion in costs related to premature mortality. In 1987, the mean per-person direct medical expenditures among individuals with COPD was US$6469 (47).

The COPD Confronting International Survey also provided estimates of the direct and indirect costs of COPD (48). The annual direct cost ranged from US$522 in France to US$4119 in the United States. Hospitalization fees represented more than half of the costs in five of the eight participating countries. The annual indirect cost of COPD was calculated from the lost productivity. Indirect costs ranged from US$47 per patient in the Italian survey sample to US$1527 per patient in the US sample (Fig. 2.6).

CONCLUSIONS

An understanding of the epidemiology of COPD is important for those associated with health care services that fund or provide care for individuals with this common condition. Accurate information on the burden of disease will enable appropriate strategies to be established, both for primary and secondary prevention and for disease management. Moreover, such data will enable the monitoring of effectiveness of care within and among different geographic jurisdictions. Such monitoring is of value both for planning health care delivery and for evaluating the clinical impact of newer management strategies. It will also facilitate the judicious use of limited resources to their best effect.

Although, in recent years, substantial progress has been made in our understanding of the need for accurate epidemiological information, as well as in the refinement of the most appropriate tools for reflecting the impact of COPD on the population, there are still many issues that complicate and challenge us to succeed in this area. One of the fundamental issues is an accepted definition of COPD, or at least a clear understanding of the differences that exist among the various countries that have published guidelines in this area. It is important to have agreement on spirometric criteria, as well as the role of reversibility, in the diagnosis of this condition and to include information, such as health status, that goes beyond the simple measurement of airflow limitation. Other issues, such as the accuracy of reporting and record-keeping within the health care system, as well as the design, precision and generalizability of population health surveys, remain to be better refined.

Notwithstanding the above, the modern realization of the importance of COPD as the fourth most common cause of mortality and morbidity in many countries has fuelled a concerted effort to improve our understanding of the epidemiology of this common condition.

Key points

- Cigarette smoking is the most important cause of chronic obstructive lung disease.
- The definition of COPD for clinical, research and epidemiological purposes may differ. The available international data suggest that the actual burden of COPD is underestimated.

Derby Hospitals NHS Foundation
Trust
Library and Knowledge Service

3

Pathophysiological basis of pulmonary rehabilitation in chronic obstructive pulmonary disease

BARTOLOME R. CELLI

Chronic obstructive pulmonary disease (COPD) currently ranks as the fourth cause of death in the United States (1). Its prevalence has increased as overall mortality from myocardial infarction and cerebrovascular accident, the two organ systems affected by the same risk factor (namely cigarette smoking), have decreased. Once diagnosed, COPD is progressive and leads to disability, usually due to dyspnoea, at a relatively early age (sixth or seventh decade) (2). Limitation to airflow occurs as a consequence of destruction of lung parenchyma or alterations in the airway itself. This chapter integrates the pathological changes of COPD with the known adaptive and maladaptive consequences of those changes. Knowledge of these factors should help us understand the rationale behind the different therapeutic strategies utilized in pulmonary rehabilitation and which are aimed at decreasing the symptoms and addressing the complications of patients with COPD.

Definition

From the expanded definition of COPD and its different pathological components, it is possible to infer the pathophysiological changes that are observed and that are responsible for the clinical presentation. COPD is defined as a disease state characterized by the presence of airflow obstruction due to emphysema or intrinsic airway disease. The airflow limitation is associated with an abnormal inflammatory response to inhaled particles or noxious gases (mainly cigarette smoking) (2). The obstruction is generally progressive, may be accompanied by airway hyperactivity and may be partially reversible. Emphysema is defined pathologically as an abnormal

permanent enlargement of the air spaces distal to the terminal bronchioles, accompanied by destruction of their walls, without fibrosis. In most patients both processes coexist simultaneously (3–5). The disease does not affect all portions of the lung to the same degree. This uneven distribution influences the physiological behaviour of different parts of the lung.

PATHOPHYSIOLOGY

Biopsy studies from the large airways of patients with COPD reveal the presence of a large number of neutrophils (6). This neutrophilic predominance is more manifest in smoking patients who develop airflow obstruction than in smoking patients without airflow limitation (7). Interestingly, biopsies of smaller bronchi reveal the presence of a large number of lymphocytes, especially of the CD8+ type (8). The same types of cells, as well as macrophages, have been shown to increase in biopsies that include lung parenchyma (8, 9). Taken together, these findings suggest that cigarette smoking induces an inflammatory process characterized by intense interaction and accumulation of cells, which are capable of releasing many cytokines and enzymes that may cause injury, as seen in Fig. 3.1. Indeed, the level of interleukin-8 (IL-8) is increased in the secretions of patients with COPD (10). This is also true for tumour necrosis factor (11) and markers of oxidative stress (12). In addition, the release of enzymes known to be capable of destroying lung parenchyma, such as neutrophilic elastase and metalloproteinases (MMPs), by many of these activated cells has been documented in patients with COPD (13, 14). Therefore, an increasing body of evidence indicates that the anatomic alterations of COPD, such as airway inflammation and dysfunction, as well as parenchymal destruction, could result from altered cellular interactions triggered by external agents such as cigarette or environmental smoke. Whatever the mechanisms, the disease distribution is not uniform, so in one single patient, areas of the lung with severe destruction may coexist with less affected areas. In addition, some of the inflammatory cytokines may spill over into the systemic circulation with possible systemic effects (15).

Functionally, COPD is characterized by decrease in airflow, which is more prominent on maximal efforts. Like the pathological distribution, the airflow limitation is not uniform in nature. This causes uneven distribution of ventilation and also of blood perfusion (16, 17). This in turn results in arterial hypoxaemia (decreased P_aO_2) and, if overall ventilation is decreased, in hypercarbia (increased P_aCO_2). In those patients with an important component of emphysema or bullous disease, total lung volume increases, resulting in hyperinflation. Each of these interrelated elements is important in the adaptive changes observed in patients with COPD, and helps to explain the clinical manifestations of the disease.

The relationship between structure and function in COPD is not well understood. Whether due to loss of attachments or tethering forces and/or due to inflammation and mucous secretion, patients with COPD have decreased airflow. In spite of this, there is no good correlation between the currently used scoring system of either emphysematous or bronchitic changes and the degree of airflow obstruction. Therefore, it is practical to describe the patient by the degree of physiologically determined airflow limitation. At present, the best predictor of morbidity and mortality in COPD is the value of

post-bronchodilator forced expiratory volume in one second (FEV_1) (18). There is an extensive literature on factors that affect mortality in COPD, the principal variables being age and FEV_1 (18, 19). The data are relatively old and, by and large, precede the advent of low-flow oxygen and mechanical ventilation. The presence of hypoxaemia and hypercapnia is also important in that they are predictive of mortality, once the patient has moderate to severe airflow limitation. The FEV_1 is the best single predictor of mortality in COPD. However, it is not until values fall below 50 per cent of predicted that mortality begins to increase (16). Once patients reach very low values of FEV_1 this measurement has little predictive value, but no other measurements have been thoroughly validated. A patient with significant hypoxaemia represents a complicated medical problem and one likely to require more resources. Similarly, the presence of hypercarbia is recognized as a significant correlate of mortality and a marker of advanced, complicated disease (20).

The cardinal symptom of COPD is dyspnoea (1, 21). This sensation is the consequence of the interaction between cognitive and non-volitional neural processes and respiratory mechanics, including airway obstruction. Dyspnoea often limits functional activity and frequently causes the patient to seek medical attention (22, 23). Recent data from Nishimura *et al.* (24) suggest that dyspnoea may actually be a better predictor of mortality than the gold standard; the FEV_1. If confirmed, this is extremely important because, conceptually, a decrease in functional dyspnoea could result in a change in outcome. This hypothesis remains to be studied.

Finally, the functional capacity to walk has been shown to be a better predictor of survival than the FEV_1 in patients with moderate to severe disease (25–27). In addition to the

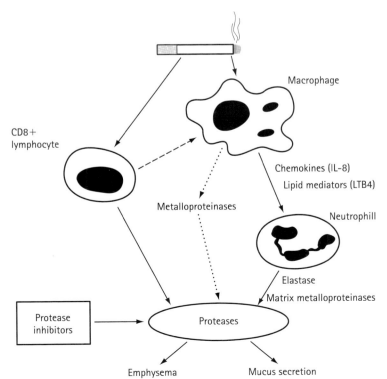

Figure 3.1 *Cigarette smoking induces inflammation. The interaction of different cells results in the release of cytokines that further perpetuate the inflammatory state and cause tissue injury.*

functional capacity to walk, a recent study has shown that the peak oxygen uptake documented during an exercise study is a better predictor of survival than the degree of airflow limitation in a cohort of patients with COPD (28). Again, these observations are extremely important, especially when considering the effects of rehabilitation, a therapeutic intervention where the benefit is more manifest in changes in the exercise capacity and functional ability. Indeed, the presence of peripheral muscle dysfunction and its improvement with exercise training remains the cornerstone of pulmonary rehabilitation, as we will explore later.

AIRFLOW LIMITATION

To move air in and out of the lungs, the bellows must force air through the conducting airways. The resistance to flow is given by the interaction of air molecules with each other and with the internal surface of the airways. Therefore, airflow resistance depends on the physical property of the gas and the length and diameter of the airways. For a constant diameter, flow is proportional to the applied pressure. This relationship holds true in normals for inspiratory flow measured at fixed lung volume. In contrast, expiratory flow is linearly related to the applied pressure only during the early portion of the manoeuvre. Beyond a certain point, flow does not increase despite further increase in driving pressure. This flow limitation is due to the dynamic compression of airways as force is applied around them during forced expirations. This can be readily understood in the commonly determined flow–volume expression of the vital capacity as shown in Fig. 3.2. As effort increases, expiratory flow increases up to a certain point (outer envelope) beyond which further efforts result in no further increase in airflow. During tidal breathing (inner tracing) only a small fraction of the maximal flow is used, and therefore flow is not limited under these circumstances. In

contrast the flow–volume loop of patients with COPD is markedly different. The expiratory portion of the curve is caved out. This shape is due to the smaller diameter of the intrathoracic airways, which decreases even more as pressure is applied around them. The flow limitation can be severe enough that maximal flow may be reached even during tidal breathing. A patient with this degree of obstruction (a not uncommon finding in clinical practice) cannot increase flow with increased ventilatory demand. As we shall review later, increased demands can only be met by increasing respiratory rate, which in turn is detrimental to the expiratory time and causes dynamic hyperinflation, a significant problem in patients with COPD.

The precise reason for the development of airflow obstruction in COPD is not entirely clear, but it is probably multifactorial (29, 30). Because airflow obstruction is physiologically evident during exhalation, COPD has been thought to be a problem of 'expiration'. Unfortunately, inspiration is also affected because inspiratory resistance is also increased and, more importantly, the inability to expel the inhaled air, coupled with parenchymal destruction, leads to hyperinflation (31).

HYPERINFLATION

As the parenchymal destruction of many patients with COPD progresses, the distal air spaces enlarge. The loss of the lung elastic recoil resulting from this destruction increases resting lung volume. In a pervasive way, the loss of elastic recoil and airway attachments narrows the already constricted airways even more. The decrease in airway diameter increases resistance to airflow and worsens the obstruction. Decreased lung elastic recoil is therefore a major contributor of airway narrowing in emphysema (32, 33). Because in most patients the distribution of emphysema is not uniform, portions of lung with low elastic recoil may coexist with portions with more normal elastic recoil properties, as depicted in Fig. 3.3. It follows

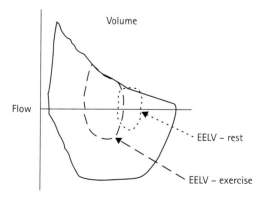

Figure 3.2 *Patients with severe COPD manifest flow limitation during tidal breathing. Increases in ventilatory demand (i.e. exercise and acute exacerbation) can only be met by an increase in breathing frequency. This results in air-trapping as expiratory time is shortened. The consequence of these changes is the development of dynamic hyperinflation and associated dyspnoea. EELV, end-expiratory lung volume.*

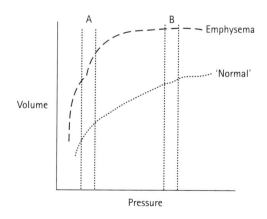

Figure 3.3 *The pressure–volume relationship in the lungs of patients with COPD can be represented as composed of two portions: one more compliant and one more normal. The same pressure applied at different lung volumes will result in unequal ventilation in the different portions of the lungs. This has profound effects on lung emptying and ventilation/perfusion match.*

that ventilation to each one of those portions will not be uniform. This helps to explain some of the differences in gas exchange. It also explains why reduction of the uneven distribution of recoil pressures by procedures that resect more afflicted lung areas results in better ventilation of the remainder of the lung and improved gas exchange.

Increased breathing frequency worsens hyperinflation (34, 35), because the expiratory time decreases, even if patients simultaneously shorten their inspiratory time. This dynamic hyperinflation can occur even during activities such as walking (36). The resulting 'dynamic' hyperinflation is very detrimental to lung mechanics and helps to explain the occurrence of dyspnoea with minimal activities. It follows that any intervention that results in decreased hyperinflation with activities should result in improvement in functional capacity through less dyspnoea at similar levels of exercise.

ALTERATION IN GAS EXCHANGE

The uneven distribution of airway disease and emphysema helps to explain the change in blood gases. The lungs of patients with COPD can be considered as consisting of two portions: one more emphysematous and the other one more normal (Fig. 3.3). The pressure–volume curve of the emphysematous portion is displaced up and to the left compared with that of the more normal lung. At low lung volume the emphysematous (more compliant) portion undergoes greater volume changes than the more normal lung. In contrast, at higher lung volume the emphysematous lung is overinflated and accepts less volume change, per unit of pressure change, than the normal lung. Therefore, the distribution of ventilation is non-uniform, and overall, the emphysematous areas of the lung are underventilated compared with the more normal lung. Because perfusion is even more compromised than ventilation in the emphysematous areas, they have a high ventilation/perfusion ratio and behave as dead space. Indeed, this wasted portion of ventilation (V_D/V_T) corresponding to approximately 0.3–0.4 of the tidal breath of a normal person has been measured to be much higher in patients with severe emphysema (37). At the same time, narrower bronchi in other areas may not allow appropriate ventilation to reach relatively well-perfused areas of the lung. This low ventilation/perfusion ratio will contribute to venous admixture ($\dot{V}/\dot{Q}$) and hypoxaemia (38, 39). The overall result is the simultaneous coexistence of high V_D/V_T regions with regions of low $\dot{V}/\dot{Q}$ match. Both increase the ventilatory demand, thereby taxing the respiratory system of these patients even more.

As ventilatory demand increases, so does the work of breathing, as the patient with COPD must attempt to increase ventilation in order to maintain an adequate delivery of oxygen. Alveolar ventilation must also be sufficient to eliminate the CO_2 produced. If this does not occur, P_aCO_2 will increase. Indeed, the arterial blood gas changes over time in patients with COPD in parallel with this sequence. Initially P_aO_2 progressively decreases, but is compensated with increased ventilation. When the ventilation is insufficient, the P_aCO_2 rises (40,

41). This is consistent with the observation that patients with COPD who develop severe hypoxaemia and hypercarbia have a very poor prognosis (19).

CONTROL OF VENTILATION

For gas exchange to occur it is necessary to move air in and out of the lung. This is achieved by the respiratory pump, which is composed of the respiratory centres, the nerves that carry the signals from those centres, the respiratory muscles that are the pressure-generating structures and the rib cage and abdomen. These components are linked and ordinarily function in a well-orchestrated manner whereby ventilation goes unnoticed and utilizes very little energy (42, 43).

The central controller or respiratory centre is located in the upper medulla and integrates input from the periphery and other parts of the nervous system (44). The output of this generator is not only modulated by mechanical, cortical and sensory inputs, but also by the state of oxygenation (P_aO_2), CO_2 concentration (P_aCO_2) and acid–base status (pH). Once generated, the output is distributed by the conducting nerves to the respiratory muscles, which shorten, deform the rib cage and abdomen, and generate intrathoracic pressures. These pressure changes displace volume, and air moves in and out depending on the direction of the pressure changes.

The relation between 'drive' and inspiratory pressure or volume is referred to as 'coupling'. Coupling is usually smooth and occurs with minimal effort. This is why breathing is perceived as effortless. The act of breathing that requires effort, which is perceived as 'work', is the unpleasant sensation known as dyspnoea. The interaction between the central drive (controller output) and the final output (ventilation) is complex and involves many components (45, 46). This complexity renders it very difficult to ascribe dyspnoea to a dysfunction in any individual portion of the system. The ventilatory control can be assessed at different levels. The simplest is the minute ventilation (V_E), which reflects the final effectiveness of the ventilatory drive. Further insight can be obtained by measuring the two contributors to V_E, the tidal volume (V_T) represented by the volume of air inhaled in a breath and the respiratory frequency.

Analysis of these variables in COPD reveals that as the disease progresses, V_E increases (47). This is expected, as the need to keep oxygen uptake and CO_2 removal constant is challenged by the changes in lung mechanics and ventilation perfusion. The increase in V_E is achieved first by an increase in V_T; but as the resistive work due to airflow obstruction worsens tidal volume decreases. The respiratory rate responds in a more linear fashion, increasing as the obstruction progresses (48). The V_E can also be expressed in terms of the mean inspiratory flow rate. This is obtained by relating the V_T to the inspiratory time (V_T/T_i) and the fractional duration of inspiration or (T_i/T_{tot}). V_T/T_i reflects drive and T_i/T_{tot} reflects timing. In COPD, both are altered by the need to increase V_E. The T_i/T_{tot}, which normally has values of close to 0.38, shortens somewhat while the V_T/T_i increases more, in order to accommodate the increase in respiratory rate and shortened T_i/T_{tot}.

A relatively non-invasive way to measure central drive is the mouth occlusion pressure measured 0.1 s after the onset of inspiration ($P_{0.1}$) (49). With increased central drive, the increase in $P_{0.1}$ is higher than that of V_T/T_i (49, 50). This is due to airflow impedance that decreases mean inspiratory flow measured at the mouth while air is moving. The $P_{0.1}$ is much less affected in COPD, because it is measured in conditions of no airflow, as the airway is temporarily obstructed. Mouth occlusion pressure, or $P_{0.1}$, has been shown to increase as the degree of obstruction worsens, irrespective of the alteration in arterial blood gases. The central drive increases as the degree of air-flow obstruction progresses, reaching its maximum in patients in respiratory failure (50). The drive is effectively 'coupled' to increased V_T in the early stages of obstruction, but V_T actually drops as the work to move air becomes very high. The only alternative is to increase respiratory rate. This also occurs, but as determined by the flow limitation characteristics of these patients, these adaptive phenomena may result in further hyperinflation. As described earlier, hyperinflation displaces diseased portions of lung higher in their pressure–volume relationship. This effectively turns many portions of the lung into 'restrictive' tissue. At this point, respiration is less demanding (in terms of work or pressure changes) when a fast and shallower ventilatory pattern is adopted. Indeed, this is the observed breathing strategy in patients with the most severe COPD (47, 51).

RESPIRATORY MUSCLES

As noted before, breathing depends on the coordinated action of different groups of muscles. The respiratory muscles can be divided into those that help inflate the lungs (inspiratory) and those that have an expiratory action. In addition, there are upper airway muscles (tongue, muscles of the palate, pharynx and vocal cords), the function of which is to contract at the beginning of inspiration and hold the upper airways open throughout inhalation. Although very important in normal function, they play a limited role in pure COPD and will not be discussed further.

The diaphragm and the other inspiratory muscles are inner-vated by a wide array of motor neurons that range from cranial nerve 11 (C-11), which provides neuronal input to the sterno-mastoid, to lumbar roots L2–L3, which innervate abdominal muscles. The respiratory cycle is regulated by a complex series of centrally organized neurons, which maintain rhythmic breathing that usually goes unnoticed and which can be vol-untarily overridden by the cortex.

The most important inspiratory muscle is the diaphragm (52). It is well suited to perform its work due to its anatomic arrangement and histochemical composition. Its long fibres extend from the non-contractile central tendon, and are directed down and outwards to insert circumferentially in the lower ribs and upper lumbar spine. This concave shape allows the muscle its lifting action as it contracts. The diaphragm can shorten up to 40 per cent between full expiration and end

inspiration (53, 54). During quiet breathing, it accounts for most of the force needed to displace the rib cage. Other inspiratory muscles are also agonists during quiet breathing and contribute to inspiratory effort. They are the scalene and parasternal intercostal muscles. There are yet other muscles (truly accessory in nature) that are not active during quiet breathing in normals but which may contribute to ventilation in situations of increased demand, e.g. the sternomastoid, pectoralis minor, latissimus dorsi and trapezius, which are truly 'accessory' muscles (43, 45, 47). The abdominal muscles are expiratory in action, since their contractions will decrease lung volume (55). In as much as they also provide tone to the abdominal wall, they help the diaphragm because they con-tribute to the generation of the gastric pressure needed for diaphragmatic contraction to be effective.

It has been postulated that the automatic and voluntary ventilatory pathways are different and that the respiratory and tonic functions of these muscles are driven from different central nervous areas and integrated at the spinal level. In patients in whom some of these muscles are participating in respiration, to perform non-ventilatory work they must main-tain a high degree of coordination. Either because of the load or because of competing central integration, muscle function may become uncoordinated and result in dysfunction. We have shown that this occurs in patients with COPD who per-form unsupported arm exercise (56). This type of exercise leads to early fatigue of the muscles involved in arm positioning and to dyssynchrony between rib cage and diaphragm–abdomen. This could also be caused by competing outputs of the various driving centres that control rhythmic respiratory and tonic activities of the accessory ventilatory muscles and the diaphragm. This dyssynchrony may be perceived as dysp-noea. Its occurrence has been observed in normal subjects breathing against resistive loads and in patients with COPD breathing during voluntary hyperventilation (57). Likewise, it has been observed in patients immediately after disconnection from ventilators but before evidence of contractile fatigue (58). This suggests that dyssynchrony is a consequence of the load and not an indication of fatigue itself. Whatever the reason, this breathing pattern is ineffective and associated with dyspnoea.

DYSPNOEA

Many patients with COPD stop exercising because of dys-pnoea, and dyspnoea is the dominant symptom during acute exacerbations of the disease (59–61). Recent studies have shown that, in COPD, dyspnoea with exercise correlates bet-ter with the degree of dynamic hyperinflation (35, 36, 62) than with changes in airflow indices or blood gas exchange. Dyspnoea also correlates better with respiratory muscle func-tion than with airflow obstruction (62). Studies in normals have shown that dyspnoea increases as the ratio between the pressure needed to ventilate and the maximal pressure that the muscles can generate ($P_{breath}/P_{i\,max}$) increases. Dyspnoea also worsens in proportion to the duration of the inspiratory contraction (T_i/T_{tot}) and respiratory frequency. These are also the factors that are associated with electromyographic (EMG) evidence of respiratory muscle fatigue (63, 64). Therefore, it has been suggested that patients with COPD develop dynamic hyperinflation which compromises ventilatory muscle function and that this is the main determinant of dyspnoea in these patients. Although respiratory muscle fatigue has been reasonably well documented in patients with COPD suffering from acute decompensation (65), its presence in stable patients remains in doubt. It is fair to state that the respiratory muscles of patients with severe COPD are functioning at a level closer to the fatigue threshold but are not fatigued. It is possible that restoration of the respiratory muscles to a better contractile state could improve the dyspnoea of these patients. Indeed, Martinez *et al.* (66) observed that the factor that best predicted the improvement in dyspnoea reported by COPD patients after lung volume reduction surgery was the lesser dynamic hyperinflation seen during exercise after the procedure. This is consistent with similar reports from other groups (67–69) and the close association between decreased dynamic hyperinflation and dyspnoea in patents treated with bronchodilators (70–72).

Dyspnoea in patients with severe COPD may also be due to the level of resting respiratory drive, and the individual's response of the central output to different stimuli. In other words, at similar mechanical load and similar levels of respiratory muscle dysfunction, dyspnoea may result from an individual's response to the central motor output. This hypothesis is supported by work from Marin *et al.* (73), who demonstrated that the most important predictor of dyspnoea with exercise was the baseline central drive response to CO_2. The importance of this observation lies in the possibility that there may be a group of patients with COPD who manifest increased central drive, and in whom adequate manipulation of this drive may result in decreased dyspnoea. This has been shown to be the case after lung volume reduction surgery (74). Until further studies are completed, this remains just an interesting hypothesis.

PERIPHERAL MUSCLE FUNCTION

Many patients with COPD will stop exercise because of leg fatigue rather than dyspnoea. This observation has prompted renewed interest in the function of limb muscles in these patients. Perhaps the most important of these studies are those reported by Maltais *et al.* (75, 76), who performed biopsies of the vastus lateralis before and after lower extremity exercise training in patients with severe COPD. At baseline, patients with COPD have lower levels of the oxidative enzymes citric synthase (CS) and 3-hydroxy-acyl-CoA-hydrogenase (HADH) than normals. After exercise, the mitochondrial content of these enzymes increased. This was associated with an improvement in exercise endurance and decreased lactic acid production at peak exercise. These biochemical changes are in line with the observation of several groups who have suggested

the presence of a dysfunctional myopathy in patients with COPD (77, 78). However, Heijdra *et al.* (79) in our laboratory found that the oxygen kinetics and peripheral muscle strength were similar between patients with COPD and normal fat-free mass and smokers and non-smokers of a similar age. It is possible the changes observed in the peripheral muscle may be explained by disuse atrophy. However, it has been amply shown that the greatest effect of pulmonary rehabilitation occurs in the improvement in exercise capacity (80–82).

INTEGRATIVE APPROACH

The overall function of the respiratory system in COPD can be represented by the model shown in Fig. 3.4. Central to the model is the problem of airway narrowing and hyperinflation. In order to reverse the model to a normal state, it is necessary to resolve those two problems. Efforts to prevent the disease from developing (smoking cessation) must be associated with methods aimed at reversing airflow obstruction. Indeed, pharmacotherapy, including bronchodilators, antibiotics and corticosteroids, is given to improve airflow. If this were effective, hyperinflation should consequently decrease. One alternative is to resect the portion of the lungs that is severely diseased, as has been done in cases of large bullae (83). Partial resection of lesser evident emphysematous areas (lung volume reduction surgery) seems effective for a minority of patients (84). Finally, in acute exacerbations or under situations of increased ventilatory demands, the system may fail and respiratory failure with death may occur. Fortunately, the advances in non-invasive and invasive mechanical ventilation have made possible the support required to guarantee survival of most patients with acute-on-chronic respiratory failure.

Pulmonary rehabilitation through improvement in peripheral muscle function, optimization of nutrition, oxygenation and medication use, as well as implementation of adequate

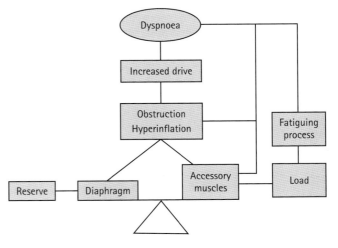

Figure 3.4 *Schematic model that integrates the different components of breathing in patients with COPD.*

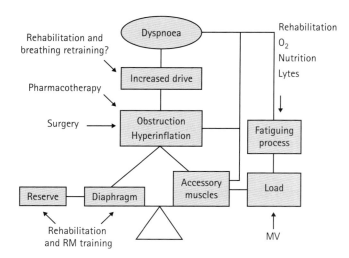

Figure 3.5 *Interventions that may be beneficial in COPD as based on the model in Fig. 3.4. MV, mechanical ventilation; RM, respiratory muscle.*

coping mechanisms, as shown in Fig. 3.5, remains the best available option because it has an impact on all of the different components of the vicious cycle of COPD. Therefore, a 'do nothing' attitude to patients with symptomatic airflow obstruction is neither appropriate nor justified.

Key points

- Most of our knowledge about the effects of pulmonary rehabilitation centres on COPD, because these patients are the ones most often studied.
- COPD is primarily an airways disease associated, to a greater or lesser degree, with parenchymal lung destruction. The extent of both events varies in different portions of the lung.
- The regional differences result in inhomogenous ventilation and perfusion and alterations in gas exchange.
- Airflow limitation, rapid breathing and lung destruction lead to hyperinflation that tends to worsen with increased ventilatory demand.
- Lung inflation hinders rib cage anatomy and respiratory muscle function.
- All of this results in increased work of breathing, decreased reserve and dyspnoea.
- In addition, COPD has important associated peripheral muscle dysfunction, which, coupled with the respiratory events, promotes a sedentary lifestyle and ever-increasing functional limitation.
- Pulmonary rehabilitation reverses many of the consequences of these pathophysiological problems and thereby improves overall outcome with little impact on airflow limitation.

REFERENCES

● 1. Mannino DM. COPD: epidemiology, prevalence, morbidity and mortality, and disease heterogeneity. *Chest* 2002; **121**: 121–6.
● 2. Pauwels RA, Buist AS, Calverley PM *et al*. Global strategy for the diagnosis, management, and prevention of chronic obstructive pulmonary disease. NHLBI/WHO Global Initiative for Chronic Obstructive Lung Disease (GOLD) Workshop summary. *Am J Respir Crit Care Med* 2001; **163**: 1256–76.
3. American Thoracic Society. Standards for the diagnosis and care of patients with chronic obstructive pulmonary disease (COPD). *Am J Respir Crit Care Med* 1995; **154**: 120–1.
4. Mitchell RS, Stanford RE, Johnson JM *et al*. The morphologic features of the bronchi, bronchioles and alveoli in chronic airway obstruction. *Am Rev Respir Dis* 1976; **114**: 137–45.
5. Thurlbeck WM. Pathophysiology of chronic obstructive pulmonary disease. *Clin Chest Med* 1990; **11**: 389–403.
6. Jeffery PK. Structural and inflammatory changes in COPD: a comparison with asthma. *Thorax* 1998; **53**: 129–36.
7. Keatings VM, Barnes PJ. Granulocyte activation markers in induced sputum: comparison between chronic obstructive pulmonary disease, asthma and normal subjects. *Am J Respir Crit Care* 1997; **155**: 449–53.
8. Saetta M, Di Stefano A, Turato G. CD8+ T-lymphocytes in peripheral airways of smokers with chronic obstructive pulmonary disease. *Am J Respir Crit Care Med* 1998; **157**: 822–6.
9. Finkelstein R, Fraser RS, Ghezzo H, Cosio MG. Alveolar inflammation and its relation to emphysema in smokers. *Am J Respir Crit Care Med* 1995; **152**: 1666–72.
10. Yamamoto C, Yoneda T, Yoshikawa M *et al*. Airway inflammation in COPD assessed by sputum level of interleukin-8. *Chest* 1997; **112**: 505–10.
11. Barnes PJ. New therapies for chronic obstructive pulmonary disease. *Thorax* 1998; **53**: 137–47.
12. Pratico D, Basili S, Vieri M *et al*. Chronic obstructive pulmonary disease is associated with an increase in urinary levels of isoprostane F$_{2a}$-111, an index of oxidant stress. *Am J Respir Crit Care Med* 1998; **158**: 1709–14.
13. Finlay GA, Driscoll LR, Russell KJ *et al*. Matrix-metalloproteinase expression and production by alveolar macrophages in emphysema. *Am J Respir Crit Care Med* 1997; **156**: 240–7.
14. Vignole AM, Riccobono L, Mirabella A *et al*. Metalloprotinase-9/tissue inhibitor of metalloprotinase-1 ratio correlates with airflow obstruction in asthma and chronic bronchitis. *Am J Respir Crit Care Med* 1998; **158**: 1945–50.
15. Delmastro M, Balbi B. Acute exacerbations of COPD: is inflammation central to prevention and treatment strategies? *Monaldi Arch Chest Dis* 2002; **57**: 293–6.
16. Berend N, Woolcock AJ, Marlin GE. Correlation between the function and the structure of the lung in smokers. *Am Rev Respir Dis* 1979; **119**: 695–702.
17. Buist AS, Van Fleet DL, Ross BB. A comparison of conventional spirometric tests and the tests of closing volume in one emphysema screening center. *Am Rev Respir Dis* 1973; **107**: 735–40.
◆ 18. Fletcher C, Peto R. The natural history of chronic airflow obstruction. Br *Med J* 1977; **1**: 1645–8.
◆ 19. Anthonisen NR. Prognosis in chronic obstructive pulmonary disease: results from multicenter clinical trials. *Am Rev Respir Dis* 1989; **133**: 95–9.

20. Hodgkin JE. Prognosis in chronic obstructive pulmonary disease. *Clin Chest Med* 1990; **11**: 555–69.

21. Sweer L, Zwillich CW. Dyspnea in the patient with chronic obstructive pulmonary disease. *Clinics in Chest Med* 1990; **11**: 417–55.

22. Mahler DA, Weinburg DH, Wells CK, Feinstein AR. The measurement of dyspnea: contents, interobserver agreement, and physiologic correlates of two new clinical indexes. *Chest* 1984; **85**: 751–8.

23. Ries A, Kaplan R, Limberg T, Prewitt L. Effects of pulmonary rehabilitation on physiologic and psychosocial outcomes in patients with COPD. *Ann Int Med* 1995; **122**: 823–32.

24. Nishimura K, Izumi T, Tsukino M, Oga T. Dyspnea is a better predictor of 5-year survival than airway obstruction in patients with COPD. *Chest* 2002; **121**: 1434–40.

25. Gerardi D, Lovett L, Benoit-Connors J, ZuWallack R. Variables related to increased mortality following outpatient pulmonary rehabilitation. *Eur Respir J* 1996; **9**: 431–5.

26. Pinto-Plata V, Cote C, Taylor J *et al.* Natural decline in the six minute walking distance (6 MWD) in COPD. *Eur Respir J*, in press.

27. Szekely L, Oelberg D, Wright C *et al.* Preoperative predictors of operative mortality in COPD patients undergoing bilateral lung volume reduction surgery. *Chest* 1997; **111**: 550–8.

28. Oga T, Nishimura K, Tsukino M *et al.* Analysis of the factors related to mortality in chronic obstructive pulmonary disease. Role of exercise capacity and health status. *Am J Respir Crit Care Med* 2002; **167**: 544–49.

29. Nagai A, Yamawaki I, Takizawa T, Thurlbeck WM. Alveolar attachments in emphysema of human lungs. *Am Rev Respir Dis* 1991; **144**: 888–91.

30. Postma DS, Slinter HJ. Prognosis of chronic obstructive pulmonary disease: the Dutch experience. *Am Rev Respir Dis* 1989; **140**: 100–5.

31. Bates DV. *Respiratory Function in Disease*, 3rd edn. Philadelphia: WB Saunders, 1989; 172–87.

32. Greaves IA, Colebatch HJ. Elastic behavior and structure of normal and emphysematous lungs postmortem. *Am Rev Respir Dis* 1980; **121**: 127–8.

33. Hogg JC, Macklem PT, Thurlbeck WA. Site and nature of airways obstruction in chronic obstructive lung disease. *N Eng J Med* 1968; **278**: 1355–9.

◆34. O'Donnell SE, Sanil R, Anthonisen NR, Younis M. Effect of dynamic airway compression on breathing pattern and respiratory sensation in severe chronic obstructive pulmonary disease. *Am Rev Respir Dis* 1987; **135**: 912–8.

◆35. O'Donnell D, Lam M, Webb K. Measurement of symptoms, lung hyperinflation and endurance during exercise in COPD. *Am J Respir Crit Care Med* 1998; **158**: 1557–65.

◆36. Marin J, Carrizo S, Gascon MS *et al.* Inspiratory capacity, dynamic hyperinflation, breathlessness and exercise performance during the 6 minute walk test in chronic obstructive pulmonary disease. *Am J Respir Cirt Care Med* 2001; **163**: 1395–400.

37. Javahari S, Blum J, Kazemi H. Pattern of breathing and carbon dioxide retention in chronic obstructive lung disease. *Am J Med* 1981; **71**: 228–34.

38. Rodriguez-Roisin R, Roca J. Pulmonary gas exchange. In: Calverly PM, Pride NB, eds. *Chronic Obstructive Pulmonary Disease*. London: Chapman & Hall, 1995; 167–84.

39. Parot S, Miara B, Milic-Emili J, Gautier H. Hypoxemia, hypercapnia and breathing patterns in patients with chronic obstructive pulmonary disease. *Am Rev Respir Dis* 1982; **126**: 882–6.

40. Begin P, Grassino A. Inspiratory muscle dysfunction and chronic hypercapnia in chronic obstructive pulmonary disease. *Am Rev Respir Dis* 1991; **143**: 905–12.

41. Montes de Oca M, Celli BR. Mouth occlusion pressure, CO_2 response and hypercapnia in severe obstructive pulmonary disease. *Eur Respir J* 1998; **12**: 666–71.

42. Flaminiano L, Celli BR. Respiratory muscle testing. *Clin Chest Med* 2001; **22**: 661–77.

43. Roussos Ch, Macklem PT. The respiratory muscles. *N Engl J Med* 1982; **307**: 786–97.

44. VonEuler C. On the central pattern generator for the basic breathing rhythmicity. *J Appl Physiol* 1983; **55**: 1647–59.

45. Derenne JP, Macklem PT, Roussos CH. The respiratory muscles: mechanics, control and pathophysiology. *Am Rev Respir Dis* 1978; **119**: 119–33, 373–90.

46. Sears TA. Central rhythm and pattern generation. *Chest* 1990; **97**: 45–7.

47. Martinez FJ, Couser JI, Celli BR. Factors influencing ventilatory muscle recruitment in patients with chronic airflow obstruction. *Am Rev Respir Dis* 1990; **142**: 276–82.

48. Murciano D, Broczkowski J, Lecocguic M *et al.* Tracheal occlusion pressure. A simple index to monitor respiratory muscle fatigue during acute respiratory failure in patients with chronic obstructive pulmonary disease. *Ann Int Med* 1988; **108**: 800–5.

49. Milic-Emili J, Grassino AE, Whitelaw WA. Measurement and testing of respiratory drive. In: Horbein TF. *Regulation of Breathing. Lung Biology in Health and Disease*. New York: Marcel Dekker, 1981; 675–743.

50. Sasoon CS, Te TT, Mahutte CR, Light R. Airway occlusion pressure. An important indicator for successful weaning in patients with chronic obstructive pulmonary disease. *Am Rev Respir Dis* 1987; **135**: 107–13.

51. Loveridge B, West P, Anthonisen NR, Krugger MH. Breathing patterns in patients with chronic obstructive pulmonary disease. *Am Rev Respir Dis* 1984; **130**: 730–3.

◆52. Rochester DF. The diaphragm contractile properties and fatigue. *J Clin Invest* 1985; **75**: 1397–402.

53. Braun NM, Arora NS, Rochester DF. The force-length relationship of the normal human diaphragm. *J Appl Physiol* 1982; **53**: 405–12.

54. Celli BR. Respiratory management of diaphragmatic paralysis. *Sem Respir Crit Care Med* 2002; **23**: 275–81.

55. DeTroyer A, Estenne M. Functional anatomy of the respiratory muscles. *Clin Chest Med* 1988; **9**: 175–93.

56. Celli BR, Rassulo J, Make B. Dyssynchronous breathing during arm but not leg exercise in patients with chronic airflow obstruction. *N Engl J Med* 1986; **314**: 1485–90.

57. Sharp JT. The respiratory muscles in emphysema. *Clin Chest Med* 1983; **4**: 421–32.

58. Tobin MJ, Perez W, Guenther SM *et al.* Does rib-cage abdominal paradox signify respiratory muscle fatigue? *J Appl Physiol* 1987; **63**: 857–60.

59. Killian K, Jones N. Respiratory muscle and dyspnea. *Clin Chest Med* 1988; **9**: 237–48.

60. LeBlanc P, Bowie DM, Summers E *et al.* Breathlessness and exercise in patients with cardiorespiratory disease. *Am Rev Respir Dis* 1986; **133**: 21–5.

61. Girish M, Pinto V, Kenney L *et al.* Dyspnea in acute exacerbation of COPD is associated with increase in ventilatory demand and not with worsened airflow obstruction. ACCP *Chest* 1998; **114**: 266S.

62. Killian K, Jones N. Respiratory muscle and dyspnea. *Clin Chest Med* 1988; **9**: 237–48.

63. Bellemare F, Grassino A. Forces reserve of the diaphragm in patients with chronic obstructive pulmonary disease. *J Appl Physiol* 1983; **55**: 8–15.

64. Breslin EH, Garroutte BC, Carrieri VK, Celli BR. Correlations between dyspnea, diaphragm and sternomastoid recruitment during inspiratory resistance breathing in normal subjects. *Chest* 1990; **98**: 298–302.

65. Cohen C, Zagelbaum G, Gross D *et al.* Clinical manifestations of inspiratory muscle fatigue. *Am J Med* 1982; **73**: 308–16.

66. Martinez F, Montes de Oca M, Whyte R *et al.* Lung-volume reduction surgery improves dyspnea, dynamic hyperinflation and respiratory muscle function. *Am J Respir Crit Care Med* 1997; **155**: 2018–23.

67. Brantigan OC, Mueller E, Kress MB. A surgical approach to pulmonary emphysema. *Am Rev Respir Dis* 1959; **80**: 194–202.

68. Cooper JD, Trulock ER, Triantafillou AN *et al.* Bilateral pneumonectomy (volume reduction) for chronic obstructive pulmonary disease. *J Thor Cardiovasc Surg* 1995; **109**: 116–19.

69. Knudson RJ, Gaensler E. Surgery for emphysema. *Ann Thor Surg* 1965; **1**: 332–62.

70. Belman M, Botnick W, Shin W. Inhaled bronchodilators reduce dynamic hyperinflation during exercise in patients with chronic obstructive pulmonary disease. *Am J Respir Crit Care Med* 1996I; **53**: 967–75.

71. Di Marco F, Milic-Emili J, Boveri B *et al.* Effect of inhaled bronchodilators on inspiratory capacity and dyspnoea at rest in COPD. *Eur Respir J* 2003; **21**: 86–94.

72. O'Donnell DE, Lam M, Webb KA. Spirometric correlates of improvement in exercise performance after anticholinergic therapy in chronic obstructive pulmonary disease. *Am J Respir Crit Care Med* 1999; **160**: 542–9.

73. Marin J, Montes De Oca M, Rassulo J, Celli BR. Ventilatory drive at rest and perception of exertional dyspnea in severe COPD. *Chest* 1999; **115**: 1293–300.

74. Celli BR, Montes de Oca M, Mendez R, Stetz J. Lung reduction surgery in severe COPD decreases central drive and ventilatory response to CO_2. *Chest* 1997; **112**: 902–6.

◆75. Maltais F, Simard A, Simard J *et al.* Oxidative capacity of the skeletal muscle and lactic acid kinetics during exercise in normal subjects and in patients with COPD. *Am J Respir Crit Care Med* 1995; **153**: 288–93.

◆76. Maltais F, LeBlanc P, Simard C *et al.* Skeletal muscle adaptation of endurance training in patients with chronic obstructive pulmonary disease. *Am J Respir Crit Care Med* 1996; **154**: 442–7.

77. Engelen MP, Schols AM, Baken WC *et al.* Nutritional depletion in relation to respiratory and peripheral skeletal muscle function in out-patients with COPD. *Eur Respir J* 1994; **7**: 1793–7.

78. Polkey MI. Muscle metabolism and exercise tolerance in COPD. *Chest* 2002; **121**: 131–5.

◆79. Heijdra Y, Pinto-Plata V, Frants R *et al.* Muscle strength and exercise kinetics in COPD patients with a normal fat-free mass index are comparable to control subjects. Chest 2003; **124**: 75–82.

80. Casaburi R, Patessio A, Ioli F *et al.* Reductions in exercise lactic acidosis and ventilation as a result of exercise training in patients with obstructive lung disease. *Am Rev Respir Dis* 1991; **143**: 9–18.

81. Goldstein RS, Gort EH, Stubbing D *et al.* Randomized controlled trial of respiratory rehabilitation. *Lancet* 1994; **344**: 1394–7.

82. Reardon J, Awad E, Normandin E *et al.* The effect of comprehensive outpatient pulmonary rehabilitation on dyspnea. *Chest* 1994; **105**: 1046–52.

83. Fitzgerald MX, Keelan PJ, Cugel DW, Gaensler EA. Long-term results of surgery for bullous emphysema. *J Thor Cardiovasc Surg* 1974; **68**: 566–87.

84. National Emphysema Treatment Trial Research Group. A randomized trial comparing lung-volume-reduction surgery with medical therapy for severe emphysema. *N Engl J Med* 2003; **348**: 2059–73.

4

The influence of tobacco smoking on lung disease

STEFANO NARDINI

GROWTH OF TOBACCO CONSUMPTION

Tobacco was imported to Europe in the early sixteenth century, after the discovery of America by Columbus. Its use spread throughout the 'civilized' world during the seventeenth and eighteenth centuries. As tobacco consumption increased, so did the ways of using it. In the eighteenth century the favourite use of tobacco was as snuff, but during the nineteenth century cigars and pipes became fashionable. The twentieth century saw massive use of the manufactured cigarette, following the invention of the cigarette machine in 1881. Tobacco consumption increased to include, at its peak, one-third of the world's adults. Currently 1.1 billion people smoke, a figure expected to rise to 1.6 billion by the year 2025.

In 1938, Ochsner reported the link between smoking tobacco and lung cancer (1). Subsequent landmark studies included reports by Wynder and Graham (2), in the USA and Doll and Hill in the UK, both in the 1950s (3, 4). In 1962, The Royal College of Physicians in the UK published their report on *Smoking and Health* (5) and in 1964 in the US Surgeon General's report was published (6). Each of these reports has contributed substantially to our understanding of the harms associated with smoking. Despite unequivocal evidence as to the harmful effects of smoking on health, overall reductions in tobacco consumption have been slow, as decreases in some countries have been overshadowed by increases in others.

TOBACCO AS A DISEASE

Epidemiology

The number of smokers on each continent varies considerably, with a global prevalence of 29 per cent (47 per cent males, 12 per cent females). Whereas in higher income societies, smoking prevalence has been decreasing since the 1980s to a current prevalence of 30 per cent (29 per cent male, 22 per cent female), in low-income societies, the prevalence has been increasing, and now stands at 29 per cent (49 per cent male, 9 per cent female) (7).

In the Americas, smoking is decreasing, while in Europe, after a decreasing trend, it is again increasing. Smoking is stable in South-east Asia, Africa and the eastern Mediterranean. In the western Pacific it is increasing. The epidemic of smoking follows a bell-shaped curve, with an initially high uptake and low quitting rate, followed by a low intake and low quitting rate, and finally a low intake and a high quitting rate (8). Male sex is a strong predictor of tobacco smoking in all parts of the world. Socioeconomic status is also a strong predictor of smoking, with more smokers among less educated people.

Smoking-related diseases

Smoking is a cause or key risk factor in a number of diseases, including all upper and lower respiratory cancers, ischaemic heart disease, cerebrovascular disease, peripheral vascular disease and chronic obstructive pulmonary disease (COPD).

In 2000, smoking deaths were second to hypertension and ahead of hypercholesterolaemia. The disease burden attributed to tobacco was ranked fourth, after malnutrition, unsafe sex and hypertension and ahead of alcohol. Tobacco-related deaths are projected to increase globally from 3.0 million/year in 1990 to 10 million/year by 2030 making smoking more important than the sum of pneumonia, diarrhoeal diseases, tuberculosis and the complications of childbirth. Globally, smoking is responsible for 1 in 10 deaths among adults, 1 in 5 in high-income countries. One-third of deaths are due to cancers (mainly lung), one-third due to respiratory diseases and one-third due to cardiovascular deaths (9, 10). Smokers have six times the risk of developing COPD and 10 times the risk of contracting lung cancer compared with non-smokers. In the US, smokers are 20 times more likely to die of lung cancer during middle age (11). As male deaths decrease in North America and Europe, female deaths continue to climb.

Aetiology

Tobacco contains noxious agents, coming directly from the plant as well as substances used for cultivation and processing. In addition to nicotine, more than 40 carcinogens have been identified in tobacco smoke (12, 13).

Nicotine addiction

Tobacco dependence is a recognized medical disorder by the WHO's International Classification of Diseases (ICD-10) (14) and the American Psychiatric Association's *Diagnostic and Statistical Manual* (DSM-IV) (15). Nearly all smokers are dependent on tobacco to some extent. A sure sign of nicotine dependence is the withdrawal syndrome, which comes when nicotine is not available for a certain period of time during usual hours. Nicotine receptors in the central nervous system, when stimulated, will trigger pleasant feelings by stimulating a reward system common to cocaine, amphetamine and other drugs, as well as modifications of mental processes that soothe anxiety and improve manual activities. These effects encourage smokers to seek nicotine (16–18). Nicotine is a simple alkaloid, a tertiary amine, capable of binding to nicotinic acetylcholinergic receptors. Nicotine receptors are freed from nicotine very quickly, so that the smoker needs to smoke again, titrating the dose by modulating the number of puffs over time, the depths of each inspiration and the number of cigarettes smoked daily. Smokers can be 'peak seekers', who smoke irregularly, seeking peak levels of nicotine to help particular situations or 'steady-state maintainers', who smoke regularly to maintain nicotine blood levels roughly constant in order to soothe the symptoms of withdrawal (19). Both the addiction to nicotine and withdrawal symptoms are obstacles to smoking cessation.

ACTIVE AND PASSIVE SMOKING AND PULMONARY DISEASE

Smoking causes lung cancer and chronic bronchitis. In 1986 (20), the first Surgeon General's report on the effects of tobacco smoke was released. In this report, distinguished physicians and scientists concluded that 'even the lower exposure to smoke received by the non-smoker carries with it a health risk'. Their conclusions are summarized in Box 4.1.

The panel reviewed studies showing the association between smoking and lung cancer, chronic respiratory disease and cardiovascular disease. They also concluded that involuntary smoking can also have small effects on pulmonary function.

Box 4.1   First statement that environmental tobacco smoke is a health hazard (20)

1. Involuntary smoking is a cause of disease, including lung cancer, in healthy non-smokers.
2. The children of parents who smoke, compared with the children of non-smoking parents, have an increased frequency of respiratory infections, increased respiratory symptoms, and slightly smaller rates of increase in lung function as the lung matures.
3. Simple separation of smokers and non-smokers within the same air space may reduce, but does not eliminate, exposure of non-smokers to environmental tobacco smoke (19).

Box 4.2   Effects of environmental tobacco smoke in the elderly (23)

- Several cross-sectional studies show an increased occurrence of chronic respiratory symptoms and deficits in ventilatory lung function in relation to environmental tobacco smoke (ETS) exposure at home or at work.
- A limited number of studies have found a significant relationship between ETS exposure and asthma, COPD, pneumococcal infections and stroke in the elderly.

A comprehensive review, published in 1998 (21), also investigated effects of involuntary smoking on adult-onset asthma and COPD. In the European Community Respiratory Health Survey, the effects of involuntary smoking on respiratory symptoms, bronchial responsiveness and lung function were investigated (22). Data from 7882 adults, aged 20–48 years, who had never smoked, were collected from 36 centres in 16 countries. The odds ratio for chronic bronchitis and for asthma was higher in subjects reporting exposure to smoke in the workplace, especially when daily exposure was over 8 hours. The effects of environmental tobacco smoke (ETS) in the elderly are summarized in Box 4.2 (23).

Environmental smoke exposure increases the risk of lung cancer and COPD (24, 25). In a prospective study of environmental smoke in Californians, the relative risk for COPD was 1.80 for men and 1.57 for women (26). The risk from ETS also includes exacerbation of pre-existent chronic respiratory conditions such as asthma. The risk is created by the particulate matter produced by the cigarette, which we have shown to exceed that of a diesel engine exhaust (27).

In conclusion, active smoking unequivocally causes several respiratory and vascular conditions. Exposure to ETS (passive smoking) should also be questioned in the diagnosis of patients with pulmonary diseases and must be addressed as part of the management of those with documented lung disease to prevent the risk of worsening the condition.

Box 4.3 Standard for tobacco control as reported by the Surgeon General (28)

- Educational strategies
- Management of nicotine addiction
- Regulatory efforts
  - advertising and promotion
  - product regulation
  - clean indoor air regulation
  - minors' access to tobacco
  - litigation approaches
- Economic approaches (increasing unit price)
- Comprehensive programmes
- Global efforts
- Elimination of health disparities

TOBACCO CONTROL

Smoking tobacco is a medical condition which needs to be treated. Although there are effective medical treatments, its control cannot be achieved solely with clinical interventions. This is why a clinician must be informed about them. The Surgeon General recently published a report examining all the possible interventions for tobacco control (28); the actions indicated in this document can be considered as the current standard (Box 4.3).

Tobacco control includes three strategies:

- helping smokers to quit
- protecting non-smokers from ETS
- protecting youngsters from tobacco smoking initiation.

According to the Surgeon General's report, achieving tobacco control should include health education, providing information regarding the effects of smoking and the best way to manage the risks from tobacco. Other important aspects of tobacco control include controlling the market through regulatory and economic measures, restricting the access of minors to tobacco products and regulating indoor air pollution.

Educational strategies

These refer to the initiatives for keeping youngsters free from tobacco and those for informing adults about the health risks associated with smoking as well as teaching them alternative behaviours to reduce those risks.

Management of nicotine addiction

This includes the diagnosis and treatment of this disorder and the available interventions for all interested people.

Regulatory efforts

Regulatory efforts include all interventions which influence tobacco production, trade and consumption through rules and laws, such as rules for the protection of non-smokers from exposure to ETS, regulations regarding the maximum levels of tar and nicotine and other substances in each cigarette, and laws limiting advertising of tobacco products and their sale to youngsters. Regulatory efforts include litigation associated with health damage due to lack of protection from passive smoking and lack of information regarding the effects of smoking.

Economic approaches

These are the interventions which, by increasing the price of tobacco products, make them less attractive to the consumer.

Comprehensive programmes

These refer to structured interventions in which educational, regulatory and economic approaches are used in combination. This is most likely to achieve significant results.

Global efforts

Global efforts emphasize the fact that tobacco production and trade are international issues. Whenever possible, international organizations such as the WHO and the European Union should work with governments towards shared programmes for more effective tobacco control.

Elimination of health disparities

Access and available treatments should be similar across different jurisdictions. A comprehensive approach is always necessary to facilitate a cultural change. In addition to regulations, medical and educational interventions, if a cultural change is obtained all actions work better.

SMOKING CESSATION

Smoking cessation is one of the most cost-effective health interventions. Even if the sustained cessation rate is modest, such as 10–20 per cent at 1 year, the results are dramatic due to the enormous prevalence of this condition. According to the 1990 report of the US Surgeon General (29), quitting smoking has effects on both mortality and morbidity of former smokers. These effects are age-independent; indeed, former smokers lived longer than those who continued to smoke. A recent update of the well-known study by British doctors Doll and Peto, comparing smokers and non-smokers, demonstrated that even quitting at the age of 60 years improves life expectancy by 3 years (30). A smoker can quit without help, but it is difficult. Long-term abstinence is improved when quitting is aided by medical treatment (31). It is especially important for patients with established respiratory conditions to quit smoking. Symptoms and signs associated with airway disease improve; the exaggerated decline of forced expiratory volume in 1s (FEV$_1$), compared with non-smokers or non-susceptible smokers, lessens (see Fig. 4.1) (32, 33).

In COPD, only smoking cessation and long term oxygen therapy have been shown to be life extending. In the Lung Health Study (34) some benefit was noted in subjects who did not succeed in sustained abstinence from smoking, but sustained quitters had the lowest prevalence of chronic cough, chronic sputum, dyspnoea and wheeze, whereas continuous smokers had the greatest prevalence of these symptoms.

Even among patients with cancer, the effects of smoking cessation are associated with increased survival. Patients with

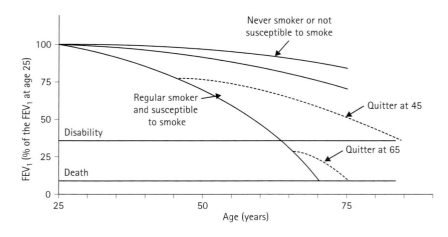

Figure 4.1 *Plot showing how the exaggerated decline of forced expiratory volume in 1 s (FEV_1), compared with non-smokers or non-susceptible smokers, lessens upon cessation of smoking, irrespective of age. After Fletcher et al. (32).*

Table 4.1 *Smoking cessation activities by classes of risk (42)*

Patients	Treatment	Staff
'Healthy' patients	Minimal advice (3 min)	Every health professional
	Over-the-counter products or pharmacotherapy	Primary care
Patients with other risk facors	Structured counselling (>30 min)	General practitioner
	Managed pharmacotherapy	Smoking cessation clinic
Patients with smoking-related conditions	Multiple pharmacotherapies	Smoking cessation clinic
	Behavioural treatment	

head and neck cancer who quit smoking had a better response to radiation therapy than those who continued to smoke (35) and patients receiving chemotherapy for limited small-cell lung cancer experienced a decreased survival if they continued to smoke (36). The issue of smoking cessation among individuals with respiratory disease raises some interesting, unresolved issues. Do side-effects of smoking cessation on mood compound the secondary impairments of mood associated with chronic respiratory disease? Is the approach to smoking cessation the same among patients with severe COPD as it is among relatively asymptomatic individuals?

In conclusion, smoking cessation is the most important therapeutic intervention for the prevention and management of COPD and should be available for all patients (37). The earlier this management is started, the more successful its effect on the underlying disease is likely to be.

Motivation to quit

The importance a person ascribes to a treatment will determine how that person manages the difficulties associated with it. In smoking cessation motivation is a key factor. Prochaska and Di Clemente (38) proposed five stages of motivation to quit: pre-contemplation, contemplation, preparation, action and maintenance. As with other respiratory conditions, such as asthma and tuberculosis, motivation to adhere to health care recommendations varies and is sometimes at its highest when the patient feels unwell. Therefore, at each encounter with a health care provider, smokers should be encouraged to quit and provided with a framework for follow-up. Although sustained quitting may not be easily achievable, a reasonable goal

for an encounter is to move the patient one step along the five Prochaska and Di Clemente stages.

Smoking reduction

The issues of smoking reduction and smoking cessation are addressed in Chapter 22. Reduction is an endpoint, if total and sustained cessation cannot be attained. As with smoking cessation, a combination of behavioural and pharmacological approaches can be used.

The role of the chest physician

Although chest physicians are key role models for smoking cessation, their training is often lacking in this area (39). This puts them and their patients at a disadvantage, given the contribution of smoking-related diseases to their practice (40). The success in smoking cessation is closely related to the time allocated to it (41). Therefore, a chest physician should be able to administer minimal interventions when encountering patients during an acute illness, as they are highly receptive to smoking cessation at that time, as well as more intensive interventions during a more stable phase of their disease. Chest physicians interested in this area can be very effective in operating smoking cessation clinics (42). Such clinics provide resources for referral by general practitioners and can participate in the evaluation of innovative modalities of care. Smoking cessation activities can be adjusted according to the smokers' risk (Table 4.1). Smoking cessation clinics utilize the 'five A's' list described by Fiore *et al.* (41), as summarized in Box 4.4.

Box 4.4   The 'five As' of smoking cessation

- **Ask** all patients if they smoke – a complete smoking history includes the age of starting smoking, the number of cigarettes smoked per day, the type of cigarette smoked, the main characteristics of routine smoking, information about previous cessation attempts. Objective measures are recorded with the Fagerstrom Tolerance Questionnaire (43) and with the measurement of exhaled carbon monoxide (44).
- **Advise** patients to quit, using personalized information from their history.
- **Assess** motivation, which is important both in predicting the likelihood of success and in establishing the intensity of management. A smoker's diary can improve motivation to the point of halving the number of cigarettes smoked. For the physician, the diary provides an important profile of the smoker.
- **Assist** in quitting through a comprehensive management approach for each smoker.
- **Arrange** follow-up after cessation to provide positive reinforcement and identify relapse-threatening issues at regular intervals. If relapse does occur, then it is necessary to assist the patient by re-contacting and initiating a management strategy to address what happened. The goal is to maintain contact.

Box 4.5   The 'five Rs' of the smoker unwilling to quit

- **Relevance** – ask why quitting can be relevant, e.g. health reasons, protection of children, economic reasons
- **Risks** – ask about the risks of continuing smoking: the acute and long-term health risks
- **Rewards** – ask about the potential benefits (rewards) of quitting
- **Roadblocks** – ask the patient to identify which issues prevent quitting smoking
- **Repetition** – repeat this motivational intervention every time the unmotivated patient comes to the clinic

It should be remembered that tobacco smoking is 'a chronic disease, which moves through multiple periods of relapse and remission. Like hypertension or COPD, smoking requires ongoing care with counselling advice, support and pharmacotherapy. Relapse is common and just reflects the chronic nature of the condition, not a failure of the physician or patient' (41). A smoker who is unable or unwilling to quit can be helped by the application of the 'five R's', as summarized in Box 4.5 (41).

Limited resources are required for a smoking cessation clinic: a room for the visit, a telephone line for contacts, a personal computer for database management, a carbon monoxide analyser, a physician, a nurse and a psychologist, often on a part-time basis, who have been trained in smoking cessation techniques (45).

FUTURE DEVELOPMENTS

The WHO has identified tobacco-related diseases as one of its two priorities for this millennium. This will require enhanced training of health care providers regarding tobacco dependence and its treatment. Key issues include the following:

- The importance of tobacco smoking should be emphasized in medical society meetings, scientific journals, scientific websites and educational programmes.
- Audits regarding the dissemination and application of guidelines on smoking cessation should be encouraged.
- Postgraduate education regarding smoking cessation should be available through professional societies.
- Medical school curricula should include tobacco control and smoking cessation.
- Granting agencies to fund research on the essentials of tobacco control.
- Improved regulations by the European Respiratory Society and other similar professional organizations should be promoted, to limit publicity of events by tobacco companies.

Efforts such as the above, and partnership with the WHO as well as other scientific societies, will result in a significant contribution to reducing the burden of diseases associated with smoking.

Key points

- The global burden of smoking on lung disease remains enormous.
- Environmental smoke exposure also increases the risk of lung disease.
- Tobacco control is best tackled by comprehensive approaches, including education, legislation and cultural changes.
- Chest physicians are key role models in smoking cessation, in terms of both their own behaviour and their role in treating smokers.
- Scientific and political partnerships between national societies, governments and the WHO will reduce the burden of lung disease associated with smoking.

REFERENCES

1. Doll R. Tobacco: a medical history. *J Urban Health* 1999; **76**: 289–313.
2. Wynder EL, Graham EA. Tobacco smoking as a possible etiologic factor in bronchogenic carcinoma. *J Am Med Assoc* 1950; **143**: 329–36.

3. Doll R, Hill AB. Smoking and carcinoma of the lung. *Br Med J* 1950; **221**: 739–48.

4. Doll R, Hill AB. A study of aetiology of carcinoma of the lung. *Br Med J* 1952; **225**: 1271–86.

5. Royal College of Physicians. *Smoking and Health*. London: Pitman Medical Publishing, 1962.

6. Centers for Disease Control. *Smoking and Health: Report of the Advisory Committee to the Surgeon General of the Public Health Service*. PHS Publication No. 1103. Washington, DC, US: Department of Health, Education, and Welfare, Centers for Disease Control, 1964.

7. Peto R, Lopez AD. Future worldwide health effects of current smoking patterns. In: Koop CE, Pearson CE, Schwarz MR, eds. *Critical Issues in Global Health*. San Francisco: Wiley, 2001; 154–61.

8. Slama K. The role of information, education and treatment in tobacco control. *Monaldi Arch Chest Dis* 2001; **56**: 546–9.

9. Boring CC, Squires TS, Tong T *et al*. Mortality trends for selected smoking-related cancers and breast cancer – United States, 1950–1990. *MMWR* 1993; **42**: 8638–66.

10. Tager IB, Segal MR, Speizer FE *et al*. The natural history of forced expiratory volumes. Effect of cigarette smoking and respiratory symptoms. *Am Rev Respir Dis* 1988; **138**: 837–49.

11. Peto R, Lopez AD, Boreham J *et al. Mortality from Smoking in Developed Countries: 1950–2000*. Oxford: Oxford University Press, 1994.

12. Wynder EL, Hoffmann D. Present status of laboratory studies on tobacco carcinogenesis. *Acta Path Microbiol Scand,* 1961 **52**: 119–32.

13. International Agency for Research on Cancer. *Monographs on the Evaluation of the Carcinogenic risk of Chemicals to Humans*. Tobacco Smoking No 38. Lyons: IARC, 1986.

14. WHO. *World Health Organization International Classification of Disease – Tenth Revision Vol. 1 F17– Mental and Behavioural Disorders due to Use of Tobacco*. Geneva: World Health Organization, 1992.

15. American Psychiatric Association. Nicotine induced disorder. *Diagnostic and Statistical Manual of Mental Disorders (DSM IV)*. Washington: American Psychiatric Association, 1994; 244–7.

16. Balfour D, Fagerström K-O. Pharmacology of nicotine and its therapeutic use in smoking cessation and neurodegenerative disorders. *Pharmacology & Therapeutics* 1996; **72**: 51–81.

17. Pickworth WB, Keenan RM, Henningfield JE. Nicotine: effects and mechanisms. In: Chang LW, Byer RS, eds. *Handbook of Neurotoxicology*. New York: Marcel Dekker, 1995; 801–24.

18. US Department of Health and Human Services. *The Health Consequences of Smoking: Nicotine Addiction. A Report of the Surgeon General*. DHHS (CDC) Publication No. 88. Washington DC: DHHS, 2004.

19. Hughes JR, Higgins ST, Hatsukami DK. Effects of abstinence for tobacco: a critical review. In: Kozlowski LT, Annis H, Cappell HD *et al*. eds. *Research Advances in Alcohol and Drug Problems*. New York: Plenum Press, 1990; 317–98.

20. US Department of Health and Human Services. *The Health Consequences of Involuntary Smoking. A Report of the Surgeon General PHS-CDC-CHPE*. Rockville, Maryland: DHHS, 1986.

21. Coultas DB. Health effects of passive smoking. Passive smoking and risk of adult asthma and COPD. In: Britton JR; Weiss ST, eds. Health effects of passive smoking. *Thorax* 1998; **53**: 381–7.

22. Janson C, Chinn S, Jarvis D *et al*. European Community Respiratory Health Survey. Effect of passive smoking on respiratory symptoms, bronchial responsiveness, lung function, and total serum IgE in the European Community Respiratory Health Survey: a cross-sectional study. *Lancet* 2001; **358**: 2103–9.

23. Jaakkola MS. Environmental tobacco smoke and health in the elderly. *Eur Respir J* 2002; **19**: 172–81.

24. Hopkins DP, Briss PA, Ricard CJ *et al*. Task Force on Community Preventive Services. Reviews of evidence regarding interventions to reduce tobacco use and exposure to environmental tobacco smoke. *Am J Prev Med* 2001; **20**: 16–66.

25. Allwright S, McLaughlin JP, Murphy D *et al. Report on the Health Effects of Environmental Tobacco Smoke (ETS) in the Workplace*. Ireland: Health and Safety Authority and the Office of Tobacco Control, 2002.

26. Enstrom JE, Kabat GC. Environmental tobacco smoke and tobacco-related mortality in a prospective study of Californians 1960–1998. *Br Med J* 2003; **326**: 1057–67.

27. Invernizzi G, Ruprecht A, Mazza R *et al*. Particulate matter from tobacco versus diesel car exhaust: an educational perspective. *Tobacco Control* 2004; **13**: 219–21.

28. US Department of Health and Human Services. *Reducing Tobacco Use. A Report of the Surgeon General – Executive Summary*. Atlanta: GEO, 2000.

29. US Department of Health and Human Services. *The Health Benefits of Smoking Cessation: A Report of the Surgeon General, 1990*. Washington, DC: US Department of Health and Human Services, 1990.

30. Doll R, Peto R, Boreham J, Sutherland I. Mortality in relation to smoking: 50 years observations on male British doctors. *Br Med J* 2004; **328**: 1519.

31. Lancaster T, Stead L, Silagy C, Sowden A. Effectiveness of interventions to help people stop smoking: findings from the Cochrane Library. *Br Med J* 2000; **321**: 355–8.

32. Fletcher C, Peto R, Tinker C *et al. The Natural History of Chronic Bronchitis and Emphysema*. London: Oxford University Press, 1976.

33. Kanner RE, Connett JE, Williams DE, Buist AS. Effects of randomized assignment to a smoking cessation intervention and changes in smoking habits on respiratory symptoms in smokers with early chronic obstructive pulmonary disease: The Lung Health Study. *Am J Med* 1999; **106**: 410–16.

34. Murray RP, Anthonisen NR, Connett JE *et al*. Effects of multiple attempts to quit smoking and relapses to smoking on pulmonary function. Lung health Study Research Group. *J Clin Epidemiol* 1998; **51**: 1317–26.

35. Browman GP, Wong G, Hodson I *et al*. Influence of cigarette smoking on the efficacy of radiation therapy in head and neck cancer. *N Engl J Med* 1993; **328**: 159–63.

36. Videtic GM, Stitt LW, Dar AR *et al*. Continued cigarette smoking by patients receiving concurrent chemoradiotherapy for limited-stage small-cell lung cancer is associated with decreased survival. *J Clin Oncol* 2003; **21**: 1544–9.

37. West R, McNeill A, Raw M. Smoking cessation guidelines for health professionals: an update. Health Education Authority. *Thorax* 2000; **55**: 987–99.

38. Prochaska JO, Di Clemente CC. Toward a comprehensive model of change. In: Miller WR, Heather N, eds. *Treating Addictive Behaviours: Processes of Change*. New York: Plenum Press, 1986; 3–27.

39. Nardini S, Bertoletti R, Rastelli V *et al*. The influence of personal tobacco smoking on the clinical practice of italian chest physicians. *Eur Respir J* 1998; **12**: 1450–3.

40. Behr J, Nowak D. Tobacco smoke and respiratory disease. *Eur Respir Mon* 2002; **21**: 161–79.

41. Fiore MC, Bailey WC, Cohen SJ *et al. Smoking Cessation: Clinical Practice Guideline No. 18*. Public health service, Agency for Health

Care Policy and Research, AHCPR Publication No. 96-0692. Rockville, MD: US Department of Health and Human Services, 1996.

42. Nardini S. The smoking cessation clinic. *Monaldi Arch Chest Dis* 2000; **55**: 495–501.

43. Heatherton TF, Kozlowsky LT, Frecker RC, Fagerstroem KO. The Fagerstroem Test for nicotine dependence: a revision of the Fagerstroem Tolerance Questionnaire. *Br J Addict* 1991; **86**: 1119–27.

44. Jarvis MJ, Russell MAH, Saloojee Y. Expired air carbon monoxide: a simple breath test of tobacco smoke intake. *Br Med J* 1980; **281**: 484–5.

45. Richmond R. Teaching medical students about tobacco. *Thorax* 1999; **54**: 70–8.

5

Genetics of airflow limitation

ANDREW J. SANDFORD, NOE ZAMEL

INTRODUCTION

It is clear that the main risk factor for airflow limitation is cigarette smoking. However, it is equally clear that exposure to cigarette smoke, by itself, is not sufficient to explain the development of this disabling condition. In their classic study, Fletcher et al. (1) estimated that only 10–20 per cent of chronic heavy smokers will develop symptomatic chronic obstructive pulmonary disease (COPD) (1). While increased exposure to cigarette smoke is associated with a more rapid decline in lung function, smoking habits (estimated by pack-years and duration of smoking) account for only ~15 per cent of the variation in FEV_1 levels (2). Therefore, other factors must contribute to the development of airflow limitation. Several environmental risk factors have been identified, such as childhood viral respiratory infections, latent adenoviral infections and air pollution (3, 4). In this chapter, we discuss the evidence for a genetic susceptibility to airflow limitation and the genes that are potentially involved in the pathogenesis of this condition (see Box 5.1 for a glossary of genetic terms).

GENETIC EPIDEMIOLOGY OF AIRFLOW LIMITATION

Family studies

A condition that is at least partially genetically determined would be expected to cluster in families, as has been shown for chronic bronchitis (5). However, familial clustering may occur due to common environment conditions rather than a common genetic susceptibility. Evidence to indicate that genetic factors are responsible for familial clustering include the results of studies where it was shown that COPD was increased in the relatives of cases compared with the relatives of controls (i.e. individuals without respiratory disease) (6, 7). This increased prevalence could not be explained by factors such as age, sex and smoking history. In addition, the prevalence of clinically diagnosed airflow limitation and correlation of lung function have been shown to decrease with increased genetic distance (e.g. in second-degree relatives versus first-degree relatives) (8, 9). In the general population unselected for airflow limitation, there was a higher correlation of lung function between parents and their children or between two siblings than between spouses (10, 11).

Twin studies

Twin studies provide a means to estimate the relative contributions of genes and environment to a trait, by comparing the correlation of the trait in monozygotic (MZ) twins with the correlation in dizygotic (DZ) twins. Once it was established by Man and Zamel (12), based on data obtained in MZ twins, that the mechanical properties of the lung in healthy non-smokers were genetically determined, tests of lung mechanics could be used to study the role of genetic factors on the susceptibility of the airways to chronic cigarette smoke exposure.

Webster et al. (13) studied 45 pairs of apparently healthy MZ twins, comparing maximum expiratory flow at 60 per cent of total lung capacity of smokers and non-smokers, and found that this test could discriminate smokers from

Box 5.1   Glossary of genetic terms

Allele	A known variation (version) of a particular gene
Association	The correlation of the occurrence of traits with alleles of genetic markers
Compound heterozygotes	Persons with different deleterious mutations in each gene of their pair of chromosomes
Dizygotic	Referring to twins derived from two eggs. Dizygotic twins form when two separate eggs are fertilized by separate sperm. Dizygotic twins are as genetically similar as other sibling pairs
Exon	A DNA sequence in a gene that codes for a gene product
Genome	The entire complement of genetic material in an organism
Genotype	The set of alleles at a single point on a pair of chromosomes
Haplotype	The alleles of a set of closely linked genetic markers present on one chromosome that tend to be inherited together
Heritability	Proportion of the variability of a trait due to genetic factors
Heterozygote	An individual who has inherited two different alleles at a particular locus
Homozygote	An individual who has inherited two identical copies of an allele at a particular locus
Linkage	The tendency for genes and other genetic markers to be inherited together because of their location near one another on the same chromosome
Locus	The position of a gene or a genetic marker on a chromosome
Mendelian inheritance	Mendelian inheritance is seen when a disorder is caused by mutations in just one gene (such as cystic fibrosis), as opposed to polygenic disorders (such as COPD), which involve the interaction of several genes. Mendelian disorders (also known as 'monogenic disorders' or 'single-gene disorders') are so called because their inheritance patterns follow the genetic laws first described by Gregor Mendel
Monozygotic	Referring to twins derived from a single egg. Monozygotic twins form when a single fertilized egg splits into two and therefore the twins are genetically identical
Mutation	Any alteration in a gene from its natural state; it may be disease-causing or a benign variant
Nucleotide	A subunit of RNA or DNA containing a base, a phosphate and a sugar; nucleotides link up to form a molecule of DNA or RNA
Phenotype	The appearance of an organism with respect to a particular character or group of characters (physical, biochemical and physiological), as a result of the interaction of its genotype and its environment
Polymorphism	Natural variations in a gene that occur with fairly high frequency in the general population
Positional cloning	Cloning a gene based simply on knowing its position in the genome without any idea of the function of that gene
Promoter	DNA sequence regulating gene expression; the nature of the promoter determines which transcription factors will stimulate or repress the gene
Segregation analysis	An analysis to determine the mode of inheritance of a disease phenotype by studying its segregation (transmission) within families
Transcription factor	A protein that binds to regulatory regions of a gene and helps to control gene expression

non-smokers, among pairs of twins in which one member smoked and the other did not. The intra-pair difference of this test in pairs where both members smoked was the same as in pairs in which both members did not smoke, supporting the view that genetic factors are important in determining the vulnerability of the airways to cigarette smoke.

As with the family studies described above, studies done in twins raised together may reflect the similar childhood environments as much as the genetic make-up of the twins. In order to overcome this overlap, Hankins et al. (14) studied 15 pairs of MZ twins and one set of MZ triplets, who were separated soon after birth and raised apart. Six twin pairs were concordant for non-smoking and six were discordant. Three pairs and the triplets were concordant for smoking. The results of this study, along with those of the previous studies of twins raised together, support the conclusion that genetic factors are important in determining susceptibility to airflow limitation from chronic cigarette smoke exposure.

The proportion of the variability of a trait due to genetic factors is known as the heritability of that trait, and for forced expiratory volume in 1 s (FEV_1) this proportion ranges from 50 to 80 per cent (15, 16). Variation in heritability estimates in

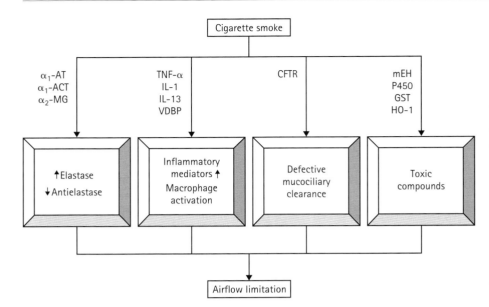

Figure 5.1 *Summary of pathways and possible candidate genes involved in the pathogenesis of COPD. α_1-AT, alpha-1-antitrypsin; α_1-ACT, alpha-1-antichymotrypsin; α_2-MG, alpha-2-macroglobulin; TNF-α, tumour necrosis factor-alpha; VDBP, vitamin D binding protein; CFTR, cystic fibrosis transmembrane regulator; IL-1,13; interleukin-1, 13; mEH, microsomal epoxide hydrolase; P450, cytochrome P450; GST, glutathione S-transferase; HO-1: haem oxygenase 1.*

these studies could be due to differences in exposure to environmental factors and/or differences in genetic make-up of the respective populations.

Segregation analyses

While twin studies provide evidence for a genetic basis to a disease, they are unable to identify the nature or number of inherited factors involved. In order to achieve this, a technique known as segregation analysis can be employed. In this approach, the level of pulmonary function is investigated in families and statistical models are fitted to the data. In this way, information regarding the mode of inheritance of a trait (dominant or recessive inheritance, the number of genes involved, etc.) can be gained. The results of such studies have confirmed a significant genetic component to pulmonary function (17, 18). Generally, the results suggest that the best model for this genetic component was that there were several genes, each with a small effect, rather than a single major gene. Most recently, Kurzius-Spencer *et al.* (19) reported the results of a study of 746 white, non-Mexican families from Tucson. Significant correlations of FEV_1 levels were observed between parents and offspring and between siblings but not between spouses. The correlations between the siblings were higher than between parents and offspring, which may reflect shared childhood environmental factors. All of the correlations were similar whether or not smoking was adjusted for, suggesting that exposure to similar levels of cigarette smoke did not account for the familial aggregation of FEV_1. As in previous studies, segregation analysis of FEV_1 showed significant familial effects with no evidence for a major gene.

In summary, results of these epidemiological studies demonstrate that COPD is a complex genetic disease, i.e. there is a genetic component to COPD but it is unlikely that there is a major susceptibility gene in the majority of families.

IDENTIFICATION OF GENES THAT INFLUENCE SUSCEPTIBILITY TO DISEASE

Two major strategies have been used to identify genes containing mutations or polymorphisms (common sequence variants) which contribute to the development of airflow limitation. The first strategy is positional cloning, which involves searching the entire human genome for disease-causing genes. The genes are identified solely on the basis of their position in the genome. The second strategy is the candidate gene approach, in which individual genes are directly tested for their involvement in a disease process. The genes selected for this approach are those which, because of their function, are plausible candidates for being the disease gene (Fig. 5.1). Traditionally, positional cloning has been performed using family data, employing a technique known as linkage analysis, whereas candidate genes have been tested by association studies of unrelated subjects.

Genome screens for COPD

To perform linkage analysis, phenotypic data and DNA are collected from affected families of at least two generations. Each family member is typed for genetic markers that are scattered throughout the genome, i.e. a genome screen. Linkage analysis determines whether any of the markers are inherited with the disease more often than predicted by chance. If so, that disease is said to be 'linked' to that marker on a certain chromosome. The next step is to identify candidate genes near that marker. An advantage of linkage analysis is that completely novel genes can be identified and implicated in the pathogenesis of a disease.

Few genome screens have been performed for COPD due to the difficulty of obtaining complete families with such a late-onset disease. Recently, a genome-wide screen was performed in a panel of 72 families with severe, early-onset COPD (20). The authors found evidence for genes that influenced spirometric measures of lung function at several locations around the

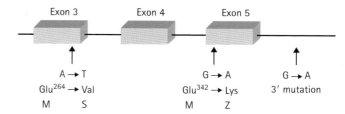

Figure 5.2 *Polymorphisms in the α_1-antitrypsin gene. Two point mutations in exon 3 and exon 5 result in amino acid substitutions at positions 264 and 342 of the protein. The third mutation occurs at the 3' end of the gene. M, S and Z refer to the name of the variants of the gene. A, adenine; T, thymine; G, guanine; Glu, glutamic acid; Val, valine; Lys, lysine.*

Box 5.2 Genes tested for an association with chronic obstructive pulmonary disease

- ABH secretor status
- ABO blood group
- Alpha-1-antichymotrypsin
- Alpha-1-antitrypsin
- Cystic fibrosis transmembrane regulator
- Cytochrome P450
- Glutathione S-transferase P1 and M1
- Haem oxygenase-1
- Human leucocyte antogen
- Human beta-defensin-1
- Interleukin-1β and interleukin-1 receptor antagonist
- Interleukin-13
- Matrix metalloproteinase-1, -9 and -12
- Microsomal epoxide hydrolase
- Tumour necrosis factor-alpha
- Vitamin D binding protein

genome, most notably on chromosomes 2 and 12. Candidate genes located in these regions include a subunit of the IL-8 receptor and microsomal glutathione S-transferase (an enzyme involved in detoxification of products found in cigarette smoke). When the same families were used in a genome screen with airflow obstruction as the outcome variable, the linkage to chromosome 12 was replicated but that with chromosome 2 was not (21).

Candidate genes for COPD

Chronic obstructive pulmonary disease is characterized by a slowly progressive irreversible airflow limitation that is primarily due to two pathophysiological changes in the lung: peripheral airway inflammation and a loss of lung elastic recoil resulting from parenchymal destruction. Many inflammatory cells, mediators and enzymes have been implicated and these offer potential targets for genetic investigations. It seems certain that there will be a complex interaction between several different genetic and environmental factors. To date, the genes that have been implicated in the pathogenesis of airflow limitation are involved in antiproteolysis, metabolism of toxic substances in cigarette smoke, antioxidation, the inflammatory response to cigarette smoke and mucociliary clearance. The genes involved or potentially involved in the pathogenesis of COPD are summarized in Box 5.2.

PROTEOLYSIS – ANTIPROTEOLYSIS

SEVERE ALPHA-1-ANTITRYPSIN DEFICIENCY

α_1-Antitrypsin (α_1-AT) is an acute-phase protein synthesized in the liver and, to a lesser extent, by alveolar macrophages. This antiprotease provides the major defence against proteolytic digestion of the lung by neutrophil elastase. It has been known since the early 1960s that individuals who have extremely low levels of α_1-AT have an increased prevalence of emphysema (22). A genetic basis for α_1-AT deficiency was demonstrated by the observation that the deficiency followed a simple Mendelian pattern of inheritance and was usually associated with the Z isoform of α_1-AT (23–25). The two most common deficiency variants of α_1-AT, S and Z, result from point mutations in the α_1-AT gene (26–28) (Fig. 5.2) and are named on the basis of their altered electrophoretic mobility on isoelectric focusing gels compared with the normal M allele (29). Homozygosity of the Z variant (which contains lysine rather than glutamic acid at amino acid position 342) results in a severe deficiency that is characterized by plasma α_1-AT levels approximately 10 per cent of the normal M allele. Individuals with the ZZ phenotype have a clearly accelerated rate of decline in lung function (30), sometimes even in the absence of smoking (31). However, the homozygous state is rare in the population (32) and thus can explain only a small percentage of the genetic susceptibility to cigarette smoke.

Despite the strong association of the ZZ genotype with early-onset COPD, the clinical course of the disease is highly variable (33) as is common with other genetic disorders. Exposure to cigarette smoke plays an important role in determining this variability (34), but nevertheless the rate of decline of lung function in ZZ subjects who are lifelong non-smokers is also highly variable (35). In studies in which index and non-index cases have been compared, many non-index ZZ subjects show normal lung function (36) and a survival similar to the normal population (33) if they are non-smokers. Therefore, the effect of the ZZ genotype in increasing the risk of clinically significant airflow limitation is likely to have been overestimated in some studies due to selection bias. It is possible that other genetic factors influence the clinical course in ZZ homozygotes. Polymorphisms in the endothelial nitric oxide synthase (NOS3) gene were shown to contribute to the development of COPD in ZZ individuals (37).

INTERMEDIATE ALPHA-1-ANTITRYPSIN DEFICIENCY

With the clear association of severe α_1-AT deficiency with COPD, it was a natural question to ask whether individuals with intermediate deficiency were also at risk for airflow limitation.

Individuals who have one copy of either the S or Z alleles are present in Caucasian populations at ∼10 and 3 per cent, respectively. These MS and MZ heterozygotes have reductions in α_1-AT levels to ∼80 and 60 per cent of normal, respectively. SZ compound heterozygotes are rare but have even lower levels, at ∼40 per cent of normal. In one study, SZ heterozygotes were shown to have an increased risk for COPD if they smoked (38). However, in a study from Spain, no association between SZ phenotype and COPD was found (39). To date, there have been no studies to demonstrate convincingly that MS heterozygotes are at increased risk of airflow limitation.

The results of many case–control studies have shown an increased prevalence of MZ heterozygotes in COPD patients compared with controls (40–44). In such studies, the odds ratio (OR) for MZ typically ranges from 1.5 to 5.0. However, in some of these studies the controls were not selected from the same population as the cases and this may lead to spurious associations of the MZ genotype with COPD due to differences in MZ frequency between populations. In addition, some of these case–control study results were not adjusted for confounding variables such as smoking history and age. Recently, the MZ genotype was investigated as a risk factor for increased rate of decline of lung function in smokers (45). The study group consisted of 283 smokers with rapid decline of lung function (mean ($FEV_1 = -154$ mL/year) and 308 smokers with no decline (mean ($FEV_1 = +15$ mL/year). Rapid decline of FEV_1 was associated with the MZ (OR $= 2.8$) and the association was stronger for a combination of a family history of COPD with MZ (OR $= 9.7$). These data suggest that the MZ genotype results in an increased rate of decline in lung function and interacts with other familial factors. Some of these familial factors could be genetic and others could be environmental.

Investigators have also assessed the risk of the MZ genotype by studying lung function in the general population (44, 46–49). In these studies, a population sample is phenotyped for α_1-AT variants and the prevalence of COPD in those with the MZ phenotype is compared with the prevalence in those with the MM phenotype. A weakness of many of these studies was that they were based on small numbers of individuals and therefore had insufficient power to detect an effect of the MZ or MS phenotype. In a recent large cohort study from Denmark, Seersholm et al. (50) compared the prevalence of obstructive pulmonary disease in 1551 MZ individuals versus 14 484 controls from the general population of unknown α_1-AT genotype. Obstructive pulmonary disease was defined as a hospital discharge diagnosis of asthma, chronic bronchitis or emphysema. The risk for obstructive pulmonary disease was significantly increased in the MZ individuals compared with the controls (relative risk $= 2.2$). However, only first-degree relatives of ZZ COPD patients had a significantly increased risk, suggesting that other genetic or environmental factors were contributing to the increased risk in these patients. Most recently Dahl et al. (51) performed a large cross-sectional study of 9187 individuals from the general population of Copenhagen in Denmark. The study subjects underwent pulmonary function testing (FEV_1 and FVC) and were genotyped for the S and Z α_1-AT variants. Only the SZ and ZZ individuals in this population showed an increased prevalence of airflow limitation (FEV_1 <80 per cent predicted). There was no association of either the MS or MZ genotype with lower level of lung function in individuals without clinically established COPD. However, among the COPD patients, FEV_1 was 655 mL less in MZ individuals compared with MM individuals ($P < 0.05$), after adjustment for confounding variables. The observation that the MZ genotype was associated with airflow limitation only in those with COPD suggests that other predisposing factors exist, consistent with the results of Seersholm et al. (50).

ALPHA$_1$–ANTITRYPSIN POLYMORPHISMS NOT ASSOCIATED WITH DEFICIENCY

There are several polymorphisms of the α_1-AT gene that are not associated with α_1-AT deficiency. The most extensively studied example is a polymorphism in the 3′ untranslated region of the α_1-AT gene that has been associated with COPD in some populations (52, 53) but not others (45, 54, 55). In vitro, this polymorphism was associated with decreased binding of a transcription factor and decreased gene expression (56). The most likely transcription factor is the nuclear factor of IL-6, which is activated by IL-6 and subsequently increases expression of α_1-AT (57). Thus, the 3′ mutation could affect the acute-phase response, leading to reduced α_1-AT synthesis in response to inflammation. However, in contrast to the in vitro data, the 3′ polymorphism was not associated with a reduced α_1-AT acute-phase response in patients undergoing open heart surgery (58) or in patients who had cystic fibrosis (59). Therefore, the role of the 3′ polymorphism in the pathogenesis of COPD remains to be determined.

Another polymorphism in the 3′ region of the α_1-AT gene has been associated with COPD (60). The polymorphism was associated with normal α_1-AT levels and was found in eight out of 70 COPD patients but in none of 52 controls. There have been no follow-up studies to confirm this association.

OTHER ANTIPROTEASE GENES

The association of airflow limitation with genetic defects in the α_1-AT gene also led to a search for genetic variants of other antiproteases that may be involved in protection against lung destruction. α_1-Antichymotrypsin (α_1-ACT) is another protease inhibitor which is secreted by the liver and alveolar macrophages. The gene contains several polymorphisms that have been associated with COPD in some studies (61, 62), whereas other investigators have found no association (55, 63). α_2-Macroglobulin is a broad-spectrum protease inhibitor that is also synthesized in hepatocytes and in alveolar macrophages. Several polymorphisms of the α_2-macroglobulin gene have been described (64). However, all of these polymorphisms in other antiproteases are rare and the evidence that they contribute to susceptibility to COPD is weak.

Matrix metalloproteinase genes

Matrix metalloproteinases (MMPs) are a structurally and functionally related family of proteolytic enzymes that play an essential role in tissue remodelling and repair associated with development and inflammation (65). Several studies in animals and humans have provided evidence that MMP1 (interstitial collagenase), MMP12 (human macrophage elastase) and MMP9 (gelatinase B) are important in airway inflammation and the development of emphysema. In 1992, D'Armiento *et al.* (66) demonstrated that transgenic mice over-expressing human *MMP1* in their lungs developed morphological changes strikingly similar to human pulmonary emphysema. *MMP12* knockout mice did not develop emphysema following exposure to cigarette smoke compared with wild-type mice (67), suggesting that the presence of MMP12 is critical in smoke-induced lung injury. Smokers with airway obstruction show increased expression of MMP1 and MMP9 compared to smokers without COPD and non-smokers (68, 69).

A promoter polymorphism in the *MMP1* gene (G-1607GG) was associated with rate of decline of lung function in smokers (70). In the same study, polymorphisms of *MMP9* and *MMP12* were not individually associated with rate of decline of lung function (70). However, combination of alleles (i.e. haplotypes) from the *MMP1* G-1607GG and *MMP12* Asn357Ser polymorphisms revealed an association with rate of decline of lung function ($P = 0.0007$). These data suggest that the polymorphisms in the *MMP1* and *MMP12* genes investigated by Joos *et al.* (70) either are causative factors in smoking-related lung injury or are associated with causative polymorphisms.

Minematsu *et al.* (71) examined the association between a *MMP9* promoter polymorphism (C-1562T) and the development of emphysema in Japanese smokers. They demonstrated that the T allele frequency was higher in subjects with distinct emphysema on chest CT scans than in those without it ($P = 0.02$). In addition, the diffusing capacity of the lung for carbon monoxide per litre of alveolar volume was lower ($P = 0.02$) and emphysematous changes were more conspicuous ($P = 0.03$) in subjects with C/T or T/T than those with the C/C genotype (71). These data are consistent with the higher level of gene expression associated with the T allele in an *in vitro* assay (72).

XENOBIOTIC METABOLIZING ENZYMES

Xenobiotic metabolizing enzymes are a class of molecules that play an important role in detoxifying potentially damaging organic compounds found in cigarette smoke (73, 74). There is considerable interindividual variation in the catalytic efficiencies of these enzymes in many, if not all, human populations. Therefore, these molecules have been studied to determine whether genetically determined deficiencies in xenobiotic metabolism may predispose an individual to the development of airflow limitation in response to cigarette smoke.

MICROSOMAL EPOXIDE HYDROLASE

Microsomal epoxide hydrolase (mEH) is an enzyme that plays a critical role in the lung's ability to metabolize highly reactive epoxide intermediates found in cigarette smoke. mEH is expressed in a variety of different cell types, including hepatocytes and bronchial epithelial cells. Two common polymorphisms occur in the mEH gene: in exon 3 (resulting in the Tyr[113]→His amino acid substitution) and exon 4 (resulting in the His[139]→Arg amino acid substitution). The polymorphisms have been shown to correlate with the level of mEH enzymatic activity *in vitro* (75), although there is some controversy surrounding these data since similar correlations were not shown in liver tissue samples (76). The slow metabolizing form of mEH was found in a higher proportion of patients with emphysema (22 per cent) and COPD (19 per cent) than in control subjects (6 per cent), yielding an odds ratio of ~5 (77). In a smaller Japanese study, the slow metabolizing form of mEH was associated with more severe disease in patients with airflow limitation (78). These results were not confirmed in a Korean population (79), but in a recent study, the slow metabolizing form of mEH was associated with rapid rate of decline of lung function in smokers (45). In the most recent study, the slow metabolizing form of mEH was associated with COPD in a group of Spanish Caucasians (80). Therefore, despite the one inconsistent study, overall these data suggest that genetic variation in the mEH gene does modify an individual's risk of airflow limitation.

GLUTATHIONE S-TRANSFERASES

Glutathione S-transferases (GSTs) are members of a family of enzymes that play an important role in detoxifying various aromatic hydrocarbons found in cigarette smoke. GSTs conjugate electrophilic substrates with glutathione and this facilitates further metabolism and excretion. One type of glutathione S-transferase, GSTM1, is expressed in the liver and the lung. Homozygous deletion of the GSTM1 gene occurs in approximately 50 per cent of Caucasians and therefore results in complete absence of this enzyme in these individuals. Homozygous deficiency for GSTM1 was associated with emphysema in Caucasian patients who had lung cancer (OR = 2.1) (81) and severe chronic bronchitis in heavy smokers (OR = 2.8) (82). However, in a Korean study, there was no association of the GSTM1 deletion with COPD (79). These discrepant results may be due to differences in the ethnicity of the study subjects. Certain genetic variants may be associated with disease only in certain ethnic groups due to interactions with population-specific environmental factors or other genetic factors.

GSTP1 is an enzyme expressed in the same cell types as GSTM1, although at a higher level (83). There is a polymorphism at position 105 (Ile[105] → Val), leading to an increased catalytic activity of the enzyme *in vitro* (84). Homozygotes for the isoleucine allele were significantly increased in Japanese patients with COPD compared with the controls (OR = 3.5) (85). However, this result was not replicated in a larger study of Korean COPD patients and controls (86).

CYTOCHROME P4501A1

Cytochrome P4501A1 (CYP1A1) also metabolizes xenobiotic compounds, enabling them to be excreted. CYP1A1 is expressed throughout the lung and may play a role in the activation of procarcinogens. A polymorphism in exon 7 of CYP1A1 causes an amino acid substitution (Ile[462] → Val) that results in increased CYP1A1 activity *in vivo* (87). The high-activity isoform (Val[462]) was associated with susceptibility to centriacinar emphysema in patients who had lung cancer (OR = 2.5) (88).

ANTIOXIDANTS

HAEM OXYGENASE-1

Haem oxygenase degrades haem to biliverdin and has been demonstrated to provide cellular protection against haem and non-haem-mediated oxidant injury (89, 90). A polymorphism consisting of variable numbers of guanine-thymine (GT) nucleotides within the haem oxygenase gene (*HMOX1*) promoter was associated with pulmonary emphysema in Japanese smokers (91). This was an association study of 100 patients with pulmonary emphysema and 101 controls. Alleles with a high number of GT repeats (≥30) were significantly more prevalent in the cases (0.21) than the controls (0.10), yielding an odds ratio of 2.4. The authors hypothesized that the reason for the association was the effect of GT repeats in promoting the formation of a conformation of DNA known as Z DNA. Z DNA has been shown to decrease gene expression (92) and therefore a high number of GT repeats in the *HMOX1* promoter may suppress expression of the gene and leave the individual susceptible to oxidant-induced lung injury. In support of this hypothesis, the authors showed that high numbers of GT repeats resulted in decreased *in vitro* gene expression in response to hydrogen peroxide.

INFLAMMATORY MEDIATORS

VITAMIN D BINDING PROTEIN

Vitamin D binding protein (VDBP) is a protein secreted by the liver, which is able to bind vitamin D, extracellular actin and endotoxin. VDBP enhances the chemotactic activity of two complement factors (C5a and C5a des-Arg) for neutrophils by one to two orders of magnitude (93). Chemoattractants such as these complement factors are believed to play an important role in the accumulation of neutrophils in lung that is seen in COPD (94). In addition, VDBP can be converted to a potent macrophage-activating factor (95). Thus, besides its vitamin D binding function, VDBP could have important influences on the intensity of the inflammatory reaction in the lung in response to cigarette smoke.

There are three major isoforms of this protein, termed 1S, 1F and 2, and these isoforms are due to two common substitutions in exon 11 of the VDBP gene. Individuals who had one or two copies of allele 2 were shown to be protected against COPD (96, 97). In addition, Horne *et al.* (96) demonstrated that 1F homozygous individuals had a significantly increased risk of developing COPD. This association was confirmed in a Japanese population (72). In contrast, no association of this genotype with accelerated decline of lung function was found (45).

Schellenberg *et al.* (97) examined whether the associations of VDBP isoforms with COPD could be due to the effect of VDBP on neutrophil chemotaxis. However, there were no significant differences between the three VDBP isoforms in their ability to enhance chemotaxis of neutrophils to C5a. It remains possible that the mechanism for the association with COPD is related to the activation of macrophages at sites of inflammation. However, no investigators have examined the influence of these genetic variants on the ability of the protein to act as a macrophage-activating factor.

TUMOUR NECROSIS FACTOR-α

Tumour necrosis factor-α (TNF-α) and TNF-β (lymphotoxin) are proinflammatory cytokines that have many effects of relevance to the pathogenesis of COPD, e.g. neutrophil release from the bone marrow and neutrophil activation. The TNF-α and TNF-β genes contain several polymorphisms, including a G→A transition in the TNF-α gene promoter (TNF-α G-308A) and an A→G transition in the first intron of the TNF-β gene (TNF-β A252G). These polymorphisms have been shown to be associated with the level of TNF-α and TNF-β production *in vitro* (98). In addition, the TNF-α -308A allele has been associated with several diseases, including cerebral malaria (99) and asthma (100, 101). An association of the TNF-α -308A allele with COPD was found in a Taiwanese population (102). The patients were selected based on the presence of chronic bronchitis and airflow limitation (FEV$_1$ <80 per cent predicted and FEV$_1$/FVC <69 per cent). The prevalence of the TNF-α -308A allele was considerably increased in the patients compared with the controls, yielding an odds ratio of 11.1 for chronic bronchitis. Recently, this association was confirmed by Sakao *et al.* in a Japanese population (103). In this study, 106 patients were selected based on an FEV$_1$ <80 per cent and an FEV$_1$/FVC <80 per cent and these individuals were compared with 110 asymptomatic smokers or ex-smokers and 129 adult blood donors. The presence of the TNF-α -308A allele (homozygotes and heterozygotes combined) was significantly increased in cases (27 per cent) compared with both control groups (12 per cent), yielding an odds ratio of 2.6. Evidence for the role of the TNF-α -308A allele in the pathogenesis of COPD was further strengthened by the observation that this allele was associated with more severe emphysema as judged by high-resolution computed tomography (CT) (104).

In contrast, no association of the -308A allele with COPD was found in a study of 53 physician-diagnosed COPD patients and 65 controls from the Japanese population (105). However, the sample size in this study was small and there were considerably fewer subjects (2 per cent) with the -308A allele than in the study by Sakao *et al.* (103). Studies of Caucasian populations have found no association of TNF-α -308A with COPD (106) or rate of decline of lung function (45). Interestingly, a study of a Caucasian population from the Netherlands also reported no association of TNF-α -308A with COPD (107). However, these authors did find an association of COPD with the presence of the A allele of another TNF-α polymorphism (TNF-α G489A). This association was only found in patients who had no evidence of emphysema based on high-resolution CT scans, consistent with the hypothesis that TNF-α polymorphisms would affect airway inflammation rather than proteolytic destruction of the lung. In summary, the role of TNF-α polymorphisms in COPD has yet to be established, but this may be another example of ethnic group-specific genetic risk factors.

IL-1 COMPLEX

The IL-1 family consists of two proinflammatory cytokines, IL-1α and IL-1β, and a naturally occurring anti-inflammatory agent, the IL-1 receptor antagonist (IL1RN). The two forms of IL-1 are the products of different genes, but they are structurally related and bind to the same receptor. IL-1α and IL-1β are synthesized by a variety of cell types, but mainly monocytes and macrophages. IL1RN is a protein that binds to the IL-1 receptor with the same affinity as IL-1 but does not possess agonist activity and therefore acts as a competitive inhibitor of IL-1 (108). The genes of the IL-1 complex are found in close proximity on the long arm of human chromosome 2 (109) and each of the genes is polymorphic. The IL-1β gene (IL1B) has a single nucleotide polymorphism in the promoter region (C-511T) (110) and the IL1RN gene has a polymorphic site in intron 2 containing two to six repeats of an 86 base-pair sequence (111). There is evidence that allele 2 of the IL1RN gene (IL1RN*2) is associated with increased susceptibility or more severe outcome in chronic inflammatory diseases such as ulcerative colitis, systemic lupus erythematosus and alopecia areata (112–114). The IL1B C-511T has been associated with inflammatory bowel disease (115) as well as plasma levels of IL1B and IL1RN (116).

In a recent study, individual IL-1 genotypes were not associated with rate of decline of lung function in smokers. However, there was a significant influence of combinations of IL1RN/IL1B alleles in these individuals (117). The association of these haplotypes with the decline of lung function may represent an interaction between the genes. A smaller study in a Japanese population found no association with individual IL1B and IL1RN genotypes and COPD (105).

INTERLEUKIN-13

In a recent study, Wong *et al.* (118) demonstrated that over expression of interleukin-13 in the adult murine lung caused emphysema, elevated mucus production, and inflammation reminiscent of human COPD. Consistent with these data, a recent study found an association of a promoter polymorphism (C-1055T) with COPD in a Caucasian population.

MUCOCILIARY CLEARANCE

The rate at which particulate matter is cleared from the lungs is highly variable between individuals (119). The trachaeobronchial clearance rate of 6–7 μm particles was studied in nine pairs of MZ and nine pairs of DZ twins (120). The intrapair correlation in clearance rates was significantly higher in the MZ twins than in the DZ twins, suggesting that genetic factors

may affect an individual's mucociliary clearance rate. This may have important implications for an individual's cumulative exposure to the compounds found in cigarette smoke.

CYSTIC FIBROSIS TRANSMEMBRANE REGULATOR

The cystic fibrosis transmembrane conductance regulator (CFTR) forms a chloride channel at the apical surface of airway epithelial cells and is involved in the control of airway secretions. In 1989, mutations in the CFTR gene were identified as the cause of cystic fibrosis (CF). CF carriers may also be predisposed to respiratory disease. CF heterozygotes had increased bronchial reactivity to methacholine (121) and increased incidence of wheeze accompanied by decreased FEV_1 and forced expiratory flow between 25 and 75 percent of vital capacity (FEF_{25-75}) (122).

The most frequent CF-causing variant is ΔF508 and heterozygosity for this mutation was increased in patients who had disseminated bronchiectasis (123, 124), and in patients who had 'bronchial hypersecretion' (125). The prevalence of ΔF508 was not increased in patients who had chronic bronchitis (124). Other CFTR mutations were increased in patients who had disseminated bronchiectasis and normal sweat chloride levels (126, 127). One of these mutations is a variable-length thymine repeat in intron 8 of the CFTR gene (IVS8). The IVS8-5T allele results in reduced CFTR gene expression. Studies of IVS8-5T as a risk factor for COPD have yielded conflicting results (126, 127). Most recently, patients with obstructive lung diseases were screened for variants in the whole CFTR coding region (128). The study compared 12 COPD patients with 52 controls, both groups from the Greek population. There was no significant increase in CF-causing mutations in the patients versus the controls. However, the frequency of the methionine allele of the Met470Val polymorphism was increased in the patients (71 per cent) compared with the controls (36 per cent). However, the Met470 variant is associated with increased CFTR chloride channel activity compared with the Val variant (129) and therefore the reason for the association with COPD is unclear.

In summary, CFTR variants have been consistently associated with disseminated bronchiectasis. This may be due to the effect of these variants on the rate of mucociliary clearance. However, it is not clear whether the patients who have disseminated bronchiectasis represent a clinically distinct group or have mild, undiagnosed CF with an unknown CFTR mutation on their other chromosome (130). In addition, all the studies described above were based on small numbers of subjects and only three (126–128) compared cases with controls. The other studies compared frequencies in the cases with published allele frequencies and therefore the results of these studies are far from definitive.

CONCLUSION

Although there is clear evidence of a genetic contribution to the pathogenesis of COPD, few specific genes have been implicated to date. Most studies have been case–control candidate gene studies and were often too small in size to be powerful enough to detect genes of modest effect. In addition, the reported studies have been mostly limited to known biologically plausible candidates. In earlier-onset diseases, such as asthma, large-scale family studies have provided clues as to the location of susceptibility genes using the technique of genome-wide screening. This technique can identify susceptibility genes irrespective of whether the biological function is known.

In the future, more information about the role of genetic risk factors in the development of COPD may be provided by large-scale family studies, genome-wide association studies and investigation of an increased number of possible candidate genes identified by the Human Genome Project.

Key points

- Chronic airflow limitation is most commonly due to exposure to cigarette smoke, but nevertheless only a minority of chronic, heavy smokers develop symptoms of airflow limitation.
- Epidemiological studies of families and twins suggest that individuals who develop airflow limitation may be genetically susceptible to the effects of cigarette smoke.
- Severe deficiency of α_1-antitrypsin is one genetic factor that leads to airflow limitation in smokers.
- Other genes that have been investigated as possible risk factors for obstructive pulmonary disease are involved in the protease/antiprotease balance, the oxidant/antioxidant balance, xenobiotic metabolism and the inflammatory response.
- Identification of genetic risk factors for chronic airflow limitation may reveal new aspects of the pathogenesis of this condition, point to new therapeutic targets and lead to treatment that is optimized for each individual patient.

REFERENCES

●1. Fletcher C, Peto R, Tinker C, Speizer FE. *The Natural History of Chronic Bronchitis. An Eight-year Study of Chronic Obstructive Lung Disease in Working Men in London.* Oxford: Oxford University Press, 1976.

2. Beck GJ, Doyle CA, Schachter EN. Smoking and lung function. *Am Rev Respir Dis* 1981; **123**: 149–55.

3. Hogg JC. Childhood viral infection and the pathogenesis of asthma and chronic obstructive lung disease. *Am J Respir Crit Care Med* 1999; **160**: S26–8.

4. Dockery DW, Pope CA 3rd, Xu X *et al.* An association between air pollution and mortality in six U.S. cities. *N Engl J Med* 1993; **329**: 1753–9.

5. Tager IB, Rosner B, Tishler PV *et al.* Household aggregation of pulmonary function and chronic bronchitis. *Am Rev Respir Dis* 1976; **114**: 485–92.

6. Speizer FE, Rosner B, Tager I. Familial aggregation of chronic respiratory disease: use of National Health Interview Survey data for specific hypothesis testing. *Int J Epidemiol* 1976; **5**: 167–72.

7. Cohen BH, Diamond EL, Graves CG *et al.* A common familial component in lung cancer and chronic obstructive pulmonary disease. *Lancet* 1977; **2**: 523–6.

8. Tager I, Tishler PV, Rosner B *et al.* Studies of the familial aggregation of chronic bronchitis and obstructive airways disease. *Int J Epidemiol* 1978; **7**: 55–62.

●9. Redline S, Tishler PV, Rosner B *et al.* Genotypic and phenotypic similarities in pulmonary function among family members of adult monozygotic and dizygotic twins. *Am J Epidemiol* 1989; **129**: 827–36.

10. Kauffmann F, Tager IB, Munoz A, Speizer FE. Familial factors related to lung function in children aged 6–10 years. Results from the PAARC epidemiologic study. *Am J Epidemiol* 1989; **129**: 1289–99.

11. Devor EJ, Crawford MH. Family resemblance for normal pulmonary function. *Ann Hum Biol* 1984; **11**: 439–48.

12. Man SFP, Zamel N. Genetic influence on normal variability of maximum expiratory flow-volume curves. *J Appl Physiol* 1976; **41**: 874–7.

13. Webster PM, Lorimer EG, Man SF *et al.* Pulmonary function in identical twins: comparison of nonsmokers and smokers. *Am Rev Respir Dis* 1979; **119**: 223–8.

14. Hankins D, Drage C, Zamel N, Kronenberg R. Pulmonary function in identical twins raised apart. *Am Rev Respir Dis* 1982; **125**: 119–21.

15. Hubert HB, Fabsitz RR, Feinleib M, Gwinn C. Genetic and environmental influences on pulmonary function in adult twins. *Am Rev Respir Dis* 1982; **125**: 409–15.

●16. Redline S, Tishler PV, Lewitter FI *et al.* Assessment of genetic and nongenetic influences on pulmonary function: a twin study. *Am Rev Respir Dis* 1987; **135**: 217–22.

17. Givelber RJ, Couropmitree NN, Gottlieb DJ *et al.* Segregation analysis of pulmonary function among families in the Framingham Study. *Am J Respir Crit Care Med* 1998; **157**: 1445–51.

18. Chen Y, Horne SL, Rennie DC, Dosman JA. Segregation analysis of two lung function indices in a random sample of young families: the Humboldt Family Study. *Genet Epidemiol* 1996; **13**: 35–47.

19. Kurzius-Spencer M, Holberg CJ, Martinez FD, Sherrill DL. Familial correlation and segregation analysis of forced expiratory volume in one second (FEV$_1$), with and without smoking adjustments, in a Tucson population. *Ann Hum Biol* 2001; **28**: 222–34.

20. Silverman EK, Palmer LJ, Mosley JD *et al.* Genome-wide linkage analysis of quantitative spirometric phenotypes in severe early-onset chronic obstructive pulmonary disease. *Am J Hum Genet* 2002; **70**: 1229–39.

●21. Silverman EK, Mosley JD, Palmer LJ *et al.* Genome-wide linkage analysis of severe, early-onset chronic obstructive pulmonary disease: airflow obstruction and chronic bronchitis phenotypes. *Hum Mol Genet* 2002; **11**: 623–32.

●22. Laurell CC, Eriksson S. The electrophoretic alpha$_1$-globulin pattern of serum in alpha$_1$-antitrypsin deficiency. *Scand J Clin Lab Invest* 1963; **15**: 132–40.

23. Eriksson S. Pulmonary emphysema and α_1-antitrypsin deficiency. *Acta Med Scand* 1964; **175**: 197–205.

24. Eriksson S. Studies in α_1-antitrypsin deficiency. *Acta Med Scand* 1965; **177**: 1–85.

25. Kueppers F, Briscoe WA, Bearn AG. Hereditary deficiency of α_1-antitrypsin. *Science* 1964; **146**: 1678–9.

26. Owen MC, Carrell RW, Brennan SO. The abnormality of the S variant of human alpha-1-antitrypsin. *Biochim Biophys Acta* 1976; **453**: 257–61.

27. Jeppsson JO. Amino acid substitution Glu leads to Lys alpha-1-antitrypsin PiZ. *FEBS Lett* 1976; **65**: 195–7.

28. Yoshida A, Lieberman J, Gaidulis L, Ewing C. Molecular abnormality of human alpha1-antitrypsin variant (Pi-ZZ) associated with plasma activity deficiency. *Proc Natl Acad Sci USA* 1976; **73**: 1324–8.

29. Brantly M, Nukiwa T, Crystal RG. Molecular basis of α_1-antitrypsin deficiency. *Am J Med* 1988; **84**: 13–31.

30. Brantly ML, Paul LD, Miller BH *et al*. Clinical features and history of the destructive lung disease associated with α_1-antitrypsin deficiency of adults with pulmonary symptoms. *Am Rev Respir Dis* 1988; **138**: 327–36.

31. Janus ED, Phillips NT, Carrell RW. Smoking, lung function, and α_1-antitrypsin deficiency. *Lancet* 1985; **1**: 152–4.

32. O'Brien ML, Buist NR, Murphey WH. Neonatal screening for alpha1-antitrypsin deficiency. *J Pediatr* 1978; **92**: 1006–10.

33. Seersholm N, Kok-Jensen A, Dirksen A. Survival of patients with severe α_1-antitrypsin deficiency with special reference to non-index cases. *Thorax* 1994; **49**: 695–8.

34. Piitulainen E, Eriksson S. Decline in FEV1 related to smoking status in individuals with severe alpha1-antitrypsin deficiency (PiZZ). *Eur Respir J* 1999; **13**: 247–51.

35. Black LF, Kueppers F. α_1-antitrypsin deficiency in nonsmokers. *Am Rev Respir Dis* 1978; **117**: 421–8.

36. Silverman EK, Pierce JA, Province MA *et al*. Variability of pulmonary function in alpha-1-antitrypsin deficiency: clinical correlates. *Ann Intern Med* 1989; **111**: 982–91.

37. Novoradovsky A, Brantly ML, Waclawiw MA *et al*. Endothelial nitric oxide synthase as a potential susceptibility gene in the pathogenesis of emphysema in alpha-1-antitrypsin deficiency. *Am J Respir Cell Mol Biol* 1999; **20**: 441–7.

38. Turino GM, Barker AF, Brantly ML *et al*. Clinical features of individuals with PI*SZ phenotype of α_1-antitrypsin deficiency. α_1-Antitrypsin Deficiency Registry Study Group. *Am J Respir Crit Care Med* 1996; **154**: 1718–25.

39. Alvarez-Granda L, Cabero-Perez MJ, Bustamante-Ruiz A *et al*. PI SZ phenotype in chronic obstructive pulmonary disease. *Thorax* 1997; **52**: 659–61.

40. Bartmann K, Fooke-Achterrath M, Koch G *et al*. Heterozygosity in the Pi-system as a pathogenetic cofactor in chronic obstructive pulmonary disease (COPD). *Eur J Respir Dis* 1985; **66**: 284–96.

41. Janus ED. α_1-antitrypsin Pi types in COPD patients. *Chest* 1988; **94**: 446–7.

42. Lieberman J, Winter B, Sastre A. α_1-antitrypsin Pi-types in 965 COPD patients. *Chest* 1986; **89**: 370–3.

43. Sandford AJ, Weir TD, Spinelli JJ, Paré PD. Z and S mutations of the α_1-antitrypsin gene and the risk of chronic obstructive pulmonary disease. *Am J Respir Cell Mol Biol* 1999; **20**: 287–91.

44. Sandford AJ, Weir TD, Paré PD. Genetic risk factors for chronic obstructive pulmonary disease. *Eur Respir J* 1997; **10**: 1380–91.

45. Sandford AJ, Chagani T, Weir TD *et al*. Susceptibility genes for rapid decline of lung function in the Lung Health Study. *Am J Respir Crit Care Med* 2001; **163**: 469–73.

46. Chan-Yeung M, Ashley MJ, Corey P, Maledy H. Pi phenotypes and the prevalence of chest symptoms and lung function abnormalities in workers employed in dusty industries. *Am Rev Respir Dis* 1978; **117**: 239–45.

47. McDonagh DJ, Nathan SP, Knudson RJ, Lebowitz MD. Assessment of alpha-1-antitrypsin deficiency heterozygosity as a risk factor in the etiology of emphysema. Physiological comparison of adult normal and heterozygous protease inhibitor phenotype subjects from a random population. *J Clin Invest* 1979; **63**: 299–309.

48. Buist AS, Sexton GJ, Azzam AM, Adams BE. Pulmonary function in heterozygotes for α_1-antitrypsin deficiency: a case-control study. *Am Rev Respir Dis* 1979; **120**: 759–66.

49. Bruce RM, Cohen BH, Diamond EL *et al*. Collaborative study to assess risk of lung disease in Pi MZ phenotype subjects. *Am Rev Respir Dis* 1984; **130**: 386–90.

●50. Seersholm N, Wilcke JT, Kok-Jensen A, Dirksen A. Risk of hospital admission for obstructive pulmonary disease in alpha(1)-antitrypsin heterozygotes of phenotype PiMZ. *Am J Respir Crit Care Med* 2000; **161**: 81–4.

●51. Dahl M, Nordestgaard BG, Lange P *et al*. Molecular diagnosis of intermediate and severe alpha(1)-antitrypsin deficiency: MZ individuals with chronic obstructive pulmonary disease may have lower lung function than MM individuals. *Clin Chem* 2001; **47**: 56–62.

52. Kalsheker NA, Watkins GL, Hill S *et al*. Independent mutations in the flanking sequence of the α_1-antitrypsin gene are associated with chronic obstructive airways disease. *Dis Markers* 1990; **8**: 151–7.

53. Poller W, Meisen C, Olek K. DNA polymorphisms of the α_1-antitrypsin gene region in patients with chronic obstructive pulmonary disease. *Eur J Clin Invest* 1990; **20**: 1–7.

54. Sandford AJ, Spinelli JJ, Weir TD, Paré PD. Mutation in the 3' region of the α_1-antitrypsin gene and chronic obstructive pulmonary disease. *J Med Genet* 1997; **34**: 874–5.

55. Bentazzo MG, Gile LS, Bombieri C *et al*. α_1-antitrypsin *Taq* I polymorphism and α_1-antichymotrypsin mutations in patients with obstructive pulmonary disease. *Respir Med* 1999; **93**: 648–54.

56. Morgan K, Scobie G, Kalsheker NA. Point mutation in a 3' flanking sequence of the α_1-antitrypsin gene associated with chronic respiratory disease occurs in a regulatory sequence. *Hum Mol Genet* 1993; **2**: 253–7.

57. Morgan K, Scobie G, Marsters P, Kalsheker NA. Mutation in an α_1-antitrypsin enhancer results in an interleukin-6 deficient acute-phase response due to loss of cooperativity between transcription factors. *Biochim Biophys Acta* 1997; **1362**: 67–76.

58. Sandford AJ, Chagani T, Spinelli JJ, Paré PD. α_1-antitrypsin genotypes and the acute-phase response to open heart surgery. *Am J Respir Crit Care Med* 1999; **159**: 1624–8.

59. Mahadeva R, Westerbeek RC, Perry DJ *et al*. α_1-antitrypsin deficiency alleles and the Taq-I G→A allele in cystic fibrosis lung disease. *Eur Respir J* 1998; **11**: 873–9.

60. Buraczynska M, Schott D, Hanzlik AJ, Holtmann B, Ulmer WT. α_1-antitrypsin gene polymorphism related to respiratory system disease. *Klin Wochenschr* 1987; **65**: 538–41.

61. Lindmark B, Svenonius E, Eriksson S. Heterozygous α_1-antichymotrypsin and PiZ α_1-antitrypsin deficiency. Prevalence and clinical spectrum in asthmatic children. *Allergy: Eur J Allergy Clin Immunol* 1990; **45**: 197–203.

62. Poller W, Faber JP, Scholz S *et al*. Mis-sense mutation of α_1-antichymotrypsin gene associated with chronic lung disease. *Lancet* 1992; **339**: 1538.

63. Sandford AJ, Chagani T, Weir TD, Paré PD. α_1-antichymotrypsin mutations in patients with chronic obstructive pulmonary disease. *Dis Markers* 1998; **13**: 257–60.

64. Poller W, Faber JP, Klobeck G, Olek K. Cloning of the human α_2-macroglobulin gene and detection of mutations in two functional domains: the bait region and the thiolester site. *Hum Genet* 1992; **88**: 313–9.

65. Kumagai K, Ohno I, Okada S *et al*. Inhibition of matrix metalloproteinases prevents allergen-induced airway inflammation in a murine model of asthma. *J Immunol* 1999; **162**: 4212–9.

66. D'Armiento J, Dalal SS, Okada Y *et al*. Collagenase expression in the lungs of transgenic mice causes pulmonary emphysema. *Cell* 1992; **71**: 955–61.

67. Hautamaki RD, Kobayashi DK, Senior RM, Shapiro SD. Requirement for macrophage elastase for cigarette smoke-induced emphysema in mice. *Science* 1997; **277**: 2002–4.

68. Finlay GA, O'Driscoll LR, Russell KJ *et al.* Matrix metalloproteinase expression and production by alveolar macrophages in emphysema. *Am J Respir Crit Care Med* 1997; **156**: 240–7.

69. Segura-Valdez L, Pardo A, Gaxiola M *et al.* Upregulation of gelatinases A and B, collagenases 1 and 2, and increased parenchymal cell death in COPD. *Chest* 2000; **117**: 684–94.

70. Joos L, He JQ, Shepherdson MB *et al.* The role of matrix metalloproteinase polymorphisms in the rate of decline in lung function. *Hum Mol Genet* 2002; **11**: 569–76.

71. Minematsu N, Nakamura H, Tateno H *et al.* Genetic polymorphism in matrix metalloproteinase-9 and pulmonary emphysema. *Biochem Biophys Res Commun* 2001; **289**: 116–19.

72. Zhang BP, Ye S, Herrmann SM *et al.* Functional polymorphism in the regulatory region of gelatinase B gene in relation to severity of coronary atherosclerosis. *Circulation* 1999; **99**: 1788–94.

73. Cohen GM. Pulmonary metabolism of foreign compounds: its role in metabolic activation. *Environ Health Perspect* 1990; **85**: 31–41.

74. Taningher M, Malacarne D, Izzotti A *et al.* Drug metabolism polymorphisms as modulators of cancer susceptibility. *Mutat Res* 1999; **436**: 227–61.

75. Hassett C, Aicher L, Sidhu JS, Omiecinski CJ. Human microsomal epoxide hydrolase: genetic polymorphism and functional expression *in vitro* of amino acid variants. *Hum Mol Genet* 1994; **3**: 421–8.

76. Kitteringham NR, Davis C, Howard N *et al.* Interindividual and interspecies variation in hepatic microsomal epoxide hydrolase activity: studies with cis-stilbene oxide, carbamazepine 10, 11-epoxide and naphthalene. *J Pharmacol Exp Ther* 1996; **278**: 1018–27.

●77. Smith CA, Harrison DJ. Association between polymorphism in gene for microsomal epoxide hydrolase and susceptibility to emphysema. *Lancet* 1997; **350**: 630–3.

78. Yoshikawa M, Hiyama K, Ishioka S *et al.* Microsomal epoxide hydrolase genotypes and chronic obstructive pulmonary disease in Japanese. *Int J Mol Med* 2000; **5**: 49–53.

79. Yim JJ, Park GY, Lee CT *et al.* Genetic susceptibility to chronic obstructive pulmonary disease in Koreans: combined analysis of polymorphic genotypes for microsomal epoxide hydrolase and glutathione S-transferase M1 and T1. *Thorax* 2000; **55**: 121–5.

80. Rodriguez F, Jardi R, Costa X *et al.* Detection of polymorphisms at exons 3 (Tyr113→His) and 4 (His139→Arg) of the microsomal epoxide hydrolase gene using fluorescence PCR method combined with melting curves analysis. *Anal Biochem* 2002; **308**: 120.

81. Harrison DJ, Cantlay AM, Rae F *et al.* Frequency of glutathione S-transferase M1 deletion in smokers with emphysema and lung cancer. *Hum Exp Toxicol* 1997; **16**: 356–60.

82. Baranova H, Perriot J, Albuisson E *et al.* Peculiarities of the GSTM1 0/0 genotype in French heavy smokers with various types of chronic bronchitis. *Hum Genet* 1997; **99**: 822–6.

83. Cantlay AM, Smith CA, Wallace WA *et al.* Heterogeneous expression and polymorphic genotype of glutathione S-transferases in human lung. *Thorax* 1994; **49**: 1010–14.

84. Sundberg K, Johansson AS, Stenberg G *et al.* Differences in the catalytic efficiencies of allelic variants of glutathione transferase P1-1 towards carcinogenic diol epoxides of polycyclic aromatic hydrocarbons. *Carcinogenesis* 1998; **19**: 433–6.

85. Ishii T, Matsuse T, Teramoto S *et al.* Glutathione S-transferase P1 (GSTP1) polymorphism in patients with chronic obstructive pulmonary disease. *Thorax* 1999; **54**: 693–6.

86. Yim JJ, Yoo CG, Lee CT *et al.* Lack of association between glutathione S-transferase P1 polymorphism and COPD in Koreans. *Lung* 2002; **180**: 119–25.

87. Cosma G, Crofts F, Taioli E *et al.* Relationship between genotype and function of the human CYP1A1 gene. *J Toxicol Environ Health* 1993; **40**: 309–16.

88. Cantlay AM, Lamb D, Gillooly M *et al.* Association between the CYP1A1 gene polymorphism and susceptibility to emphysema and lung cancer. *J Clin Pathol Mol Pathol* 1995; **48**: M210–14.

89. Otterbein LE, Lee PJ, Chin BY *et al.* Protective effects of heme oxygenase-1 in acute lung injury. *Chest* 1999; **116**: 61S–63S.

90. Choi AM, Alam J. Heme oxygenase-1: function, regulation, and implication of a novel stress-inducible protein in oxidant-induced lung injury. *Am J Respir Cell Mol Biol* 1996; **15**: 9–19.

91. Yamada N, Yamaya M, Okinaga S *et al.* Microsatellite polymorphism in the heme oxygenase-1 gene promoter is associated with susceptibility to emphysema. *Am J Hum Genet* 2000; **66**: 187–95.

92. Naylor LH, Clark EM. d(TG)n.d(CA)n sequences upstream of the rat prolactin gene form Z-Dna and inhibit gene transcription. *Nucleic Acids Res* 1990; **18**: 1595–601.

93. Kew RR, Webster RO. Gc-globulin (vitamin D-binding protein) enhances the neutrophil chemotactic activity of C5a and C5a des Arg. *J Clin Invest* 1988; **82**: 364–9.

94. Williams TJ, Jose PJ. Neutrophils in chronic obstructive pulmonary disease. *Novartis Found Symp* 2001; **234**: 136–41 (discussion, pp. 141–8).

95. Yamamoto N, Homma S. Vitamin D-binding protein (group-specific component) is a precursor for the macrophage-activating signal factor from lysophosphatidylcholine-treated lymphocytes. *Proc Natl Acad Sci USA* 1991; **88**: 8539–43.

96. Horne SL, Cockcroft DW, Dosman JA. Possible protective effect against chronic obstructive airways disease by the GC 2 allele. *Hum Hered* 1990; **40**: 173–6.

97. Schellenberg D, Paré PD, Weir TD *et al.* Vitamin D binding protein variants and the risk of COPD. *Am J Respir Crit Care Med* 1998; **157**: 957–61.

98. Bouma G, Crusius JB, Oudkerk Pool M *et al.* Secretion of tumour necrosis factor a and lymphotoxin a in relation to polymorphisms in the TNF genes and HLA-DR alleles. Relevance for inflammatory bowel disease. *Scand J Immunol* 1996; **43**: 456–63.

99. McGuire W, Hill AV, Allsopp CE *et al.* Variation in the TNF-a promoter region associated with susceptibility to cerebral malaria. *Nature* 1994; **371**: 508–10.

100. Moffatt MF, Cookson WOCM. Tumour necrosis factor haplotypes and asthma. *Hum Mol Genet* 1997; **6**: 551–4.

101. Chagani T, Paré PD, Zhu S *et al.* Prevalence of tumour necrosis factor-α and angiotensin converting enzyme polymorphisms in mild/moderate and fatal/near-fatal asthma. *Am J Respir Crit Care Med* 1999; **160**: 278–82.

102. Huang SL, Su CH, Chang SC. Tumor necrosis factor-α gene polymorphism in chronic bronchitis. *Am J Respir Crit Care Med* 1997; **156**: 1436–9.

103. Sakao S, Tatsumi K, Igari H *et al.* Association of tumor necrosis factor alpha gene promoter polymorphism with the presence of chronic obstructive pulmonary disease. *Am J Respir Crit Care Med* 2001; **163**: 420–2.

104. Sakao S, Tatsumi K, Igari H *et al.* Association of tumor necrosis factor-alpha gene promoter polymorphism with low attenuation areas on high-resolution CT in patients with COPD(*). *Chest* 2002; **122**: 416–20.

105. Ishii T, Matsuse T, Teramoto S *et al.* Neither IL-1beta, IL-1 receptor antagonist, nor TNF-alpha polymorphisms are associated with susceptibility to COPD. *Respir Med* 2000; **94**: 847–51.

106. Higham MA, Pride NB, Alikhan A, Morrell NW. Tumour necrosis factor-alpha gene promoter polymorphism in chronic obstructive pulmonary disease. *Eur Respir J* 2000; **15**: 281–4.

107. Kucukaycan M, Van Krugten M, Pennings HJ *et al.* Tumor necrosis factor-alpha +489G/A gene polymorphism is associated with chronic obstructive pulmonary disease. *Respir Res* 2002; **3**: 29.

108. Arend WP, Malyak M, Guthridge CJ, Gabay C. Interleukin-1 receptor antagonist: role in biology. *Annu Rev Immunol* 1998; **16**: 27–55.

109. Steinkasserer A, Spurr NK, Cox S *et al.* The human IL-1 receptor antagonist gene (IL1RN) maps to chromosome 2q14–q21, in the region of the IL-1 alpha and IL-1 beta loci. *Genomics* 1992; **13**: 654–7.

110. di Giovine FS, Takhsh E, Blakemore AI, Duff GW. Single base polymorphism at -511 in the human interleukin-1 b gene (IL1 b). *Hum Mol Genet* 1992; **1**: 450.

111. Tarlow JK, Blakemore AI, Lennard A *et al.* Polymorphism in human IL-1 receptor antagonist gene intron 2 is caused by variable numbers of an 86-bp tandem repeat. *Hum Genet* 1993; **91**: 403–4.

112. Mansfield JC, Holden H, Tarlow JK *et al.* Novel genetic association between ulcerative colitis and the anti-inflammatory cytokine interleukin-1 receptor antagonist. *Gastroenterology* 1994; **106**: 637–42.

113. Blakemore AI, Tarlow JK, Cork MJ *et al.* Interleukin-1 receptor antagonist gene polymorphism as a disease severity factor in systemic lupus erythematosus. *Arthritis Rheum* 1994; **37**: 1380–5.

114. Tarlow JK, Clay FE, Cork MJ *et al.* Severity of alopecia areata is associated with a polymorphism in the interleukin-1 receptor antagonist gene. *J Invest Dermatol* 1994; **103**: 387–90.

115. Nemetz A, Nosti-Escanilla MP, Molnar T *et al.* IL1B gene polymorphisms influence the course and severity of inflammatory bowel disease. *Immunogenetics* 1999; **49**: 527–31.

116. Hurme M, Santtila S. IL-1 receptor antagonist (IL-1RA) plasma levels are co-ordinately regulated by both IL-1RA and IL-1b genes. *Eur J Immunol* 1998; **28**: 2598–602.

117. Joos L, McIntyre L, Ruan J *et al.* Association of IL-1b and IL-1 receptor antagonist haplotypes with rate of decline in lung function in smokers. *Thorax* 2001; **56**: 863–6.

118. Wong ZD, Zhu Z, Homer RJ *et al.* Inducible expression of interferon-g in the lung causes pulmonary emphysema. *Am J Respir Crit Care Med* 2000; **161**: A822.

119. Philipson K, Falk R, Camner P. Long-term lung clearance in humans studied with Teflon particles labeled with chromium-51. *Exp Lung Res* 1985; **9**: 31–42.

120. Camner P, Philipson K, Friberg L. Tracheobronchial clearance in twins. *Arch Environ Health* 1972; **24**: 82–7.

121. Davis PB. Autonomic and airway reactivity in obligate heterozygotes for cystic fibrosis. *Am Rev Respir Dis* 1984; **129**: 911–4.

122. Davis PB, Vargo K. Pulmonary abnormalities in obligate heterozygotes for cystic fibrosis. *Thorax* 1987; **42**: 120–5.

123. Poller W, Faber JP, Scholz S *et al.* Sequence analysis of the cystic fibrosis gene in patients with disseminated bronchiectatic lung disease. Application in the identification of a cystic fibrosis patient with atypical clinical course. *Klin Wochenschr* 1991; **69**: 657–63.

124. Gervais R, Lafitte JJ, Dumur V *et al.* Sweat chloride and DF508 mutation in chronic bronchitis or bronchiectasis. *Lancet* 1993; **342**: 997.

125. Dumur V, Lafitte JJ, Gervais R *et al.* Abnormal distribution of cystic fibrosis DF508 allele in adults with chronic bronchial hypersecretion. *Lancet* 1990; **335**: 1340.

126. Pignatti PF, Bombieri C, Benetazzo M *et al.* CFTR gene variant IVS8-5T in disseminated bronchiectasis. *Am J Hum Genet* 1996; **58**: 889–92.

127. Bombieri C, Benetazzo M, Saccomani A *et al.* Mutational screening of the CFTR gene in 120 patients with pulmonary disease. *Hum Genet* 1998; **103**: 718–22.

128. Tzetis M, Efthymiadou A, Strofalis S *et al.* CFTR gene mutations – including three novel nucleotide substitutions – and haplotype background in patients with asthma, disseminated bronchiectasis and chronic obstructive pulmonary disease. *Hum Genet* 2001; **108**: 216–21.

129. Cuppens H, Lin W, Jaspers M *et al.* Polyvariant mutant cystic fibrosis transmembrane conductance regulator genes. The polymorphic (Tg)m locus explains the partial penetrance of the T5 polymorphism as a disease mutation. *J Clin Invest* 1998; **101**: 487–96.

130. Romano L, Padoan R, Romano C. Disseminated bronchiectasis and cystic fibrosis gene mutations. *Eur Respir J* 1998; **12**: 998–9.

6

Using the rehabilitation literature to guide patient care: a critical appraisal of trial evidence

HOLGER J. SCHÜNEMANN, GORDON H. GUYATT

INTRODUCTION

Pulmonary rehabilitation and evidence–based medicine

The need to solve clinical problems has provided the stimulus for the evolution of evidence-based medicine (EBM). In contrast to the traditional paradigm of clinical practice, EBM emphasizes that intuition, unsystematic clinical experience and pathophysiological rationale are not sufficient for making the best clinical decisions. Although EBM recognizes the importance of clinical experience, it includes the evaluation of evidence from clinical research as a prerequisite for optimal clinical decision-making (1).

In addition, EBM advocates that a formal set of rules must complement training and common sense for clinicians to interpret and apply evidence from the results of clinical research effectively. Thus, EBM places a lower value on authority than the traditional medical paradigm.

Another fundamental principle of EBM is the explicit inclusion of patients' and society's values and clinical circumstances in the clinical decision-making process (2). Patients, their proxies, or, if a parental approach to decision-making is desirable, the clinician as decision-maker, must always weigh up the benefits, harm and costs associated with alternative treatment strategies. Values and preferences always bear on those trade-offs.

For clinicians, integration of research evidence in their practice requires an understanding of what represents higher versus lower quality evidence. EBM teaches us that our confidence in research results should be greatest when systematic error, known as bias, is lowest and that it should fall when bias is more likely. Study design is a fundamental issue in appraising

the quality of evidence and in avoiding bias. Randomization is the most certain – although not perfect – method to avoid bias when comparing interventions. Therefore, randomized controlled studies constitute the highest quality of evidence, while observational studies bear a greater risk of bias and provide lower quality evidence.

Outcomes of importance to the patient

The objective of pulmonary rehabilitation is to improve outcomes that are important to patients. Patients are less interested in variables that clinicians often use to make judgments about effectiveness, such as FEV_1. Clinicians should not rely primarily on physiological measures because they often correlate only weakly with the patients' experience of their disease and its impact on their life. Therefore, studies in pulmonary rehabilitation should focus on outcomes that are of importance to the patient (3). These 'patient-important' outcomes are:

- improvement in health-related quality of life (HRQL)
- exercise capacity if it directly correlates with how patients are functioning (physical functioning is a domain included in many HRQL instruments)
- exacerbations (the impact of which may also be measured with HRQL instruments)
- survival.

The goal of this chapter is to provide an overview of how to ask the proper clinical question and how to appraise the evidence for pulmonary rehabilitation as an intervention designed to improve outcomes in patients with chronic respiratory disease. Other chapters in this book focus on the disease-specific topics relevant to pulmonary rehabilitation and the efficacy of the interventions used to treat them; this chapter focuses on how those interested in evaluating evidence can become confident in their appraisals.

Asking the right clinical question

Appraising the evidence and obtaining an answer to a clinical problem, such as that posed in Case Study 6.1, should begin by asking the right question. Box 6.1 presents a framework for asking clinical questions (4). Clinical questions should include defining the population, the intervention, the comparison intervention and the outcome. A question based on Case Study 6.1 might be as follows: 'In patients with severe chronic obstructive pulmonary disease (COPD), does respiratory rehabilitation compared to standard care improve patients' survival or quality of life or exercise capacity or reduce exacerbations?'

Case Study 6.1   Pulmonary rehabilitation vs. usual care

A 71-year-old man with severe chronic obstructive pulmonary disease (COPD) is considering participation in a respiratory rehabilitation programme. After many years of heavy smoking, the patient finally quit, but was left with severely impaired pulmonary function (FEV$_1$ = 35 per cent predicted) and dyspnoea on minimal activity. He feels tired all the time and is often frustrated as well as anxious. Participation in a rehabilitation programme would disrupt his routine and involve over an hour of driving, on most days, for 8 weeks. He is wondering whether the programme is worth the inconvenience and effort. 'Doctor,' he asks the chest physician responsible for his care, 'does this really

work and, if so, how much benefit will I get from a rehabilitation programme? It seems I will be away all this time from my family.'

EVALUATING RESEARCH EVIDENCE IN PULMONARY REHABILITATION

The proper study design

The question framed in the previous section is one of therapy and there are a variety of ways to address such questions. The most appropriate study design addressing a question of therapy is a randomized controlled trial (RCT) that compares two or more alternative management strategies. However, a number of trials compared pulmonary rehabilitation with usual care, the question raised by our case study. A clinician would ask the question: 'Which of the available studies should I trust and consider for decision-making?'.

Even for clinicians trained in critical appraisal, evaluating all available studies would be a time-intensive solution. Because clinicians are busy and often overwhelmed by the amount of information available, they traditionally rely on review articles or text books by authorities in the field. However, experts may be unsystematic in their approach to summarizing the evidence. Unsystematic approaches to identification and collection of evidence risks biased ascertainment. That is, treatment effects may be underestimated or, more commonly, overestimated, and side-effects may be exaggerated or ignored.

Even if the evidence has been identified and collected in a systematic fashion, if reviewers are unsystematic in the way they summarize the collected evidence, they run similar risks of bias. Oxman and Guyatt (5) showed that self-rated expertise was inversely related to the methodological rigour of the review. The result of unsystematic approaches may be recommendations advocating harmful treatment; in other cases, there may be a failure to encourage effective therapy.

Much of the evidence exploring interventions in pulmonary rehabilitation comes from RCTs. Thus, the appraisal of RCTs and of systematic summaries of RCTs, such as a systematic review, should be part of the standard repertoire for clinicians and researchers in pulmonary rehabilitation. As it turns out, systematic reviews exist for many interventions in pulmonary rehabilitation and many of the outcomes described relate to HRQL.

Systematic reviews

Systematic reviews are rigorous evaluations of the evidence on a given topic (6, 7) and, for interested specialists, will often be the first source for answering a specific clinical question. A systematic review attempts to address a focused clinical question using methods that reduce the likelihood of bias. Thus, high-quality systematic reviews will provide the summaries for clinicians who want more than a quick answer, but who

---

Box 6.1   Formulating the clinical question

Population

Who are the relevant patients?

Interventions or exposures

What are the management strategies clinicians are interested in (e.g. exercise training, a diagnostic test, drugs, nutrients, surgical procedures)?
What are the exposures leading to a specific outcome (e.g. smoking or workplace or air pollution exposure)?

Comparison (or control) intervention or exposures

What is the comparison, control or alternative intervention clinicians or patients are interested in? For questions about therapy or harm there will always be a comparison or control (including doing nothing, placebo, alternative active treatment or routine care). For questions about diagnosis there may be a comparison diagnostic strategy.

Outcome

What are the patient-important consequences of the intervention or exposure clinicians are interested in?

cannot critically appraise every single study that addresses the question. We will not describe in detail how one should conduct a systematic review of the literature; for the readers of this book we will focus on how to appraise a systematic review critically.

Of the numerous systematic reviews about the efficacy of pulmonary rehabilitation, three were published in 2003 alone and focused on pulmonary rehabilitation in COPD (8–10). This abundance of available reviews underlines the need for critical appraisal skills by clinicians in the field of pulmonary rehabilitation. These reviews used similar methodology and thus include similar studies. We will use the systematic review by Lacasse *et al.* (8) to lead the reader through the process of critical appraisal.

This systematic review appeared in the Cochrane Database of Systematic Reviews (8). The Cochrane Collaboration, an international organization dedicated to making up-to-date and accurate information about the effects of health care readily available worldwide, maintains this database. The collaboration has provided important insights into the conduct of systematic reviews and meta-analyses that inform clinicians' and patients' choices. It produces and disseminates systematic reviews of health care interventions and promotes the search for evidence (www.cochrane.org). We will appraise the review using the commonly applied critical appraisal tool shown in Box 6.2 (6).

Critical appraisal of a systematic review

We will first explore whether the results of a systematic review are valid. If we find that a systematic review has limited validity, then there would be little reason to trust the results or to apply the results of a systematic review to patient care.

Box 6.2 Users' guides for an article about systematic reviews

---

Are the results of the study valid?

- Did the review explicitly address a sensible clinical question?
- Was the search for relevant studies detailed and exhaustive?
- Were the primary studies of high methodological quality?
- Were assessments of studies reproducible?

What are the results?

- Were the results similar from study to study?
- What are the overall results of the review?
- How precise were the results?

Will the results help me in caring for my patients?

- How can I best interpret the results to apply them to the care of patients in my practice?
- Were all clinically important outcomes considered?
- Are the benefits worth the costs and potential risks?

DID THE REVIEW EXPLICITLY ADDRESS A SENSIBLE CLINICAL QUESTION?

The evaluation of validity begins with answering the above question. Consider a systematic review that pooled results from all rehabilitation modalities, ranging from 2-day education or psychological support to an 8-week comprehensive rehabilitation programme including exercise training, to generate a single estimate of the impact on mortality. Let us also consider a systematic review that pooled results from all randomized trials that compared rehabilitation, including at least 4 weeks of systemic exercise training, in patients with COPD in comparison to usual (community) care. Most clinicians would not find the first of these reviews useful, because it addresses an overly broad question. Most clinicians, however, would be comfortable with the second question.

What makes a systematic review too broad or too narrow? We have argued above that identifying the population, the interventions or exposures and the outcomes of interest is a useful way of structuring a clinical question (11). When deciding if the question posed in the review is sensible, clinicians need to ask themselves whether the underlying biology is such that they would expect the same treatment effect across the range of patients included. Readers of systematic review should ask the parallel question about the other components of the study question. For example, is the underlying biology (or psychology if one opts to separate these issues) such that, across the range of interventions and outcomes included, they expect more or less the same treatment effect?

The reason clinicians reject a systematic review that pools across all modalities of rehabilitation is that their understanding of the biology suggests that rehabilitation intervention effects are likely to vary across modes and intensities of intervention. Combining the results of these studies would yield an estimate of effect that may not be applicable to any of the interventions. Clinicians have to decide whether, across a range of patients, interventions and outcomes, it is plausible that the intervention will have a similar effect.

To facilitate this decision, authors of systematic reviews have to describe clearly what range of patients, interventions and outcomes they include. These explicit criteria help readers to decide whether the question was sensible, but also reduce the likelihood for selected inclusion of studies by the authors. Lacasse *et al.* (8) specified clear inclusion and exclusion criteria for their systematic review. The authors clearly described the types of participant (clinical diagnosis of COPD, FEV_1/FVC ratio <0.7 or FEV_1 <70 per cent of the predicted value) and the type of intervention, namely any in-patient, outpatient or home-based rehabilitation programme of at least 4 weeks' duration, including exercise therapy with or without education or psychological support delivered to patients with exercise limitation from COPD; they also described the type of outcome (HRQL and/or exercise capacity, measured either during exercise or during walk tests). Thus, the authors defined a specific clinical question.

WAS THE SEARCH FOR RELEVANT STUDIES DETAILED AND EXHAUSTIVE?

Having defined the clinical question, the next question a reader of a systematic review should ask is: 'Was the search for relevant studies detailed and exhaustive?' Authors of a systematic review should conduct a thorough search for all studies that meet their inclusion criteria. The search should include the use of bibliographic databases, such as Medline, Embase, the Cochrane Controlled Trials Register (containing more than 300 000 RCTs), and other databases of current research. In addition, they should check the reference lists of the retrieved articles and seek personal contact with experts in the area. It may also be important to examine recently published abstracts presented at scientific meetings and to look at less frequently used databases, including those that summarize doctoral theses and ongoing trials.

Listing these sources, it becomes evident that a search of Medline alone may not be satisfactory. Unless the authors tell readers how they located relevant studies, readers cannot assess whether relevant studies were missed. Contacting experts may help to identify studies that are overlooked or those that are unpublished. These strategies help to detect publication bias, which occurs when the publication of research depends on the direction of the study results and whether they are statistically significant. Investigators sometimes refrain from publishing the results of a study if the intervention is not found to be effective. As a result, systematic reviews that fail to include unpublished studies may overestimate the true effect of an intervention.

Lacasse *et al.* systematically searched for all studies that investigated pulmonary rehabilitation compared with usual care by randomizing patients to one of the two alternatives. They searched the electronic databases Medline and CINAHL and identified additional RCTs by searching the Cochrane Airways Group COPD trial registry. The authors also reviewed the reference lists of relevant articles, and retrieved any potential additional citation. Finally, they reviewed the abstracts presented at international meetings (American Thoracic Society, 1980–2000; American College of Chest Physicians, 1980–2000; and European Respiratory Society, 1987–2000) and contacted the authors of studies included in the meta-analysis and experts in the field of pulmonary rehabilitation inquiring about unpublished material. The reader can deduce that the authors used a comprehensive strategy that identified all available RCTs in this field.

WERE THE PRIMARY STUDIES OF HIGH METHODOLOGICAL QUALITY?

Even if a review article includes only RCTs, knowing whether they were of good quality is important. Unfortunately, peer review does not guarantee the validity of published research and, therefore, the quality of a systematic review is only as good as the quality of the original studies. Therefore, a reader of a systematic review should ask whether the primary studies were of high methodological quality. Disparities in study methodology might explain important differences among the results. For example, less rigorous studies tend to overestimate the effectiveness of therapeutic and preventive interventions (12). Even if the results of different studies are consistent, determining their validity is still important. Consistent results are less compelling if they come from weak studies than if they come from strong studies. In observational studies, physicians may systematically select patients with a good prognosis to receive therapy. This pattern of practice may be consistent over time and geographic setting.

There is no single correct way to assess the quality of studies, although in the context of a systematic review, the focus should be on validity and users should therefore be cautious about the use of scales to assess the quality of studies. Some investigators use long checklists to evaluate methodological quality of primary studies, whereas others focus on three or four key aspects of the study. The primary criteria for evaluating RCTs include: (i) an assessment of whether investigators blinded patients, care providers, outcome adjudicators, statisticians and those interpreting the results; (ii) concealment of the randomization; and (iii) the proportion of patients followed up.

In their systematic review, Lacasse *et al.* used several methods to assess the quality of the original RCTs. They evaluated whether randomization was concealed, whether study personnel were blinded as well as the rate of follow-up and dropout. Although summary scores have limitations in the assessment of study quality, they also used a summary score developed by Jadad (13). Because blinding of participants in studies of pulmonary rehabilitation is impossible, it is very important in these studies that trialists make efforts to blind other individuals involved in the experiment. In particular, outcome adjudicators should remain blind to the treatment assignment of the subjects. It is possible that more rigorous methods, such as blinding of statisticians and manuscript authors, are important to provide unbiased results of the findings in the highly supervised setting of pulmonary rehabilitation (14–16).

Laccase *et al.* included a total of 23 RCTs in the last update of their systematic review (8). They found that only one trial did not meet the inclusion criteria of the meta-analysis, because it was a crossover trial. They also found that the randomization process was appropriate in all trials but one, and that the author of one trial could not provide details regarding the randomization process used in his study. In 11 studies, those who assessed the clinical outcomes were blinded to the treatment received by the participants. In two other studies, the primary outcome assessor, quality of life (QoL) was blinded, whereas the secondary outcome assessor (exercise capacity) was not. In one study the cycle ergometer test was blinded, whereas the 6-min walk test was not. Conversely, in another trial, the cycle ergometer test was not blinded, whereas the 12-min walk test was. Obviously, none of the trials included blinding of study participants. This situation demonstrates the limited usefulness of generic scales, such as Jadad's scale, in discriminating trials according to the quality of their report when blinding of patients becomes implausible.

WERE ASSESSMENTS OF STUDIES REPRODUCIBLE?

Authors of systematic review articles must decide which studies to include, how valid they are and what data to extract. These decisions require judgment by the reviewers, which may be subject to both mistakes (i.e. random errors) and bias (i.e. systematic errors). Participation of two or more people in each decision protects against errors; if there is good agreement beyond chance between the reviewers, the clinician can have more confidence in the results of the systematic review. Thus, readers of systematic reviews should ask whether the assessments of studies were reproducible.

Lacasse *et al.* retrieved 522 publications from the computerized search and reduced this list to 68 potentially eligible papers. They measured the agreement for the initial exclusion of studies from the more comprehensive list. Several measures of agreement beyond chance exist (11). One that is commonly used is called kappa and described in other texts (11). The magnitude of kappa (0.53; 95 per cent CI = 0.45–0.61) in the systematic review indicated good agreement. The two primary reviewers agreed to include 17 papers in the meta-analysis (quadratic kappa = 0.89; 95 per cent CI = 0.65–1.00). The other six RCTs included in the meta-analysis were retrieved from the references of a prior meta-analysis and not assessed for agreement.

Overall, the methods of the systematic review by Lacasse *et al.* were strong and the methodological quality of the trials included in the systematic review was satisfactory.

DID THE RESULTS PROVE SIMILAR FROM STUDY TO STUDY?

Most systematic reviews describe important differences in patients, interventions, outcome measures and research methods among studies. Consequently, the most common answer to the initial question as to whether one can expect similar results across the range of patients, interventions and outcomes is 'perhaps'. Fortunately, one can resolve this unsatisfactory situation. Having completed the review, investigators should present the results in a way that allows readers to check the validity of the initial assumption that the results were similar from study to study.

Readers should consider two things when deciding whether the results are similar enough to warrant making a single estimate of treatment effects that can be applied across the populations, interventions and outcomes studied. First, how similar are the best estimates of the treatment effect (i.e. the point estimates) from the individual studies? The more discrepant they are, the more clinicians should question the decision to pool results across studies. Second, to what extent are differences among the results of individual studies greater than one would expect by chance? Users can make an initial assessment by examining the extent to which the confidence intervals (CIs) overlap. The greater the overlap, the more comfortable one is with pooling results. Widely separated CIs indicate the presence of important variability in results, which requires explanation.

Readers can also look to formal statistical analyses, called tests of heterogeneity, which assess the degree of difference or variance among samples, groups or populations. When the

P-value associated with the test of heterogeneity is small (e.g. <0.05 or <0.10), chance becomes an unlikely explanation for the observed differences in the size of the effect. However, a higher *P*-value (0.1, or even 0.3) does not entirely rule out important heterogeneity. The reason for this is that when the number of studies and their sample sizes are both small, the test of heterogeneity is not very powerful. Thus, large differences between the point estimate of the treatment effect between studies dictates caution in interpreting the overall findings, even in the face of a non-significant test of heterogeneity. Conversely, if the differences in results across studies are not clinically important, then heterogeneity is of little concern, even if it is statistically significant. Another measure of heterogeneity is called I^2 (17). I^2 describes the proportion of total variation in study estimates that is due to heterogeneity rather than sampling error (chance). I^2 ranges from 0 to 100 per cent and a value greater than 50 per cent may be considered substantial heterogeneity (17).

However, authors of systematic reviews should try to explain any between-study variability in their findings. Possible explanations include differences between patients, such as mild-versus-severe COPD, or between interventions, such as short-versus-long exercise programmes. Other differences might be between outcome measurements, such as HRQL versus exercise capacity, or 1 versus 12 months of follow-up, or differences in methodology; for example, the effect may be smaller in blinded trials or in those with more complete follow-up.

Because one can almost always *imagine* a way to explain heterogeneity between study results, explanations of heterogeneity are more credible if the authors described a priori hypotheses explaining potential heterogeneity. Lacasse *et al.* defined several a priori hypotheses on which sensitivity analyses were to be based. They surmised that treatment effects might vary according to the population, i.e. by severity of the disease. They hypothesized that patients with severe disease and minimal respiratory reserve may be too physically impaired to participate significantly in and benefit from the programme. The authors also thought that the intervention could explain differences in the effect. They suggested that the more comprehensive and the longer the duration of rehabilitation, the larger the effect size. Finally, they hypothesized that the methodological quality of the studies would influence the results, in particular whether those assessing outcomes were blind to the allocation of subjects between control or intervention groups.

When they analysed the results, the authors found heterogeneity among study results that none of their a priori hypotheses could explain. Other sources of heterogeneity that were not considered in the definition of subgroups must have been responsible for this heterogeneity. If residual heterogeneity in study results remains unexplained, there are ways to deal with these differences. We will describe strategies in our discussion of the applicability of the results of the systematic review.

In clinical research, investigators collect data from individual patients and use statistical methods to summarize and analyse them. In systematic reviews, investigators collect data from individual studies. Investigators must also summarize these data and, increasingly, they are relying on quantitative methods to do so. Some understanding of the methods used to pool data across studies helps in answering the question: 'What are the overall results of the review and how precise are the results?'

Typically, meta-analysis weighs studies according to their size, with larger studies receiving more weight. Thus, the overall results represent a weighted average of the results of the individual studies. Occasionally studies are also given more or less weight depending on their quality. Poorer-quality studies might be given a weight of zero, i.e. they are excluded either in the primary analysis or in a secondary, sensitivity analysis that tests the extent to which different assumptions lead to different results.

Readers should look at the overall results of a systematic review in the same way that they look at the results of primary studies. In a systematic review of a therapeutic question, when the outcome measure is dichotomous, one should look for the relative risk and the relative risk reduction, or the odds ratio.

Sometimes the outcome measures that investigators have used in different studies are similar but not identical, or they are measured on a continuous scale. For example, different trials might measure functional status using different instruments. If the patients and the interventions are reasonably similar, estimating the average effect of the intervention on functional status might still be worthwhile. One way of doing this is to summarize the results of each study as an effect size. The effect size is the difference in outcomes between the intervention and control groups divided by the standard deviation. The effect size summarizes the results of each study in terms of the number of standard deviations of difference between the intervention and control groups. Investigators can then calculate a weighted average of effect sizes from studies that measured a given outcome in different ways.

In the same way that it is possible to estimate the average effect across studies, it is possible to estimate a confidence interval around that estimate. The CI is a range of values with a specified probability (typically 95 per cent) of including the true effect. Evaluating the CI helps our understanding of the precision of the estimates. The narrower the CI, the greater is one's confidence that the true effect is close to the point estimate obtained from the analysis.

Lacasse *et al.* restricted their analysis of the effect on HRQL to the CRQ, because it was the most widely used questionnaire, used in eight of the trials that met the inclusion criteria of the meta-analysis. They reported the results of the CRQ (dyspnoea, fatigue, emotional function and mastery domains; see Chapter 16) on a seven-point scale. For instance, for the fatigue domain of the CRQ they obtained a weighted mean difference of 0.9 (95 per cent CI = 0.7–1.1), indicating a mean change of 0.9 on the seven-point scale as a result of pulmonary rehabilitation.

For each outcome, the common effect size exceeded the minimal important difference (MID) 0.5 points on the seven-point scale (18). In brief, the MID is 'the smallest difference in score in the outcome of interest that informed patients or informed proxies perceive as important, either beneficial or harmful, and which would lead the patient or clinician to

consider a change in the management' (19). The boundary of the confidence intervals suggested the smallest effect exceeded the MID for dyspnoea, fatigue and mastery dimensions, but for the emotional function domain it included the MID, which raised questions about the importance of the effect on the emotional function domain.

There is guidance in the literature as to how users of evidence can evaluate whether HRQL outcomes are valid outcome measures and how readers can interpret the results (11), evaluating whether the investigators have measured aspects of patients' lives that the patients themselves consider important and whether the instrument works in the intended way (validity). The CRQ measures HRQL in domains that have been carefully developed, based on areas of HRQL that patients with COPD describe as important. Furthermore, the CRQ has been shown, in numerous studies, to be valid, i.e. it truly measures HRQL in the areas that it intends to cover and is responsive, i.e. it is able to measure change in HRQL if this change has occurred (see Chapter 16). With regard to evaluating the results, the guide suggests evaluating whether readers can interpret the magnitude of the effects. For the CRQ, there is ample evidence that a mean change of 0.5 on each of the domains on the CRQ is what patients judge to be an important change, the MID (see Chapter 16).

The meta-analysis of the 14 trials that used the incremental cycle ergometer test as the outcome showed a common effect (weighted mean difference) of a 5.46-watt (95 per cent CI = 0.49–10.23) increase as a result of pulmonary rehabilitation. For the meta-analysis of the 10 trials that used the 6-min walk test as an outcome, the common effect (weighted mean difference) was 49 m (95 per cent CI = 26–72). The estimate of the MID for the walk test is approximately 50 m. Because the lower limit of the confidence interval around the pooled effect (26–72 m) lies beyond the limit of the confidence interval around the estimate of the MID for the 6-min walk test, the importance of the result obtained from the meta-analysis remains uncertain. The interpretation of the results is somewhat further limited because the results of the latter analysis indicated the presence of heterogeneity ($P = 0.09$).

In summary, the results of the meta-analysis showed statistically significant and patient-important benefits for all CRQ domains, indicating important improvements for patients undergoing pulmonary rehabilitation. It also indicated that patients experienced important improvements in their exercise capacity. The pooled estimate for the improvement in functional exercise came with some uncertainty and a relatively wide CI that overlapped with the estimate for the MID for the 6-min walk distance.

HOW CAN I BEST INTERPRET THE RESULTS TO APPLY THEM TO THE CARE OF PATIENTS IN MY PRACTICE?

Having evaluated the results of the systematic review, users should ask themselves how the results might be interpreted so as to apply them to patient care. One issue in interpretation is the extent to which one should believe subgroup analyses. The play of chance will inevitably cause observed results between studies to differ, and naive interpretations of these differences may lead to spurious inferences. For example, a study with older patients may happen, by chance, to be the one with the smallest treatment effects. An author of a systematic review may erroneously conclude that the treatment is less effective in elderly patients. The more subgroup analyses the reviewer undertakes, the greater is the risk of a spurious conclusion.

The user of the review can apply a number of criteria to distinguish subgroup analyses that are credible from those that are not. Criteria that make a hypothesized difference in subgroups more credible include the following:

- conclusions drawn on the basis of within-study rather than between-study comparisons
- a large difference in treatment effect across subgroups
- a highly statistically significant difference in treatment effect (e.g. the lower the P-value on the comparison of the different effect sizes in the subgroups, the more credible the difference)
- a hypothesis that was made before the study began and that was one of only a few that were tested
- consistency across studies
- indirect evidence in support of the difference (e.g. 'biologic plausibility').

The results of a subgroup analysis are less likely to be trustworthy if these criteria are not met. The reader should assume that the overall effect across all patients and all treatments, rather than the subgroup effect, applies to the patient at hand and to the treatment under consideration.

Lacasse *et al.* did not observe heterogeneity in the studies they evaluated for the outcome HRQL and maximal exercise capacity. Thus, assuming generalizability across the groups of patients studied appears reasonable for these outcomes. However, none of the subgroup analyses they proposed explained statistical heterogeneity in the results of the functional exercise capacity test.

What are readers of the review to do if subgroup analyses fail to provide an adequate explanation for unexplained heterogeneity in study results? A question that users want to address in studies focusing on HRQL outcomes is whether the studies simulated clinical practice. Treatments affect HRQL both by reducing disease symptoms and consequences and by creating new problems: side-effects. In fact, side-effects may make the cure worse than the disease. Clinicians conducting clinical trials involving medications try to maintain patients on the study medication for as long as possible. Thus, the design of the clinical trial may create an artificial situation, with misleading estimates of the impact of treatment on HRQL. This issue is of less concern for patients participating in pulmonary rehabilitation. The trials of pulmonary rehabilitation are likely to have simulated clinical practice. COPD is serious enough and its symptoms troubling enough that if pulmonary rehabilitation is beneficial and patients tolerate it well, they are likely to continue with the treatment despite minor side-effects. If patients are experiencing problems similar to those of the trial patients, and if those problems are important to them, they are likely to achieve comparable benefit to patients enrolled in the trial.

WERE ALL IMPORTANT OUTCOMES CONSIDERED AND WERE THE BENEFITS WORTH THE COST?

Before making a final decision whether to apply the results of the systematic review to a patient, users of a review should look for answers to two additional and related questions: 'Were all important outcomes considered, and were the benefits worth the cost?'

Because they are focused on specific clinical questions, systematic review articles are more likely to provide valid results. However, this does not mean that readers should ignore outcomes that are not included in a review. For example, the potential benefits of pulmonary rehabilitation include improved HRQL and improved exercise capacity, but potential down-sides may include an increased risk of injuries during exercise training, absence from the home environment, burden of travel and increased cost. Focused reviews of the evidence are more likely to provide valid results of the impact of pulmonary rehabilitation on each of these four outcomes, but a clinical decision requires consideration of all of them.

In addition, systematic reviews frequently do not report the adverse effects of therapy. One reason is that the individual studies often measure these adverse effects either in different ways or not at all, making pooling, or even effective summarizing, difficult. Cost is an outcome that is often absent from systematic reviews.

Finally, both clinicians and patients must weigh the expected benefits against costs and potential risks. Although this is most obvious when deciding whether to use a therapeutic intervention or a preventive one, providing patients with information about causes of disease or prognosis can also have both benefits and risks. For example, during educational sessions, informing patients with COPD about their increased risk of dying from their disease as compared to the general population might cause anxiety or make their lives less convenient.

Although a valid review article provides the best possible basis for quantifying the expected outcomes, these outcomes must still be considered in the context of the patient's values and concerns. Trading off benefits and risks will involve value judgments which, whenever possible, should reflect the views of the patient. For example, patients should be involved in evaluating whether small but important increments in HRQL and exercise capacity are worth the trouble of being away from their home and family, or the transportation cost to a rehabilitation facility. Many, if not most, patients would value the former more than the latter. However, it is only by engaging the patients in the decision-making process that clinicians can make sure they provide optimal care for their patients (20). In some instances, termed the parental approach, patients request that the clinician makes the decision for them. In other instances, patients and clinicians make the decision together after exchanging information (shared decision-making), and in yet other instances patients want to make the decision independently after having received all the necessary information (informed decision-making).

RESOLUTION OF THE SCENARIO

Overall, the results of the systematic review by Lacasse *et al.* appear applicable to clinical practice. Therefore, clinicians can use this review to guide patient care. A reasonable approach to solving the scenario in Case Study 6.1 would be to explain to the patient that most participants in a pulmonary rehabilitation programme experience important and noticeable improvements in their HRQL. They will experience fewer feelings of dyspnoea and improved mastery of their disease. Many patients will improve their exercise capacity. The patient should know that he will have to weigh these benefits against the possible disadvantages and that he may want to take a week or two to make his choice. Finally, society has to weight the benefits of pulmonary rehabilitation against the cost (see Chapter 17).

SUMMARY

We have described how clinicians and investigators in pulmonary rehabilitation can assess the quality of the research evidence. Systematic reviews have become the mainstay of information in guiding practice. Simple tools to assess their validity, results and application into practice exist. They can also use simple tools to assess studies that deal with HRQL. Clinicians should use these tools to provide the best care to patients.

Key points

- Critical appraisal is an important part of a clinician's repertoire in the field of pulmonary rehabilitation.
- Studies evaluating the efficacy of pulmonary rehabilitation should include outcomes of importance to patients as end-points.
- High-quality evidence shows that, on average, COPD patients receive some benefits from respiratory rehabilitation.
- The main benefit is an improvement in health-related quality of life.

REFERENCES

1. Guyatt G. Introduction. In: Guyatt G, Rennie D, eds. *Users' Guide to the Medical Literature: A Manual for Evidence-based Clinical Practice.* Chicago: AMA Press, 2002; 3–13.

◆2. Haynes RB, Devereaux PJ, Guyatt GH. Clinical expertise in the era of evidence-based medicine and patient choice. *ACP Journal Club* 2002; **136**: A11.

3. Guyatt G, Montori V, Devereaux PJ *et al.* Patients at the center: in our practice, and in our use of language. *ACP Journal Club* 2004; **140**: A11–2.

◆4. McKibbon A, Hunt D, Richardson SW *et al.* Finding the evidence. In: Guyatt G, Rennie D, eds. *Users' Guides to the Medical Literature: A Manual for Evidence-based Clinical Practice.* Chicago: AMA Press, 2002; 16.

5. Oxman A, Guyatt G. The science of reviewing research. *Ann N Y Acad Sci* 1993; **703**: 125–33 (discussion, pp. 133–4).

6. Oxman A, Guyatt G, Cook D, Montori V. Summarizing the evidence. In: Guyatt G, Rennie D, eds. *Users' Guide to the Medical Literature: A Manual for Evidence-based Clinical Practice.* Chicago: AMA Press, 2002; 155–73.

7. Egger M, Davey Smith G, Altman D. Meta-analysis in context. In: Egger M DSG, Altman DG, eds. *Systematic Reviews in Health Care.* London: BMJ Books, 2000.

◆8. Lacasse Y, Brosseau L, Milne S *et al.* Pulmonary rehabilitation for chronic obstructive pulmonary disease [see comment]. *Cochrane Database Syst Rev* 2004; **3**: CD003793.

9. Sin DD, Man S, Paul M. Why are patients with chronic obstructive pulmonary disease at increased risk of cardiovascular diseases?: the potential role of systemic inflammation in chronic obstructive pulmonary disease. *Circulation* 2003; **107**: 1514–19.

10. Salman GF, Mosier MC, Beasley BW, Calkins DR. Rehabilitation for patients with chronic obstructive pulmonary disease: meta-analysis of randomized controlled trials. *J Gen Intern Med* 2003; **18**: 213–21.

11. Guyatt G, Naylor C, Juniper E *et al.* Quality of Life. In: Guyatt G, Rennie D, eds. *Users' Guides to the Medical Literature: A Manual for Evidence-based Clinical Practice.* Chicago: American Medical Association Press, 2002; 309–27.

12. Balk EM, Bonis PA, Moskowitz H *et al.* Correlation of quality measures with estimates of treatment effect in meta-analyses of randomized controlled trials. [comment]. *J Am Med Assoc* 2002; **287**: 2973–82.

13. Moher D, Pham B, Jones A, Cook DJ *et al.* Does quality of reports of randomised trials affect estimates of intervention efficacy reported in meta-analyses? [comment]. *Lancet* 1998; **352**: 609–13.

14. Gotzsche P. Blinding during data analysis and writing of manuscripts. *Contr Clin Trials* 1996; **17**: 285–90.

15. Schünemann H, Armstrong D, Fallone C *et al.* A randomized multi-center trial to evaluate simple utility elicitation techniques in patients with gastro esophageal reflux disease. 2004; **4**: 1132–42.

16. Schünemann H, Goldstein R, Mador J *et al.* Do marker states improve measurement properties of utility instruments: a randomized multi-center trial in patients with chronic respiratory disease. *Qual Life Res*, invited for resubmission.

17. Higgins JP, Thompson SG. Quantifying heterogeneity in a meta-analysis. *Stat Med* 2002; **21**: 1539–58.

18. Jaeschke R, Singer J, Guyatt GH. Measurement of health status. Ascertaining the minimal clinically important difference. *Control Clin Trials* 1989; **10**: 407–15.

19. Schünemann H, Puhan M, Goldstein R *et al.* Measurement properties and interpretability of the Chronic Respiratory Disease Questionnaire (CRQ). *J COPD* 2005, in press.

◆20. Charles C, Whelan T, Gafni A. What do we mean by partnership in making decisions about treatment? *Br Med J* 1999; **319**: 780–2.

PART **2**

Outcome measurement

7

Lung function and respiratory mechanics assessment

LORENZO APPENDINI, MARTA GUDJÓNSDÓTTIR, ANDREA ROSSI

The Greek physician Miltus (570 BC) stated that *pneuma*, or breath, was the essence of all things (1). It took a millennium before we understood that its primary purpose is that of gas exchange. Assessments of lung function focus on defining the properties of the respiratory system. The respiratory muscles form part of the pump, together with the lungs and the chest wall (2). By contracting, they change the chest wall configuration, displacing its components, so that air can move in and out of the lungs (2). The respiratory muscles must overcome the mechanical properties of the pump for ventilation to be effective, at a bearable energy cost (2). In this chapter we will review lung function and respiratory mechanics that are relevant to pulmonary rehabilitation.

LUNG FUNCTION ASSESSMENT

Over the last 50 years, spirometry has become so generally used as to be considered part of the complete physical examination in the rehabilitation setting. Spirometry is an inexpensive test that is widely available. However, it is an effort-dependent manoeuvre that requires understanding, coordination and cooperation by the patient with a trained technician (3, 4). Computer-assisted methods have enhanced the speed and sophistication of the calculations. Standards of testing and interpretation are available in the USA (3) and Europe (4). Basic measurements are based on flow and volume recordings, during either slow or forced respiratory manoeuvres. Graphic tracings must also be available, as they are essential to appreciate the technical test quality as well as the characteristic patterns of disease.

Spirometry has been used to measure vital capacity (VC) since Hutchinson developed the first spirometer more than

150 years ago. Nearly 100 years later, a method to time the forced vital capacity (FVC) was described (5). Subsequently, spirometry has become the standard for defining the presence of airway obstruction by means of the progressive loss of forced expiratory volume in 1 s (FEV_1). Basic spirometry measures the volume of air exhaled by force over a time period (Fig. 7.1). The VC is the difference between the total lung capacity (TLC) and the residual volume (RV). The TLC is the volume at which the tension generated by the diaphragm and the other inspiratory muscles is balanced by the elastic recoil of the lungs and the chest wall. Reduced compliance of the chest wall (e.g. in the presence of kyphoscoliosis) or of the

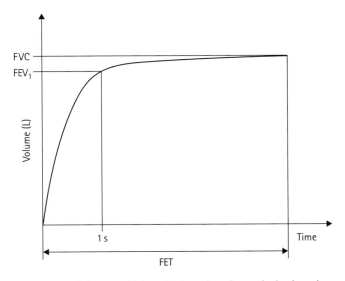

Figure 7.1 *Spirogram. Volume is plotted on the vertical axis and time on the horizontal axis. FEV_1, forced expired volume in 1 s; FET, forced expiratory time; FVC, forced vital capacity.*

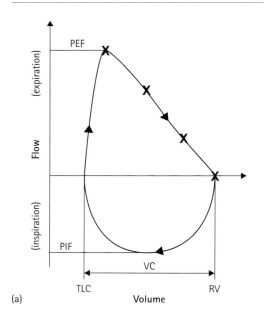

(a)

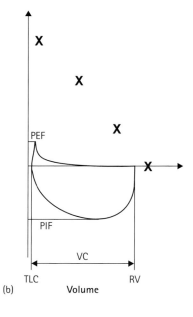

(b)

Figure 7.2   *Flow–volume loop of normal (a) and pathological (b) size and shape due to severe airflow obstruction. Expiratory and inspiratory flows are plotted on the vertical axes and volume on the horizontal axes. Arrows indicate the direction of the loop; crosses indicate reference values. PEF, peak expiratory flow; PIF, peak inspiratory flow; RV, residual volume; TLC, total lung capacity; VC, vital capacity.*

lungs (e.g. in the presence of interstitial diseases of the lungs), weakness of the respiratory muscles (e.g. in the presence of Duchenne's dystrophy, amyotrophic lateral sclerosis, etc.) or their submaximal activation (e.g. in the presence of chest pain, fatigue and poor effort) all lead to a reduced TLC and VC compared with reference values.

In young adults the RV is determined mainly by the compliance of the respiratory system and by the limits of the expiratory muscles. Small airway closure prevents further alveolar emptying of dependent regions of the lungs at low lung volumes, becoming an important RV determinant in older people. As the lung elastic recoil diminishes, the small airways close at higher lung volumes (6). Finally, airway narrowing and expiratory dynamic airway compression can reduce expiratory flow and prolong expiratory time (see also below) for as long as expiratory effort can be maintained (7). RV is more hypothetical than real in older adults and in most individuals with obstructive lung disease, depending on dynamic rather than on static characteristics of the respiratory system. To minimize dynamic determinants of VC in such conditions, expiratory effort should be continued for at least 6 and preferably for 10 s to obtain valid measurements of the expiratory VC.

In chronic obstructive lung disease (COPD), RV increases with increasing severity, whereas TLC only increases slightly. Therefore the VC is diminished (Figs 7.2 and 7.3). In other pathological states, such as congestive heart failure, VC is reduced by a combination of increased intrathoracic blood volume, increased heart size, reduced alveolar distensibility and small airway closure.

FEV_1 is the physiological variable that characterizes COPD severity and correlates with mortality (8). Many guidelines stage the severity of airflow obstruction by FEV_1 and its ratio to FVC (FEV_1/FVC ratio) (9, 10). Initially the FEV_1 is above 80 per cent of predicted, but the FEV_1/FVC ratio reduces to below 70 per cent. As the severity of the obstruction increases, the FEV_1 and FVC fall and the shape of the flow volume loop

changes (Fig. 7.2). Recently it has been suggested that the forced expiratory volume at 6 s of exhalation (FEV_6) may be a better screen for airway obstruction in COPD as it is much more repeatable than VC or FVC (11).

More sophisticated spirometers plot expiratory and inspiratory flow against the volume of air to form a flow volume loop (Fig. 7.2a). In addition to FVC and FEV_1 the overall shape of the loop is helpful in detecting airflow obstruction (Fig. 7.2b) as well as extrathoracic obstruction (12). During forced expiration, the driving pressure to exhale air from the lungs is the alveolar pressure, equal to the sum of the pleural pressure and the static elastic recoil pressure. The intraluminal pressure in the airways falls progressively as the distance from the alveoli increases, until it equals the pleural pressure (the so-called 'equal pressure point') (13). The greater the resistance of the peripheral airways, the more distally the equal pressure point will be located. If the equal pressure points are within the thorax, the 'downstream' airways will tend to collapse during forced expiration. Greater expiratory effort will increase both the pleural and the alveolar pressures, but since the increment is transmitted equally inside and outside the airways, the equal pressure points do not change their position. Once the resistance of the small airways causes the intraluminal pressure to fall below the pleural pressure, the effective driving pressure for expiration is the static elastic recoil pressure. At high lung volumes the static elastic recoil pressure is sufficient to prevent compression of the intrathoracic airways, thus permitting expiratory flow to be effort-dependent (i.e. the stronger the expiratory muscle contraction, the higher the resulting expiratory flow). At low lung volumes, after perhaps 75–80 per cent of the VC has been exhaled, 'dynamic compression' occurs, so that forced expiratory flow becomes independent of effort and depends only on the recoil pressure (Fig. 7.2a). Since the recoil pressure diminishes with decreasing lung volume, flow falls progressively as forced expiration continues (Fig. 7.2a).

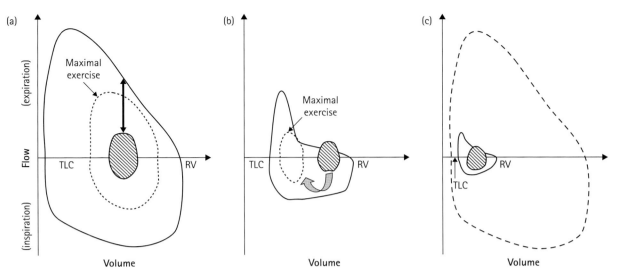

Figure 7.3   *Flow–volume loops at rest (dashed areas) and at maximal exercise (dotted loops) superimposed on maximal flow–volume loops (black loops) in normal subjects (a) and in patients with chronic obstructive pulmonary disease (COPD) with moderate (b) to severe (c) expiratory flow limitation. Dashed flow–volume loop in (c), theoretical normal maximal flow–volume loop; TLC, total lung capacity; RV, residual volume; vertical thick arrow in (a), reserve expiratory flow; curvilinear thick arrow in (b), shift of the end-expiratory lung volume (EELV) closer to TLC, decreasing the inspiratory capacity (IC) at maximal exercise. Note the high reserve of expiratory flow in normal subjects at rest (panel a) as the expiratory flow at maximal exercise is still submaximal. In contrast, expiratory flow is supramaximal at rest in COPD patients with moderate (panel b) and severe (panel c) expiratory flow limitation. In moderate COPD, the increase of EELV allows the increase of expiratory flow and, hence, of minute ventilation during exercise. In severe expiratory flow limitation, the expiratory flow is maximal at rest and the EELV is already close to TLC (panel c), thus precluding the possibility of significantly increasing both expiratory flow and minute ventilation.*

In COPD the resistance of the small airways is increased and the static recoil pressure may be reduced, so that dynamic compression occurs at a relatively high lung volume. Forced expiratory flow is reduced due to a reduced driving pressure and a loss of expiratory flow effort dependence (Figs 7.2b and 7.3b and c). Patients with markedly reduced lung elastic recoil may show 'negative effort dependence' such that flow decreases with increasing the expiratory muscle effort (Fig. 7.3b and c). The above characteristics of forced expiratory flow have a profound impact on exercise limitation in COPD patients (14), which is discussed below.

The FEV_1 correlates poorly with symptoms such as dyspnoea (breathlessness) and exercise performance (14). Other physiological outcome variables have been proposed, based on a better understanding of the mechanism of dyspnoea and exercise limitation. COPD patients, particularly those with severe obstruction, are likely to have dynamic compression of the airways and flow limitation during quiet breathing, which leads to dynamic hyperinflation of the lungs (DH). The DH is present at rest and worsens as ventilation increases (15). This results in an inability to expand tidal volume in response to the increased respiratory drive of exercise, which contributes importantly to dyspnoea and exercise intolerance in COPD (14, 15) (Fig. 7.3). Inspiratory capacity (IC = tidal volume plus inspiratory reserve volume) has been used to estimate the dynamic hyperinflation, i.e. the increase in end-expiratory lung volume (EELV), at rest and during exercise (15, 16). Assuming a constant TLC, a decrease in IC indicates an increase in EELV (Fig. 7.3). IC measurements need simple

equipment and can be performed easily during exercise in a pulmonary function laboratory (14).

ASSESSMENT OF RESPIRATORY MECHANICS

Action of the respiratory muscles

Resting breathing consists of active inspiration, using power provided by the inspiratory muscles, and passive expiration using energy stored in the elastic recoil of the lungs and chest wall (17, 18). The expiratory muscles provide the force necessary for an effective cough, but are also recruited when the ventilatory drive increases, particularly during exercise. Our understanding of respiratory muscle action has been advanced by the simultaneous recording of oesophageal (P_{oes}) and gastric (P_{ga}) pressures using the double balloon technique (Figs 7.4 and 7.5), as a way to partition ventilatory muscle recruitment patterns (19).

The P_{oes}–P_{ga} diagram shown in Fig. 7.5 reflects the relative contributions of the diaphragm, rib cage inspiratory muscles and abdominal muscles to ventilation (20). Pressure is measured using balloon-tipped catheters connected to differential pressure transducers, usually three, that measure P_{oes}, P_{ga} and airway opening pressures (P_{ao}), respectively (Fig. 7.4). Transpulmonary (P_L) and transdiaphragmatic (P_{di}) pressures are obtained by subtraction of P_{oes} from P_{ao} and P_{ga}, respectively. The relationship between P_{oes} and P_{ga} during relaxation

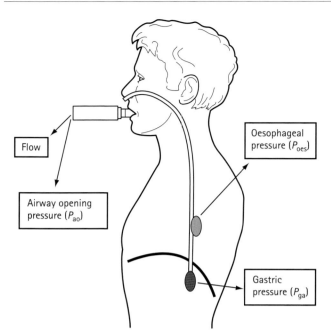

Figure 7.4 *Positioning of the oesophageal and gastric balloon-tipped catheters, which are inserted via the nose after topical anaesthesia. Changes of pressure are measured in the stomach (P_{ga}), in the oesophagus (P_{oes}), and at the airway opening (P_{ao}).*

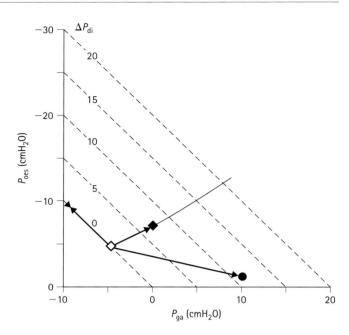

Figure 7.5 *Plot of oesophageal pressure (P_{oes}) against gastric pressure (P_{ga}). Open square: beginning of inspiration. Isopleths for different levels of transdiaphragmatic pressure (P_{di}) are shown as dashed diagonal lines. The curvilinear line crossing the transdiaphragmatic isopleths represents the P_{oes}/P_{ga} relationship during relaxed exhalation. Arrows indicate simultaneous changes in P_{oes} and P_{ga} during the contraction of different groups of respiratory muscles starting from the relaxation volume (end-expiratory lung volume with all respiratory muscles relaxed). Closed square: end of inspiration during normal quiet breathing. The middle arrow indicates the negative change in P_{oes} accompanied by an opposite (in sign) change in P_{ga} induced by the diaphragm contraction during inspiration. Note that during normal quiet breathing, pressure changes lie close to the relaxation pressure line. Closed circle: end of a contraction of the abdominal muscles alone (diaphragm relaxed). Abdominal muscle contraction produces an increase in P_{ga} and less negative P_{oes}, as indicated by displacement of the $P_{oes}-P_{ga}$ plot down and to the right (right arrow). The associated passive stretching of diaphragm results in an increase in P_{di} (the arrow crosses P_{di} isopleths). Closed triangle: end of an inspiratory effort obtained by the contraction of the rib cage muscles alone (diaphragm relaxed). The plot moves up and to the left along the isopleth for $P_{di} = 0$, indicating diaphragm relaxation during the manoeuvre in the absence of passive stretching (left arrow).*

must first be established, i.e., the $P_{oes}-P_{ga}$ relaxation line. Excursions in P_{oes} and P_{ga} are referred to the relaxation line, and departures from this relationship are used to infer the recruitment of various respiratory muscle groups. As the diaphragm contracts, the plot moves upwards and to the right, crossing the P_{di} isopleths, signalling an increase in P_{di}. During normal inspiration, the changes in P_{oes} (becoming more negative) and P_{ga} (becoming more positive) occur along the relaxation line, indicating little distortion of the respiratory system (19, 20). At the same time P_{di} increases, indicating the diaphragm contraction (middle arrow in Fig. 7.5). In general, left-sided shifts of the $P_{oes}-P_{ga}$ diagram from the relaxation line indicate predominant activation of inspiratory accessory muscles, as occurs in the inspiratory phase during heavy exercise, whereas right-sided shifts indicate predominant activation of expiratory muscles, as occurs in the expiratory phase during heavy exercise. Breathing changes in P_{oes} and P_{ga} occurring along a P_{di} isopleth indicate the absence of diaphragm contraction and is seen in patients with bilateral diaphragmatic paralysis (21) or those with COPD with ineffective diaphragmatic function (22).

Relaxation of the expiratory muscles causes P_{ga} to become abruptly less positive and P_{oes} to become abruptly more negative, generating passive inspiration due to the elastic energy stored in the chest wall (23). A typical example of this condition is seen in the early inspiratory phase during heavy exercise, in which several muscle groups (diaphragm, accessory inspiratory muscles and expiratory muscles) participate in the increased inspiratory energy demands. Pure inspiratory rib cage contraction causes inward abdominal displacement, whereas abdominal muscles relaxation causes the abdomen to expand outward.

The preceding discussion of the $P_{oes}-P_{ga}$ plots addresses the activity of a single respiratory muscle group. However, in COPD, several muscle groups are recruited during a single

respiratory cycle, making the interpretation of the $P_{oes}-P_{ga}$ diagrams more complicated (20).

Respiratory muscle function

Respiratory muscles generate more force as they lengthen, until an optimal length is reached (20), after which further stretching is associated with decreased strength until the muscle fibre breaks. As the resting length of a muscle shortens, during lung hyperinflation, the force-generating capacity for a given electrical stimulus decreases. Respiratory muscles compensate by increasing the motor output of the central nervous system, to recruit more muscle fibres (24).

As the velocity of respiratory muscle contraction increases (e.g. increased respiratory rate), the capacity to generate tension decreases. This relationship becomes clinically relevant in patients with rapid rates or short inspiratory times. At rest, the velocity of contraction and the inspiratory muscle force generated are about 5 per cent of maximum. Up to 50 per cent of maximal force or velocity can be sustained for several hours. Below these thresholds, ventilation can be sustained indefinitely and represents the safe boundaries that protect respiratory muscles (25).

There are several ways to assess respiratory muscle function. Volitional methods measure maximal respiratory pressures and non-volitional methods measure respiratory muscle electrical activity (power spectral analysis, integrated electrical activity or some combination of these two). Other tests that measure the force-generating capacity of the diaphragm independently of the central control mechanism, such as bilateral phrenic nerve stimulation and P_{di} frequency curves (20) are beyond the aims of this chapter.

CONTROL OF BREATHING

The role of the respiratory control system is to adjust ventilation in order to maintain adequate gas exchange at as low a cost as possible. This system consists of (26, 27):

- arterial and central chemoreceptors
- airway, lung and chest wall mechanoreceptors
- respiratory muscle force and length sensors
- a system to relay information to a network of neurons in the medulla.

Additional inputs are transmitted via cardiovascular and other receptors in the viscera. Output is generated by a medullary network in which chemical and mechanical signals determine the depth and frequency of each breath (27).

In healthy subjects, breathing occurs effortlessly until exertion increases the metabolic demand for greater respiration (26, 28). The respiratory muscles are also subject to voluntary control from the cortex, allowing the breath to be held as well as actions other than breathing (29). Autonomic control coordinates the sequencing of the contraction of the thoracic, abdominal and upper airway muscles to maintain ventilation despite changes in the environment, metabolic rate or force-generating ability of the respiratory muscles.

Alveolar ventilation is measured by the level of arterial P_{CO_2} (partial pressure of carbon dioxide), which, when increased, signifies alveolar hypoventilation (e.g. respiratory centre depression or respiratory muscle impairment). In the face of impaired gas exchange in the lung or suboptimal performance of the respiratory muscles, control system attempts to adjust ventilation can lead to dyspnoea (28). Dyspnoea may also occur in control system malfunction if ventilation is driven beyond the requirements of gas exchange (26, 28).

Measurements of volume, flow, pressure or muscle electrical activity are used as indirect measurements of global respiratory output (30). In healthy subjects, the increase in minute ventilation in response to hypercapnic or hypoxic stimulation will provide an assessment of the respiratory control system. However, in patients with increased respiratory resistance or decreased compliance, the ventilatory response may be decreased despite a normal or increased respiratory centre output (31). Diaphragmatic electromyography (EMG) activity does reflect a change in motor neuron discharge, but such recordings are difficult to standardize.

Occlusion pressure measurements

The negative pressure generated by contraction of the inspiratory muscles against an occluded airway is directly related to its neural stimulus, as reflected by the diaphragmatic EMG (30). In practice, the airway is occluded for 0.1 s, without warning, and the resulting change in airway pressure (termed $P_{0.1}$) is measured before the subject recognizes and reacts to the occlusion (31). Although the $P_{0.1}$ is a negative pressure, it is reported as a positive unit (normal $P_{0.1}$ = 0.93 ± 0.48 (SD) cmH$_2$O with a coefficient of variation of 50 per cent) (32). High $P_{0.1}$ values indicate that ventilatory failure is not due to insufficient ventilatory drive but rather to inadequate transformation of that drive into ventilatory output (33). This may be useful in predicting weaning outcomes.

Breathing pattern analysis

Breathing pattern analysis can provide valuable information regarding the respiratory system. Minute ventilation ($\dot{V}_E$) is the product of tidal volume (V_T) and breathing frequency (f) (32):

$$\dot{V}_E = V_T f \tag{1}$$

In healthy subjects, f is approximately 17 breaths/min and V_T is approximately 0.4 L making $\dot{V}_E$ = 6.8 L/min (34).

Arterial partial pressure of carbon dioxide (P_aCO_2) is determined by the relationship between alveolar ventilation ($\dot{V}_A$) and CO$_2$ production ($\dot{V}CO_2$) according to equation:

$$P_aCO_2 = K(\dot{V}CO_2/\dot{V}_A) \tag{2}$$

where K is a constant of proportionality. Since $\dot{V}_A = \dot{V}_E - \dot{V}_D$, where $\dot{V}_D$ is dead space ventilation this equation can be rewritten as follows (35):

$$P_aCO_2 = K[\dot{V}CO_2/(\dot{V}_E - \dot{V}_D)] \tag{3}$$

or

$$P_aCO_2 = K\{\dot{V}CO_2/[\dot{V}_E(1 - V_D/V_T)]\} \tag{4}$$

where V_D is the dead space and V_T is the tidal volume.

High $\dot{V}_E$ in the presence of hypercapnia indicates increased dead space ventilation and/or increased CO$_2$ production (35). Conversely, hypercapnia associated with low minute ventilation indicates decreased respiratory drive, structural abnormality of the thoracic cage or respiratory muscle dysfunction.

An elevated breathing frequency is often the earliest sign of impending respiratory failure (36). Patients who fail a weaning trial show increased frequency and reduced V_T. Combining these two factors into an index of rapid shallow breathing (RSB) (37) gives the following:

$$\text{RSB index} = f/V_T \tag{5}$$

If the RBS index is above 100 breaths/min per L, rapid shallow breathing is present (37, 38).

Additional information on respiratory centre function can be obtained from breathing pattern analysis. Equation (1) can be rearranged, as respiratory frequency is equal to 60 divided by the time of a total respiratory cycle (T_{TOT}) or single breath, as follows:

$$\dot{V}_E = V_T 60/T_{TOT} \tag{6}$$

and 60 can be deleted from the equation:

$$\dot{V}_E = V_T \times [1/T_{TOT}] \tag{7}$$

Dividing V_T by inspiratory time (T_I) while multiplying $1/T_{TOT}$ by T_I gives:

$$\dot{V}_E = [V_T/T_I] \times [T_I/T_{TOT}] \tag{8}$$

V_T/T_I is mean inspiratory flow and T_I/T_{TOT} has been termed fractional inspiratory time or duty cycle.

Mean inspiratory flow has been widely used to evaluate respiratory drive (31). It reflects the mechanical transformation of respiratory neural activity and is related to standard indices of respiratory centre output, such as $P_{0.1}$. In the presence of abnormal pulmonary mechanics, even an elevated V_T/T_I may underestimate the increase in respiratory drive.

Fractional inspiratory time (also known as duty cycle) also determines the stress placed on the respiratory muscles (39). However, although a reduction in T_I/T_{TOT} is a useful strategy for decreasing the risk of muscle fatigue, patients rarely display a meaningful change in this index, in clinical practice (40).

Respiratory workload

Given that the respiratory system is essentially a pump that moves gases in and out the body, it follows that the act of breathing requires work to be performed against several impediments (41):

- elastic forces (lungs and chest wall as volume is increased)
- resistive forces (gas flow through conducting airways)
- viscoelastic forces (stress adaptation of units within the lung and chest wall)
- plastoelastic forces (differences in static elastic recoil pressure between inflation and deflation)
- inertial forces (depend on the mass of gases and tissues)
- gravitational forces (included in the measurement of elastic forces)

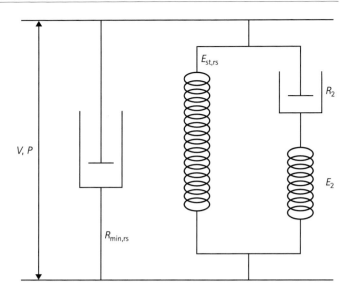

Figure 7.6 *Respiratory system consists of interrupter (viscous) resistance (R_{rs}), in parallel with static elastance ($E_{st,rs}$) and series spring and dashpot bodies (E_2, R_2) representing viscoelastic elements. The distance between the two bars and the tension between the bars are analogous to lung volume (V) and pressure applied to the respiratory system (P).*

- compressibility of intrathoracic gas
- distortion of the chest wall from its passive (relaxed) configuration

Figure 7.6 illustrates a simplified linear viscoelastic model for the interpretation of respiratory mechanics. The dynamics of breathing have been represented by a single-compartment model consisting of a rigid tube and a compliant balloon (1, 41). In this mechanical model, pressure, airflow and volume are related by the equation of motion of the relaxed respiratory system:

$$P = E_{rs}V + R_{rs}\dot{V} \tag{9}$$

In this equation, P is the pressure applied to inflate the respiratory system, E_{rs} is the elastance and R_{rs} is the resistance of the respiratory system, V is the volume of the lung above end-expiratory volume and $\dot{V}$ is the flow. To breathe, pressure must be applied to the respiratory system to generate flow and displace volume. Expiration is driven by the elastic recoil pressure stored in the respiratory system as a result of the preceding lung inflation and the total flow resistance is the opposing force at the end of inspiratory activity, before the expiratory muscles are active (41).

The mechanical properties of the respiratory system are essentially resistive and elastic. Flow is measured using meters at the mouth or trachea and volume is calculated from integrating flow. Pressure is measured as described in Fig. 7.4. In Fig. 7.7, tracings of flow, volume, P_{ao}, P_{oes} and P_{ga} are shown, as well as calculations of transpulmonary pressure (P_L) and transdiaphragmatic pressure (P_{di}).

$$E_{st,w} = E_{st,rs} - E_{st,L} \qquad (12)$$

$$E_{st,rs} = E_{st,L} + E_{st,w} \qquad (13)$$

where P_L is the transpulmonary pressure, i.e. the pressure difference between the airway opening (P_{ao}) and the pleural pressure (P_{pl}), and P_{oes} is the oesophageal pressure that provides an estimate of P_{pl}.

Compliance (C) is the inverse of elastance ($C = 1/E$), measured as the change in lung volume per unit change in applied static pressure (elastic recoil pressure). Therefore equations (4) and (6) become, respectively:

$$C_{st,rs} = \Delta V/\Delta P_{el,rs} \qquad (14)$$

$$1/C_{st,rs} = 1/C_{st,L} + 1/C_{st,w} \qquad (15)$$

$C_{st,rs}$ amounts to about $0.100 \, \text{L/cmH}_2\text{O}$, while $C_{st,L}$ and $C_{st,w}$ amount to approximately $0.200 \, \text{L/cmH}_2\text{O}$ each (42).

The lung and the chest wall display different pressure–volume relationships (43). The resulting pressure–volume relationship of the respiratory system is sigmoidal in shape, and compliance is greatest in the mid-volume range, where breathing normally occurs. At the relaxed static equilibrium volume of the respiratory system, elastic recoil of the lung and the chest wall exactly balance each other. Also at this point, compliances of the lung and chest wall are approximately equal in normal subjects. The point where the opposing elastic forces of the lungs and chest wall are equal is the elastic equilibrium volume, also called relaxation volume (V_r), of the total respiratory system and is normally coincident with functional residual capacity (FRC), which is the amount of gas in the lungs and airways at the end of a tidal expiration (43).

In the mid-volume range, the elastic work of breathing and fluctuations in transpulmonary pressure are minimized (43). Compliance of the respiratory system is decreased both at high lung volumes, as the pressure–volume curve of the lung flattens and becomes fully distended, and at low lung volumes, due to stiffening of the chest wall resulting from the volume restriction imposed by obesity of abdominal distension. The slope of the pressure–volume curve of the respiratory system is altered by changes in the lung or chest wall. Lung recoil is decreased in emphysema and increased in interstitial fibrosis, oedema and pneumonectomy. The chest wall is stiffer in patients with kyphoscoliosis, ankylosing spondylitis, obesity and massive ascites (44). As lung compliance is reduced, as in emphysema, expiratory flow will also be abnormally limited (44).

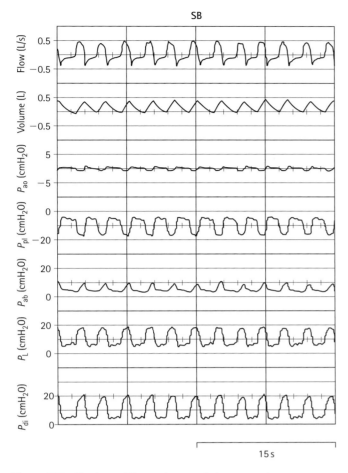

Figure 7.7 *Tracings of flow, volume and airway opening, oesophageal and gastric pressures [P_{ao}, P_{pl} (or P_{oes}) and P_{ab} (or P_{ga}) respectively]. Transpulmonary (P_L) and transdiaphragmatic (P_{di}) pressures are obtained by subtracting P_{pl} from P_{ao} and P_{ab}, respectively. The volume is calculated from numerical integration of the flow signal.*

ELASTANCE AND COMPLIANCE

Elastance (E), namely the change in pressure per unit change of volume is commonly used to describe the elastic properties of the respiratory system (E_{rs}) and is usually expressed in $\text{cmH}_2\text{O/L}$:

$$E_{rs} = \Delta P_{el,rs}/\Delta V \qquad (10)$$

where $\Delta P_{el,rs}$ and ΔV are the changes in elastic transrespiratory pressure and volume, respectively (42). In the upright adult, the static respiratory elastance $E_{st,rs}$ is $10 \, \text{cmH}_2\text{O/L}$. Pressure applied to the airway is first transmitted to the lung, after which a reduced pressure is transferred to the chest wall. The pressure to distend the respiratory system is the sum of the pressures required to distend the lung and chest wall (42). Thus, the static elastance of the respiratory system ($E_{st,rs}$) is the sum of static lung elastance ($E_{st,L}$) and static chest wall elastance ($E_{st,w}$), each amounting approximately to $5 \, \text{cmH}_2\text{O/L}$:

$$E_{st,L} = \Delta P_L/\Delta V \qquad (11)$$

RESISTANCE

Flow ($\dot{V}$) through a pipe requires a driving pressure to overcome frictional resistance. The magnitude of flow depends on the difference in pressure (ΔP) across the pipe and the resistance (R) offered by the pipe itself (44):

$$\dot{V} = \Delta P/R \qquad (16)$$

Flow resistance is proportional to the length (44) of the pipe and varies inversely with the fourth and fifth powers of the radius (r) for laminar and turbulent flow, respectively, as described by the Poiseuille's law:

$$R = 8\eta L/\pi r^4 \qquad (17)$$

where η represents the viscosity of the gas and $8/\pi$ is a constant (44).

In normal subjects, the $P/\dot{V}$ relationship is linear during quiet breathing and, hence, airway resistance can be expressed as a single number, 2–4 cmH$_2$O/L per s (42). Airway resistance (R_{aw}) is only one component of the total respiratory system's resistance (R_{rs}), which also includes tissue resistance of the lung (R_{TL}), thus giving the total pulmonary resistance (R_L) and chest wall resistance (R_w) (44). In the case of the respiratory system, resistance is rarely linear, and the relationship between pressure and flow is usually expressed by Rohrer's equation (44):

$$P_{res} = K_1\dot{V} + K_2\dot{V}^2 \qquad (18)$$

where K_1 and K_2 are constants. Respiratory pressure–flow relationships may also be described by the following exponential function (41):

$$P = a\dot{V}^b \qquad (19)$$

where a is the resistance when flow equals 1 L/s, and b is constrained to vary between 1 and 2, depending on the relative amounts of laminar and turbulent flow.

Resistance varies throughout the respiratory cycle (41) with turbulence changing lung volume and (especially in COPD) the phase of respiration (41). Resistance may be overestimated during expiration, especially when elastic recoil is lost and expiratory flow is limited, as in patients with emphysema (42).

Endotracheal tubes.   In ventilator-dependent patients, a significant component of the total flow resistance is provided by endotracheal tubes, which have highly curvilinear flow-resistance properties (42). The flow resistance for adult endotracheal tube diameters has been determined experimentally (42). This resistance increases markedly with increasing flow and varies with the size of the tube (42).

INTRINSIC POSITIVE END-EXPIRATORY PRESSURE

In normal subjects, expiratory flow stops before the onset of the next inspiration and FRC corresponds to the elastic equilibrium volume of the total respiratory system (44). If the end-expiratory volume exceeds the predicted FRC, there is an elevation of the static recoil pressure of the respiratory system and thus alveolar pressure (18, 42, 45). This positive recoil pressure has been termed intrinsic positive end-expiratory pressure (PEEP$_i$) (18).

Increased flow resistance
Increased flow resistance, often associated with expiratory flow limitation, leads to DH in airway obstruction, mechanical

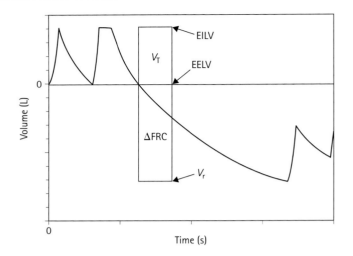

Figure 7.8   *Volume/time relationship with a complete relaxed expiration following a brief end-inspiratory occlusion in a ventilator-dependent patient. EILV, end-inspiratory lung volume; V$_T$, tidal volume; EELV, end-expiratory lung volume; ΔFRC, differences in volume from EELV to the relaxed functional capacity (FRC) or relaxation volume (V$_r$).*

ventilation and acute respiratory failure (ARF) (18). Expiration cannot be completed within the time available, so that inspiration starts before full decompression of the lungs. The FRC stabilizes above the V_r. The usual end-expiratory pause is replaced by a change in flow direction from expiration to inspiration (18) (Fig. 7.8).

Expiratory flow limitation
In patients with advanced COPD, destruction of lung parenchyma causes loss of alveolar septal attachments (46). Poorly supported small airways that are dynamically compressed during expiration give rise to expiratory flow limitation (47), resulting in air trapping, a major determinant of DH and PEEP$_i$ in COPD patients.

The measurement of PEEP$_i$ is much easier during controlled mechanical ventilation than during assisted ventilation, weaning and spontaneous breathing, since the respiratory muscles are increasingly recruited in these latter conditions. When the respiratory muscles are relaxed, the pressure at the airway opening during airway occlusion reflects the mean alveolar pressure. This principle has been used to compute PEEP$_i$ from end-expiratory airway occlusion (EEO) (42). During the EEO, the pressure in the airways increases until a plateau is reached, usually between 1 and 5 s after the occlusion (18), and PEEP$_i$ is the difference between the end-expiratory plateau pressure during airway occlusion and atmosphere.

PEEP$_i$ is measured in actively breathing patients, using an oesophageal balloon to measure changes in P_{pl} (48). The method is valid provided that the expiratory muscles are relaxed at the end of expiration (Fig. 7.9a). If they are not, part of the decrease in P_{pl} in early inspiration could be due to expiratory muscle relaxation rather than to inspiratory muscle contraction (49, 50) (Fig. 7.9b).

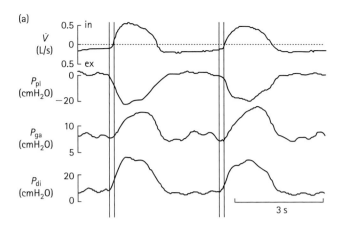

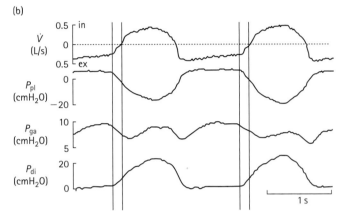

Figure 7.9   *Determination of PEEP$_{i,dyn}$. P$_{pl}$, pleural pressure, estimated from oesophageal pressure. The first vertical line indicates the point corresponding to the onset of the inspiratory effort (P$_{di}$ swing). The second vertical line indicates the point corresponding to the start of the inspiratory flow. The dotted horizontal line represents zero flow (V̇) where 'in' is inspiratory flow and 'ex' is expiratory flow. (a) Expiratory flow ends abruptly before inspiration, whereas the P$_{di}$ and P$_{pl}$ swings have already begun and P$_{ga}$ has remained constant during that interval. In this case, PEEP$_{i,dyn}$ can be measured as the negative deflection in P$_{pl}$ between the point corresponding to the onset of the P$_{di}$ swing and the point of zero flow. (b) P$_{ga}$ increases throughout most of the expiration, and becomes less positive from the onset of the inspiratory effort indicated by the start of positive P$_{di}$ swing to the start of inspiratory flow. In this case PEEP$_{i,dyn}$ is measured as the negative P$_{pl}$ deflection between the point corresponding to the onset of the P$_{di}$ swing and the point of zero flow subtracted by the amount of P$_{ga}$ negative deflection observed in that interval. Reproduced with permission from Appendini et al. (49).*

WORK OF BREATHING

The work of breathing (WOB) is the mechanical work performed, to expand the respiratory system, by the respiratory muscles. Mechanical work (W) implies that the applied force or pressure (P) produces some displacement of the system,

i.e., volume (V), according to the formula:

$$W = P \times V = \int P \Delta V \qquad (20)$$

which represents the area subtended by the volume–pressure curve.

Work per minute (power), or work rate, is designated by the symbol W' and is calculated by multiplying the work of one breath by the respiratory frequency. The most popular units of work are kilogram metre (kg m) and joules (J). In general, 0.1 kg m approximates 1 J, and this can be thought of as the energy that is needed to move 1 L through a 10 cmH$_2$O pressure gradient (44). While breathing through the nose, the normal resting WOB is 3.9 J/min or 0.47 J/L (51). For a given level of ventilation (60–70 L/min), work ranges from 49 to 196 J/min (51, 52). Patients with COPD have a high WOB because of their low compliance and high resistance.

Pressure–time product

The pressure–time product (PTP) correlates with oxygen consumption (53) and can be used as an index of inspiratory muscle energy expenditure. Changes in inspiratory muscle effort can be estimated from changes in the pressure–time product for the inspiratory muscles (PTP$_{pl}$) and for the diaphragm (PTP$_{di}$), obtained from the area under the P_{pl} and P_{di} versus time curves, respectively, and expressed as the value over 1 min (45).

Efficiency

The efficiency of the respiratory muscles is the ratio of mechanical work to the energy expenditure, as follows:

Efficiency = mechanical work/energy expenditure

The energy expenditure during breathing can be determined by measuring O$_2$ consumption at rest and during hyperventilation. The oxygen cost of breathing is approximately 1 mL/L of ventilation (less than 5 per cent of the total oxygen consumption of the body). The efficiency of the respiratory muscles is 5–10 per cent, less in the presence of lung or chest wall disease (2). Patients with emphysema have low efficiencies, as some inspiratory muscles contract isometrically and therefore do not perform work (i.e. there is no shortening even though energy is consumed). They also breathe at a mechanical disadvantage, such that a more forceful contraction is required to produce a given pressure change. Also, a greater degree of excitation is required to develop a given force, as the muscles are operating on an inefficient part of their force–length relationship. Both the greater excitation and the stronger contraction increase the energy consumption for a given pressure.

Load/capacity balance of the respiratory muscles

A normal ventilatory pump has enough reserve to handle major increases in load during exercise. Ventilatory failure and CO$_2$ retention occurs with

- reduced central neuromuscular drive
- inadequate ventilatory muscle force-generating capacity
- excessive respiratory load.

If the respiratory load is in excess of the respiratory muscle capacity (39, 54) the ventilatory pump may fail. When the transdiaphragmatic pressure developed with each inspiration is greater than 40 per cent of the subject's maximum P_{di} the endurance time limit (T_{lim}) falls to below 60 min. Since the diaphragm contracts during inspiration, the duration of inspiration (T_I) to the duration of the total respiratory cycle (T_{TOT}), i.e. the duty cycle, should be an important determinant of diaphragmatic dysfunction. By combining the diaphragmatic pressure (mean $P_{di}/P_{di,max}$) with the duty cycle (T_I/T_{TOT}), the tension-time index of the diaphragm (TT_{di}) is obtained:

$$TT_{di} = [\text{mean } P_{di}/P_{di,max}] \times [T_I/T_{TOT}] \qquad (21)$$

As the TT_{di} increases, T_{lim} shortens (39). Breathing below a TT_{di} of 0.15 can be sustained indefinitely, but above 0.18 it cannot be tolerated for more than 30–60 min. The TT_{di} in healthy subjects at rest is 0.02, and in stable patients with COPD it is 0.05 (range 0.01–0.12) (54). The major limitation of TT_{di} is the velocity of inspiratory muscle contraction (55), so that tolerable TT_{di} decreases with increasing flow rate (20). Irrespective of the breathing pattern, the TT_{di} cannot exceed 15 per cent of $P_{di,max}$, as with any striated muscle without dysfunction (56). During exercise, increasing circulating metabolites originating in the contraction of locomotor muscles and compromising blood flow to the diaphragm also contribute to the muscular dysfunction (57).

CONCLUSIONS

By characterizing the load/capacity balance of the respiratory pump, we can track a system that adapts to increasing workloads by shifting its power output towards its maximum. In healthy subjects, the respiratory system has a substantial reserve. Increases of respiratory workload and/or impairment of neuromuscular function, reduce the ability of the respiratory system to cope with increased ventilatory demands. Pharmacological intervention, surgical correction by volume reduction or improved fitness of peripheral muscles will reduce the inspiratory workload. If adequate resting ventilation cannot be maintained, mechanical ventilation may be necessary. Assessing ventilatory mechanics will be invaluable in the management of patients with chronic respiratory conditions.

Key points

- Assessment of respiratory mechanics enables us to understand ventilatory function better.
- The respiratory system is a pump in which the respiratory muscles are the engine, the chest wall and

the lungs the elastic compartments and the airways the resistive compartment. Respiratory system tissues also have viscoelastic properties.

- The respiratory pump functions well, unless the force-generating capacity of the respiratory muscles falls below the required work of breathing. This results in functional impairment and ultimately ventilatory failure.
- Modelling of the respiratory system allows us to quantify the extent of the respiratory impairment.
- Respiratory mechanics are sensitive to the changes in ventilatory function and exercise tolerance associated with respiratory rehabilitation.
- Assessing respiratory mechanics will help with therapeutic and rehabilitation interventions, as well as providing basic outcome measurement tools.

REFERENCES

1. Colice GL. Historical perspective on the development of mechanical ventilation. In: Tobin MJ, ed. *Principles and Practice of Mechanical Ventilation*. New York: McGraw-Hill Inc, 1994; 1–35.
◆ 2. Roussos C, Macklem PT. The respiratory muscles: medical progress. *N Engl J Med* 1982; **307**: 786–97.
3. American Thoracic Society. Standardization of spirometry: 1994 update. *Am J Respir Crit Care Med* 1995; **152**: 1107–36.
4. Quanjer PhH, Tammeling GJ, Cotes JE *et al*. Lung volumes and forced ventilatory flows. Official statement of the European Respiratory Society. *Eur Respir J* 1993; **6**: 5–40.
5. Ruppel GL. Spirometry and Related Tests. In: Gregg L, Ruppel GL, eds. *Manual of Pulmonary Function Testing*. Missouri: Mosby-Year Book Inc, 1998; 27–68.
6. Engel LA, Grassino A, Anthonisen NR. Demonstration of airway closure in man. *J Appl Physiol* 1975; **38**: 1117–25.
7. Leith DE, Mead J. Mechanisms determining residual volume of the lungs. *J Appl Physiol* 1967; **23**: 221–7.
8. Crapo RO, Jensen RL, Hargreave FE. Airway inflammation in COPD: physiological outcome measures and induced sputum. *Eur Respir J* 2003; **21**(Suppl. 41): 19–28.
● 9. Pauwels RA, Buist AS, Ma P *et al*. Global strategy for the diagnosis, management, and prevention of chronic obstructive pulmonary disease: NHLBI/WHO Global Initiative for Chronic Obstructive Lung Disease (GOLD) Workshop Summary. *Am J Respir Crit Care Med* 2001; **163**: 1256–76.
10. American Thoracic Society. Statement. Standards for the diagnosis and care of patients with COPD. *Am J Respir Crit Care Med* 1995; **152**: 77–120.
●11. Hankinson JL, Crapo RO, Jensen RL. Spirometric reference values for the 6-s FVC maneuver. *Chest* 2003; **124**: 1805–11.
12. Dakin JH, Kourteli EN, Winter RJD. *Making Sense of Lung Function Testing*. London: Arnold, 2003; 9–36.
13. Mead J, Turner JM, Macklem PT, Little JB. Significance of the relationship between lung recoil and maximum expiratory flow. *J Appl Physiol* 1967; **22**: 95–108.

14. Milic-Emili J. Inspiratory capacity and exercise tolerance in chronic obstructive pulmonary disease. *Can Respir J* 2000; **7**: 282–5.

15. O'Donnell DE, Revill SM, Webb K. Dynamic hyperinflation and exercise intolerance in chronic obstructive pulmonary disease. *Am J Respir Crit Care Med* 2001; **164**: 770–7.

16. Dolmage TE, Goldstein R. Repeatability on inspiratory capacity during incremental exercise in patients with severe COPD. *Chest* 2002; **121**: 708–14.

◆17. DeTroyer A. Respiratory muscle function. In: Cherniack NS, Altose MD, Homme I, eds. *Rehabilitation of the Patient with Respiratory Disease.* New York: McGraw-Hill, 1999; 21–32.

◆18. Rossi A, Polese G, Brandi G, Conti G. Intrinsic positive end-expiratory pressure (PEEPi). *Intensive Care Med* 1995; **21**: 522–36.

●19. Macklem PT, Gross D, Grassino A, Roussos C. Partitioning of the inspiratory pressure swings between diaphragm and intercostal/accessory muscles. *J Appl Physiol* 1978; **44**: 200–8.

◆20. Tobin MJ, Laghi F. Monitoring of respiratory muscle function. In: Tobin MJ, ed. *Principles and Practice of Intensive Care Monitoring.* New York: McGraw-Hill, 1998; 497–544.

21. Hillman DR, Finucane KE. Respiratory pressure partitioning during quiet inspiration in unilateral and bilateral diaphragmatic weakness. *Am Rev Respir Dis* 1988; **137**: 1401–5.

22. Martinez FJ, Couser JI, Celli BR. Factors influencing ventilatory muscle recruitment in patients with chronic airflow obstruction. *Am Rev Respir Dis* 1990; **142**: 276–82.

●23. Dodd DS, Brancatisano T, Engel LA. Chest wall mechanics during exercise in patients with severe chronic airflow obstruction. *Am Rev Respir Dis* 1984; **129**: 33–8.

24. Rochester DF. The diaphragm: Contractile properties and fatigue. *J Clin Invest* 1985; **75**: 1397–402.

25. Martin J, Moreno R, Pare P, Pardy R. Measurement of inspiratory muscle performance with incremental threshold loading. *Am Rev Respir Dis* 1987; **135**: 919–23.

26. Schwartzstein RM. Pathophysiology of dyspnea. *N Engl J Med* 1995; **333**: 1547–53.

27. Blanche A, Denavit-Saubie M, Champagnat J. Neurobiology of the central control of breathing in mammals; neuron circuitry, membrane properties and neurotransmitters involved. *Physiol Rev* 1995; **751**: 1–45.

28. Cherniack NS. Respiratory sensation as a respiratory controller. In: Adams L, Guz A, eds. *Respiratory Sensation,* vol. 90. New York: Marcel Dekker, 1996; 213–30.

◆29. Cherniack NS. The impact of abnormalities in the control of breathing on pulmonary rehabilitation. In: Cherniack NS, Altose MD, Homme I, eds. *Rehabilitation of the Patient with Respiratory Disease.* New York: McGraw-Hill, 1999; 163–8.

30. Lopata M, Lourenco RV. Evaluation of respiratory control. *Clin Chest Med* 1980; **1**: 33–45.

◆31. Milic-Emili J. Recent advances in clinical assessment of control of breathing. *Lung* 1982; **160**: 1–17.

32. Tobin MJ, Laghi F, Walsh JM. Monitoring of respiratory neuromuscular function. In: Tobin MJ, ed. *Principles and Practice of Mechanical Ventilation.* New York: McGraw-Hill, 1994; 945–66.

●33. Murciano D, Boczkowski J, Lecocguic Y et al. Tracheal occlusion pressure: a simple index to monitor respiratory muscle fatigue during acute respiratory failure in patients with chronic obstructive pulmonary disease. *Ann Intern Med* 1988; **108**: 800–5.

34. Tobin JJ, Chadha TS, Jenouri G et al. Breathing patterns: Part I. Normal subjects. *Chest* 1983; **84**: 202–5.

35. Wasserman K, Hansen JE, Sue DY et al. *Principles of Exercise Testing and Interpretation,* 2nd edn. Malvern: Lea & Febiger, 1994; 1–479.

36. Gravelyn TR, Weg JR. Respiratory rate as an indicator of acute respiratory dysfunction. *J Am Med Assoc* 1980; **244**: 1123–5.

●37. Yang K, Tobin MJ. A prospective study of indexes predicting the outcome of trials of weaning from mechanical ventilation. *N Engl J Med* 1991; **324**: 1445–50.

38. Roussos C. Ventilatory muscle fatigue governs breathing frequency. *Bull Eur Physiopathol Respir* 1984; **20**: 445–1.

39. Bellemare F, Grassino A. Effect of pressure and timing of contraction on human diaphragm fatigue. *J Appl Physiol* 1982; **53**: 1190–5.

40. Tobin JJ, Chadha TS, Jenouri G et al. Breathing patterns: Part II. Diseased subjects. *Chest* 1983; **84**: 286–94.

◆41. Rodarte JR, Rehder K. Dynamics of respiration. In: Macklem PT, Mead J, eds. *Handbook of Physiology,* Section 3. *The Respiratory System.* Bethesda, MD: American Physiological Society, 1986; 131–44.

◆42. Rossi A, Polese G, Milic-Emili J. Monitoring respiratory mechanics in ventilator-dependent patients. In: Tobin MJ, ed. *Principles and Practice of Intensive Care Monitoring.* New York: McGraw-Hill, 1998; 553–96.

43. Agostoni E, Hyatt RE. Static behaviour of the respiratory system. In: Fishman P, ed. *Handbook of Physiology: the Respiratory System,* vol. 3. Bethesda, MD: American Physiologic Society, 1986; 113–44.

◆44. Tobin MJ, Van De Graaf WB. Monitoring of lung mechanics and work of breathing. In: Tobin MJ, ed. *Principles and Practice of Mechanical Ventilation.* New York: McGraw-Hill, 1994; 967–1003.

●45. Petrof BJ, Legaré M, Goldberg P et al. Continous positive airway pressure reduces work of breathing and dyspnea during weaning from mechanical ventilation in severe chronic obstructive pulmonary disease. *Am Rev Respir Dis* 1990; **141**: 281–9.

46. Saetta M, Ghezzo H, Kim VD et al. Loss of alveolar attachment in smokers. *Am Rev Respir Dis* 1985; **132**: 894–900.

●47. Gay P, Rodarte JR, Hubmayr RD. The effects of positive expiratory pressure on isovolume flow and dynamic hyperinflation in patients receiving mechanical ventilation. *Am Rev Respir Dis* 1989; **139**: 621–6.

◆48. Zin WA, Milic-Emili J. Esophageal pressure measurement. In: Tobin MJ, ed. *Principles and Practice of Intensive Care Monitoring.* New York: McGraw-Hill, 1998; 545–52.

●49. Appendini L, Patessio A, Zanaboni S et al. Physiologic effects of positive end-expiratory pressure and mask pressure support during exacerbations of chronic obstructive pulmonary disease. *Am J Respir Crit Care Med* 1994; **149**: 1069–76.

50. Ninane V, Yernault JC, DeTroyer A. Intrinsic PEEP in patients with chronic obstructive pulmonary disease. *Am Rev Respir Dis* 1993; **148**: 1037–42.

51. Roussos C, Campbell EJM. Respiratory muscle energetics. In: Macklem PT, Mead J, eds. *Handbook of Physiology,* Section 3. *The Respiratory System,* vol. 3. *Mechanics of Breathing.* Bethesda, MD: American Physiological Society, 1986; 481–509.

52. Fritts HN, Filler J, Fishman AP, Cournand A. The efficiency of ventilation during voluntary hyperapnea. *J Clin Invest* 1959; **38**: 1339–48.

●53. Field S, Grassino A, Sanci S. Respiratory muscle oxygen consumption estimated by the diaphragm pressure-time index. *J Appl Physiol* 1984; **57**: 44–51.

●54. Bellemare F, Grassino A. Force reserve of the diaphragm in patients with chronic obstructive pulmonary disease. *J Appl Physiol* 1983; **55**: 8–15.

55. McCool FD, McCann DR, Leith DE, Hoppin FG Jr. Pressure-flow effects on endurance of inspiratory muscles. *J Appl Physiol* 1986; **60**: 299–303.

56. Appendini L, Donner CF. Tension-time index for the diaphragm (TTdi), revisited. *Eur Respir J* 2000; **16**: 35 (abstract).

57. Babcock MA, Pegelow DF, McClaran SR *et al*. Contribution of diaphragmatic power output to exercise-induced diaphragm fatigue. *J Appl Physiol* 1995; **78**: 1710–9.

8

Respiratory muscle assessment in pulmonary rehabilitation

THIERRY TROOSTERS, FABIO PITTA, MARC DECRAMER

INTRODUCTION

Respiratory muscle weakness is an important clinical feature. Inspiratory muscle weakness may partially explain dyspnoea, exercise intolerance and orthopnoea. In addition, reduced respiratory muscle weakness has been shown to be an important predictive factor for poor survival in chronic obstructive lung disease (COPD) (1), cystic fibrosis (2) and congestive heart failure (3). In advanced stages, the functional consequence of respiratory muscle weakness is a reduction of the operational lung volume. Expiratory muscle weakness may lead to problems with speech, and mucus retention due to impaired cough efficacy.

Measurement of respiratory muscle function is important in the diagnosis of respiratory muscle disease (4–6) and respiratory muscle dysfunction (7). It may also may be helpful in the assessment of the impact of chronic diseases (8–12) or their treatment (13–15) on the respiratory muscles.

The present chapter aims to provide clinicians with some aspects of respiratory muscle testing. More detailed, excellent reviews are, however, available for the interested reader (16, 17). Indications, techniques commonly used in clinical practice, and interpretation and selection of patients for respiratory muscle training are the main focuses of this chapter.

INDICATIONS

Measurements of respiratory muscle function should always be performed as part of a more complete diagnostic process. Measurements of respiratory muscle strength or endurance should never be over-interpreted. A relatively low inspiratory or expiratory muscle strength without clinical context has relatively poorly defined clinical consequences. The clinician may encounter two possibilities that would prompt for careful assessment of respiratory muscle function: (i) clinical signs or symptoms that are suggestive of respiratory muscle weakness; or (ii) a pathological condition where respiratory muscle weakness may occur and assessment of the respiratory muscles is advised in the screening, prevention or follow-up of these patients.

Clinical signs of respiratory muscle weakness

Clinical signs and symptoms that can be suggestive of respiratory muscle weakness are summarized in Box 8.1. It should be noted that respiratory muscle weakness is often advanced before these symptoms occur. This follows from the relatively low respiratory muscle force that is required to overcome most respiratory tasks. For example, in healthy 30-year-old male subjects, Wanke and co-workers reported an oesophageal pressure (P_{oes}) of 46 cmH_2O during maximal exercise. The maximal P_{oes} was 106 cmH_2O in these patients. With this value of 43 per cent of the maximal pressure, the healthy volunteers generated a ventilation of 141 L/min, and a power output of 296 watts. Therefore, the data by Mador and co-workers, who could not detect diaphragm fatigue after exhaustive whole-body exercise (18) are not surprising. It can be concluded that the respiratory muscles are not a limiting factor of exercise capacity in sedentary, healthy sedentary subjects.

Symptoms only poorly relate to measurements of respiratory muscle strength or endurance. In patients with neuromuscular disease, for instance, hypercapnia only modestly relates to respiratory muscle strength (5, 19). This is due to the fact that symptoms generally only occur in the presence of an imbalance between the load on the respiratory pump and its capacity.

Box 8.1   Clinical findings that would prompt assessment of respiratory muscles

- Unexplained reduction in vital capacity
- CO_2 retention while awake or during sleep, specifically in the absence of severe airflow obstruction
- Shortness of breath
- Orthopnoea (shortness of breath while supine) or dyspnoea during bathing or swimming
- Short sentences during speech
- Tachypnoea
- Paradoxical movement of abdominal or thoracic wall
- Problems with cough (and recurrent infections)
- Generalized muscle weakness

Box 8.2   Situations where repeated measurements of respiratory muscle strength can be advised

- Known disease which affects the respiratory muscles
- Dyspnoea after thoracic operation (n. phrenicus paresis)
- Progressive lung diseases with uncertain impact on respiratory muscle function
- Patients to be treated with high doses of corticosteroids
- Patients following specific respiratory muscle training
- Patients weaning or recovering from mechanical ventilation

The capacity of the pump, one side of this balance, is determined by respiratory muscle strength, endurance, central neural drive and the substrates provided to the muscle at work (nutritional and oxygen) (20). Abnormally high load on the respiratory muscles, imposed by hyperventilation, increased lung or chest wall compliance (due to concurrent interstitial lung disease, chest wall deformities or obesity), airflow obstruction or hyperinflation, may also contribute to a variable extent to the clinically observed symptoms.

When respiratory muscle strength is moderately to severely reduced, discrete clinical symptoms may occur, and this may prompt for assessment of the respiratory muscles to help in the diagnostic process. The cardinal symptom of respiratory muscle weakness is dyspnoea. Dyspnoea may first be present in situations where the demand on the respiratory muscles is increased. Typically, this is during exercise. Another situation that increases the work of breathing is immersion. Reid *et al.* (21) showed an increase of the abdominal pressure upon immersion. Lastly, changes in body position, and hence gravitational and postural changes, may impact on the work of breathing, or may elicit symptoms like dyspnoea in patients with compromised respiratory muscle function. Abrupt dyspnoea is observed when patients with bilateral diaphragm paralysis are put in the recumbent position, and is perhaps the most typical example of this. In congestive heart failure, orthopnoea is often present and is related to increased diaphragmatic load (22).

When muscle weakness becomes more obvious, symptoms may occur at rest; dyspnoea, hypercapnia and/or speech problems disable the patient. In the case of severe expiratory muscle weakness, reduced cough efficiency may become an important handicap. Only in severe respiratory muscle dysfunction is vital capacity generally reduced as a consequence of the respiratory muscle weakness and this may become a better predictor of morbidity than measurements of respiratory muscle strength (23).

Pathological conditions where assessment of respiratory muscle force is indicated

Theoretically, any situation where the respiratory pump is at risk of imbalance invites follow-up of respiratory muscle function. In these cases the measurements are not necessary to achieve a diagnosis, but when respiratory muscle function is reduced compared with previous measures, preventive action should be considered. These actions may be either unloading the respiratory pump intermittently (e.g. with non-invasive mechanical ventilation) or improving the respiratory muscle function by respiratory muscle training. Situations where repeated measurements of respiratory muscle force may be indicated, even in the absence of symptoms, are summarized in Box 8.2.

It is important that clinicians recognize the opportunities to undertake preventive action, rather than waiting until symptoms occur. Unfortunately, evidence-based guidelines as to when to start respiratory muscle training or non-invasive mechanical ventilation are lacking. Decisions are often taken on clinical judgment (see below). For example, in patients receiving relatively high doses of oral corticosteroids, the follow-up of respiratory muscle force may be useful in the early detection of corticoid-induced myopathy, and inspiratory muscle training may be an effective treatment option to prevent force loss during glucocorticoid treatment (24, 25). Nava *et al.* (26) recently showed that even a short course of oral corticosteroids may have deleterious effects on respiratory muscle function. If the steroids are prescribed to alleviate airflow obstruction, a careful trade-off between optimal relief of bronchial constriction and/or inflammation, on the one hand, and prevention of respiratory muscle weakness due to steroid-induced myopathy on the other is often a difficult clinical dilemma.

RESPIRATORY MUSCLE ASSESSMENT: THEORETICAL CONSIDERATIONS

Measurement of respiratory muscle strength is nothing new in the lung function laboratory (27) and is nowadays routinely performed in clinical practice. However, some aspects, described below, make the interpretation of measurements of respiratory muscle strength somewhat more complex than most other measurements of skeletal muscle strength.

In clinical practice, respiratory muscle force is indirectly measured through the pressure generated during inspiration or expiration. Respiratory muscle force is generally expressed as kilopascals (kPa) or cm of water (cmH$_2$O). These pressures are not absolute, but reflect pressure changes against atmospheric pressure. The pressure is generated by all the muscles under investigation (inspiratory or expiratory) and is hence not muscle-specific. In addition, reduced respiratory muscle force may result from cerebral, spinal cord, anterior horn, peripheral (i.e. phrenic) nerve, neuromuscular junction or muscle fibre dysfunction, and should not be attributed to a respiratory muscle dysfunction *per se*. The pressures measured largely depend on the geometry of the thorax in which the pressure is generated. For instance, the pressure generated by the diaphragm is dependent on its *in vivo* three-dimensional shape (taking into account the Laplace law), the relative degree to which it is apposed to the rib cage, and its length–force properties (28). In stable patients with emphysema, the flattened diaphragm often fails to generate normal pressure, although the diaphragm muscle is generally believed to be well 'trained' (29–32). Interesting preliminary data from a Canadian group showed that, although $P_{I,max}$ was reduced in patients with COPD, inspiratory muscle strength measured *in vitro* was not abnormal (33).

Another variable influencing the outcome of the inspiratory and expiratory pressure measurement is the relative lung volume at which it is obtained. Like all skeletal muscles, the respiratory muscles have a well defined length–tension relationship. If the diaphragm is shortened below its optimal length (L_o, the length at which a maximal tension is obtained) it can generate less tension. This obviously has repercussions during acute hyperinflation. The length–tension relationship has important consequences for the technique of measuring inspiratory and expiratory muscle force. Indeed, when applying these measurements, the lung volume at which the measurement is performed is crucial and should be properly standardized.

Another factor influencing the pressure measured during maximal inspiratory or expiratory manoeuvres is the elastic recoil of the lungs and chest wall. This is depicted schematically in Fig. 8.1. At functional residual capacity, the net result of the two components is zero. Consequently, at these lung volumes, pressures measured during inspiration or expiration are independent of elastic recoil. At lower lung volumes, the maximal inspiratory pressure is the resultant of the pressure developed by the inspiratory muscles and the pressure developed by the thorax (which at this point is larger than the lung recoil). Conversely, when maximal expiratory pressure is measured at total lung capacity, the pressure obtained is the result of the elastic lung recoil, the recoil of the chest wall and the expiratory pressure developed by the expiratory muscles.

Combining all these factors, clinicians should be aware that the respiratory pressures obtained in patients or healthy subjects are not a 'clean' measure of the strength of the respiratory muscles. They are the net result of the tension (force) generated by the muscle, which is dependent on the lung volume at which the manoeuvre is obtained. In addition, the pressures are dependent on the chest wall and lung mechanics. Elastic recoil is also dependent on the lung volume, but may also be altered by the disease (e.g. lung fibrosis, emphysema).

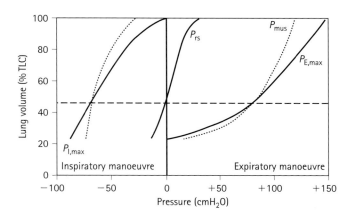

Figure 8.1 *Theoretical summary of the pressures developed by the respiratory system (resultant of chest wall and lung compliance, P$_{rs}$) and the pressures developed by the inspiratory and expiratory muscles (P$_{mus}$, dashed line). The solid lines accompanying the P$_{mus}$ line represent the pressures that can be monitored during static inspiratory or expiratory manoeuvres at the mouth. Hence, for example, P$_{E,max}$ represents the pressure measured at the mouth during a maximal expiration from total lung capacity (TLC) and represents the P$_{mus}$ plus the positive pressure generated by the recoil of lungs and chest wall at this lung volume.*

The resulting pressures are, on the other hand, a good reflection of the functional reserve of the respiratory pump, since the net pressure generated is needed to drive the ventilation.

MEASURING RESPIRATORY MUSCLE FORCE

Measurements of respiratory muscle function are generally obtained from measuring pressures achieved by volitional activation or electrical or magnetic stimulation. Pressure can be measured in the nose, at the mouth, in the oesophagus or across the diaphragm (measuring the pressure above, in the oesophagus, and below the diaphragm, in the stomach). The different places where pressure measurements can be carried out are shown in Fig. 8.2.

Routine clinical investigations

MAXIMAL VOLUNTARY RESPIRATORY PRESSURES MEASURED AT THE MOUTH

Technique

Maximal voluntary inspiratory ($P_{I,max}$) and expiratory ($P_{E,max}$) pressures (MIP and MEP) are probably the most frequently reported non-invasive estimates of respiratory muscle force. Ever since Black and Hyatt (27) reported this non-invasive technique in the late 1960s, it has been widely used in patients, healthy control subjects across all ages and sportsmen. Pressure is recorded at the mouth during a quasi-static, short (few seconds) maximal inspiration (Müller manoeuvre) or expiration (Valsalva manoeuvre). The manoeuvre is generally performed at residual volume (RV) for $P_{I,max}$, and at total lung capacity (TLC) for $P_{E,max}$. Although functional residual capacity would

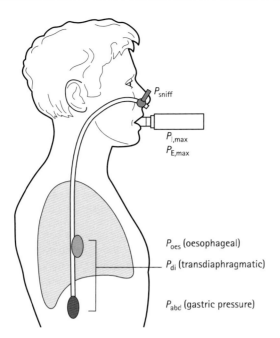

Figure 8.2 *Respiratory muscle strength can be measured at the nose (inspiratory muscles), at the mouth, in the oesophagus or in the stomach.*

In the figure:
- P_{sniff}
- $P_{I,max}$
- $P_{E,max}$
- P_{oes} (oesophageal)
- P_{di} (transdiaphragmatic)
- P_{abd} (gastric pressure)

theoretically be more appropriate, as lung and chest wall compliance are neutralized, and the pressure theoretically would better reflect the tension developed by the respiratory muscles (P_{mus}), patients find it easier and more straightforward to perform the manoeuvres from RV and TLC. Only a few contraindications exist for these measurements (Box 8.3) and these can be summarized as pathological conditions where relatively large pressure swings in the thorax or abdomen should be avoided.

Although the technique appears simple at first sight and hardware and software became available to make these measurements easily accessible in the pulmonary function laboratory, there are some technical pitfalls that may influence the obtained results and make the results more variable than most other lung function measurements. Some critical aspects in the methodology are summarized in Box 8.4.

Quality control of the measurements can only be obtained from inspection of the pressure/time curves. The peak pressure should be obtained in the very beginning of the manoeuvre. The pressure maintained for at least 1 s is generally reported as the $P_{I,max}$ or $P_{E,max}$. Measurements are obtained preferentially in the sitting position. Although body posture has no significant influence on the result of the measurement in healthy subjects (34), and even in convalescent neonates (35), in COPD patients, changes in body posture may significantly impact on the obtained result. Leaning forward, for example, may result in higher inspiratory pressures (36), while measurements obtained in the recumbent position may lead to lower pressures (37).

To avoid pressure generation by the muscles of the cheeks and buccal muscles, a small leak should be present in the equipment. The leak described by Black and Hyatt is 15 mm

---

Box 8.3 Some relative or absolute contraindications for measurements of maximal respiratory muscle strength

- Unstable cardiac disease
- Uncontrolled hypertension
- Hernia nucleus pulposus
- Hernia inguinalis
- Aneurysm
- Recent pneumothorax
- Recent abdominal or thoracic surgery (not consolidated)
- Severe osteoporosis of the back
- Kahler's disease

Box 8.4 Important aspects of standardization of the measurements of maximal voluntary inspiratory ($P_{I,max}$) and expiratory ($P_{E,max}$) pressures

- Leak provided
- Mouthpiece (preferably not flanged)
- Lung volume at which manoeuvre is performed
- Volume history (smooth deep inspiration or expiration should proceed manoeuvre)
- Position (seated/standing)
- Nose clip (especially for $P_{I,max}$)
- Sufficient number of repetitions
- Time pressure is sustained (1 s is advised)

---

long and has an internal diameter of 2 mm. Using this leak, the glottis should be opened to generate pressures for longer than 1 s, and the pressure obtained reflects the pressure generated by the respiratory muscles. When a leak is absent, the recorded pressures may erroneously reflect the pressure generated in the mouth by the cheeks and buccal muscles. A final technical point of attention concerns the mouthpiece. It has been reported that flanged mouthpieces (the ones generally used for lung function testing) result in pressures inferior to those obtained when a rigid mouthpiece is sealed against the mouth. Especially for the expiratory pressures, flanged mouthpieces may result in underestimated pressures due to additional leaks that appear with the increased pressure in the mouth.

Tests should be performed by an experienced technician. Since Valsalva manoeuvres or Müller manoeuvres are unfamiliar to patients, the manoeuvre should be carefully explained. There has been some debate on the number of repetitions that need to be done before a result can be considered valid (38–40). Our experience, shared by others (41), suggests that a minimum of five manoeuvres should be performed, and reproducibility should be within 5–10 per cent. Increasing the number of measurements is time-consuming and tedious. In case of questionable effort, a sniff nasal pressure manoeuvre (see below) may give additional information.

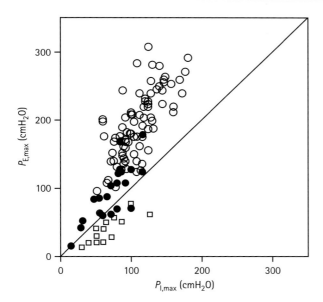

Figure 8.3 *Maximum inspiratory ($P_{I,max}$) and expiratory ($P_{E,max}$) pressures measured in 85 healthy subjects (open circles), 21 patients with multiple sclerosis (MS, closed circles) tested in our centre (108), and 13 patients with spinal cord injury (SCI, open squares) (109). As can be observed, in healthy subjects, $P_{E,max}$ exceeds $P_{I,max}$ in every single case. In MS, $P_{I,max}$ may be larger than $P_{E,max}$, and in SCI, $P_{I,max}$ is typically larger than $P_{E,max}$.*

Equipment

A recent statement of the American Thoracic Society and European Respiratory Society advises the use of a metal membrane or piezoelectric transducers with an accuracy of 0.5 cmH$_2$O (0.049 kPa) in a pressure range of ± 200 cmH$_2$O (19.6 kPa). When healthy subjects are tested, higher expiratory pressures may be obtained. In a cohort of 85 healthy subjects, aged >50 years, the maximum inspiratory and expiratory pressures obtained were −180 and 308 cmH$_2$O, respectively.

It is preferred that the signal of pressure versus time is recorded and is available to the technician for immediate inspection. Calibration of the manometer should be done regularly, and can be done easily using a water column.

Interpretation and normal values

In absolute numbers, the $P_{E,max}$ is roughly double the $P_{I,max}$. When the Black and Hyatt technique is used with a rigid mouthpiece, it is very rare to find $P_{E,max}$ inferior to $P_{I,max}$, when both values are expressed in natural units. This is illustrated in Fig. 8.3. In some diseases, however (e.g. spinal cord injury, below C3–5, multiple sclerosis), $P_{E,max}$ is typically more reduced than $P_{I,max}$, and the value of $P_{E,max}$ may be smaller than $P_{I,max}$ in natural units (Fig. 8.3).

Many authors have reported normal values for maximal inspiratory and expiratory pressures. Impressive differences are observed between the normal values (41–50) reported in the literature. This is largely due to the previously described differences in methodology (lung volume, mouthpiece, number of repetitions). It is advised that a cohort of healthy subjects is tested and consequently the most appropriate reference values

are chosen. In addition, it has to be noted that in all models of maximal inspiratory and expiratory pressures, the explained variance is low, reflecting large interindividual differences even when age, gender and anthropometric values are taken into account.

INSPIRATORY PRESSURE MEASURED AT THE NOSE (P_{sniff})

Technique

Maximal inspiratory pressure measured at the nostril during a sniff manoeuvre is a relatively newly developed technique (51) to measure inspiratory muscle function. Pressure is measured in an occluded nostril during a forced sniff. The unoccluded nostril serves as a variable resistance, prohibiting flow from exceeding 30 L/min, and the pressures measured at the nose reflect those obtained in the oesophagus during sniff manoeuvres (51). Since there is more airflow compared with the $P_{I,max}$ manoeuvre, these sniff manoeuvres are not static. Generally the sniff nasal pressures are as high as $P_{I,max}$ (or even slightly higher) (52). Maillard *et al.* (53) reported a $P_{sniff}/P_{I,max}$ ratio of 1.03 $\pm$ 0.17, and reported equal and good within-session reproducibility. Although infrequently seen in routine clinical practice, this technique has been shown to be extremely useful in the diagnosis and follow-up of respiratory muscle weakness in children (54, 55), and patients with neuromuscular disease (56, 57) where sniff nasal pressures were reported to be higher than $P_{I,max}$. In patients with low $P_{I,max}$, the addition of sniff nasal pressures further improved the diagnostic process and some patients were consequently classified with normal respiratory muscle force (58). The two techniques should hence be considered complementary, rather than interchangeable. Normal values for the sniff nasal pressure are available (52). It should be noted that sniff measurements may be problematic in patients with significant upper airway disease.

Equipment

Essentially the equipment can consist of the same pressure transducer as the one used in the assessment of $P_{I,max}$. A perforated plug with a tube is used to occlude the nostril. The tube is connected to the pressure transducer and the pressure–time curve is recorded for inspection and quality control. The peak pressure is reported after a series of maximal sniffs separated by normal breathing. A plateau is generally obtained after five to 10 sniffs. Currently these devices and accompanying software are commercially available.

MEASUREMENT IN OESOPHAGUS OR STOMACH

In rare clinical cases, and to answer specific research questions, it may be useful to measure pressures in the oesophagus or gastric area. In the oesophagus the pressure (P_{oes}) is a reflection of the pleural pressure (P_{pl}), while the gastric pressure reflects the abdominal pressure (P_{abd}). The difference between these two pressures is the 'transdiaphragmatic pressure', which is a more specific measure of diaphragmatic function.

To obtain these pressures, a latex balloon catheter should be put in place. Generally this is done by swallowing a balloon catheter introduced in the nose, after application of a local anaesthetic spray to the nasal mucosa and the pharynx. These tests are perceived by many patients as rather uncomfortable, but the results give probably the best estimate of the pressures generated by the respiratory muscles during normal breathing, during exercise or during static manoeuvres or sniffs. When the balloon is positioned in the stomach, gastric pressure can also be recorded during cough. Hence 'cough' pressure is recorded (P_{cough}) (59). In healthy subjects, P_{cough} was reported to be greater than $P_{E,max}$, and the lower limit of normal is set at 132 cmH$_2$O for males and 97 cmH$_2$O for females. Recently cough pressures were found to be a useful addition in the diagnosis of expiratory muscle weakness. In a significant number of patients with low $P_{E,max}$, P_{cough} was reported normal. By contrast only few patients with normal $P_{E,max}$ exhibited low P_{cough} (59).

NON-VOLITIONAL TESTS OF RESPIRATORY MUSCLE FUNCTION

Measurements of maximal voluntary inspiratory or expiratory pressures at the mouth, nose or even using balloon catheters to measure oesophagus or gastric pressures are biased by the motivation of the patient to collaborate with the tests. Maximal effort is sometimes difficult to ascertain because of lack of patient motivation, anxiety, pain or discomfort, submaximal central activation, poor mental status or difficulties in understanding the manoeuvres.

To overcome the issue of submaximal (voluntary) activation, investigation of the diaphragmatic function can be done through electrical (60) or magnetic (61) stimulation of the phrenic nerve. The diaphragm is exclusively innervated by the phrenic nerve (left and right). This nerve passes superficially in the neck and can be stimulated relatively easily. In addition, EMG of the costal diaphragm can be done. In the latter case, the phrenic nerve latency can be studied (62, 63), which allows the detection of lesions of the phrenic nerve. Pressures developed after twitch stimulation of the phrenic nerve can be measured transdiaphragmatically or at the mouth. Although this technique is not routinely used in the clinic, there are specific situations in which it may provide useful and unique information (64).

RESPIRATORY MUSCLE ENDURANCE

Although maximal inspiratory and expiratory muscle strength gives important information on respiratory muscle function, the respiratory muscles (especially the inspiratory muscles) should be able to cope with endurance tasks. Measurements of respiratory muscle endurance, therefore, give clinicians further insight into the function of the respiratory pump, and may unmask early task failure. In the authors' opinion, measurements of inspiratory muscle endurance are especially helpful when inspiratory muscle weakness is discrete, and its clinical consequence is unclear. In the clinic, respiratory muscle endurance is generally assessed using one of the following techniques.

Maximal sustainable ventilation

The maximum ventilation that can be sustained by patients is measured, or estimated, from protocols with incremental ventilation. The achieved sustainable ventilation is then reported as a fraction of the actually measured 12-s maximum voluntary ventilation, and/or as a fraction of the predicted maximum voluntary ventilation (MVV). Maximal sustainable ventilation (MSV) should be roughly 60–80 per cent of the 12-s MVV. This test can be considered as a test of inspiratory and expiratory muscles, but it is relatively sensitive to changes in airway obstruction, and needs careful control and adjustment of expiratory CO$_2$. In addition, in patients with severe airflow obstruction, MVV may be low due to important dynamic compression of the airways during the vigorous 12-s manoeuvre. Therefore MSV/MVV may be relatively high in these patients, whereas other measurements of endurance showed reduced respiratory muscle endurance in COPD (65). In a variant of this test, proposed for COPD patients, patients are asked to sustain a ventilation of 66–75 per cent of their MVV (66). This test allows comparison within one subject, but normal values are not available.

Incremental threshold loading

Patients are asked to breathe against increasing inspiratory loads. The inspiratory load is increased every 2 min (67). The test can be compared to an incremental exercise test. Generally patients should be able to reach a pressure equivalent to 75–80 per cent of $P_{I,max}$. Johnson et al. (68) reported that the $P_{max}/P_{I,max}$ was dependent on age. Important learning curves are reported for this test, and the test should be repeated at least two to three times (69, 70). Due to the incremental nature of the test, however, it can be criticized as a clean measure of endurance. Alternatively the maximum sustainable threshold load can be determined. The sustainable load is the load that can be sustained for >10 min. This technique reflects better the concept of 'endurance', but it is time-consuming.

In the authors' hospital, respiratory muscle endurance is assessed only when inspiratory muscle force is impaired, by recording the time patients can sustain an inspiratory load equivalent to 60 per cent of $P_{I,max}$. If the subjects can sustain this load for 10 min, inspiratory muscle endurance is considered normal.

Recently an expiratory incremental threshold loading test was developed, and used in healthy subjects and COPD (71). Interestingly, the authors reported that the expiratory pressure that was achieved following an incremental protocol was only 44 per cent of $P_{E,max}$ in COPD. In healthy subjects, 87 per cent of $P_{E,max}$ was reached. The clinical consequences of these findings may be illustrated by the recent finding that expiratory muscle training in COPD may be a successful training strategy to improve exercise capacity and dyspnoea in patients with COPD (72). Further studies, however, should be conducted to assess the usefulness of such an intervention on a larger scale.

ASSESSMENT OF RESPIRATORY MUSCLE FUNCTION: SOME TYPICAL REHABILITATION SCENARIOS

COPD

In COPD, respiratory pressures are reduced in a significant number of patients (8, 73). The reduced maximal pressures generated by the respiratory muscles may be due to several factors, including treatment with corticosteroids (13), malnutrition (74), inflammation and concomitant heart failure. The consequences of reduced respiratory pump capacity are impaired exercise capacity (75), reduced health-related quality of life (76) and dyspnoea (77, 78).

Although the respiratory muscles may adapt to chronic hyperinflation by dropping sarcomeres, dynamic hyperinflation, which may occur during exercise, significantly impairs contractility (79). In patients with COPD, therefore, one has to distinguish between respiratory pump failure due to dynamic hyperinflation and that due to intrinsic respiratory muscle weakness. The latter may be the case in COPD patients who are clearly malnourished (80), who receive high doses of glucocorticoids (13) or who were mechanically ventilated (81).

Dynamic hyperinflation can be tackled by optimal bronchodilatation (82), lung volume reduction surgery (83) reducing the ventilatory requirements for a given workload by exercise training (84, 85), or oxygen supplementation (86). Intrinsic respiratory muscle weakness in COPD can be treated with specific respiratory muscle training. The latter can be done using resistive breathing or threshold loading with a load that exceeds 30–40 per cent of $P_{I,max}$ (87, 88). Inspiratory muscle training in COPD seems only useful when inspiratory muscle strength is less then 60 cmH$_2$O (15). Specific inspiratory muscle training should not be advised as the sole intervention in COPD, but should always be an integrated part of a pulmonary rehabilitation programme, also including whole-body exercise (89–91). Whole-body exercise training may also increase respiratory muscle function (84, 92), and the addition of inspiratory muscle training does not necessarily improve the outcome of pulmonary rehabilitation (93). Since inspiratory muscle training is not expensive, the addition of inspiratory muscle training in selected patients (with severe inspiratory muscle weakness) can be defended, but clearly further studies are warranted (15). The flow chart in Fig. 8.4 presents a strategy for prescribing respiratory muscle training, balancing experience, the available evidence, and the fact that respiratory muscle training should be restricted to those patients who may benefit most from it. Prospective validation of this flowchart, however, should be provided.

Neuromuscular disorders

In patients with neuromuscular disorders, measurements of respiratory muscle strength are useful in the context of rehabilitation and decision-making. When neuromuscular disease is progressive, respiratory muscles may become

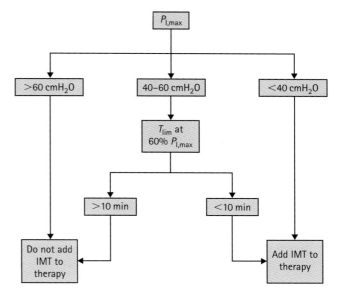

Figure 8.4 *Flow chart for inspiratory muscle training (IMT) in COPD based on a recent meta-analysis (15), and trying to limit the number of measurements (i.e. endurance, which is time-consuming and tedious to patients and health care providers) to a minimum. The cut-off of 40 cmH$_2$O is arbitrary. However, during maximal exercise the mean oesophageal pressure was reported to be 19.9 ± 7 cmH$_2$O (110). Hence it is rather unlikely that patients would need inspiratory pressures larger than 20–30 cmH$_2$O to overcome tasks of daily life. Therefore, if they are able to sustain pressures of 60 per cent of 40 cmH$_2$O (24 cmH$_2$O) they are not likely to be limited in their exercise performance primarily by inspiratory muscle weakness. Prospective validation of this chart, however, is warranted.*

involved at a given point. A careful review of respiratory muscle involvement in neuromuscular disease is presented in Lieberman et al. (94). Inspiratory muscle force alone does not predict alveolar hypoventilation accurately. Other factors, such as lung and chest wall compliance or breathing pattern, may also contribute to it (95). Although not perfect, hypercapnia could be estimated with an accuracy of approximately 80 per cent in amyotrophic lateral sclerosis, using a cut-off for $P_{I,max}$ of 32 per cent of predicted (57). When $P_{I,max}$ becomes as low as 30–40 per cent of predicted, sleep-disordered breathing is prevalent in most neuromuscular disorders (96). As mentioned above, in severe disease, vital capacity may better reflect respiratory pump function. In mild to moderate disease, however, lung function changes are relatively insensitive.

Reduced lung and chest wall compliance (due to microatelectasis or scoliosis), observed in patients with severe neuromuscular disorders, further impairs the already compromised respiratory muscle pump function. When alveolar hypoventilation is present, and patients become hypercapnic, (non-) invasive mechanical ventilation may become necessary and should be discussed with patients and their family. In some neuromuscular diseases, attempts have been made to train the respiratory muscles. In multiple sclerosis, small studies showed that inspiratory (97, 98) and expiratory muscle training (99) can potentially be used as therapeutic tools. Also, in patients with Duchenne's dystrophy (100, 101), inspiratory muscle training was feasible. In less severe disease, respiratory muscle training could be useful (102). In patients with neuromuscular disease already suffering from respiratory failure, there is no evidence to support respiratory muscle training. Mobilizing the chest wall using passive techniques and mechanical hyper-inflation may help to improve compliance and, hence, may reduce the work of breathing in these severely impaired patients (103, 104).

In patients with spinal cord injury, respiratory muscle training has been shown to result in improved respiratory muscle force (105, 106). In these patients, the remaining innervated muscles are essentially normal, and respiratory muscle training may improve the function of these muscles. Estenne *et al.* (107) even showed an effect on expiratory muscle function in these patients by specific training of the pectoralis muscle.

Key points

● Respiratory muscle weakness may contribute to respiratory symptoms such as dyspnoea.
● There is not a strong relationship between respiratory muscle weakness and clinical symptoms.
● Symptoms generally occur only in advanced stages of respiratory muscle weakness.
● For clinical purposes, respiratory muscle force can be measured non-invasively by measuring the maximal pressures generated at the mouth or nose.
● Respiratory muscle endurance testing is a useful addition in the assessment of respiratory muscle dysfunction.
● Respiratory muscle training may be a specific treatment option to tackle respiratory muscle weakness, in selected patients.

REFERENCES

1. Gray-Donald, Gibbons KL, Shapiro SH *et al*. Nutritional status and mortality in chronic obstructive pulmonary disease. *Am J Respir Crit Care Med* 1996; **153**: 961–6.
2. Ionescu AA, Chatham K, Davies CA *et al*. Inspiratory muscle function and body composition in cystic fibrosis. *Am J Respir Crit Care Med* 1998; **158**: 1271–6.
3. Meyer FJ, Borst MM, Zugck C *et al*. Respiratory muscle dysfunction in congestive heart failure: clinical correlation and prognostic significance. *Circulation* 2001; **103**: 2153–8.
4. Black LF, Hyatt RE. Maximal static respiratory pressures in generalized neuromuscular disease. *Am Rev Respir Dis* 1971; **103**: 641–50.
5. Braun NM, Arora NS, Rochester DF. Respiratory muscle and pulmonary function in polymyositis and other proximal myopathies. *Thorax* 1983; **38**: 616–23.
6. Rochester DF, Esau SA. Assessment of ventilatory function in patients with neuromuscular disease. *Clin Chest Med* 1994; **15**: 751–63.
7. Vantrappen G, Decramer M, Harlet R. High-frequency diaphragmatic flutter: symptoms and treatment by carbamazepine. *Lancet* 1992; **339**: 265–7.
8. Decramer M, Demedts M, Rochette F *et al*. Maximal transrespiratory pressures in obstructive lung disease. *Bull Eur Physiopathol Respir* 1980; **16**: 479–90.
9. Stassijns G, Lysens R, Decramer M. Peripheral and respiratory muscles in chronic heart failure. *Eur Respir J* 1996; **9**: 2161–7.
10. De Troyer A, Estenne M, Yernault JC. Disturbance of respiratory muscle function in patients with mitral valve disease. *Am J Med* 1980; **69**: 867–73.
11. De Troyer A, Yernault JC. Inspiratory muscle force in normal subjects and patients with interstitial lung disease. *Thorax* 1980; **35**: 92–100.
12. Baydur A, Alsalek M, Louie SG, Sharma OP. Respiratory muscle strength, lung function, dyspnea in patients with sarcoidosis. *Chest* 2001; **120**: 102–8.
13. Decramer M, Lacquet LM, Fagard R, Rogiers P. Corticosteroids contribute to muscle weakness in chronic airflow obstruction. *Am J Respir Crit Care Med* 1994; **150**: 11–16.
14. Weiner P, Waizman J, Magadle R *et al*. The effect of specific inspiratory muscle training on the sensation of dyspnea and exercise tolerance in patients with congestive heart failure. *Clin Cardiol* 1999; **22**: 727–32.
15. Lötters F, Van Tol B, Kwakkel G, Gosselink R. Effects of controlled inspiratory muscle training in patients with COPD: a meta-analysis. *Eur Respir J* 2002; **20**: 570–6.
16. American Thoracic Society/European Respiratory Society. ATS/ERS statement on respiratory muscle testing. *Am J Respir Crit Care Med* 2002; **166**: 518–624.
17. Laghi F, Tobin MJ. Disorders of the respiratory muscles. *Am J Respir Crit Care Med* 2003; **168**: 10–48.
18. Jeffery MM, Kufel TJ, Pineda LA. Quadriceps and diaphragmatic function after exhaustive cycle exercise in the healthy elderly. *Am J Respir Crit Care Med* 2000; **162**: 1760–6.
19. Begin P, Mathieu J, Almirall J, Grassino A. Relationship between chronic hypercapnia and inspiratory-muscle weakness in myotonic dystrophy. *Am J Respir Crit Care Med* 1997; **156**: 133–9.
20. Vassilakopoulos T, Zakynthinos S, Roussos C. The conventional approach to weaning from mechanical ventilation. *Eur Respir Monograph* 1998; **3**: 266–98.
21. Reid MB, Loring SH, Banzett RB, Mead J. Passive mechanics of upright human chest wall during immersion from hips to neck. *J Appl Physiol* 1986; **60**: 1561–70.
22. Nava S, Larovere MT, Fanfulla F *et al*. Orthopnea and inspiratory effort in chronic heart failure patients. *Respir Med* 2003; **97**: 647–53.
23. Mellies U, Ragette R, Schwake C *et al*. Daytime predictors of sleep disordered breathing in children and adolescents with neuromuscular disorders. *Neuromuscul Disord* 2003; **13**: 123–8.
24. Weiner P, Azgad Y, Weiner M. Inspiratory muscle training during treatment with corticosteroids in humans. *Chest* 1995; **107**: 1041–4.
25. Decramer M, de Bock V, Dom R. Functional and histologic picture of steroid-induced myopathy in chronic obstructive pulmonary disease. *Am J Respir Crit Care Med* 1996; **153**: 1958–64.
26. Nava S, Fracchia C, Callegari G *et al*. Weakness of respiratory and skeletal muscles after a short course of steroids in patients with acute lung rejection. *Eur Respir J* 2002; **20**: 497–9.
27. Black LF, Hyatt RE. Maximal respiratory pressures: normal values and relationship to age and sex. *Am Rev Respir Dis* 1969; **99**: 696–702.

28. Gauthier AP, Verbanck S, Estenne M et al. Three-dimensional reconstruction of the in vivo human diaphragm shape at different lung volumes. J Appl Physiol 1994; 76: 495–506.

29. Ribera F, Guessan BN, Zoll J et al. Mitochondrial electron transport chain function is enhanced in inspiratory muscles of patients with chronic obstructive pulmonary disease. Am J Respir Crit Care Med 2003; 167: 873–9.

30. Levine S, Gregory C, Nguyen T et al. Bioenergetic adaptation of individual human diaphragmatic myofibers to severe COPD. J Appl Physiol 2002; 92: 1205–13.

31. Levine S, Kaiser L, Leferovich J, Tikunov B. Cellular adaptations in the diaphragm in chronic obstructive pulmonary disease. N Engl J Med 1997; 337: 1799–1806.

32. Orozco-Levi M, Gea J, Lloreta JL et al. Subcellular adaptation of the human diaphragm in chronic obstructive pulmonary disease. Eur Respir J 1999; 13: 371–8.

33. Doucet M, Debigare R, Cote CG et al. In vitro contractile properties of the diaphragm muscle in COPD-preliminary data. Am J Med Sports 2003; 5: 183.

34. Fiz JA, Texido A, Izquierdo J et al. Postural variation of the maximum inspiratory and expiratory pressures in normal subjects. Chest 1990; 97: 313–14.

35. Dimitriou G, Greenough A, Pink L et al. Effect of posture on oxygenation and respiratory muscle strength in convalescent infants. Arch Dis Child Fetal Neonatal Ed 2002; 86: 147–50.

36. O'Neill S, McCarthy DS. Postural relief of dyspnoea in severe chronic airflow limitation: relationship to respiratory muscle strength. Thorax 1983; 38: 595–600.

37. Heijdra YF, Dekhuijzen PN, van Herwaarden CL, Folgering HT. Effects of body position, hyperinflation, blood gas tensions on maximal respiratory pressures in patients with chronic obstructive pulmonary disease. Thorax 1994; 49: 453–8.

38. Wen AS, Woo MS, Keens TG. How many manoeuvers are required to measure maximal inspiratory pressure accurately? Chest 1997; 111: 802–7.

39. Fiz JA, Montserrat JM, Picado C et al. How many manoeuvres should be done to measure maximal inspiratory mouth pressure in patients with chronic airflow obstruction? Thorax 1989; 44: 419–21.

40. Larson JL, Covey MK, Vitalo CA et al. Maximal inspiratory pressure. Learning effect and test-retest reliability in patients with chronic obstructive pulmonary disease. Chest 1993; 104: 448–53.

41. Enright PL, Kronmal RA, Manolio TA et al. Respiratory muscle strength in the elderly. Correlates and reference values. Cardiovascular Health Study Research Group. Am J Respir Crit Care Med 1994; 149: 430–8.

42. Bruschi C, Cerveri I, Zoia MC et al. Reference values of maximal respiratory mouth pressures: a population-based study. Am Rev Respir Dis 1992; 146: 790–3.

43. Rochester DF, Arora NS. Respiratory muscle failure. Med Clin North Am 1983; 67: 573–97.

44. Vincken W, Ghezzo H, Cosio MG. Maximal static respiratory pressures in adults: normal values and their relationship to determinants of respiratory function. Bull Eur Physiopathol Respir 1987; 23: 435–9.

45. Ringqvist T. The ventilatory capacity in healthy subjects. An analysis of causal factors with special reference to the respiratory forces. Scand J Clin Lab Invest Suppl 1966; 88: 5–179.

46. Wilson SH, Cooke NT, Edwards RH, Spiro SG. Predicted normal values for maximal respiratory pressures in caucasian adults and children. Thorax 1984; 39: 535–8.

47. Leech JA, Ghezzo H, Stevens D, Becklake MR. Respiratory pressures and function in young adults. Am Rev Respir Dis 1983; 128: 17–23.

48. McElvaney G, Blackie S, Morrison NJ et al. Maximal static respiratory pressures in the normal elderly. Am Rev Respir Dis 1989; 139: 277–81.

49. Hautmann H, Hefele S, Schotten K, Huber RM. Maximal inspiratory mouth pressures (PIMAX) in healthy subjects – what is the lower limit of normal? Respir Med 2000; 94: 689–93.

50. Neder JA, Andreoni S, Lerario MC, Nery LE. Reference values for lung function tests. II. Maximal respiratory pressures and voluntary ventilation. Braz J Med Biol Res 1999; 32: 719–27.

51. Heritier F, Rahm F, Pasche P, Fitting JW. Sniff nasal inspiratory pressure. A noninvasive assessment of inspiratory muscle strength. Am J Respir Crit Care Med 1994; 150: 1678–83.

52. Uldry C, Fitting JW. Maximal values of sniff nasal inspiratory pressure in healthy subjects. Thorax 1995; 50: 371–5.

53. Maillard JO, Burdet L, van Melle G, Fitting JW. Reproducibility of twitch mouth pressure, sniff nasal inspiratory pressure, maximal inspiratory pressure. Eur Respir J 1998; 11: 901–5.

54. Rafferty GF, Leech S, Knight L et al. Sniff nasal inspiratory pressure in children. Pediatr Pulmonol 2000; 29: 468–75.

55. Fauroux B. Respiratory muscle testing in children. Paediatr Respir Rev 2003; 4: 243–9.

56. Fitting JW, Paillex R, Hirt L et al. Sniff nasal pressure: a sensitive respiratory test to assess progression of amyotrophic lateral sclerosis. Ann Neurol 1999; 46: 887–93.

57. Lyall RA, Donaldson N, Polkey MI et al. Respiratory muscle strength and ventilatory failure in amyotrophic lateral sclerosis. Brain 2001; 124: 2000–13.

58. Hughes PD, Polkey MI, Kyroussis D et al. Measurement of sniff nasal and diaphragm twitch mouth pressure in patients. Thorax 1998; 53: 96–100.

59. Man WD, Kyroussis D, Fleming TA et al. Cough gastric pressure and maximum expiratory mouth pressure in humans. Am J Respir Crit Care Med 2003; 168: 714–7.

60. Aubier M, Farkas G, De Troyer A et al. Detection of diaphragmatic fatigue in man by phrenic stimulation. J Appl Physiol 1981; 50: 538–44.

61. Similowski T, Fleury B, Launois S et al. Cervical magnetic stimulation: a new painless method for bilateral phrenic nerve stimulation in conscious humans. J Appl Physiol 1989; 67: 1311–8.

62. Aubier M, Murciano D, Lecocguic Y et al. Bilateral phrenic stimulation: a simple technique to assess diaphragmatic fatigue in humans. J Appl Physiol 1985; 58: 58–64.

63. Chen R, Collins S, Remtulla H et al. Phrenic nerve conduction study in normal subjects. Muscle Nerve 1995; 18: 330–5.

64. Rafferty GF, Greenough A, Manczur T et al. Magnetic phrenic nerve stimulation to assess diaphragm function in children following liver transplantation. Pediatr Crit Care Med 2001; 2: 122–6.

65. Morrison NJ, Richardson J, Dunn L, Pardy RL. Respiratory muscle performance in normal elderly subjects and patients with COPD. Chest 1989; 95: 90–4.

66. Scherer TA, Spengler CM, Owassapian D et al. Respiratory muscle endurance training in chronic obstructive pulmonary disease: impact on exercise capacity, dyspnea, quality of life. Am J Respir Crit Care Med 2000; 162: 1709–14.

67. Martyn JB, Moreno RH, Pare PD, Pardy RL. Measurement of inspiratory muscle performance with incremental threshold loading. Am Rev Respir Dis 1987; 135: 919–23.

68. Johnson PH, Cowley AJ, Kinnear WJ. Incremental threshold loading: a standard protocol and establishment of a reference range in naive normal subjects. *Eur Respir J* 1997; **10**: 2868–71.

69. Hopp LJ, Kim MJ, Larson JL, Sharp JT. Incremental threshold loading in patients with chronic obstructive pulmonary disease. *Nurs Res* 1996; **45**: 196–202.

70. Eastwood PR, Hillman DR, Morton AR, Finucane KE. The effects of learning on the ventilatory responses to inspiratory threshold loading. *Am J Respir Crit Care Med* 1998; **158**: 1190–6.

71. Ramirez-Sarmiento A, Orozco-Levi M, Barreiro E *et al*. Expiratory muscle endurance in chronic obstructive pulmonary disease. *Thorax* 2002; **57**: 132–6.

72. Weiner P, Magadle R, Beckerman M *et al*. Specific expiratory muscle training in COPD. *Chest* 2003; **124**: 468–73.

73. Gosselink R, Troosters T, Decramer M. Distribution of muscle weakness in patients with stable chronic obstructive pulmonary disease. *J Cardiopulm Rehabil* 2000; **20**: 353–60.

74. Schols AM, Soeters PB, Mostert R *et al*. Physiologic effects of nutritional support and anabolic steroids in patients with chronic obstructive pulmonary disease. A placebo-controlled randomized trial. *Am J Respir Crit Care Med* 1995; **152**: 1268–74.

75. Gosselink R, Troosters T, Decramer M. Peripheral muscle weakness contributes to exercise limitation in COPD. *Am J Respir Crit Care Med* 1996; **153**: 976–80.

76. Mahler DA, Mackowiak JI. Evaluation of the short-form 36-item questionnaire to measure health-related quality of life in patients with COPD. *Chest* 1995; **107**: 1585–9.

77. Mahler DA, Harver A. A factor analysis of dyspnea ratings, respiratory muscle strength, lung function in patients with chronic obstructive pulmonary disease. *Am Rev Respir Dis* 1992; **145**: 467–70.

78. Mahler DA, Tomlinson D, Olmstead EM *et al*. Changes in dyspnea, health status, lung function in chronic airway disease. *Am J Respir Crit Care Med* 1995; **151**: 61–5.

79. Polkey MI, Kyroussis D, Hamnegard CH *et al*. Diaphragm strength in chronic obstructive pulmonary disease. *Am J Respir Crit Care Med* 1996; **154**: 1310–17.

80. Engelen MP, Schols AM, Baken WC *et al*. Nutritional depletion in relation to respiratory and peripheral skeletal muscle function in out-patients with COPD. *Eur Respir J* 1994; **7**: 1793–7.

81. Nava S. Rehabilitation of patients admitted to a respiratory intensive care unit. *Arch Phys Med Rehabil* 1998; **79**: 849–54.

82. O'Donnell DE, Lam M, Webb KA. Spirometric correlates of improvement in exercise performance after anticholinergic therapy in chronic obstructive pulmonary disease. *Am J Respir Crit Care Med* 1999; **160**: 542–9.

83. Martinez FJ, de Oca MM, Whyte RI *et al*. Lung-volume reduction improves dyspnea, dynamic hyperinflation, respiratory muscle function. *Am J Respir Crit Care Med* 1997; **155**: 1984–90.

84. Troosters T, Gosselink R, Decramer M. Short- and long-term effects of outpatient rehabilitation in patients with chronic obstructive pulmonary disease: a randomized trial. *Am J Med* 2000; **109**: 207–12.

85. Casaburi R, Patessio A, Ioli F *et al*. Reductions in exercise lactic acidosis and ventilation as a result of exercise training in patients with obstructive lung disease. *Am Rev Respir Dis* 1991; **143**: 9–18.

86. Snider GL. Enhancement of exercise performance in COPD patients by hyperoxia: a call for research. *Chest* 2002; **122**: 1830–6.

87. Goldstein RS. Pulmonary rehabilitation in chronic respiratory insufficiency. 3. Ventilatory muscle training. *Thorax* 1993; **48**: 1025–33.

88. Grassino A. Inspiratory muscle training in COPD patients. *Eur Respir J Suppl* 1989; **7**: 581–6.

89. Lacasse Y, Guyatt GH, Goldstein RS. The components of a respiratory rehabilitation program: a systematic overview. *Chest* 1997; **111**: 1077–88.

90. Wanke T, Formanek D, Lahrmann H *et al*. Effects of combined inspiratory muscle and cycle ergometer training on exercise performance in patients with COPD. *Eur Respir J* 1994; **7**: 2205–11.

91. Weiner P, Azgad Y, Ganam R. Inspiratory muscle training combined with general exercise reconditioning in patients with COPD. *Chest* 1992; **102**: 1351–6.

92. O'Donnell DE, McGuire M, Samis L, Webb KA. General exercise training improves ventilatory and peripheral muscle strength and endurance in chronic airflow limitation. *Am J Respir Crit Care Med* 1998; **157**: 1489–97.

93. Larson JL, Covey MK, Wirtz SE *et al*. Cycle ergometer and inspiratory muscle training in chronic obstructive pulmonary disease. *Am J Respir Crit Care Med* 1999; **160**: 500–7.

94. Lieberman SL, Shefner JM, Young RR. Neurological disorders affecting respiration. In: Roussos C, ed. *The Thorax*, 2nd edn. New York: Marcel Dekker, 1995; 2135–75.

95. Misuri G, Lanini B, Gigliotti F *et al*. Mechanism of CO(2) retention in patients with neuromuscular disease. *Chest* 2000; **117**: 447–53.

96. Ragette R, Mellies U, Schwake C *et al*. Patterns and predictors of sleep disordered breathing in primary myopathies. *Thorax* 2002; **57**: 724–8.

97. Klefbeck B, Hamrah NJ. Effect of inspiratory muscle training in patients with multiple sclerosis. *Arch Phys Med Rehabil* 2003; **84**: 994–9.

98. Gosselink R, Kovacs L, Ketelaer P *et al*. Respiratory muscle weakness and respiratory muscle training in severely disabled multiple sclerosis patients. *Arch Phys Med Rehabil* 2000; **81**: 747–51.

99. Smeltzer SC, Lavietes MH, Cook SD. Expiratory training in multiple sclerosis. *Arch Phys Med Rehabil* 1996; **77**: 909–12.

100. Wanke T, Toifl K, Merkle M *et al*. Inspiratory muscle training in patients with Duchenne muscular dystrophy. *Chest* 1994; **105**: 475–82.

101. Koessler W, Wanke T, Winkler G *et al*. 2 years' experience with inspiratory muscle training in patients with neuromuscular disorders. *Chest* 2001; **120**: 765–9.

102. McCool FD, Tzelepis GE. Inspiratory muscle training in the patient with neuromuscular disease. *Phys Ther* 1995; **75**: 1006–14.

103. Bach JR. Noninvasive ventilation is more than mask ventilation. *Chest* 2003; **123**: 2156–7.

104. Kang SW, Bach JR. Maximum insufflation capacity. *Chest* 2000; **118**: 61–5.

105. Gross D, Ladd HW, Riley EJ *et al*. The effect of training on strength and endurance of the diaphragm in quadriplegia. *Am J Med* 1980; **68**: 27–35.

106. Huldtgren AC, Fugl-Meyer AR, Jonasson E, Bake B. Ventilatory dysfunction and respiratory rehabilitation in post traumatic quadriplegia. *Eur J Respir Dis* 1980; **61**: 347–56.

107. Estenne M, Knoop C, Vanvaerenbergh J *et al.* The effect of pectoralis muscle training in tetraplegic subjects. *Am Rev Respir Dis* 1989; **139**: 1218–22.

108. Buyse B, Demedts M, Meekers J *et al.* Respiratory dysfunction in multiple sclerosis: a prospective analysis of 60 patients. *Eur Respir J* 1997; **10**: 139–45.

109. Van Houtte S, Vanlandewijck Y, Kiekens C, Gosselink R. Respiratory muscle endurance in patients with spinal cord injury, a pilot study. *Eur Respir J* 2003; **22**: 332s.

110. Hayot M, Ramonatxo M, Matecki S *et al.* Noninvasive assessment of inspiratory muscle function during exercise. *Am J Respir Crit Care Med* 2000; **162**: 2201–7.

9

Role of peripheral muscle function in rehabilitation

DIDIER SAEY, FRANÇOIS MALTAIS

INTRODUCTION

Exercise intolerance is a common feature of chronic obstructive pulmonary disease (COPD) and it has a profound impact on quality of life. Exercise intolerance in patients with COPD results from a complex interplay of central (dyspnoea-ventilation) and peripheral muscle factors. Early dyspnoea and limitations in ventilation and gas exchange are important causes of exercise intolerance (1). Peripheral muscle fatigue may also contribute to exercise limitation (2), and it is increasingly recognized that skeletal muscle dysfunction is common in patients with COPD (3, 4). From a physiological perspective, a therapy allowing the improvement of pulmonary function, reduction of ventilatory requirement and decrease in leg fatigue during exertion would be the best strategy to ameliorate functional status in COPD. While the first therapeutic objective could be reached by pharmacological treatment, the latter two could only be obtained with exercise training. Several studies confirm the beneficial effects of exercise training on peripheral muscle function, providing a strong physiological rationale for this intervention. A comprehensive management strategy incorporating pharmacological and rehabilitative elements will provide the best chance for an optimal functional and health status in patients with symptomatic COPD.

OBJECTIVES

The general objective of this chapter is to familiarize physicians and health care professionals with the impact of peripheral muscle dysfunction on exercise tolerance in patients with COPD and also with the use of exercise training to improve muscle function in this population.

After reading this chapter, physicians and health care professionals should: (i) be able to recognize the general and specific benefits of exercise training on peripheral function and exercise tolerance in patients with COPD; (ii) understand the principles of exercise training in patients with COPD; (iii) recognize the indications of exercise training in patients with COPD; and (iv) be able to design an effective and safe exercise training programme for patients with COPD.

PERIPHERAL MUSCLE ADAPTATION IN COPD

Evidence of peripheral muscle adaptation in COPD

Exercise limitation is multifactorial in COPD. Recognized contributing factors include:

- ventilatory limitation due to impaired respiratory system mechanics and ventilatory muscle dysfunction (5)
- gas exchange abnormalities (6)
- cardiac impairment
- unpleasant exertional symptom perception (2)
- peripheral muscle dysfunction (3).

The predominant limiting factors to exercise may vary, not only among patients with COPD, but also in a given patient from time to time. As the disease progresses, a growing number of these factors come into play in a complex integrative manner. The first part of this chapter will focus on the peripheral component of exercise limitation.

Peripheral muscle abnormalities described in patients with COPD have been discussed at length in recent reviews (7–12). Muscle atrophy, weakness and fatigability, alteration in fibre-type distribution and decreased metabolic capacity have been described in this disease (Box 9.1). Independently of the impairment in lung function, alteration in peripheral muscle structure, metabolism and function have been associated with exercise intolerance (13), poor quality of life (14, 15), greater utilization of health care resources (16) and poor survival (17). The presence of peripheral muscle dysfunction may also help in identifying candidates who are more likely to benefit from exercise training (18). As opposed to patients with clear ventilatory limitation and normal muscle strength, patients with muscle weakness may benefit more from exercise training in terms of quality of life and exercise tolerance (18).

PERIPHERAL MUSCLE WASTING

Although muscle wasting has long been recognized by clinicians, its relevance to patients' outcome and management has been overlooked. Available information suggests that muscle wasting is present in a high proportion of patients with COPD (19–21), a reduced body weight being reported in approximately 50 per cent of 253 patients with COPD involved in pulmonary rehabilitation (19). Importantly, the disproportionately greater reduction in thigh muscle cross-sectional area than body weight (20) indicates a preferential loss of muscle

---

Box 9.1   Evidence of peripheral muscle dysfunction in COPD

- Muscle atrophy
- Weakness
- Fatigability
- Morphological change
  - $\downarrow$ proportion of type I fibres
  - $\uparrow$ proportion of type IIb fibres
  - atrophy of type I and IIa fibres
  - $\downarrow$ capillarization
- Altered metabolic capacity
  - $\downarrow$ intra-muscular pH
  - $\downarrow$ ATP concentration
  - $\uparrow$ muscle lactate concentration
  - $\uparrow$ ionosine monophosphate
  - $\downarrow$ mitochondrial enzyme activities

---

tissue over other body compartments (Fig. 9.1). Low muscle mass in COPD is associated with weaker peripheral muscles, impaired functional status (20) and poor health-related quality of life (15) and has a strong impact on mortality in patients with severe COPD (17). Based on these findings, improving muscle mass through rehabilitation appears to be a reasonable therapeutic target.

PERIPHERAL MUSCLE FIBRE TYPE, SIZE AND CAPILLARIZATION

The fibre-type profile of the vastus lateralis muscle, an important determinant of the muscle metabolic capacity (22), has been assessed in patients with moderate to severe COPD. Type I fibres have a slow contraction speed and develop a relatively small tension but, because of their reliance on aerobic metabolism, are fatigue-resistant. In contrast, type II fibres have fast contraction speed and develop larger tensions but are susceptible to fatigue because their energy is mostly derived from glycolytic metabolism. Probably the most consistent muscle adaptation in COPD is the shift in fibre composition of peripheral muscle with a reduction in the proportion of type I fibres and a reciprocal increase in type IIb fibres (Fig. 9.2) (23–27). Although this fibre-type shift may be useful to preserve strength, it could increase susceptibility to fatigue.

Atrophy of type I and IIa fibres has also been found in COPD (20, 24, 25, 28–30) and, with the reduction in type I and IIa fibre cross-sectional area being proportional to the reduction in mid-thigh cross-sectional area (20), the loss in muscle mass would appear to be mostly due to a specific type I-IIa fibre-type atrophy. In contrast, some studies reported type IIb fibre atrophy in some patients with COPD (27, 31), perhaps a consequence of systemic steroid exposure (7, 27). Lastly, the capillarization of the vastus lateralis, an important determinant of muscle aerobic capacity, is also reduced when compared with age-matched healthy subjects (24).

PERIPHERAL MUSCLE ENERGY METABOLISM

The energy metabolism of the peripheral muscles has been studied extensively in COPD over the past 10–15 years.

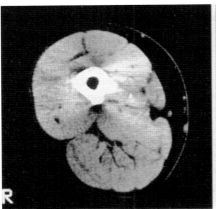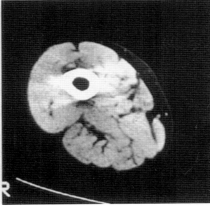

Figure 9.1 *Computed tomography of one healthy subject (left panel) and one patient with COPD (right panel). The mid-thigh muscle cross-sectional area (CSA) was considerably reduced in the COPD patient compared with that of the healthy subject, amounting to 80 cm² and to 119 cm², respectively. Reproduced with permission from Bernard et al. (20).*

Although the *in vitro* enzymatic activities in muscle energy metabolism do not necessarily reflect the physiological situation, since only maximal activities under the optimal circumstances are evaluated, they do provide an indication of the enzymatic adaptations of various metabolic pathways. In line with the fibre-type profile described above, low activity of two mitochondrial enzymes, citrate synthase (CS) and 3-hydroxyacyl-CoA dehydrogenase (HADH), in the vastus lateralis muscle have been reported in COPD (32, 33). These two enzymes, which are respectively involved in the citric acid cycle and β-oxidation of fatty acids, are good markers of muscle oxidative capacity. In keeping with these enzymatic changes, the substrate and co-factor levels in the peripheral muscles indicate that the muscle energy metabolism is impaired at rest and during exercise in COPD. Low intracellular pH, reduced glycogen, phosphocreatine (PCr) and adenosine triphosphate (ATP) contents, and increased lactate, pyruvate and ionosine monophosphate concentrations have been found in the vastus lateralis muscle of these individuals (28, 32, 34–37). Using nuclear magnetic resonance spectroscopy (^{31}P-NMR) to study

the oxidative metabolism of the skeletal muscle during dynamic contraction, a greater decline in intracellular pH and in phosphocreatine/inorganic phosphate ratio (PCr/Pi) has been reported in patients with chronic lung disease compared with healthy subjects (37–41). These findings are indicative of an impaired oxidative phosphorylation and ATP resynthesis, with a high reliance on anaerobic glycolysis within the contracting muscles (37–41). In addition, a slower recovery of phosphocreatine muscle levels (37) and prolonged acidosis (37, 38, 40, 42) were observed after exercise in patients with COPD. These peripheral muscle metabolic abnormalities may be worsened by hypoxaemia and can be partially reversed with oxygen supplementation (37, 41, 43) but they are not necessarily related to reduction in peripheral O_2 delivery (44, 45). This last finding suggests that the altered muscle metabolism during exercise in COPD is related, at least in part, to a poor muscle oxidative capacity or an abnormal metabolic regulation (46) and that rephosphorylation of high-energy phosphates is less efficient in these patients during and after exercise. Because the anaerobic energy metabolism yields far less ATP compared with complete oxidative glucose degradation, the lower capacity for muscle aerobic metabolism may influence exercise tolerance in several fashions. Premature muscle acidosis, a contributory factor to muscle fatigue and early exercise termination in healthy subjects (47–49) may be an important mechanism contributing to exercise intolerance in COPD (44). Increased lactic acidosis for a given exercise work rate, which is a common finding in COPD (6, 50–53), could enhance the ventilatory needs by increasing non-aerobic CO_2 production (6, 54, 55), imposing an additional burden on the respiratory muscles already facing an increased work of breathing (Fig. 9.3).

MUSCLE STRENGTH AND ENDURANCE

Strength and endurance are two fundamental characteristics of muscle performance. Strength is defined as the capacity of the muscle to produce maximal force, and endurance as the capacity of the muscle to maintain a given level of force for a given period of time. Loss in either one of these muscle characteristics results in impaired muscle performance.

Quadriceps strength is decreased on average by 30 per cent in patients with moderate to severe COPD but there is considerable interindividual variability (13, 20, 56, 57). This observation is clinically relevant since peripheral muscle strength is an important determinant of exercise capacity in patients with COPD, correlating with peak oxygen uptake and 6-min walking distance (13). The perception of leg fatigue, a common exercise symptom limiting patients with COPD during exercise, is inversely correlated to muscle strength (56).

A significant reduction in quadriceps endurance has also been reported in patients with COPD (58, 59) and may be another important factor in exercise limitation, as it may lead to premature muscle fatigue. Contractile fatigue is usually defined as a reversible reduction in the force generated by the muscle for a given neural input. In patients with COPD, it was initially thought that exercise termination would occur proximal

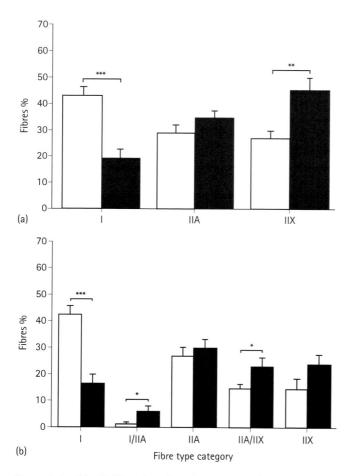

Figure 9.2 *Myofibrillar adenosine triphosphatase (mATPase) (a) and combination of mATPase and myosin heavy chain fibre-type categories (b) in the vastus lateralis. White bars, control; black bars, COPD patients. Significance of difference between the groups: *P < 0.05; **P < 0.01; ***P < 0.001. Reproduced with permission from Gosker et al. (31).*

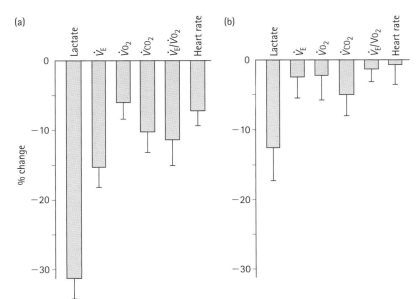

Figure 9.3 *Changes in physiological responses to an identical exercise task (high constant work rate test) produced by two exercise training strategies in patients with COPD. (a) High work rate training group (n = 11). (b) Low work rate training group (n = 8). Note that patients performed the same total work in their training programme irrespective of group assignment. Percent change is calculated from the average change in response at the time the pre-training study ended. Vertical lines represent 1 standard error mean (SEM). Decreases in blood lactate, ventilation, O_2 uptake, CO_2 output, ventilatory equivalent for O_2, and heart rate were observed for both training regimens, but decreases were appreciably greater for the high work rate training group. Reproduced with permission from Casaburi et al. (6).*

to muscle fatigue. This notion was addressed recently by using magnetic stimulation of the femoral nerve which provides a non-volitional measure of muscle strength (60–65). Consistent with the alteration in muscle metabolism and with the greater proportion of fatigue-susceptible fibres, approximately half of patients with moderately severe COPD displayed quadriceps fatigue after a cycle exercise despite a severely reduced exercise capacity (60). Interestingly, patients with severe disease were as likely to develop exercise-induced quadriceps fatigue as those with milder disease. Using the same methodology, it was also concluded that the quadriceps of patients with severe COPD is more fatigable than those of age-matched healthy controls. The impact of leg fatigue on the exercise response to acute bronchodilation in patients with COPD was also recently evaluated (64). In line with the above findings, it was found that the exercise response to bronchodilation was modulated by the presence of leg fatigue; acute bronchodilation failed to improve exercise tolerance in patients who developed leg fatigue during exercise. This study provides further evidence of the role of peripheral muscle fatigue in exercise limitation in COPD.

Aetiology of peripheral muscle adaptation in COPD

The most obvious potential cause of peripheral muscle dysfunction in COPD is chronic inactivity and muscle deconditioning. Despite the improvement in muscle function with exercise training, there is some evidence suggesting that chronic inactivity and muscle deconditionning may not be sufficient to explain all muscle changes found in this disease. Several other factors have been evoked to explain the occurrence of muscle dysfunction in COPD, and their relative importance is likely to vary among patients. Nutritional imbalance (21, 66), systemic corticosteroid use (67), hypoxaemia (28, 30), systemic

inflammation with increased circulating levels of proinflammatory cytokines (68), electrolyte disturbances (69), low anabolic hormone levels (70, 71) and oxidative stress (59) have all been suggested as potential contributors to poor peripheral muscle function in COPD and are described in detail in recent reviews (8, 10, 72).

Summary

We have seen how peripheral muscles adapt in patients with COPD and how this may influence their functional status. It is therefore reasonable to assume that an important objective of pulmonary rehabilitation and exercise training should be to improve peripheral muscle function in this disease.

EXERCISE TRAINING AND PERIPHERAL MUSCLE

Exercise training can be divided into two broad categories: aerobic/endurance training and strength/resistive training.

Effects of aerobic exercise on muscle function in healthy subjects

Aerobic training enhances health status and fitness. It is now clear that the level of activity necessary to improve health status is lower than what is required to improve fitness and induce a physiological response to exercise training (73). While low-intensity exercise such as self-paced walking may be sufficient to heighten health status, at least two weekly training sessions of moderately intense exercise are required to induce an adaptative response to training (73).

The physiological response to training consists of structural changes in the cardiovascular and peripheral muscle systems; this accounts for an improvement in the capacity to transport oxygen, and in the respiratory capacity of the trained peripheral muscles (22, 74). As a result, peak $\dot{V}O_2$ will be improved with aerobic training. Important structural changes take place within the trained peripheral muscles, which explains why their ability to extract oxygen is enhanced with aerobic training. In general, endurance training is associated with a greater oxidative enzyme capacity and capillary density and fibre-type transformation (75). Endurance training reduces the proportion of type IIb fibres with a reciprocal increase in type IIa fibres. Switch from II fibre to I fibre with endurance exercise is less common and, when it occurs, it involves only a modest proportion of fibres (76–79). The volume of type I fibres and the mitochondrial numbers are expanded; also, the activities of the mitochondrial enzymes such as CS and HADH are enhanced (22, 80–82). Improved muscle capillarization and increased myoglobin levels also occur, which, in turn, facilitate oxygen delivery and extraction (83, 84). These structural muscle changes are associated with important modifications in muscle metabolism during exercise, such as a lower blood lactate concentration and less CO_2 production for a given level of exercise. These changes in muscle metabolism are thought to contribute to the greater tolerance to submaximal exercise (22), which may be particularly relevant to activities of daily living. However, endurance training may result in fibre atrophy and eventually weakness when performed over the course of several years (85), suggesting that strength muscle training should be an integral part of any long-term training programme (73).

Effects of strength training on muscle function in healthy subjects

MUSCLE STRENGTH TRAINING

Strength is an essential characteristic of the muscle, having an impact not only on functional status but also on the general health condition status. Speed, balance and coordination may also be positively enhanced when the muscle is stronger (86). Strength training may induce hypertrophy and is an effective way to increase muscle fibre size and, consequently, strength (87). These benefits can be safely obtained by individualizing

the training programme (88, 89). Interestingly, strength begins to improve before muscle hypertrophy, a finding attributed to a better neuromechanical coupling (90), an increase in the number and size of myofibrils in muscle protein (especially myosin) per muscle cell and stronger connective tendinous and ligamentous tissues. Later, when fibre hypertrophy occurs, the capillary density tends to decrease despite new capillary growth (91). This would suggest that muscle strength training should not be used alone. The question of whether programmes of strength training induce fibre-type switch is still controversial.

When prescribing strength training, the load is generally estimated from the maximum charge which can be lifted only once over the full range of motion without compensation (1 RM). Based on the recommendations of the American College of Sports Medicine (86), the characteristics of specific strength training programmes are summarized in Table 9.1. Both concentric and eccentric muscle exercises using single and multiple joints exercise are recommended. In order to gain pure strength, a few repetitions (1–8) of near maximal loads (80–100 per cent of 1 RM) should be used. It is recommended that 2–10 per cent increase in load be applied when the trainee can perform the current workload for one to two repetitions over the desired number. Based on better training outcome when long versus short rest periods are used between set exercises (92), resting periods of at least 2–3 min are recommended. The optimal training frequency is four to five times per week, but 1–2 days per week is a sufficient maintenance strategy for individuals already engaged in a resistance training programme (86).

MUSCLE STRENGTH/ENDURANCE TRAINING

It has been suggested that the total work involved with traditional strength training may not maximize hypertrophy (93). To maximize this, a moderate load (70–85 per cent of 1 RM) for eight to 12 repetitions per set for one to three sets per exercise using 1–2 min rest periods is recommended (86). This training strategy may also result in improved muscle oxidative capacity. Indeed, the effects of strength training on maximal oxygen consumption and some of its determinants were studied by Frontera et al. (94). After 12 weeks of training, there was a small but significant improvement in quadriceps size

Table 9.1 *Optimal characteristics of strength training programmes*

	Strength	Strength-endurance	Endurance
Loading	80–100% of 1 RM	70–85% of 1 RM	30–60% of 1 RM
Volume	1–3 sets of 1–8 repetitions	3 sets of 8–12 repetitions	1–3 sets of 20–30 repetitions
Rest intervals	2–3 min	1–2 min	1 min
Frequency	4–6 days/week	2–4 days/week (maintenance 1–2 days/week)	2–4 days/week
Progression	2–10% increase	Beginners: 60–70% of 1 RM	
Expected benefits	Improvement in muscle mass and strength, and in bone density	Hypertrophy, improvement in muscle mass and strength, and in bone density Improvement in muscle endurance and exercise capacity	Improvement in muscle oxidative capacity and capillarization Improvement in muscle endurance and in exercise capacity

1 RM, maximum charge which can be lifted only once over the full range of motion without compensation.

and in maximal oxygen consumption (6 per cent). Moreover, biopsies of the vastus lateralis showed a 25 per cent increase in mean fibre area, a 15 per cent increase in capillaries per fibre, and a 38 per cent improvement in CS activity. The optimal training strategy is two to four times per week, but as for pure strength training, 1–2 days per week is a sufficient maintenance strategy for individuals already engaged in a resistance training (86) (see Table 9.1).

MUSCLE ENDURANCE TRAINING

Muscle endurance can be improved when strength training is performed at a low intensity (30–60 per cent of 1 RM) for 20–30 repetitions using short (10–15 s) resting periods (see Table 9.1). High-volume (multiple sets) programmes are superior for endurance enhancement and the frequency recommended is similar to that of strength training. Faster training velocity (i.e. 180°/s) is more effective than a slow training velocity (i.e. 30°/s) for improving local muscle endurance (86).

Effects of exercise in patients with COPD

AEROBIC TRAINING

Regardless of disease severity, patients with COPD show multiple benefits from aerobic training (see Box 9.2). Improvements in dyspnoea (95–99), maximal and submaximal exercise capacity (6, 95, 96, 100–106), neuromuscular coordination (5) and functional abilities in activities of daily living (107) have been noted, translating into enhanced quality of life (95, 98, 99, 101, 108) and reduced health care utilization (96, 109).

At moderate to high training intensity, aerobic training reduces exercise-induced lactic acidosis and improves skeletal muscle aerobic capacity and bioenergetics (6, 104, 105). ^{31}P magnetic resonance spectroscopy was used to study the skeletal muscle physiological adaptation to aerobic training in patients with COPD (105). A reduced creatine-phosphate half-time recovery and improved cellular bioenergetics during submaximal exercise were noted. In addition to these peripheral effects, aerobic training provides a modest but significant central cardiorespiratory training effect with a decreased heart rate and ventilation for a given submaximal workload (110). The likelihood of obtaining physiological benefits from an aerobic training programme appears related

---

Box 9.2   Benefits of exercise training in patients with chronic obstructive pulmonary disease (COPD)

- Lessened dyspnoea (95–97, 99, 124)
- Increased exercise capacity (6, 95, 96, 100–103, 124)
- Improved muscle oxidative capacity, strength endurance and function (6, 104–106, 115–117)
- Improved neuromuscular coordination (5)
- Improved functional activity (107)
- Enhanced quality of life (95, 99, 101, 108, 115, 125)
- Decreased health care use (96, 109)

---

more to the patient's ability to engage in more intense and prolonged exercises than to the disease severity (6, 110–113). This is particularly the case in patients with advanced COPD who may gain substantial physiological improvements in cardiovascular, respiratory and musculoskeletal systems despite the severity of their disease.

The general guidelines used to prescribe aerobic training in healthy subjects are also applicable to patients with pulmonary impairment. As for healthy subjects, the frequency, duration and intensity of training are all thought to be important. The intensity of training that should be used in COPD has been the subject of many studies. In general, a greater physiological training response and larger improvement in submaximal exercise tolerance have been obtained from training at high intensity (80 per cent of maximal work rate) rather than at low intensity (below 50 per cent of maximal work rate) (6, 113). However, as shown in a recent randomized clinical trial, these additional physiological benefits of a high-intensity training programme, as compared with low-intensity exercises, do not necessarily translate into additional gains in quality of life (113). Therefore, the training intensity should be selected on the basis of the training objectives. It is generally recommended that aerobic training includes three weekly 30-min exercise sessions for 8–12 weeks. In the most disabled patients, interval training, where 2–3 min of high-intensity exercise are interspersed with lower intensity exercise or even rest periods, may allow the patient to reach an adequate training goal (114). Aerobic training intensity can be prescribed and monitored by measuring the work rate and by monitoring heart rate and/or dyspnoea. In healthy individuals, the intensity of training is most commonly determined and monitored using a fixed proportion of the maximal heart rate, or of the heart rate reserve (73). This approach is not recommended in patients with COPD who are exercise-limited before they reach their predicted peak heart rate.

PERIPHERAL MUSCLE TRAINING

Compared with aerobic training, strength training has received relatively less attention as a rehabilitative strategy in patients with COPD. Some studies showed that a greater muscle strength is associated with less muscle fatigue, a common limiting symptom during exercise in patients with COPD (2, 56). Strength training, by promoting muscle growth and strength, represents a helpful adjunct to whole-body aerobic training in COPD patients. Furthermore, strength exercises may induce less dyspnoea than aerobic exercise and, as a result, are usually well tolerated (106, 115). In patients with COPD, an 8-week training programme including three sessions of different exercises (one for the arms and two for the legs) performed at high intensity (up to 85 per cent of the maximal strength) induced an improvement in muscle strength ranging from 16 to 40 per cent depending on the muscle group (115). This improvement was associated with improved endurance to submaximal exercise capacity and quality of life (115). Similar benefits have been reported in mild COPD (116). In a subsequent study, a 12-week low-intensity peripheral muscle conditioning programme performed at home under the supervision of a physiotherapist was evaluated in a group of patients with COPD (117). After the study period, isotonic muscle endurance and strength were increased in the training group, for both lower and upper body extremities. The authors reported a highly significant change in local and whole-body endurance capacity in the training group. This low-intensity peripheral muscle training programme was well tolerated, simple and easy to perform at home. This strategy may be helpful in patients with COPD for whom high-intensity training is difficult to achieve.

These improvements in peripheral muscle function with low-intensity exercise may not necessarily reflect a true physiological muscle response to training and could simply be due to better motivation or neuromuscular coupling. As is the case with aerobic training, a greater training intensity will increase the likelihood of obtaining an improvement in muscle function *per se*. The question of whether further improvement in muscle function and exercise capacity could be obtained by supplementing aerobic training with strength training was recently addressed (106). Greater improvements in quadriceps and pectoralis major muscle strength and in muscle mass were obtained by combining both training modalities (aerobic training combined with 45 min of strength training performed at 80 per cent of 1 RM) than by endurance training alone (Fig. 9.4). However, these additional gains in muscle strength and mass in the combined training group did not translate into further improvement in exercise tolerance.

The authors concluded that the addition of strength training to aerobic training in patients with COPD is associated with significantly greater increases in muscle strength and mass but it did not provide additional improvement in exercise capacity or quality of life in their study.

When comparing the efficacy of aerobic and strength training, Spruit *et al.* (118) surprisingly found a similar improvement in peripheral muscle strength, exercise performance and health-related quality of life with both training strategies. Their study suggests that resistance training may be a good alternative in patients in whom whole-body exercise training would be difficult to perform. Lastly, the effects of strength training (four sets of eight repetitions at 80 per cent of 1 RM), aerobic training (40 min cycling exercise at 70 per cent of maximal oxygen consumption) and a combination of the two (halving each training modality) were recently compared in a randomized study (119). As expected, the gain in submaximal exercise capacity was significantly greater in the aerobic group than in the strength group. Conversely, increases in strength were greater in the strength group than in the endurance group. Combining both training modalities provided similar improvement in exercise capacity and in strength, in contrast to endurance or strength training, respectively.

In addition to its beneficial effects on peripheral muscle, strength training may also help to increase bone density (120, 121), a potentially interesting effect for patients with COPD in whom osteoporosis is highly prevalent (122). As in other elderly individuals, the experience indicates that strength

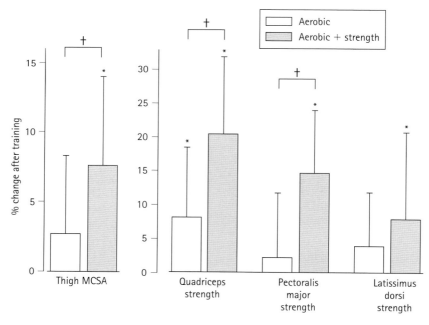

Figure 9.4 *Mean ± SD per cent change in bilateral mid-thigh muscle cross-sectional area (MCSA) and in the strength of the quadriceps, pectoralis major and latissimus dorsi muscles before and after training in the aerobic and aerobic + strength groups. The improvement in bilateral mid-thigh MCSA and in the strength of the three muscle groups was statistically significant in the aerobic + strength group. Quadriceps strength also showed a significant increase in the aerobic group. As can be seen, the magnitude of the changes in mid-thigh MCSA and in the strength of the quadriceps and pectoralis major muscles was significantly greater in the aerobic + strength group than in the aerobic group. (*P < 0.05 for pre- versus post-training within each study group; †P < 0.05 for the aerobic group versus the aerobic + strength group.) Reproduced with permission from Bernard et al. (106).*

training can also be performed safely in patients with COPD (106, 115, 117, 123). Because patients with COPD are often elderly, a careful pre-programme evaluation and the individualization of the training regimen are critical to minimize the risk of strength training. Strength training should also be used cautiously in patients with musculoskeletal disorders and/or severe osteoporosis to avoid injury such a bone fracture.

CONCLUSIONS

Exercise training is the best available strategy to enhance peripheral muscle function in patients with COPD, providing a strong physiological rationale for its use in the long-term management of these individuals. The choice of type and intensity of training should be based primarily on the patient's functional status, symptoms, needs, preferences and long-term goals. If the goal is to improve peripheral muscle function, the combination of strength and aerobic training seems a more physiologically complete approach. When tolerated, high-intensity training may lead to greater improvement in aerobic fitness and muscle function than low-intensity training, but this is not absolutely necessary to ameliorate exercise endurance or quality of life.

Key points

- Peripheral muscle dysfunction is a common feature of COPD and it has a profound impact on functional status and quality of life.
- Exercise training is the cornerstone of pulmonary rehabilitation and is one of the most effective strategies to improve exercise tolerance and quality of life in patients with COPD.
- The combination of strength and aerobic training seems to be a physiologically complete approach to treat peripheral muscle dysfunction in COPD.
- High-intensity training may lead to greater improvement in aerobic fitness and muscle function than low-intensity training but this is not absolutely necessary to ameliorate exercise endurance or quality of life.

REFERENCES

1. Gallagher CG. Exercise and chronic obstructive pulmonary disease. *Med Clin North Am* 1990; **74**: 619–41.
2. Killian KJ, Leblanc P, Martin DH *et al.* Exercise capacity and ventilatory, circulatory, and symptom limitation in patients with airflow limitation. *Am Rev Respir Dis* 1992; **146**: 935–40.
◆3. American Thoracic Society/European Respiratory Society. Skeletal muscle dysfunction in chronic obstructive pulmonary disease. *Am J Respir Crit Care Med* 1999; **159**: 1–40.

●4. Palange P, Wagner PD. The skeletal muscle in chronic respiratory diseases: summary of the ERS research seminar in Rome, Italy, February 11–12 1999. *Eur Respir J* 2000; **15**: 807–15.
5. Belman MJ. Exercise in patients with chronic obstructive pulmonary disease. *Thorax* 1993; **48**: 936–46.
●6. Casaburi R, Patessio A, Ioli F *et al.* Reductions in exercise lactic acidosis and ventilation as a result of exercise training in patients with obstructive lung disease. *Am Rev Respir Dis* 1991; **143**: 9–18.
7. Decramer M, de Bock V, Dom R. Functional and histologic picture of steroid-induced myopathy in chronic obstructive pulmonary disease. *Am J Respir Crit Care Med* 1996; **153**: 1958–64.
●8. Gosker HR, Wouters EF, van der Vusse GJ, Schols AM. Skeletal muscle dysfunction in chronic obstructive pulmonary disease and chronic heart failure: underlying mechanisms and therapy perspectives. *Am J Clin Nutr* 2000; **71**: 1033–47.
●9. Maltais F, Leblanc P, Jobin J, Casaburi R. Peripheral muscle dysfunction in chronic obstructive pulmonary disease. *Clin Chest Med* 2000; **21**: 665–77.
10. Mador MJ, Bozkanat E. Skeletal muscle dysfunction in chronic obstructive pulmonary disease. *Respir Res* 2001; **2**: 216–24.
11. Debigaré R, Côté CH, Maltais F. Peripheral muscle wasting in chronic obstructive pulmonary disease; clinical relevance and mechanisms. *Am J Respir Crit Care Med* 2001; **164**: 1712–17.
12. Rassier DE, Macintosh BR. Coexistence of potentiation and fatigue in skeletal muscle. *Braz J Med Biol Res* 2000; **33**: 499–508.
13. Gosselink R, Troosters T, Decramer M. Peripheral muscle weakness contributes to exercise limitation in COPD. *Am J Respir Crit Care Med* 1996; **153**: 976–80.
14. Oga T, Nishimura K, Tsukino M *et al.* Relationship between different indices of exercise capacity and clinical measures in patients with chronic obstructive pulmonary disease. *Heart Lung* 2002; **31**: 374–81.
15. Mostert R, Goris A, Weling-Scheepers C *et al.* Tissue depletion and health related quality of life in patients with chronic obstructive pulmonary disease. *Respir Med* 2000; **94**: 859–67.
16. Decramer M, Gosselink R, Troosters T *et al.* Muscle weakness is related to utilization of health care resources in COPD patients. *Eur Respir J* 1997; **10**: 417–23.
17. Marquis K, Debigaré R, Lacasse Y *et al.* Midthigh muscle cross-sectional area is a better predictor of mortality than body mass index in patients with chronic obstructive pulmonary disease. *Am J Respir Crit Care Med* 2002; **166**: 809–13.
18. Troosters T, Gosselink R, Decramer M. Exercise training in COPD: how to distinguish responders from nonresponders. *J Cardiopulm Rehab* 2001; **21**: 10–7.
19. Schols AMWJ, Soeters PB, Dingemans MC *et al.* Prevalence and characteristics of nutritional depletion in patients with stable COPD eligible for pulmonary rehabilitation. *Am Rev Respir Dis* 1993; **147**: 1151–6.
●20. Bernard S, Leblanc P, Whittom F *et al.* Peripheral muscle weakness in patients with chronic obstructive pulmonary disease. *Am J Respir Crit Care Med* 1998; **158**: 629–34.
21. Engelen MPKJ, Schols AMWJ, Baken WC *et al.* Nutritional depletion in relation to respiratory and peripheral skeletal muscle function in out-patients with COPD. *Eur Respir J* 1994; **7**: 1793–7.
22. Holloszy JO, Coyle EF. Adaptations of skeletal muscle to endurance exercise and their metabolic consequences. *J Appl Physiol* 1984; **56**: 831–8.
23. Jobin J, Maltais F, Doyon JF *et al.* Chronic obstructive pulmonary disease: capillarity and fiber type characteristics of skeletal muscle. *J Cardiopulm Rehab* 1998; **18**: 432–7.

●24. Whittom F, Jobin J, Simard PM et al. Histochemical and morphological characteristics of the vastus lateralis muscle in COPD patients. Comparison with normal subjects and effects of exercise training. Med Sci Sports Exerc 1998; 30: 1467–74.

25. Maltais F, Sullivan MJ, Leblanc P et al. Altered expression of myosin heavy chain in the vastus lateralis muscle in patients with COPD. Eur Respir J 1999; 13: 850–4.

●26. Gosker HR, Kubat B, Schaart G et al. Myopathological features in skeletal muscle of patients with chronic obstructive pulmonary disease. Eur Respir J 2003; 22: 280–5.

27. Gosker HR, Engelen MP, van Mameren H et al. Muscle fiber type IIX atrophy is involved in the loss of fat-free mass in chronic obstructive pulmonary disease. Am J Clin Nutr 2002; 76: 113–19.

28. Jakobsson P, Jorfeldt L, Brundin A. Skeletal muscle metabolites and fibre types in patients with advanced chronic obstructive pulmonary disease (COPD), with and without chronic respiratory failure. Eur Respir J 1990; 3: 192–6.

29. Satta A, Migliori GB, Spanevello A et al. Fibre types in skeletal muscles of chronic obstructive pulmonary disease patients related to respiratory function and exercise tolerance. Eur Respir J 1997; 10: 2853–60.

30. Hildebrand IL, Sylvén C, Esbjornsson M et al. Does hypoxaemia induce transformations of fiber types? Acta Physiol Scand 1991; 141: 435–9.

31. Gosker HR, van Mameren H, van Dijk PJ et al. Skeletal muscle fibre-type shifting and metabolic profile in patients with chronic obstructive pulmonary disease. Eur Respir J 2002; 19: 617–25.

●32. Jakobsson P, Jorfeldt L, Henriksson J. Metabolic enzyme activity in the quadriceps femoris muscle in patients with severe chronic obstructive pulmonary disease. Am J Respir Crit Care Med 1995; 151: 374–7.

33. Maltais F, Simard AA, Simard C et al. Oxidative capacity of the skeletal muscle and lactic acid kinetics during exercise in normal subjects and in patients with COPD. Am J Respir Crit Care Med 1996; 153: 288–93.

34. Gertz I, Hedenstierna G, Hellers G, Wahren J. Muscle metabolism in patients with chronic obstructive lung disease and acute respiratory failure. Clin Sci Mol Med 1977; 52: 395–403.

35. Fiaccadori E, Del Canale S, Vitali P et al. Skeletal muscle energetics, acid-base equilibrium and lactate metabolism in patients with severe hypercapnia and hypoxia. Chest 1987; 92: 883–7.

36. Pouw EM, Schols AMWJ, van der Vusse GJ, Wouters EFM. Elevated inosine monophosphate levels in resting muscle of patients with stable chronic obstructive pulmonary disease. Am J Respir Crit Care Med 1998; 157: 453–7.

37. Payen JF, Wuyam B, Levy P et al. Muscular metabolism during oxygen supplementation in patients with chronic hypoxia. Am Rev Respir Dis 1993; 147: 592–8.

38. Wuyam B, Payen JF, Levy P et al. Metabolism and aerobic capacity of skeletal muscle in chronic respiratory failure related to chronic obstructive pulmonary disease. Eur Respir J 1992; 5: 157–62.

39. Tada H, Kato H, Misawa T et al. ^{31}P-nuclear magnetic resonance evidence of abnormal skeletal muscle metabolism in patients with chronic lung disease and congestive heart failure. Eur Respir J 1992; 5: 163–9.

●40. Kutsuzawa T, Shioya S, Kurita D et al. ^{31}P-NMR study of skeletal muscle metabolism in patients with chronic respiratory impairment. Am Rev Respir Dis 1992; 146: 1019–24.

41. Lévy P, Wuyam B, Pépin JL et al. Anomalies des muscles squelettiques des BPCO en insuffisance respiratoire. Apport de la spectroscopie RMN ^{31}P. Rev Mal Resp 1996; 13: 183–91.

42. Thompson CH, Davies RJO, Kemp GJ et al. Skeletal muscle metabolism during exercise and recovery in patients with respiratory failure. Thorax 1993; 48: 486–90.

43. Mannix ET, Boska MD, Galassetti P et al. Modulation of ATP production by oxygen in obstructive lung disease as assessed by ^{31}P-MRS. J Appl Physiol 1995; 78: 2218–27.

44. Maltais F, Jobin J, Sullivan MJ et al. Metabolic and hemodynamic responses of the lower limb during exercise in patients with COPD. J Appl Physiol 1998; 84: 1573–80.

45. Roca J, Agusti AGN, Alonso A et al. Effects of training on muscle O_2 transport at VO_2 max. J Appl Physiol 1992; 73: 1067–76.

46. Putman CT, Jones NL, Lands LC et al. Skeletal muscle pyruvate dehydrogenase activity during maximal exercise in humans. Am J Physiol 1995; 269: E458–68.

47. Mainwood GW, Renaud JM. The effect of acid-base balance on fatigue of skeletal muscle. Can J Physiol Pharmacol 1985; 63: 403–16.

48. Hultman E, Carale S, Sjoholm H. Effect of induced metabolic acidosis on intracellular pH, buffer capacity and contraction force of human skeletal muscle. Clin Sci 1985; 69: 505–10.

49. Westerblad H, Lee JA, Lannergren J, Allen DG. Cellular mechanisms of fatigue in skeletal muscle. Am J Physiol 1991; 261: 195–209.

50. Shuey CB, Peirce AK, Johnson RL. An evaluation of exercise tests in chronic obstructive lung disease. J Appl Physiol 1969; 27: 256–61.

51. Jones NL, Jones GL, Edwards RHT. Exercise tolerance in chronic airway obstruction. Am Rev Respir Dis 1971; 103: 477–91.

52. Engelen MP, Schols AM, Does JD et al. Exercise-induced lactate increase in relation to muscle substrates in patients with chronic obstructive pulmonary disease. Am J Respir Crit Care Med 2000; 162: 1697–1704.

53. Maltais F, Bernard S, Jobin J et al. Lactate kinetics during exercise in chronic obstructive pulmonary disease. Can Respir J 1997; 4: 251–7.

54. Beaver WL, Wasserman K, Whipp BJ. Bicarbonate buffering of lactic acid generated during exercise. J Appl Physiol 1986; 60: 472–86.

55. Jones NL, Heigenhauser GJF. Getting rid of carbon dioxide during exercise. Clin Sci 1996; 90: 323–35.

●56. Hamilton AL, Killian KJ, Summers E, Jones NL. Muscle strength, symptom intensity and exercise capacity in patients with cardiorespiratory disorders. Am J Respir Crit Care Med 1995; 152: 2021–31.

57. Man WDC, Soliman MGG, Nikoletou D et al. Non-volitional assessment of skeletal muscle strength in patients with chronic obstructive pulmonary disease. Thorax 2003; 58: 665–9.

58. Serres I, Gautier V, Varray AL, Préfaut CG. Impaired skeletal muscle endurance related to physical inactivity and altered lung function in COPD patients. Chest 1998; 113: 900–5.

59. Couillard A, Maltais F, Saey D et al. Exercise-induced quadriceps oxidative stress and peripheral muscle dysfunction in patients with chronic obstructive pulmonary disease. Am J Respir Crit Care Med 2003; 167: 1664.

60. Mador MJ, Kufel TJ, Pineda L. Quadriceps fatigue after cycle exercise in patients with chronic obstructive pulmonary disease. Am J Respir Crit Care Med 2000; 161 (2 Pt 1): 447–53.

61. Kufel TJ, Pineda LA, Mador MJ. Comparison of potentiated and unpotentiated twitches as an index of muscle fatigue. Muscle Nerve 2002; 25: 438–44.

62. Mador MJ, Kufel TJ, Pineda LA et al. Effect of pulmonary rehabilitation on quadriceps fatiguability during exercise. Am J Respir Crit Care Med 2001; 163: 930–5.

Derby Hospitals NHS Foundation Trust Library and Knowledge Service

63. Guleria R, Lyall R, Hart N et al. Central fatigue of the diaphragm and quadriceps during incremental loading. Lung 2002; **180**: 1–13.

64. Saey D, Debigaré R, LeBlanc P et al. Contractile leg fatigue after cycle exercise: A factor limiting exercise in patients with chronic obstructive pulmonary disease. Am J Respir Crit Care Med 2003; **168**: 425–30.

65. Mador MJ, Deniz O, Aggarwal A, Kufel TJ. Quadriceps fatigability after single muscle exercise in patients with chronic obstructive pulmonary disease. Am J Respir Crit Care Med 2003; **168**: 102–8.

66. Schols AMWJ, Soeters PB, Mostert R et al. Physiologic effects of nutritional support and anabolic steroids in patients with chronic obstructive pulmonary disease. A placebo-controlled randomized trial. Am J Respir Crit Care Med 1995; **152**: 1268–74.

67. Decramer M, Lacquet LM, Fagard R, Rogiers P. Corticosteroids contribute to muscle weakness in chronic airflow obstruction. Am Rev Respir Dis 1994; **150**: 11–6.

68. Schols AMWJ, Buurman WA, Staal-van den Brekel AJ et al. Evidence for a relation between metabolic derangements and increased levels of inflammatory mediators in a subgroup of patients with chronic obstructive pulmonary disease. Thorax 1996; **51**: 819–24.

69. Fiaccadori E, Coffrini E, Ronda N et al. Hypophosphatemia in course of chronic obstructive pulmonary disease. Prevalence, mechanisms, and relationships with skeletal muscle phosphorus content. Chest 1990; **97**: 857–68.

70. Casaburi R, Goren S, Bhasin S. Substantial prevalence of low anabolic hormone levels in COPD patients undergoing rehabilitation. Am J Respir Crit Care Med 1996; **153**: 128.

71. Kamischke A, Kemper DE, Castel MA et al. Testosterone levels in men with chronic obstructive pulmonary disease with or without glucocorticoid therapy. Eur Respir J 1998; **11**: 41–5.

72. Maltais F, Leblanc P, Jobin J, Casaburi R. Peripheral muscle dysfunction in chronic obstructive pulmonary disease. Rev Mal Respir 2002; **19**: 444–53.

◆73. American College of Sports Medicine. The recommended quantity and quality of exercise for developing and maintaining cardiorespiratory and muscular fitness, and flexibility in healthy adults. Med Sci Sport Exerc 1998; **30**: 975–91.

74. Casaburi R. Physiologic responses to training. Clin Chest Med 1994; **15**: 215–27.

75. Fitts RH, Costill DL, Gardetto PR. Effect of swim exercise training on human muscle fiber function. J Appl Physiol 1989; **66**: 465–75.

76. Howald H, Hoppeler H, Claassen H et al. Influences of endurance training on the ultrastructural composition of the different muscle fiber types in human. Pfluegers Arch 1985; **403**: 369–76.

77. Adams GR, Hather BM, Baldwin KM, Dudley GA. Skeletal muscle myosin heavy chain composition and resistance training. J Appl Physiol 1993; **74**: 911–5.

78. Simoneau JA, Lortie G, Bonlay MR et al. Human skeletal muscle fibre type alteration with high-intensity intermittent training. Eur J Appl Physiol 1985; **54**: 250–3.

79. Baumann H, Jäggi M, Soland F et al. Exercise training induces transitions of myosin isoform subunits within histochemically typed human muscle fibers. Pflügers Arch 1987; **409**: 349–60.

80. Rogers MA, Evans WJ. Changes in skeletal muscle with aging: effects of exercise training. In: Holloszy JO, ed. Exercise and Sports Sciences Reviews. Philadelphia: Williams and Wilkins, 1993; 65–102.

●81. Holloszy JO. Adaptation of skeletal muscle to endurance exercise. Med Sci Sports 1975; **7**: 155–64.

82. Saltin B, Gollnick PD. Skeletal muscle adaptability: significance for metabolism and performance. In: Peachey LD, ed. The Handbook of Physiology: The Skeletal Muscle System. Bethesda, MD: American Physiological Society, 1982; 555–631.

83. Pattengale PK, Holloszy JO. Augmentation of skeletal muscle myoglobin by a program of treadmill running. Am J Physiol 1967; **213**: 783–5.

84. Saltin B, Henriksson J, Nygaard E et al. Fiber types and metabolic potentials of skeletal muscles in sedentary man and endurance runners. Ann NY Acad Sci 1977; **301**: 3–29.

85. Widrick JJ, Trappe SW, Blaser CA et al. Isometric force and maximal shortening velocity of single muscle fibers from elite master runners. Am J Physiol 1996; **271** (2 Pt 1): C666–75.

◆86. Kraemer WJ, Adams K, Cafarelli E et al. American College of Sports Medicine position stand. Progression models in resistance training for healthy adults. Med Sci Sports Exerc 2002; **34**: 364–80.

87. Staron RS, Leonardi MJ, Karapondo DL et al. Strength and skeletal muscle adaptations in heavy-resistance-trained women after detraining and retraining. J Appl Physiol 1991; **70**: 631–40.

88. McCartney N. Acute responses to resistance training and safety. Med Sci Sports Exerc 1999; **31**: 31–7.

89. Widrick JJ, Stelzer JE, Shoepe TC, Garner DP. Functional properties of human muscle fibers after short-term resistance exercise training. Am J Physiol Regul Integr Comp Physiol 2002; **283**: 408–16.

90. Fitts RH, Widrick JJ. Muscle mechanics: adaptations with exercise-training. Exerc Sport Sci Rev 1996; **24**: 427–73.

91. Tesch PA. Skeletal muscle adaptations consequent to long-term heavy resistance exercise. Med Sci Sports Exerc 1988; **20** (5 Suppl.): S132–4.

92. Pincivero DM, Lephart SM, Karunakara RG. Effects of rest interval on isokinetic strength and functional performance after short-term high intensity training. Br J Sports Med 1997; **31**: 229–34.

93. Marcinik EJ, Potts J, Schlabach G et al. Effects of strength training on lactate threshold and endurance performance. Med Sci Sports Exerc 1991; **23**: 739–43.

94. Frontera WR, Meredith CN, O'Reilly KP, Evans WJ. Strength training and determinants of VO$_2$ max in older men. J Appl Physiol 1990; **68**: 329–33.

●95. Goldstein RS, Gort EH, Stubbing D et al. Randomised controlled trial of respiratory rehabilitation. Lancet 1994; **344**: 1394–7.

●96. Ries AL, Kaplan RM, Limberg TM, Prewitt LM. Effects of pulmonary rehabilitation on physiologic and psychosocial outcomes in patients with chronic obstructive pulmonary disease. Ann Intern Med 1995; **122**: 823–32.

●97. O'Donnell DE, McGuire M, Samis L, Webb KA. The impact of exercise reconditioning on breathlessness in severe chronic airflow limitation. Am J Respir Crit Care Med 1995; **152**: 2005–13.

98. Lacasse Y, Wong E, Guyatt GH et al. Meta-analysis of respiratory rehabilitation in chronic obstructive pulmonary disease. Lancet 1996; **348**: 1115–19.

◆99. Lacasse Y, Brosseau L, Milne S et al. Pulmonary rehabilitation for chronic obstructive pulmonary disease. Cochrane Database Syst Rev 2002; CD003793.

100. Cockcroft AE, Saunders MJ, Berry G. Randomised controlled trial of rehabilitation in chronic respiratory disability. Thorax 1981; **36**: 200–3.

101. Wijkstra PJ, van Altena R, Kraan J et al. Quality of life in patients with chronic obstructive pulmonary disease improves after rehabilitation at home. Eur Respir J 1994; **7**: 269–73.

102. Lake FR, Henderson K, Briffa T et al. Upper-limb and lower-limb exercise training in patients with chronic airflow obstruction. Chest 1990; **97**: 1077–82.

103. Strijbos JH, Postma DS, van Altena R et al. A comparison between an outpatient hospital-based pulmonary rehabilitation

program and a home-care pulmonary rehabilitation program in patients with COPD. A follow-up of 18 months. *Chest* 1996; **109**: 366–72.

●104. Maltais F, Leblanc P, Simard C *et al.* Skeletal muscle adaptation to endurance training in patients with chronic obstructive pulmonary disease. *Am J Respir Crit Care Med* 1996; **154**: 442–7.

105. Sala E, Roca J, Marrades RM *et al.* Effects of endurance training on skeletal muscle bioenergetics in chronic obstructive pulmonary disease. *Am J Respir Crit Care Med* 1999; **159**: 1726–34.

●106. Bernard S, Whittom F, Leblanc P *et al.* Aerobic and strength training in patients with COPD. *Am J Respir Crit Care Med* 1999; **159**: 896–901.

107. Bendstrup KE, Ingemann Jensen J, Holm S, Bengtsson B. Out-patient rehabilitation improves activities of daily living, quality of life and exercise tolerance in chronic obstructive pulmonary disease. *Eur Respir J* 1997; **10**: 2801–6.

108. Wijkstra PJ, Ten Vergert EM, van Altena R *et al.* Long term benefits of rehabilitation at home on quality of life and exercise tolerance in patients with chronic obstructive pulmonary disease. *Thorax* 1995; **50**: 824–8.

109. Griffiths TL, Burr ML, Campbell IA *et al.* Results at 1 year of outpatient multidisciplinary pulmonary rehabilitation: a randomised controlled trial. *Lancet* 2000; **355**: 362–8.

110. Maltais F, Leblanc P, Jobin J *et al.* Intensity of training and physiologic adaptation in patients with chronic obstructive pulmonary disease. *Am J Respir Crit Care Med* 1997; **155**: 555–61.

●111. Casaburi R, Porszasz J, Burns MR *et al.* Physiologic benefits of exercise training in rehabilitation of patients with severe chronic obstructive pulmonary disease. *Am J Respir Crit Care Med* 1997; **155**: 1541–51.

112. Belman MJ, Kendregan BA. Exercise training fails to increase skeletal muscle enzymes in patients with chronic obstructive lung disease. *Am Rev Respir Dis* 1981; **123**: 256–61.

113. Puente-Maestu L, Sanz ML, Sanz P, Cubillo JM *et al.* Comparison of effects of supervised versus self-monitored training programmes in patients with chronic obstructive pulmonary disease. *Eur Respir J* 2000; **15**: 517–25.

114. Coppoolse R, Schols AMWJ, Baarends EM *et al.* Interval versus continuous training in patients with severe COPD: a randomized clinical trial. *Eur Respir J* 1999; **14**: 258–63.

115. Simpson K, Killian K, McCartney N *et al.* Randomised controlled trial of weightlifting exercise in patients with chronic airflow limitation. *Thorax* 1992; **47**: 70–5.

●116. Clark CJ, Cochrane LM, Mackay E, Paton B. Skeletal muscle strength and endurance in patients with mild COPD and the effects of weight training. *Eur Respir J* 2000; **15**: 92–7.

●117. Clark CJ, Cochrane L, Mackay E. Low intensity peripheral muscle conditioning improves exercise tolerance and breathlessness in COPD. *Eur Respir J* 1996; **9**: 2590–6.

118. Spruit MA, Gosselink R, Troosters T *et al.* Resistance versus endurance training in patients with COPD and peripheral muscle weakness. *Eur Respir J* 2002; **19**: 1072–8.

●119. Ortega F, Toral J, Cejudo *et al.* Comparison of effects of strength and endurance training in patients with chronic obstructive pulmonary disease. *Am J Respir Crit Care Med* 2002; **166**: 669–74.

120. Heinonen A, Kannus P, Sievanen H *et al.* Randomised controlled trial of effect of high-impact exercise on selected risk factors for osteoporotic fractures. *Lancet* 1996; **348**: 1343–7.

121. Evans WJ. Exercise training guidelines for the elderly. *Med Sci Sport Exerc* 1999; **31**: 12–17.

122. McEvoy CE, Ensrud KE, Bender E *et al.* Association between corticosteroid use and vertebral fractures in older men with chronic obstructive pulmonary disease. *Am J Respir Crit Care Med* 1998; **157**: 704–9.

123. Debigaré R, Maltais F, Whittom F *et al.* Feasibility and efficacy of home exercise training before lung volume reduction. *J Cardiopulm Rehab* 1999; **19**: 235–41.

124. Grobois J-M, Douay B, Fortin F *et al.* Effets de la réhabilitation respiratoire en ambulatoire sur la tolérance et la qualité de vie des patients atteints de bronchopneumopathie chronique obstructive. *Rev Mal Resp* 1996; **13**: 61–7.

125. Guyatt GH, Berman LB, Townsend M. Long-term outcome after respiratory rehabilitation. *Can Med Assoc J* 1987; **137**: 1089–95.

Assessment of respiratory function during sleep in chronic lung disease

WALTER T. McNICHOLAS

INTRODUCTION

Sleep has many effects on breathing, mostly negative, which can have an adverse impact on ventilation and gas exchange in sleeping patients with chronic lung disease. The assessment of respiratory function during sleep in clinical practice is generally done by non-invasive means, and needs to be as non-intrusive as possible in order to minimize adverse effects on sleep quality from the measurements themselves. Prior to a detailed discussion of the various techniques employed in clinical practice, it is appropriate to briefly review the various effects of sleep on respiratory function in health and disease.

EFFECTS OF SLEEP ON RESPIRATION

Sleep is a complex process associated with recurring cycles of non-rapid eye movement (non-REM) and REM sleep, each cycle lasting 90–120 min. Electroencephalographic (EEG) signals differ from wakefulness, particularly during non-REM sleep. The exact function of sleep is unclear, but there is no doubt that it is an essential restorative process, as is evident from experiments that have examined the physical and behavioural consequences of sleep deprivation.

The effects of sleep on breathing include a mild degree of hypoventilation with consequent hypercapnia, and a diminished responsiveness to respiratory stimuli, which in normal individuals have no adverse impact. However, in patients with chronic lung disease such as chronic obstructive pulmonary disease (COPD), these physiological changes during sleep may have a detrimental effect on gas exchange, and episodes of profound hypoxaemia may develop, particularly during REM sleep (1), which may predispose to death at night, particularly during exacerbations (2). Furthermore, COPD has an adverse impact on sleep quality itself (3), which may contribute to the complaints of fatigue and lethargy that are well recognized features of the condition (4).

Sleep is associated with a number of effects on respiration, including changes in central respiratory control, airways resistance and muscular contractility.

Central respiratory effects

The onset of sleep is associated with a diminished responsiveness of the respiratory centre to chemical and mechanical inputs, and to a major reduction in the stimulant effects of cortical inputs (5,6). These effects are more pronounced as sleep deepens, particularly during REM sleep. Ventilatory responsiveness to both hypoxia and hypercapnia is diminished. Furthermore, the respiratory muscles' responsiveness to respiratory centre outputs are also diminished during sleep, particularly REM sleep, although the diaphragm is less affected than the accessory muscles in this regard. There is a decrease in minute ventilation ($\dot{V}_E$) during non-REM sleep (7), predominantly due to a reduction in tidal volume, which is associated with a rise in end-tidal $P\text{CO}_2$. However, part of this hypoventilation during sleep is probably a response to the lower metabolic rate during sleep, since oxygen consumption and carbon dioxide production diminish during sleep compared with wakefulness (8). During REM sleep, both tidal volume and respiratory frequency are much more variable than in non-REM sleep, particularly during phasic REM, when there are bursts of rapid eye movement, as opposed to tonic REM where eye movements tend to be absent (7). Minute ventilation is lower during phasic REM than during tonic REM sleep.

These physiological changes are not associated with any clinically significant deterioration in gas exchange among normal subjects, but may produce profound hypoxaemia in patients with respiratory insufficiency such as COPD (1). This finding is principally due to the fact that normal subjects have P_aO_2 levels on the flat portion of the oxyhaemoglobin dissociation curve, and thus modest falls in P_aO_2 as a consequence of hypoventilation during sleep are not associated with significant falls in S_aO_2. However, COPD patients tend to have P_aO_2 levels at or near the steep portion of the oxyhaemoglobin dissociation curve, particularly during acute exacerbations. Thus, equivalent modest falls in P_aO_2 during sleep may result in clinically significant falls in S_aO_2 (9). The drop in S_aO_2 during sleep in COPD is further compounded by the increased work of breathing associated with chronic airflow limitation, which probably also aggravates the effects of the reduction in respiratory drive during sleep.

Airway resistance

Upper airway resistance increases during sleep compared with wakefulness (10), which predisposes to upper airway occlusion and obstructive sleep apnoea in susceptible individuals. In addition, lower airway patency may be compromised during sleep. The majority of normal subjects have circadian changes in airway calibre with mild nocturnal bronchoconstriction (11), which may be exaggerated in patients with obstructive airways disease, particularly asthma (12). Furthermore, cholinergic tone has a normal circadian rhythm, with higher levels during the sleeping hours, which may contribute to this nocturnal bronchoconstriction.

Rib cage and abdominal contribution to breathing

In the supine resting state, breathing is predominantly a function of diaphragmatic contraction (13). During non-REM sleep there is an increased rib cage contribution to breathing and an associated increase in the respiratory electromyographic (EMG) activity of intercostal muscles (14), with respiratory activity of the diaphragm being little increased or unchanged. The resulting expansion of the rib cage may improve mechanical efficiency of diaphragmatic contraction by optimizing the length and/or radius of curvature of the diaphragm (15). This increased efficiency of the diaphragm is reflected in an increase in the transdiaphragmatic pressure developed for a given level of diaphragmatic EMG activity.

In contrast, a reduction in rib cage contribution to breathing has been reported during REM sleep compared with wakefulness, due to a marked reduction in intercostal muscle activity (16). Diaphragmatic EMG activity is substantially increased, while transdiaphragmatic pressure falls significantly, which implies a decrease in diaphragmatic efficiency, a pattern opposite to that seen during non-REM sleep.

Neuromuscular changes during sleep

The loss of stimulant input from the cerebral cortex is an important contributor to the hypoventilation of sleep described above, but in addition, during REM sleep, there is a marked loss of tonic activity in the upper airway and intercostal muscles. There appears to be supraspinal inhibition of gamma motoneurons (and, to a lesser extent, alpha motoneurons), in addition to pre-synaptic inhibition of afferent terminals from muscle spindles. The diaphragm, being driven almost entirely by alpha motoneurons and with far fewer spindles than intercostal muscles, has little tonic (postural) activity and, therefore, escapes reduction of this particular drive during REM sleep (5). This helps to explain the increase in abdominal contribution to breathing in REM sleep.

The fall in intercostal muscle activity assumes particular clinical significance in patients who are particularly dependent on accessory muscle activity to maintain ventilation, such as those with COPD (17), since hyperinflation of the lungs results in flattening of the diaphragm and an associated reduction in the efficiency of diaphragmatic contraction. Diaphragmatic efficiency is further compromised by the supine posture since the pressure of abdominal contents against the diaphragm by gravitational forces contrasts with the effect of gravity in the erect posture, which tends to move abdominal contents away from the diaphragm. This pressure impairs diaphragmatic contraction during inspiration, since this moves the diaphragm in a caudal direction to produce lung expansion. Patients with neuromuscular weakness are also adversely affected by these physiological effects of sleep, and profound desaturation during sleep is common in such patients. REM sleep tends to be suppressed in these patients as an adaptive response to minimize desaturation and prognosis is particularly poor in patients with involvement of the diaphragm (18).

Functional residual capacity

A modest, but statistically significant, fall in functional residual capacity (FRC) has been noted in healthy sleeping adults in both non-REM and REM sleep (19). This fall is not considered sufficient to cause significant ventilation/perfusion mismatching in healthy subjects, but could do so, with resulting hypoxaemia, in patients with chronic lung disease. Possible mechanisms responsible for this reduction in FRC include respiratory muscle hypotonia, cephalad displacement of the diaphragm, and a decrease in lung compliance. This fall in FRC probably contributes to the fall in S_aO_2 seen in patients with COPD through a worsening of ventilation/perfusion

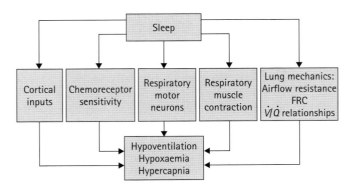

Figure 10.1 *Schematic diagram of the effects of sleep on respiration. In each case, sleep has a negative influence, which has the overall impact of producing hypoventilation and/or hypoxaemia and hypercapnia. FRC, functional residual capacity; $\dot{V}/\dot{Q}$, ventilation/perfusion ratio.*

relationships, which assumes particular significance during acute exacerbations where such relationships are already compromised.

Overall effects during sleep

The above account illustrates the complex effect of sleep on respiratory function, with the overall trend being a reduction in ventilation compared with wakefulness. In normal individuals, arterial blood gases change little from wakefulness to sleep. However, when subjects with daytime hypoxaemia, due to underlying respiratory disease, develop abnormal breathing patterns during sleep, life-threatening hypoxaemia may occur. This partly results from the fact that a similar drop in P_aO_2 will be associated with a much greater drop in S_aO_2, when the subject is already hypoxaemic and on the steep part of the oxyhaemoglobin dissociation curve. Furthermore, the changes in rib cage and abdominal contribution to breathing, and the changes in FRC, may result in worsening ventilation/perfusion relationships, which will also aggravate any tendency to hypoxaemia. In addition, the reduction in ventilatory drives and changes in breathing pattern during sleep attenuate the compensatory hyperventilation seen during wakefulness in these patients. This effect on ventilation is particularly seen during periods of REM sleep. A schematic outline of the effects of sleep on respiration is given in Fig. 10.1.

SLEEP IN SOME SPECIFIC CHRONIC DISORDERS ASSOCIATED WITH RESPIRATORY IMPAIRMENT

Chronic obstructive pulmonary disease

Patients with COPD are adversely affected by sleep in different ways. First, as indicated above, the physiological changes that occur during sleep predispose to abnormalities in ventilation

and gas exchange. Second, sleep quality is impaired in patients with COPD, which probably represents a significant factor in the complaints of fatigue and lethargy frequently exhibited by these patients.

Sleep-related hypoxaemia and hypercapnia are well recognized in COPD, particularly during REM sleep, and may contribute to the development of cor pulmonale (20) and nocturnal death (2). These abnormalities are most common in 'blue-bloater' type patients, who also have a greater degree of awake hypoxaemia and hypercapnia than 'pink-puffer' type patients. A previous report from this department demonstrated that patients who die in hospital with an exacerbation of COPD are significantly more likely to die at night, in contrast to patients who die from stroke or neoplasm (2). The excess nocturnal mortality was particularly seen in patients with severe hypoxaemia and hypercapnia. Many patients with awake P_aO_2 levels in the mildly hypoxaemic range can also develop substantial nocturnal oxygen desaturation, which appears to predispose to the development of pulmonary hypertension (21).

The principal mechanism of disordered gas exchange during sleep in COPD is the hypoventilation, a normal feature of sleep, which has a disproportionate effect in hypoxaemic patients because of their position on the oxyhaemoglobin dissociation curve (22, 23). In addition, the physiological reduction in accessory muscle contribution to breathing, particularly during REM sleep, decreases FRC, worsens ventilation/perfusion relationships, and further aggravates hypoxaemia.

The mechanisms of hypoxaemia during sleep in COPD contrast with those during exercise, where the normal physiological increase in ventilation and in lung volumes during exercise are limited in COPD because of the effects of increased airflow resistance, inadequate ventilatory response and lack of reduction in dead space. These factors combine to cause relative hypoventilation and $\dot{V}/\dot{Q}$ disturbances, leading to hypoxaemia in some patients (24).

Patients with COPD desaturate more than twice as much during sleep than during maximal exercise (22), which contrasts with the findings in patients with interstitial lung disease, who develop greater desaturation during exercise than sleep (25). This greater O_2 desaturation during sleep supports the finding that in patients with COPD, the demand for coronary blood flow during episodes of nocturnal hypoxaemia can be transiently as great as during maximal exercise (26). This increased myocardial oxygen demand may be a factor in the nocturnal arrhythmias (27) and the higher nocturnal death rate among patients with COPD (2), particularly since the level of exercise achieved during these studies was much greater than patients would normally reach during daily activities.

Sleep quality is impaired in patients with COPD (3), which is likely to be an important factor in the chronic fatigue, lethargy and overall impairment in quality of life described by these patients (4). Sleep tends to be fragmented, with frequent arousals and diminished amounts of slow-wave and REM sleep. Unfortunately, sleep impairment is an aspect of COPD that is frequently ignored by many physicians, even in research protocols designed to assess the impact of COPD on quality of life (28, 29). This aspect assumes particular importance in the context of assessing the impact of pharmacological therapy on quality of life in patients with COPD (30), since pharmacological agents that improve sleep quality in COPD (31) are likely to have a beneficial clinical impact over and above that simply associated with improvements in lung mechanics and gas exchange, particularly in terms of fatigue and overall energy levels.

Thoracic cage disorders

The maintenance of effective ventilation is dependent on adequate lung expansion in response to diaphragmatic contraction. Disorders of the thoracic cage may interfere with this process, resulting in hypoventilation, particularly during sleep. Thoracic cage disorders which have been associated with respiratory insufficiency include kyphoscoliosis (32) and thoracoplasty (33). Oxygen desaturation is most pronounced during REM sleep, because of the marked reduction of accessory muscle contribution to breathing, and night-time saturation levels closely parallel the awake levels, similar to COPD. Sleep apnoea is an uncommon cause of hypoxaemia during sleep in these patients.

Factors that contribute to respiratory insufficiency in kyphoscoliosis include ventilation/perfusion inequality, alveolar hypoventilation, increased work of breathing and reduced surface area for gas diffusion. Thoracoplasty causes an additional restrictive ventilatory defect as a consequence of pleural thickening and thoracic cage deformity, and is associated with a variable degree of scoliosis. Furthermore, airflow obstruction has been reported as a common long-term consequence of thoracoplasty, which does not appear to be related to smoking history (34). The mechanism of this airflow obstruction is uncertain, but may relate to diffuse bronchial wall fibrosis and/or emphysema.

Thoracic cage disorders also appear to have an adverse effect on respiratory muscle contractility, since effective therapy of the hypoventilation and associated respiratory insufficiency have been shown to improve respiratory muscle strength (35). However, this phenomenon may be a consequence of chronic hypoxaemia and hypercapnia, rather than a primary feature of the condition.

Neurologic and neuromuscular disorders

A variety of neurological disorders have been associated with respiratory insufficiency, particularly during sleep. These disorders can affect the brainstem respiratory centre, as outlined above, or alternatively could affect the peripheral nervous system, resulting in impaired transmission of the respiratory centre output to the muscles of respiration, particularly the diaphragm. Neurological disorders that can affect the brainstem include stroke (36), and those involving the peripheral nervous system include multiple sclerosis, polio, traumatic

paralysis such as cervical spine fracture, and motor neuron disease (37–40). Each condition is associated with a variable degree of hypoventilation, which is exacerbated by sleep because of the physiological effects of sleep on ventilation as outlined above.

Neuromuscular disorders, particularly Duchenne's and other forms of muscular dystrophy, are also typically associated with hypoventilation, which becomes more severe as the disease progresses, particularly during sleep (41, 42). Muscular dystrophy produces respiratory insufficiency because of progressive degeneration of the muscles of respiration, and respiratory failure is the major cause of death in this condition, although cardiomyopathy due to degeneration of cardiac muscle is also a common finding (43). The deterioration in awake blood gases has been found in some reports to parallel the decline in lung function as measured by spirometry and maximum inspiratory pressures (44). Although a progressive and ultimately fatal condition, patients with Duchenne's muscular dystrophy can be kept alive for many years by appropriate modalities of assisted ventilation once respiratory failure has developed.

Sleep-related hypoxaemia in muscular dystrophy is predominantly found in REM sleep, because of the loss of accessory muscle contribution to breathing in the setting of diaphragmatic weakness. REM-related desaturation is also frequently associated with recurring apnoea and hypopnoea. These apnoeas are most commonly central in nature, but obstructive apnoea could develop if upper airway muscle contraction was impaired (42). Traditional non-invasive methods of distinguishing obstructive from central apnoeas in this condition may be inadequate because of the reduced respiratory effort associated with muscle weakness, and it is possible that some apparently central apnoeas are obstructive in origin, but appear central because of poor respiratory effort. Coexisting sleep apnoea is particularly likely in obese patients, and diagnostic sleep studies may be necessary to characterize the aetiology of sleep-related hypoxaemia, depending on the clinical features.

ASSESSMENT OF RESPIRATORY FUNCTION DURING SLEEP

The assessment of respiratory function during sleep should take into account the changes in ventilation and lung mechanics outlined above in addition to the consequent effects on gas exchange. In selected cases, an assessment of sleep stages may also be indicated in order to relate changes in respiratory function to particular sleep stages. Consideration should also be given to the intrusiveness of particular recordings since the more intrusive the measurement, the greater the likelihood of sleep disturbance, which lessens the value of the measurement as an indicator of sleep-related changes. For example, precise measurements of ventilation during sleep can be obtained from a pneumotachograph linked to a tight-fitting facemask. However, this technique is both uncomfortable and cumbersome and is generally reserved for research studies where an accurate measurement of ventilation is essential.

Gas exchange

OXYGEN SATURATION (S_aO_2)

The simplest and most widely used assessment of respiration during sleep is oxygen saturation (S_aO_2). Oximeter devices are now commonplace in most hospital settings and are suitable for use in the home setting. S_aO_2 recordings can frequently distinguish the underlying cause of oxygen desaturation during sleep, particularly hypoventilation and recurring apnoea. Sleep apnoea produces a typical sawtooth pattern of oxygen desaturation (Fig. 10.2), where apnoea-associated desaturation is followed immediately by resaturation during post-apnoeic hyperventilation. Sleep-induced hypoventilation, on the other hand, is associated with periods of sustained oxygen desaturation, particularly during REM sleep. However, assessment of these desaturation patterns generally requires a printout of the S_aO_2 record over a period of time. Several reports have demonstrated that overnight S_aO_2 recording is relatively accurate in assessing the presence and severity of sleep apnoea (45–47), but this accuracy diminishes considerably with oximeters that have a relatively long averaging time for storing S_aO_2 data, since such averaging may obscure the typical pattern of oxygen desaturation and resaturation that is typical of sleep apnoea.

CARBON DIOXIDE TENSION (P_{CO_2})

P_{CO_2} is more difficult to monitor during sleep than S_aO_2 and is generally done by means of a transcutaneous device. Such devices provide a reasonably accurate determination of arterial P_{CO_2} (P_aCO_2), but the transcutaneous P_{CO_2} ($P_{tc}CO_2$) is higher than the P_aCO_2 (48). Transcutaneous capnometers must be used with caution during overnight sleep monitoring since many can cause skin burns if the recording electrode is left in place for more than 4–6 hours. This potential side-effect is less likely with the latest monitoring devices.

Ventilation and lung mechanics

A wide variety of measures have been employed in monitoring ventilation and lung mechanics during sleep in patients with chronic lung disease, ranging from pneumotachography to intrathoracic pressure recordings and diaphragmatic EMG. However, most of these recordings are more appropriate to research studies because of their invasiveness. A number of non-invasive techniques are available and widely used in clinical sleep studies.

Airflow can be estimated from oronasal recordings of changes in temperature, CO_2 or nasal pressure. All of these measures are qualitative, rather than quantitative, although recordings of pressure changes give some reasonable estimate of quantitative airflow (49). Movements of the rib cage and abdomen can also be monitored non-invasively, usually by inductance plethysmography, and some such devices, when suitably calibrated, can give a measurement of tidal volume (50).

ASSESSMENT OF SLEEP QUALITY

Sleep stages are assessed by polysomnography (PSG), which requires continuous recording of EEG, eye movements and chin EMG (51). These recordings are particularly useful in relating changes in gas exchange to sleep state, particularly REM sleep. Such recordings require the resources of a full sleep laboratory and are labour-intensive, and should thus be reserved for selected cases. Full PSG sleep studies are not routinely indicated in patients with COPD or other chronic respiratory disorder associated with respiratory insufficiency, particularly since the awake P_aO_2 level provides a good indicator of the likelihood of nocturnal oxygen desaturation (52). Sleep studies are only indicated where there is a clinical suspicion of an associated sleep apnoea syndrome or manifestations of hypoxaemia not explained by the awake P_aO_2 level, such as cor pulmonale or polycythaemia. In most situations where sleep studies are indicated, a limited study focusing on respiration and gas exchange should be sufficient.

CONCLUSION

Chronic respiratory disorders are commonly associated with deterioration in gas exchange during sleep, to an extent greater than that during maximum exercise. Thus, it is important to consider this possibility in all patients with chronic respiratory insufficiency and to perform appropriate monitoring during sleep. In most such cases, limited monitoring that focuses primarily on gas exchange should be sufficient and full PSG should only be required in highly selected cases.

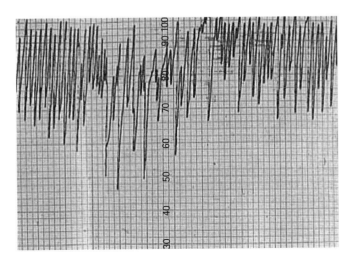

Figure 10.2 *Continuous tracing of oxygen saturation (S_aO_2) in a patient with sleep apnoea syndrome. Note the repetitive dips in S_aO_2 during sleep, which is typical of recurring apnoeas.*

Key points

- Sleep has many effects on breathing, mostly negative, which can have an adverse impact on ventilation and gas exchange in patients with chronic lung disease.
- Patients may experience deterioration in gas exchange during sleep to an extent greater than during maximum exercise.
- It is important to consider this possibility in all patients with chronic respiratory insufficiency and to perform appropriate monitoring during sleep when sleep-related breathing disturbances are suspected.
- In most such cases, limited monitoring that focuses primarily on gas exchange should be sufficient and full polysomnography should only be required in highly selected cases.
- The assessment of respiratory function during sleep in clinical practice is generally done by non-invasive means.
- Overnight monitoring of oxygen saturation (S_aO_2) provides very useful information and can often distinguish between sleep apnoea and hypoventilation, particularly when the recording device provides a continuous printout of the S_aO_2.

REFERENCES

1. Douglas NJ, Calverley PMA, Leggett RJE et al. Transient hypoxaemia during sleep in chronic bronchitis and emphysema. Lancet 1979; 1: 1–4.
2. McNicholas WT, Fitzgerald MX. Nocturnal death among patients with chronic bronchitis and emphysema. Br Med J 1984; 289: 878.
3. Cormick W, Olson LG, Hensley MJ, Saunders NA. Nocturnal hypoxaemia and quality of sleep in patients with chronic obstructive lung disease. Thorax 1986; 41: 846–54.
4. Breslin E, Van der Schans C, Breubink S et al. Perception of fatigue and quality of life in patients with COPD. Chest 1998; 114: 958–64.
5. Phillipson EA. Control of breathing during sleep. Am Rev Respir Dis 1978; 118: 909–39.
6. Phillipson EA, Duffin J, Cooper JD. Critical dependence of respiratory rhythmicity on metabolic CO_2 load. J Appl Physiol 1981; 50: 45–54.
7. Stradling JR, Chadwick GA, Frew AJ. Changes in ventilation and its components in normal subjects during sleep. Thorax 1985; 40: 364–70.
8. White DP, Weil JV, Zwillich CW. Metabolic rate and breathing during sleep. J Appl Physiol 1985; 59: 384–91.
9. Caterall JR, Calverley PMA, McNee W et al. Mechanism of transient nocturnal hypoxemia in hypoxic chronic bronchitis and emphysema. J Appl Physiol 1985; 59: 1698–703.
10. Hudgel DW, Martin RJ, Johnson BJ, Hill P. Mechanics of the respiratory system and breathing pattern during sleep in normal humans. J Appl Physiol 1984; 56: 133–7.
11. Kerr HD. Diurnal variation of respiratory function independent of air quality. Arch Environ Health 1973; 26: 144–53.
12. Hetzel MR, Clark TJH. Comparison of normal and asthmatic circadian rhythms in peak expiratory flow rate. Thorax 1980; 35: 732–8.
13. Sharp JT, Goldberg NB, Druz WS, Danon J. Relative contributions of rib cage and abdomen to breathing in normal subjects. J Appl Physiol 1975; 39: 608–18.
14. Lopes JM, Tabachnik E, Muller NL et al. Total airway resistance and respiratory muscle activity during sleep. J Appl Physiol 1983; 54: 773–7.
15. Goldman MD, Grassino A, Mead J, Sears TA. Mechanics of the human diaphragm during voluntary contraction: dynamics. J Appl Physiol 1978; 44: 840–8.
16. Tusiewicz K, Moldofsky H, Bryan AC, Bryan MH. Mechanics of the ribcage and diaphragm during sleep. J Appl Physiol 1977; 43: 600–2.
17. Johnson MW, Remmers JE. Accessory muscle activity during sleep in chronic obstructive pulmonary disease. J Appl Physiol 1984; 57: 1011–17.
18. Arnulf I, Similowski T, Salachas F et al. Sleep disorders and diaphragmatic function in patients with amyotrophic lateral sclerosis. Am J Respir Crit Care Med 2000 March; 161(3 Part 1): 849–56.
19. Hudgel DW, Devadetta P. Decrease in functional residual capacity during sleep in normal humans. J Appl Physiol 1984; 57: 1319–22.
20. Demarco FJJR, Wynne JW, Block AJ et al. Oxygen desaturation during sleep as a determinant of the 'blue and bloated' syndrome. Chest 1981; 79: 621–5.
21. Fletcher EC, Luckett RA, Miller T et al. Pulmonary vascular hemodynamics in chronic lung disease patients with and without oxyhemoglobin desaturation during sleep. Chest 1989; 95: 757–66.
●22. Mulloy E, McNicholas WT. Ventilation and gas exchange during sleep and exercise in patients with severe COPD. Chest 1996; 109: 387–94.
23. Stradling JR, Lane DJ. Nocturnal hypoxaemia in chronic obstructive pulmonary disease. Clin Sci 1983; 64: 213–22.
24. Gallagher CG. Exercise and chronic obstructive pulmonary disease. Med Clin North Am 1990; 74: 619–41.
25. Midgren B, Hansson L, Erikkson L et al. Oxygen desaturation during sleep and exercise in patients with interstitial lung disease. Thorax 1987; 42: 353–6.
26. Shepard JW, Schweitzer PK, Kellar CA et al. Myocardial stress. Exercise versus sleep in patients with COPD. Chest 1984; 86: 366–74.
27. Flick MR, Block AJ. Nocturnal vs. diurnal arrhythmias in patients with chronic obstructive pulmonary disease. Chest 1979; 75: 8–11.
28. Tsukino M, Nishimura K, Ikeda A et al. Physiological factors that determine the health-related quality of life in patients with COPD. Chest 1996; 110: 896–903.
29. Ketelaars CAJ, Schlosser MAG, Mostert R et al. Determinants of health-related quality of life in patients with chronic obstructive pulmonary disease. Thorax 1996; 51: 29–43.
30. Jones PW, Bosh TK. Quality of life changes in COPD patients treated with salmeterol. Am J Respir Crit Care Med 1997; 155: 1283–9.
31. Martin RJ, Bucher BL, Smith P et al. Effect of ipratropium bromide treatment on oxygen saturation and sleep quality in COPD. Chest 1999; 115: 1338–45.
32. Sawicka EH, Branthwaite MA. Respiration during sleep in kyphoscoliosis. Thorax 1987; 42: 801–8.
33. Jackson M, Smith I, King M, Shneerson J. Long term non-invasive domiciliary assisted ventilation for respiratory failure following thoracoplasty. Thorax 1994; 49: 915–19.
34. Philips MS, Miller MR, Kinnear WJM et al. Importance of airflow obstruction after thoracoplasty. Thorax 1987; 42: 348–52.
35. Goldstein RS, De Rosie JA, Avendano MA, Dolmage TE. Influence of noninvasive positive pressure ventilation on inspiratory muscles. Chest 1991; 99: 408–15.
36. Vingerhoets F, Bogousslavsky J. Respiratory dysfunction in stroke. Clin Chest Med 1994; 15: 729–37.

37. Howard RS, Wiles CM, Hirsch NP *et al*. Respiratory involvement in multiple sclerosis. *Brain* 1992; **115**: 479–94.

38. Bach JR. Management of post-polio respiratory sequelae. *Ann N Y Acad Sci* 1995; **753**: 96–102.

39. Loh LC, Hughes JMB, Newsom-Davis J. Gas exchange problems in bilateral diaphragm paralysis. *Bull Europ Physipat Respir* 1979: **15**(Suppl.): 137–43.

●40. Howard RS, Wiles CM, Loh L. Respiratory complications and their management in motor neuron disease. *Brain* 1989; **112**: 1155–70.

41. Smith PE, Calverley PMA, Edwards RH. Hypoxaemia during sleep in Duchenne muscular dystrophy. *Am Rev Respir Dis* 1988; **137**: 884–8.

42. Smith PEM, Calverley PMA, Edwards RHT *et al*. Practical problems in the respiratory care of patients with muscular dystrophy. *N Engl J Med* 1987; **316**: 1197–205.

43. Gilroy J, Cahalan JL, Berman R, Newman R. Cardiac and pulmonary complications in Duchenne's progressive muscular dystrophy. *Circulation* 1963; **27**: 484–93.

44. Baydur A, Gilgoff I, Prentice W *et al*. Decline in respiratory function and experience with long-term assisted ventilation in advanced Duchenne's muscular dystrophy. *Chest* 1990; **97**: 884–9.

45. Levy P, Pepin JL, Deschaux C *et al*. Accuracy of oximetry for detection of respiratory disturbances in sleep apnea syndrome. *Chest* 1996; **109**: 395–9.

46. Gyulay S, Olson LG, Hensley MJ *et al*. A comparison of clinical assessment and home oximetry in the diagnosis of obstructive sleep apnea. *Am Rev Respir Dis* 1993; **147**: 50–3.

47. Epstein LJ, Dorlac GR. Cost-effectiveness analysis of nocturnal oximetry as a method of screening for sleep apnea–hypopnea syndrome. *Chest* 1998; **113**: 97–103.

48. McLellan PA, Goldstein RS, Ramcharan V, Rebuck AS. Transcutaneous carbon dioxide monitoring. *Am Rev Respir Dis* 1981; **124**: 199–201.

49. Montserrat J, Farre R, Ballester E *et al*. Evaluation of nasal prongs for estimating nasal flow. *Am J Respir Crit Care Med* 1997; **155**: 211–15.

50. Chadha TS, Watson H, Birch S *et al*. Validation of respiratory inductive plethysmography using different calibration procedures. *Am Rev Respir Dis* 1982; **125**: 644–9.

51. Rechtschaffen A, Kales A 1968 *A Manual of Standardized Terminology, Techniques and Scoring System for Sleep Stages of Human Subjects*. Washington, DC: US Government Printing Office, Public Health Service.

●52. Connaughton JJ, Caterall JR, Elton RA *et al*. Do sleep studies contribute to the management of patients with severe chronic obstructive pulmonary disease? *Am Rev Resp Dis* 1988; **138**: 341–4.

11

Cardiopulmonary interaction during sleep

MATTHEW T. NAUGHTON

INTRODUCTION

As we need 8–9 h sleep per night, ~30 per cent of our life is spent asleep. During this time, marked changes in physiology occur which can be captured with sleep monitoring. As such, a greater understanding of the mechanisms responsible for the circadian aspects of common disorders such as asthma, chronic obstructive pulmonary disease (COPD), congestive heart failure (CHF), ischaemic heart disease (IHD) and stroke is possible. Indeed, sleep places a greater burden upon the cardiopulmonary function than exercise (1) in such disease groups. Sleep is a time of greatest mortality in COPD (2). Cardiovascular events occur with greatest frequency within the hours of sleep, at around 9am (3), in those in whom underlying sleep-disordered breathing is present (4) or an effect of sleep state upon cardiac event is suspected (5). Shift work is associated with increased cardiovascular risk (6). Thus sleep has an important role in cardiopulmonary function.

NORMAL SLEEP

Sleep is a state of neurocardiopulmonary interaction accompanied by a fall in body temperature of ~1°C (which allows monitoring of the sleep–wake 'circadian' pattern) and elevated plasma melatonin levels. Darkness sensed by the suprachiasmic nucleus via the optic nerve causes the release of melatonin and the cascade of hormonal and neuroendocrine changes that characterize sleep (7).

Sleep can be further staged by polysomnography (PSG) into six characteristic levels: non-rapid eye movement (non-REM) stages 1–4 and phasic and tonic REM.

Changes from wake to sleep result in muscle hypotonia and endocrine changes (e.g. rises in plasma histamine and growth hormone and falls in cortisol and catecholamines). Skeletal muscle hypotonia, greatest in REM, affects mainly the muscles of posture and is under the control of the locus coeruleus nucleus.

Normal ventilation during sleep

During wakefulness, respiration is integrated to allow complex activities such as speech and swallowing and to respond to increased demands such as exercise. Such wakefulness control is due to waking neural, cortical and metabolic-chemical (effects of P_aCO_2, pH and P_aO_2 on chemoreceptors) drives. During non-REM sleep, respiration is controlled by the metabolic-chemical drive. During REM sleep, metabolic and cortical drives contribute.

From the upright to the supine position, when awake, the ventilatory response to hypoxia diminishes and the response to hypercapnia increases (8). Thus the body is controlled more by hypercapnia and is permissive of mild hypoxaemia when supine (8).

At sleep onset, with the transition from wakefulness to non-REM sleep, the hypoxic and hypercapnic ventilatory responses are diminished (9, 10), thereby elevating the threshold of metabolic drive required to stimulate ventilation (1–2 mmHg rise in P_aCO_2), and upper airway resistance increases (11). Tidal volume falls from being awake to non-REM to REM sleep (0.55 to 0.43 to 0.43 L) as does minute ventilation (from 6.8 to 6.1 to 6.6 L/min), whereas respiratory rate is unchanged (12). Functional residual capacity falls and mild hypoxaemia and hypercapnia result.

Bronchial diameter (and thus markers of airflow obstruction, e.g. peak expiratory flow rate) have a minimal diameter at around 4am and maximal diameter at around 6pm (13). The supine posture has an additional effect of reducing end-expiratory lung volume (EELV) and increasing airway resistance (14).

Normal cardiac autonomic control

The nucleus tractus solitarius receives input from chemo- and baroreceptors to control efferent autonomic and cardiopulmonary activity. It also influences changes in activity from wakefulness to sleep.

From wakefulness to non-REM sleep, sympathetic nervous activity (SNA) is reduced and parasympathetic nervous activity (PNA) is increased (15). From non-REM to REM sleep, SNA to skeletal muscles increases to waking levels (15). Low-frequency power, measured by ECG spectral analysis, indicative of cardiac SNA, is reduced with the transition from wakefulness to non-REM sleep, and increases in REM sleep. High-frequency power and baroreceptor sensitivity, indicative of PNA, are increased with the transition from wakefulness to non-REM sleep, and reduced again in REM sleep (16, 17).

Overall, there is an approximately 10–15 per cent reduction in stroke volume, heart rate and systemic blood pressure during non-REM sleep compared with wakefulness (18). Regional blood flow is altered such that, during REM sleep, blood flow is negligible to peripheral skeletal muscles but greatest to the brain (19).

Trinder et al. (20) described PNA being mostly influenced by the circadian system and SNA by the sleep/wake system. Thus, PNA increases during the evening despite the state of sleep (e.g. during a night shift) whereas SNA is only withdrawn with sleep onset.

Effects of exercise on normal sleep

In a questionnaire-based study of 1600 middle-aged healthy subjects, exercise was named the most important factor that promoted sleep, above reading, bathing and psychological factors (21), particularly if early (4–8pm) rather than late (after 8pm). In addition, those subjects who reported poor sleep quality exercised less than once per week, whereas those reporting good sleep quality exercised more than three times per week. Comparisons of trained athletes with sedentary controls has shown an increase in slow-wave sleep in the athletes (22). Whether an 'exercise intervention' is sufficient to improve sleep objectively remains contentious (23).

SLEEP DEPRIVATION

Loss of sleep (e.g. <5 h per night regularly) is an important cause of impaired mood and cognitive performance (24, 25). Neuropsychological skills following 18 h of sleep deprivation are equivalent to those performed with a blood alcohol reading of 0.08 g/dL (26).

Sleep deprivation has been associated with impaired growth hormone release (27) and insulin resistance (28). In healthy humans, $\dot{V}_{O_2,peak}$ during exercise is reduced (~7 per cent) following 64 h of sleep deprivation (29). Sleep deprivation in rats (3–4 weeks) causes elevations in SNA, anabolic status, sepsis, CHF and premature death (30). Fragmented sleep, as opposed to pure sleep deprivation, is similarly detrimental (31).

SLEEP-DISORDERED BREATHING

The term sleep-disordered breathing (SDB) is used to encompass abnormal breathing patterns during sleep due to:

- an obstructed upper airway (e.g. snoring, obstructive sleep apnoeas [OSAs])
- respiratory pump failure (e.g. myopathies)
- disorders of respiratory control (e.g. periodic breathing and non-hypercapnic central sleep apnoea).

Obstructive sleep–disordered breathing

A spectrum of obstructive SDB exists from socially disturbing snoring through to life-threatening OSA with hypercapnia. Snoring is a sound generated in the oropharynx, whereas a hypopnoea is a reduction in ventilation for at least 10 s sufficient to cause a drop in S_pO_2 (2–4 per cent) and/or an arousal from sleep. An obstructive apnoea is defined as the absence of ventilation for at least 10 s.

AETIOLOGY

Between the hard palate and the epiglottis, there is an absence of structural bony or cartilaginous support, such that collapse may occur on inspiration (when the airway is sucked closed) or on expiration (when the airway is passively closed) whilst vigorous yet futile inspiratory efforts occur. Bony or soft tissue anatomical abnormalities plus functional abnormalities contribute to collapse.

Bony abnormalities include retrognathia, micrognathia, high arched palate, narrow maxilla, maxillary insufficiency and small mouth opening (e.g. <2.5 cm). Soft tissue abnormalities include nasal turbinate hypertrophy (smoking, allergic rhinitis), tonsillar and adenoid hypertrophy, macroglossia (weight gain, obesity, hypothyroidism, Down's syndrome, amyloid) and epiglottic chondromalacia.

Functional abnormalities of the upper airway include the effects of drugs (alcohol, sedatives, steroids, anti-epileptic agents, analgesics), sleep deprivation and either selective upper airway muscle weakness (e.g. polio, stroke), upper airway sensory neuropathy (32) or inspiratory incoordination of upper airway and respiratory pump musculature (e.g. polio, stroke, diabetes).

PATHOPHYSIOLOGY

There are three physiologically important consequences of obstructive SDB: first, hypoxaemia, hypercapnia and acidosis lead to increased SNA (33) via the carotid body stimulation (34), vasoconstriction, a rise in blood pressure, stiffening of

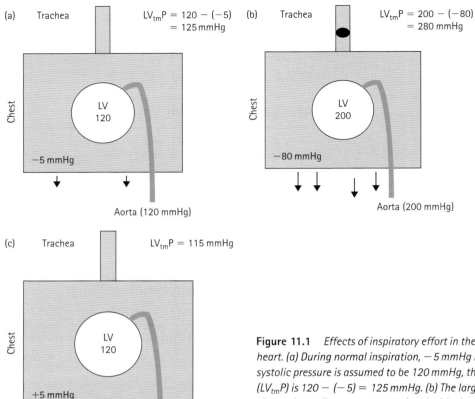

Figure 11.1 *Effects of inspiratory effort in the chest and single chamber ventricle of the heart. (a) During normal inspiration, − 5 mmHg intrathoracic pressure is generated. If systolic pressure is assumed to be 120 mmHg, the left ventricular transmural pressure ($LV_{tm}P$) is 120 − (− 5) = 125 mmHg. (b) The large negative intrathoracic pressures and elevated systolic pressures associated with obstructive sleep apnoea result in $LV_{tm}P$ of 200 − (− 80) = 280 mmHg. (c) With the application of 10 cm H_2O continuous positive airway pressure (CPAP), the intrathoracic pressure rises to + 5 mmHg and the systemic blood pressure falls to normal (120 mmHg), such that $LV_{tm}P$ is now 120 − (+5) = 115 mmHg.*

the ventricular wall (35) and increased platelet activity (36). At the end of the apnoea, a brief period of hyperventilation occurs, at which time oxygen radical damage to the vascular wall may take place and thus cause atherosclerosis (37).

Second, large negative intrathoracic pressure swings occur as a result of vigorous inspiratory efforts. Under normal circumstances, inspiratory negative intrathoracic pressures are around −5 cmH_2O (Fig. 11.1a). With OSA, values such as −80 cmH_2O (∼62 mmHg) have been recorded (Fig. 11.1b). Such large negative pressures impact upon all structures within the chest (heart and aortic arch baroreceptors). The pressure gradient across the left ventricle increases, which is well tolerated acutely by a normal ventricle, but poorly tolerated in CHF and leads to significantly reduced stroke volume (38). Increased left ventricular wall stress leads to the release of atrial natriuretic peptide, which contributes to nocturia. Continuous positive airway pressure (CPAP) significantly reduces transmural pressure (39, 40) (Fig. 11.1c).

Chronic exposure of a normal left ventricle to large negative intrathoracic pressures has been shown to contribute to a reduced left ventricular systolic contraction in a canine model (41). Increased venous return with leftward shift of the intraventricular septum impedes left ventricular filling and thus aggravates diastolic filling. Baroreflex sensitivity is thought to be reduced (42) or shifted rightward (43), due to the increased

transmural pressure gradients experienced, such as to allow higher intravascular pressures. Thus it is thought that awake systemic hypertension results in part due to the resetting of baroreflex control. Importantly, reversal of obstructive SDB has been shown to improve baroreflex control (44).

The third important consequence of obstructive SDB is the arousal from sleep that terminates the apnoea. The precise mechanism responsible for the arousal is not well understood but is thought to relate to hypoxaemia, hypercapnia and upper airway trauma. Supplemental oxygen in patients with obstructive SDB does not abolish arousals, nor does anaesthesia of the upper airway (32). Acute elevations in blood pressure and elevations in SNA occur in parallel with arousal. However, some of these effects are counteracted by the resumption of ventilation and its associated sympatholytic activity.

SYMPTOMS

Symptoms of obstructive SDB include snoring, witnessed apnoeas, dry or sore mouth, enuresis, nocturnal choking, dreaming of drowning or suffocation, excessive daytime sleepiness, mood changes, reduced higher mental functioning, early morning headache and reduced sexual performance (see Box 11.1). A recent report described 62 per cent of 331 patients with OSA having symptoms of nocturnal gastro-oesophageal

Box 11.1   Symptoms and signs suggestive of sleep apnoea

Symptoms

- Excessive sleepiness despite 8 h sleep
- Snoring >2 nights per week
- Witnessed apnoeas
- Nocturnal dyspnoea
- Nocturnal wheeze
- Personality change

Signs

- Systemic hypertension
- Tachy-bradycardia
- Intermittent atrial fibrillation
- Nocturnal pulmonary oedema
- Pulmonary hypertension
- Hypercapnia
- Large neck circumference (>43 cm)
- Difficult to intubate

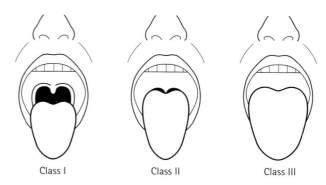

Class I   Class II   Class III

Figure 11.2 *Classification of upper airway based upon the position of the uvula (soft palate) in relation to the tongue and visibility of posterior pharyngeal wall. Note the visibility of the base of the palate in class I, which is lost in class II. Visibility of the posterior pharyngeal wall is maintained in class II, but lost in class III. Redrawn from an original description by Mallampati et al., 1985 (52).*

reflux, with a 48 per cent improvement in symptoms upon treatment of OSA with CPAP (45).

Daytime sleepiness may be sufficiently severe to cause sleepiness whilst engaged in activities such as driving (46), or subtle, so as to cause sleepiness during passive situations such as post-lunch meetings in darkened environments. The Epworth Sleepiness Scale is a commonly used and simple questionnaire which can aid in the assessment of sleepiness (47). Importantly, obstructive SDB is well recognized as a cause of occupational accidents (48) and premature death (49).

INCIDENCE

Snoring is thought to occur occasionally in ~60 per cent of the middle-aged population and regularly in 30 per cent (50). SDB, defined as more than five apnoeas and hypopnoeas per hour of sleep (apnoea hypopnoea index, AHI), occurs in 21 per cent of males and 8 per cent females; for AHI >15/h, the figures are 6 and 3 per cent, respectively, and for AHI >15/h plus symptoms, they are 4 and 2 per cent, respectively (51).

EXAMINATION

Examination of patients with obstructive SDB should include height, weight, neck circumference, nasal patency, soft palate or uvula (Mallampati index; see Fig. 11.2) (52), hard palate (high arched, narrow maxilla), dentition, mandible, temporo-mandibular joint, systemic and pulmonary blood pressure and general appearance (e.g. plethora of polycythaemia).

End organ impairment from obstructive SDB includes systemic or pulmonary hypertension, polycythaemia, systolic or diastolic heart failure, sleep-related cardiac arrhythmias (tachy-brady syndrome, intermittent atrial fibrillation), stroke and peripheral neuropathy (53).

INVESTIGATION

Given the high prevalence of snoring, significance should be given to snoring if it is frequent (> two nights per week), loud (audible in other rooms), upsetting to bed partner, associated with apnoeas or choking, or associated with symptoms or signs of end-organ impairment.

Investigation of patients with suspected obstructive SDB should include sleep monitoring of all, or some, of the following: brain (EEG, electro-oculogram [EOG], EMG), gas exchange (airflow, respiratory effort, S_pO_2, CO_2), ECG (heart rhythm, rate and ST change) and blood pressure. Limited channel monitoring (S_pO_2 and heart rate) is usually sufficient in patients with high pre-test probability for OSA (Fig. 11.3).

Full PSG (Fig. 11.4) is usually performed in patients with low pre-test probability of OSA or in those patients in whom additional monitoring (ECG, transcutaneous CO_2, detailed respiratory effort) is required, such as patients with heart, lung or neurological disease. In particular, PSG can link periods of asystole to respiratory events (Fig. 11.5) and also help resolve causes of tachy-bradycardic syndromes (Fig. 11.6).

Additional investigations that can be considered include flexible nasopharyngoscopy, echocardiogram (given the 50 per cent systemic hypertension and greater chance of left ventricular diastolic dysfunction), fasting blood glucose (54), lateral cephalograms, CT and MR scans (55, 56).

TREATMENT

Treatment for obstructive SDB can be divided into four categories: lifestyle, positive airway pressure, dental devices and surgery (see Box 11.2).

Changes to lifestyle

Although no randomized controlled trials exist for lifestyle advice, few doubt the impact that changes in weight (57) and alcohol intake (58) have on the severity of obstructive SDB.

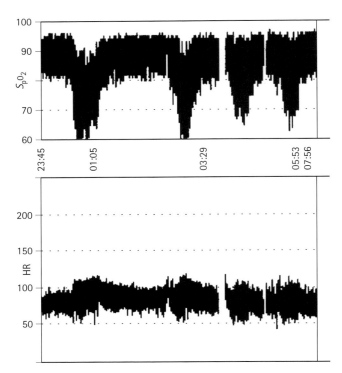

Figure 11.3 *Example of oximetry recording overnight from a patient with severe OSA. Note that oxygen saturation returns to normal after each apnoea. HR, heart rate.*

Weight loss should be stressed for all subjects, and consideration be given for medical/surgical interventions that assist weight reduction. These include gastrointestinal lipase inhibitors (e.g. Orlistat), central serotonin and noradrenaline reuptake inhibitors (e.g. Sibutramine), very low-energy diets (e.g. Modifast), or surgery to limit capacity (e.g. gastric banding surgery) or absorption (e.g. intestinal bypass).

Alcohol should be avoided (or reduced), as well as medications that can precipitate upper airway instability (e.g. anti-epileptic drugs, glucocorticoids, sedatives, codeine and narcotic-containing analgesics). Cigarette smoking is associated with increased snoring (59), probably through the mechanisms of increased nasal resistance, and thus patients should be counselled of the hazards of smoking. Other lifestyle measures include the avoidance of sleep deprivation and nasal steroids to reduce nasal resistance.

Positive airway pressure

Positive airway pressure is the mainstay of treatment and works via pneumatically splinting the upper airway. Continuous and auto-adjusting positive airway pressure (CPAP, APAP) are highly effective in symptomatic patients with SDB, with clear benefits including improved quality of life, lower systemic blood pressure, lower catecholamine activity and compliance of up to 90 per cent in specially selected patients.

Auto-adjusting devices, of which several are on the market, vary in the algorithm used to determine the change in pressure

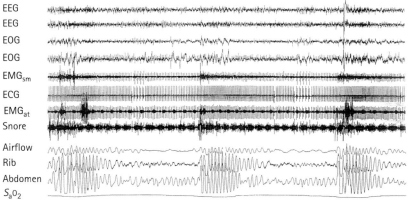

Figure 11.4 *A 4-min polysomnogram highlighting the absence of airflow (apnoea) associated with ongoing respiratory effort (rib and abdominal movement) associated with hypoxaemia and arousal. The arousal is recognized by increased activity of anterior tibialis and submental electromyography (EMG) and electroencephalography (EEG) plus tachycardia.*

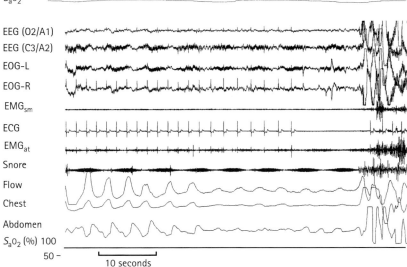

Figure 11.5 *A 30-s polysomnogram showing 13 s of ventricular standstill associated with an OSA.*

(60). Therefore each auto-titrating device needs to have validation testing prior to use. Nevertheless, there appears to be an advantage in using an auto-adjusting device when pressures with CPAP are in excess of 10 cmH$_2$O (60).

Mask technology has advanced such that there are nasal, oral and oronasal masks and nasal pillows available. Humidification can be added to prevent oronasal dryness, which often occurs when excessive oral leak occurs with a nasally delivered CPAP (61).

Upper airway surgery

Upper airway surgery may consist of jaw and hyoid advancement, widening of the maxilla, stiffening of the uvula, excision of the uvula, tonsillectomy, adenoidectomy, nasal turbinectomy, polypectomy or submucosal resection. Patient awareness of potential surgical complications is essential.

Only a modest reduction in snoring and AHI was reported in a recent trial of uvulopalatoplasty in mild OSA, and negative symptoms were reported by about 45 per cent of patients, with 20 per cent suffering from long-term dysphagia (62).

Dental devices

Dental devices which assist in protruding the mandible forward, and thus the tongue, are helpful, and randomized controlled data are now available in support (63), although patient selection is important. It would appear that suitable patients are sufficiently dentate, without dental or gum disease or temporomandibular joint disease and have mild to moderate obstructive SDB.

SYSTEMIC HYPERTENSION

Nocturnal arterial blood pressure is increased in obstructive SDB (64). Awake systemic hypertension occurs in ~50 per cent of patients with snoring and OSA (65); conversely, about 40 per cent patients with systemic hypertension have OSA (66). Although there are a number of characteristics similar to the patient with hypertension and SDB, such as obesity, male gender and alcohol, which indicate the possibility of two common diseases coexisting, a clear epidemiological relationship exists between SDB and systemic hypertension independent of these confounding factors (67, 68).

The largest cross-sectional study to date ($n = 6132$ subjects aged >40 years) has shown SDB to have an independent effect upon systemic blood pressure (67). A study of 709 subjects, of similar age, who underwent prospective sleep studies (baseline and repeated at 4 years) and detailed physiological measures, also supports the significant relationship between obstructive SDB and systemic hypertension (68).

Box 11.2   Treatment of obstructive sleep

Conservative

- Weight loss
- Avoidance of alcohol, sedatives, anti-epileptics, steroids, codeine
- Reduce nasal resistance (local steroids, surgery)
- Smoking cessation
- Sleep in non-supine position
- Avoid sleep deprivation

Positive airway pressure

- Continuous
- Automated
- Humidified

Dental splint

- Mandibular advancement
- Jaw closure
- Tongue advancement

Surgical

- Soft tissue (nasal, tonsil, adenoid, uvula)
- Bony tissue (maxilla, mandible)
- Gastric (banding, intestinal bypass)

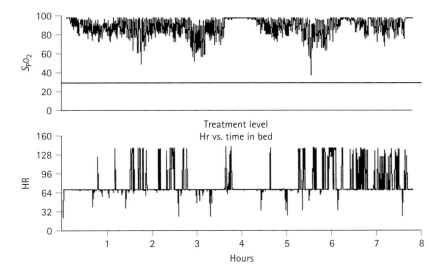

Figure 11.6 *An overnight summary of oxygen saturation (S_pO_2) and heart rate (HR) which illustrates tachy-bradycardia associated with OSA.*

Mean systemic blood pressure rises by about 3.5 mmHg with several weeks of either brief episodic hypoxia in rats (34) or simulated OSA in dogs (69). Elevated SNA (70), reduced (or reset) intrathoracic baroreceptor function (42) or abnormal endothelial function (71) may play a role in the development of systemic hypertension.

Most importantly, obstructive SDB treatment with CPAP is associated with a fall in blood pressure in those subjects with systemic hypertension. A fall in 24-h mean systemic blood pressure of ~3.3 mmHg, with ambulatory automated cuff measurements, is observed after 1 month of CPAP in unselected patients with obstructive SDB (72), with similar results obtained in an Edinburgh study (73). Recently, a greater (~10 mmHg) fall in 24-h mean systemic blood pressure was observed with CPAP in a group of mainly hypertensive patients over a longer period of time (2 months) using a continuous non-invasive blood pressure measuring device which does not cause arousals during sleep (74). Obstructive SDB is now recognized as a cause of systemic hypertension (75).

HEART FAILURE

Over the past 50 years the incidence of CHF remains at 1 per cent of the entire adult population and doubles for every decade above 60 years. The mortality has changed little over the past 50 years, with a 5-year mortality of about 50 per cent (76). Systemic hypertension (76), obesity (77) and IHD (76) appear to be the major risk factors responsible for the development of CHF. Approximately 50 per cent of patients with CHF, due to either systolic or diastolic disease, will have SDB (see Table 11.1).

Forty per cent of patients presenting with acute pulmonary oedema have pure diastolic dysfunction (78), an inability of the left ventricle to relax and allow sufficient filling. Apart from constrictive pericardial disease or myopathic conditions (e.g. amyloid, hypertrophic obstructive cardiomyopathy), diastolic dysfunction usually results from systemic hypertension (79), hypoxaemia (35) and tachycardia (80). These physiological events occur commonly in patients with OSA. Simulated OSA in dogs causes elevation of end-diastolic pressures and eventually leads to reduced systolic contractile activity (41), supporting the theory that OSA contributes to diastolic dysfunction.

Systolic CHF occurs when there is failure of left ventricular contraction. Approximately 8 per cent of general SDB patients have evidence of systolic failure (81). Obesity is an independent risk factor for the development of CHF: for every rise of 1 unit of body mass index (BMI), there are 5 and 7 per cent increases in prevalence of heart failure in males and females, respectively (77). The mechanisms are not fully elucidated, although high BMI is associated with diabetes mellitus, systemic hypertension and IHD as well as OSA.

Epidemiological data support a link between OSA and heart failure. Children who have OSA have thicker ventricular walls compared with non-snoring controls (82). Fifty-five per cent of patients with diastolic dysfunction have obstructive SDB (83). The Sleep Heart Health Study has identified a significant relationship between OSA and self-reported CHF (84).

Mechanisms that link OSA and CHF are hypoxaemia, tachycardia related to arousals and sympathetic activity, and negative intrathoracic pressure (85), thus increasing left ventricular transmural pressure. Treatment of OSA with CPAP has been shown to augment left ventricular systolic function (86, 87).

VASCULAR DISEASE

In addition to systemic hypertension, there is evidence that obstructive SDB is associated with insulin resistance (54), IHD (88) and stroke (89). Proposed mechanisms include oxygen radical formation and vascular wall injury, which result from the repeated deoxygenation/reoxygenation with apnoeic/hypopnoeic events (37).

Significant epidemiological data suggest a relationship between OSA and ST changes on ECG recordings during sleep (90), myocardial infarction (91), nocturnal angina (92) and IHD (93). Importantly, data suggest that cardiovascular mortality (94) and all-cause mortality (49) are increased if OSA is left untreated. The 10-year mortality is significantly greater (~7 vs. ~2 per cent $P = 0.007$) in male snorers with excessive sleepiness compared with non-sleepy non-snorers (49).

STROKE

Sleep-disordered breathing and stroke appear to have a complex relationship. On one hand there is epidemiological evidence that SDB may contribute as an independent risk factor for the development of stroke (84) via the mechanisms of increased systemic blood pressure and blood coagulability (36). Greater frequency of atheromatous calcified plaques in the carotid arteries has been observed in patients with SDB (95), perhaps reflecting the increased shear force or possibly the effects of snoring-related vibration. Increased levels of fibrinogen have also been reported in SDB, thus predisposing patients to stroke (96).

Stroke, however, may contribute to impaired upper airway muscle activity and thus instability of the upper airway muscles. It has been estimated that 50–75 per cent of patients presenting with stroke (either haemorrhagic or ischaemic) will have SDB, mainly obstructive in type (97), and that after 3 months the prevalence falls by 50 per cent (98).

Importantly, the prognosis from stroke is worse in those patients with untreated SDB than in those without SDB (99)

Table 11.1 *Obstructive versus central apnoea in heart failure*

	Obstructive	Central
Weight	Excessive	Normal
Snorer	Usual	Occasional
Orthopnoea	Occasional	Usual
Diastolic failure	Likely	Unlikely
Systolic failure	Possible	Likely
Pulmonary pressures (awake)	Normal	Elevated
P_aCO_2	Normal	Elevated
Response to medical treatment	Unlikely	Likely

and data are beginning to emerge that treatment of SDB in such patients reduces fibrinogen levels (96) and improves depression and functional outcome (88, 98, 100). However, success in CPAP treatment appears to be difficult in those patients with little dexterity and therefore alternative treatments, such as altered body position (supine to lateral), may prove to be an inexpensive means of dealing with a huge problem with limited resources.

Non-hypercapnic central sleep apnoea

This disorder is characterized by central apnoea interspersed with periods of hyperventilation (101) and is due to heart failure (when it is termed central sleep apnoea with Cheyne–Stokes respiration [CSA-CSR]), high altitude, premature neonates, drugs (e.g. methadone) and possibly stroke.

The pathophysiological process is hyperventilation, which in non-REM sleep allows $P_a CO_2$ levels to drop transiently below the apnoea threshold until levels return to stimulate the peripheral and central chemoreceptors (carotid body and medulla, respectively). If the 'gain' in response to CO_2 is high, hyperventilation will recur and result in a greater fall in $P_a CO_2$ below the apnoea threshold, resulting in further central apnoeas. Continuation of this pattern will result in periodic breathing.

The change in $P_a CO_2$ from eupnoea to apnoea levels is narrower in patients with CHF and CSA, compared with CHF patients without CSA (103). Thus fluctuations in $P_a CO_2$ need only be small to precipitate CSA in CHF patients with CSA, whereas CHF patients without spontaneous CSA may have induced CSA if large fluctuations in CO_2 occur.

The causes of increased ventilatory responses are poorly understood; however, elevated plasma norepinephrine (adrenaline) (104) and loss of carotid body nitric oxide (105) are thought to be responsible in heart failure, hypoxaemia in high altitude central apnoeas and unknown in neonates. Chronic narcotic use can be associated with non-hypercapnic CSA, independent of pulmonary or cardiac disease (106), probably as a result of selective impairment of one of several chemoreceptors. Similarly high-flow oxygen can be associated with central apnoeas in newborn lambs (107) and humans (108) probably through selective damping of peripheral chemoreceptors.

In adult practice, non-hypercapnic central apnoea will occur most commonly in CHF (Fig. 11.7), and less commonly due to chronic narcotic analgesia or as a result of frontal stroke. Acute cardiogenic pulmonary oedema is due to left ventricular systolic failure in 60 per cent and diastolic failure in 40 per cent. Systolic CHF relates to impaired forward pumping of cardiac output usually associated with a dilated and poorly contractile (global or segmental) left ventricle. Approximately 30 per cent of patients will have atrial fibrillation. Systemic hypertension, obesity, valvular disease, ischaemia and drugs are common risk factors.

Approximately 30 per cent of patients with CHF (due to systolic failure) will have CSA-CSR. Such patients complain of orthopnoea, paroxysmal nocturnal dyspnoea, insomnia, fatigue, with snoring often absent. Patients with CSA have much greater awake total body and cardiac-specific norepinephrine (adrenaline) spillover (109) and overnight urinary norepinephrine (104), to a level greater than that seen with OSA (110). Hypoxaemia and arousals plus severity of CHF significantly correlate with the urinary norepinephrine (adrenaline) levels (104, 109, 110). Thus, a diagnosis of CSA in CHF is likely to portend a greater risk of mortality (111).

A PSG will reveal a waxing and waning pattern of ventilation during stages 1 and 2 non-REM sleep, with an arousal at peak ventilation, followed by a period of apnoea with absence of respiratory effort. REM sleep and slow-wave sleep are spared of CSA. Cycles of CSA can be triggered by an arousal and an acute rise in ventilation. The ventilation and apnoea cycle length and the ventilation:apnoea length ratio for CSA-CSR due to CHF are 45–90 s and >1, respectively. In comparison, the cycle length and ventilation:apnoea length ratio are <30 s and <1.0 in CSA due to high altitude, neonatal immaturity, narcotics or idiopathic non-hypercapnic CSA (112). The cycle length is inversely correlated with left ventricular ejection fraction (LVEF) (112).

Ventilatory responses to CO_2 are increased in CSA-CSR due to CHF and the idiopathic CSA groups (113). In CHF, the central (medullary) ventilatory response correlates with resting $P_a CO_2$ and the peripheral (carotid body) response correlates

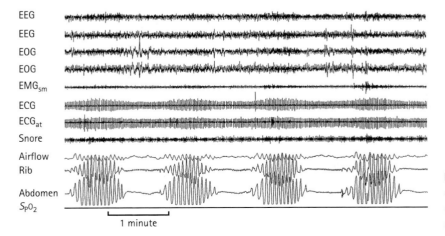

EEG	
EEG	
EOG	
EOG	
EMG$_{sm}$	
ECG	
ECG$_{at}$	
Snore	
Airflow	
Rib	
Abdomen	
S_pO_2	

1 minute

Figure 11.7 *A 4-min polysomnogram showing central sleep apnoea with a Cheyne–Stokes pattern of respiration. Note: Cheyne–Stokes breathing, S_pO_2 92% drops to 89%, P_aCO_2 32 mmHg.*

with periodicity of CSA. Moreover, the severity of CSA in CHF correlates closely with the severity of heart failure as measured by pulmonary capillary wedge pressure (PCWP) (114). As the most reliable clinical features that assist the clinician in determining the severity of CHF are the presence and absence of orthopnoea (102), a symptom of CSA, recognition of CSA-CSR in patients with CHF is indicative of worse cardiac function. In comparison, pulmonary rales, jugular venous pressure and peripheral oedema are insensitive markers of CHF severity.

Whether CSA is detrimental in itself to the underlying CHF is contentious. Arousals and hypoxaemia during sleep alter quality of life and contribute to fragmented sleep and paroxysmal nocturnal dyspnoea. Continuous hyperventilation and the associated increase in work of breathing also increase the requirement upon cardiac output significantly (115).

However, CSA may be a cost-effective way of dealing with an increased respiratory workload (due to oedematous lungs) with reduced cardiac output. A waxing and waning ventilatory pattern, akin to the cyclist in a *peleton*, is a technique to reduce the overall expenditure of work (116). Second, the hyperventilation phase may augment stroke volume through the small rhythmical unobstructed respiratory efforts (117). Third, the hyperventilation phase is associated with an increase in EELV (118). Fourth, lung inflation associated with hyperventilation is associated with bronchial dilatation and attenuation of sympathetic activity (119). Fifth, compared with acidosis, alkalosis is a more favourable environment for hypoxic greater cardiac muscle contraction. Therefore, CSA in the setting of CHF may simply represent a compensatory response to severe CHF, at the expense of mild hypoxaemia and fragmented sleep.

TREATMENT

Initial treatment of CSA should be with medical therapy aimed at improving cardiac failure with diuretics, digoxin and vasodilators. Medical therapy alone improves severity of CSA associated with improved cardiac function (120), although there has not been a formally conducted randomized controlled trial of medical intervention. Acetazolamide has been shown to be effective (114). Whether CSA is abolished with correction of CHF, with successful cardiac transplantation, has been shown in only 70 per cent of patients (121). The balance have persistent CSA, albeit more mild with a shorter cycle length and ventilation:apnoea length ratio of <1.0 (121).

Second-line treatment of CSA with CHF is CPAP. The principles by which CPAP works are similar to those which explain its success as first-line treatment for the management of acute cardiogenic pulmonary oedema (122) (Fig. 11.8). CPAP results in stabilization of the upper airway, an increase in EELV (118), elevation in alveolar pressure, assistance of the inspiratory muscles, a reduction in the pressure gradient across the left ventricular wall (123) and a fall in left ventricular diameter and reduction in mitral regurgitant fraction (44). As a secondary response, cardiac function improves (123), the circulatory delay and hypoxaemia diminish, as do the elevated noradrenaline levels, both acutely (124) and chronically (104), and associated arrhythmias.

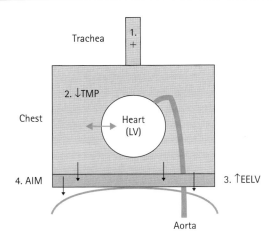

Figure 11.8 *The chest and single chamber heart illustrating some of the mechanisms by which CPAP works in heart failure. Note the pneumatic stabilization of the upper airway, reduction in left ventricular transmural pressure (TMP), increase in EELV and assistance of inspiratory muscles (AIM).*

An alternative delivery system of CPAP, incorporating a servocontrolled ventilator, 'Autoset CS', designed to deliver maximal CPAP with ventilatory assistance during the central apnoea, and lower CPAP without ventilatory support during the hyperventilation process, has been described (125). This group reported the Autoset CS to be more efficacious in improving sleep (more slow-wave and REM sleep, reduced arousals) than CPAP, bi-level PAP or oxygen (125).

Third-line management of CSA and CHF is supplemental oxygen. Supplemental oxygen, up to 0.5 F_iO_2, attenuates CSA (126) but should be used with caution due to reduced cardiac output (120, 127) and the paradoxical worsening of CSA (107, 108).

THE EFFECT OF NORMAL SLEEP IN PATIENTS WITH PULMONARY DISEASE

Asthma

There is a definite circadian influence on peak expiratory flow rate, regardless of whether the patient is awake or asleep (128). Factors contributing are thought to be multifactorial: reductions in temperature, increases in plasma histamine, reductions in cortisol and catecholamines, increased exposure to allergens in the bedding, gastro-oesophageal reflux and snoring (129). Treatment of snoring results in improved asthma control (129).

COPD

Sleep is the greatest recurring physiological stress placed upon patients with COPD (1). Patients with COPD have shorter and more fragmented periods of sleep, and less REM sleep, possibly due to tobacco, medications (e.g. theophylline), hypoxaemia, hypercapnia or SDB (130). Poor-quality sleep is considered a major factor in the reduced quality of life of such patients (131).

Patients with COPD are dependent upon accessory as well as intercostal muscles and diaphragm to maintain ventilation. Disturbance to this delicate balance is illustrated during sleep when ventilation is reduced significantly, particularly during REM sleep. Becker *et al.* (12) recently assessed falls in minute volume of ventilation by 16 per cent from wakefulness to non-REM sleep, and by 32 per cent from wakefulness to REM sleep in a group of patients with COPD. Reductions in ventilation were due to falls in tidal volume with little change in respiratory rate. Hypoxaemia is further aggravated by alterations in ventilation/perfusion matching and the greater oxygen demands of REM sleep.

Physiological responses to the loads placed upon patients with COPD determine whether they are to become a 'pink puffer' or 'blue bloater'. The loads placed upon COPD patients include upper airway obstruction, chest wall mass, abdominal mass and drug effects, including alcohol (132), upon respiratory drive and muscle function. Dietary and electrolyte disturbances are important, as is the degree of airflow obstruction.

Sleep desaturation is associated with reduced survival (133) and sleep is the greatest time of arrhythmias (134) and death for patients with COPD (2). In a study of 34 patients with stable COPD (mean $FEV_1 = 42$ per cent) nearly half had significant sleep-related hypoxaemia (mean hypoxaemia time was 28 per cent of the night) (135). They observed a significant relationship between hypoxaemia and daytime S_aO_2, FEV_1 and inspiratory muscle strength.

More recently, Sanders *et al.* (136) reported the relationship between COPD and SDB in a study which involved home PSG and lung function testing. Of a total population of 5954 adults living in the community, 19 per cent had COPD (defined as FEV_1/FVC <70 per cent), albeit mild, with a mean FEV_1/FVC value of 64 per cent and only 3.8 per cent having FEV_1/FVC <60 per cent. The prevalence of SDB (defined by AHI >10 events/h) was 29 per cent without COPD and 22 per cent with COPD, thus indicating that SDB is no more common in patients with COPD than in those without. However, they did also report the total sleep time spent hypoxaemic (defined as >5 per cent total sleep time with S_pO_2 <90 per cent) to be 6.3 per cent in non-COPD, non-SDB patients, 11.4 per cent in COPD patients without SDB, and 42.9 per cent of COPD patients with SDB. The odds ratios were 1.0, 1.8 (1.33–2.45) and 8.28 (5.78–11.86), respectively, for the three groups.

Given the relationship between hypoxaemia, pulmonary hypertension, nocturnal arrhythmias (134) and death (2), documentation and treatment of sleep-related hypoxaemia should be considered.

Quadriplegia

Quadriplegic patients have an increased chance of developing sleep-related hypoventilation. Predisposing factors are paralysis of intercostal or abdominal muscles, and, in the case of C5 injury, phrenic nerve damage and resultant diaphragm weakness (unilateral or bilateral). Additionally, drugs required to treat the underlying pain or muscle spasm (e.g. benzodiazepines and baclofen) may impair respiratory drive.

In a study of 90 quadriplegics, aged 18–60 years, with spinal injury of >6 months' duration, 65 replied to a questionnaire, of whom 40 took part in detailed sleep and ventilation monitoring (137). Of this group of 40 patients, 30 per cent had an AHI >5 events/h, mainly obstructive in type. Non-invasive ventilatory support during sleep can result in a marked improvement in ventilation both during sleep and when awake and also in quality of life.

Kyphoscoliosis

Hypoventilation during sleep commonly occurs in this group (138) due to a need for increased accessory muscle use, (which is abolished during REM sleep), reduced lung volume and thus surface area for gas exchange, and increased work of breathing. This group responds favourably to non-invasive ventilatory support (139).

Neuromuscular disease

Several neuromuscular disorders are associated with sleep-related breathing disorders, such as multiple sclerosis, polio and motor neuron disease.

Motor neuron disease affects 6 per 100 000, and over 80 per cent of patients have evidence of respiratory muscle weakness at the time of presentation. Median survival is 2–3 years, with death particularly due to respiratory failure. Impaired quality of life correlates most significantly with markers of respiratory failure (140). Most have sleep-related hypoventilation, which responds favourably to avoidance of tracheostomy, control of excessive saliva (anticholinergic drugs or radiation) and non-invasive ventilatory support (141).

SUMMARY

The measurement of sleep has provided a new avenue not only to explore and explain symptoms to patients, but, more importantly, to initiate better treatments directed towards sleep-related aspects of underlying disease. Clinicians with sufficient suspicion to initiate further investigations and management of sleep-related disorders will be rewarded by satisfied patients and improved clinical care.

Key points

- Sleep quality and quantity are important when optimizing exercise capacity.
- Sleep contributes to greater hypoxic stress than does exercise.
- The term 'sleep-disordered breathing' encompasses snoring, obstructive and central sleep apnoea and sleep-related hypoventilation.

- Patients with obesity, systemic hypertension or underlying cardiac, pulmonary or neurological disease are at risk of sleep-disordered breathing.
- Symptoms of sleep-disordered breathing include excessive daytime sleepiness, morning headache, dry throat and altered mood.
- Obstructive sleep apnoea is an important and reversible cause of systemic hypertension and heart failure and probably stroke.
- Non-hypercapnic central sleep apnoea (Cheyne–Stokes respiration) is indicative of severe congestive heart failure.
- Treatment options for sleep-disordered breathing include conservative, dental splints, surgical options and various forms of positive airway pressure, each of which can be highly effective in improving quality of life, mood, alertness and reduced health care costs.

REFERENCES

1. Mulloy E, McNicholas WT. Ventilation and gas exchange during sleep and exercise in patients with severe COPD. *Chest* 1996; **109**: 387–94.
2. McNicholas WT, Fitzgerald MX. Nocturnal death among patients with chronic bronchitis and emphysema. *Br Med J* 1984; **289**: 878.
●3. Muller JE, Stone PH, Turi ZG et al. Circadian variation in the frequency of onset of acute myocardial infarction. *N Engl J Med* 1985; **313**: 1315–22.
4. Aboyans V, Cassat C, Lacroix P et al. Is the morning peak of acute myocardial infarction's onset due to sleep-related breathing disorders? *Cardiology* 2000; **94**: 188–92.
5. Lavery CE, Mittleman MA, Cohen MC et al. Non-uniform night-time distribution of acute cardiac events. A possible effect of sleep states. *Circulation* 1997; **96**: 3321–27.
6. Knutsson A, allqvist J, Reuterwall C et al. Shift work and myocardial infarction: a case controlled study. *Occup Environ Med* 1999; **56**: 46–50.
◆7. Brzezinski A. Mechanisms of disease: melatonin in humans. *N Engl J Med* 1997; **336**: 186–95.
8. Xie A, Takasaki Y, Popkin J et al. Influence of body position on pressure and airflow generation during hypoxia and hypercapnia in man. *J Physiol (Lond)* 1993; **465**: 477–87.
9. Douglas NJ, White DP, Weil JV et al. Hypoxic ventilatory response decreases during sleep in normal men. *Am Rev Respir Dis* 1982; **125**: 286–9.
10. Douglas NJ, White DP, Weil JV et al. Hypercapnic ventilatory responses in sleeping adults. *Am Rev Respir Dis* 1982; **126**: 758–62.
11. Hudgel DW, Martin RJ, Johnston BJ, Hill P. Mechanics of the respiratory system and breathing pattern during sleep in normal humans. *J Appl Physiol: Respir Environ Exer Physiol* 1984; **56**: 133–7.
12. Becker HF, Piper AJ, Flynn WE et al. Breathing during sleep in patients with nocturnal desaturation. *Am J Respir Crit Care Med* 1999; **159**: 112–18.
13. Hetzel MR, Clark TJH. Comparison of normal and asthmatic circadian rhythms in peak expiratory flow rate. *Thorax* 1980; **35**: 732–8.

14. Moreno F. Lyons HA. Effect of body posture on lung volumes. *J Appl Physiol* 1961; **16**: 27–9.
●15. Somers VK, Dyken ME, Mark AL, Abboud FM. Sympathetic nervous system activity during sleep in normal subjects. *N Engl J Med* 1993; **328**: 303–7.
16. Vaughn BV, Quint SR, Messenheimer JA, Robertson KR. Heart period variability in sleep. *Electroencephalogr Clin Neurophysiol* 1995; **94**: 155–62.
17. Conway J, Boon N, Jones JV, Sleight P. Involvement of the baroreceptor reflexes in the changes in blood pressure with sleep and mental arousal. *Hypertension* 1983; **5**: 746–8.
◆18. Khatri IM, Freis ED. Hemodynamic changes during sleep. *J Appl Physiol* 1967; **22**: 867–73.
19. Verrier RL, Dickerson LW. Autonomic nervous system and coronary blood flow changes related to emotional activation and sleep. *Circulation* 1991; **83**: 81–9.
20. Trinder J, Kleiman J, Carrington M et al. Autonomic activity during human sleep as a function of time and sleep stage. *J Sleep Res* 2001; **10**: 253–64.
21. Vuori I, Urponen H, Hasan J, Partinen M. Epidemiology of exercise effects on sleep. *Acta Physiol Scand* 1988; **133**: 574.
22. Griffin SJ, Trinder J. Physical fitness, exercise and human sleep. *Psychophysiol* 1978; **15**: 447–50.
23. Chandler WL, Schwartz RS, Stratton JR, Vitello MV. Effects of endurance training on the circadian rhythm of fibrinolysis in males and females. *Med Sci Sport Exer* 1996; **28**: 647–55.
●24. Dinges DF, Pack F, Williams K et al. Cumulative sleepiness, mood disturbance and psychomotor vigilance performance decrements during a week of sleep restricted to 4–5 hours per night. *Sleep* 1997; **20**: 267–77.
●25. Taffinder NJ, McManus IC, Gul Y et al. Effect of sleep deprivation on surgeons' dexterity on laparoscopic simulator. *Lancet* 1998; **352**.
●26. Dawson D, Reid K. Fatigue, alcohol and performance impairment. *Nature* 1997; **388**: 235.
27. Brandenberger G, Gronfier C, Chapotot F et al. Effect of sleep deprivation on overall 24 h growth-hormone secretion. *Lancet* 2000; **356**: 1408.
28. Spiegel K, Leproult R, Van Cauter E. Impact of sleep debt on metabolic and endocrine function. *Lancet* 1999; **354**: 1435–9.
29. Martin BJ. Sleep loss and subsequent exercise performance. *Act Physiol Scand Suppl* 1988; **574**: 28–32.
●30. Bergman BM, Everson CA, Kushida CA et al. Sleep deprivation in the rat, V. Energy use and mediation. *Sleep* 1989; **12**: 31–41.
31. Bowes G, Woolf GM, Sullivan CE et al. Effect of sleep fragmentation on ventilatory and arousal responses of sleeping dogs to respiratory stimuli. *Am Rev Respir Dis* 1980; **122**: 899–908.
32. Kimoff RJ, Sforza E, Champagne V et al. Upper airway sensation in snoring and obstructive sleep apnea. *Am J Respir Crit Care Med* 2001; **164**: 250–5.
◆33. Somers VK, Dyken ME, Clry MP, Abboud FM. Sympathetic neural mechanisms in obstructive sleep apnea. *J Clin Invest* 1995; **96**: 1897–1904.
34. Fletcher EC, Lesske J, Behm R et al. Carotid chemoreceptors, systemic hypertension, and chronic episodic hypoxia mimicking sleep apnea. *J Appl Physiol* 1992; **72**: 1978–84.
35. Cargill RI, Keily DG, Lipworth BJ. Adverse effects of hypoxaemia on diastolic filling in humans. *Clin Sci* 1995; **89**: 165–9.
36. Bokinski G, Miller M, Ault K et al. Spontaneous platelet activation and aggregation during OSA and its response to therapy with CPAP. A preliminary investigation. *Chest* 1995; **108**: 625–30.

37. Prabhakar NR. Sleep apnea: an oxidative stress? *Am J Respir Crit Care Med* 2002; **176**: 859–60.

●38. Scharf SM, Bianco JA, Tow DE, Brown R. The effects of large negative intrathoracic pressure on left ventricular function in patients with coronary artery disease. *Circulation* 1981; **63**: 871–5.

39. Naughton MT, Rahman MA, Hara K, *et al*. Cardiothoracic effects of CPAP in patients with CHF. *Circulation* 1995; **91**: 1725–31.

40. Tkacova R, Liu PP, Naughton MT, Bradley TD. Effect of CPAP on mitral regurgitant fraction and atrial natriuretic peptide in patients with CHF. *J Am Coll Cardiol* 1997; **30**: 739–45.

●41. Parker JD, Brooks D, Kozar LF *et al*. Acute and chronic effects of airway obstruction on canine left ventricular performance. *Am J Respir Crit Care Med* 1999; **160**: 1888–96.

42. Carlson JT, Hedner JA, Sellgren J *et al*. Depressed baroreflex sensitivity in patients with OSA. *Am J Respir Crit Care Med* 1996; **154**: 1490–6.

43. Brooks D, Horner RL, Floras JS *et al*. Baroreflex control of heart rate in a canine model of OSA. *Am J Respir Crit Care Med* 1999; **159**: 1293–7.

44. Tkacova R, Dajani HR, Rankin F *et al*. CPAP improves nocturnal baroreflex sensitivity of patients with CHF and OSA. *J Hypertens* 2000; **18**: 1257–62.

45. Green BT, Broughton WA, O'Connor JB. Marked improvement in nocturnal gastroesophageal reflux in a large cohort of patients with OSA treated with CPAP. *Arch Intern Med* 2003; **163**: 41–5.

●46. Teran-Santos J, Jimenez-Gomez A, Cordero-Guevara J and the co-operative group Grugos-Santander. The association between sleep apnea and the risk of traffic accidents. *N Engl J Med* 1999; **340**: 847–51.

●47. Johns MW. A new method for measuring daytime sleepiness: the Epworth sleepiness scale. *Sleep* 1991; **14**: 540–5.

48. Lindberg E, Carter N, Gislason T, Janson C. Role of snoring and daytime sleepiness in occupational accidents. *Am J Respir Crit Care Med* 2001; **164**: 2031–35.

●49. Lindberg E, Janson C, Svardsudd K *et al*. Increased mortality among sleepy snorers: a prospective population-based study. *Thorax* 1998; **53**: 631–7.

50. Koskenvou M, Kaprio J, Telakivi T *et al*. Snoring as a risk factor for IHD and stroke in men. *Br Med J* 1987; **294**: 16–9.

●51. Young T, Palta M, Dempsey J *et al*. The occurrence of sleep-disordered breathing among middle aged adults. *N Engl J Med* 1993; **32**: 1230–5.

52. Mallampati SR, Gatt SP, Gugino LD *et al*. A clinical sign to predict difficult intubation: a prospective study. *Can Anaesth J* 1985; **32**: 429–4.

53. Mayer P, Dematteis M, Pepin JL *et al*. Peripheral neuropathy in sleep apnea. A tissue marker of the severity of nocturnal desaturation. *Am J Respir Crit Care Med* 1999; **159**: 213–19.

54. Ip MSM, Lam B, Ng MMT *et al*. OSA is independently associated with insulin resistance. *Am J Respir Crit Care Med* 2002; **165**: 670–6.

55. Dempsey JA, Skatrud JB, Jacques AJ *et al*. Anatomic determinants of sleep-disordered breathing across the spectrum of clinical and non-clinical male subjects. *Chest* 2002; **122**: 840–51.

56. Macey PM, Henderson LA, Macey KE *et al*. Brain morphology associated with OSA. *Am J Respir Crit Care Med* 2002; **166**: 1382–7.

57. Grunstein RR, Wilcox I, Yang TS *et al*. Snoring and sleep apnoea in men: association with central obesity and hypertension. *Int J Obes Relat Metab Disord* 1993; **17**: 533–40.

58. Scanlan MF Roebuck T, Little PJ *et al*. Effect of moderate alcohol upon OSA. *Eur Respir J* 2000; **16**: 909–13.

59. Wetter DW, Young TB, Bidwell TR, *et al*. Smoking as a risk factor for sleep-disordered breathing. *Arch Intern Med* 1994; **154**: 2219–24.

60. Massie CA, McArdle N, Hart RW *et al*. Comparison between automatic and fixed positive airway pressure therapy in the home. *Am J Respir Crit Care Med* 2003; **167**: 20–3.

61. Massie CA, Hart RW, Peralez K, Richards GN. Effects of humidification on nasal symptoms and compliance in sleep apnea patients using CPAP. *Chest* 1999; **16**: 403–8.

62. Ferguson KA, Heighway K, Ruby RRF. A randomised controlled trial of laser-assisted uvuloplatoplasty in the treatment of mild OSA. *Am J Respir Crit Care Med* 2003; **167**: 15–19.

63. Mehta A, Qian J, Petocz P *et al*. A randomised controlled study of a mandibular advancement splint for OSA. *Am J Respir Crit Care Med* 2001; **163**: 1457–61.

64. Jennum P, Wildschiodtz G, Christensen NJ *et al*. Blood pressure, catecholamines and pancreatic polypeptide in OSA with and without nasal CPAP treatment. *Am J Hypertens* 1989; **2**: 847–52.

65. Gislason T, Areng H, Taube A. Snoring and systemic hypertension: an epidemiological study. *Acta Med Scand* 1987; **222**: 415–21.

66. Worsnop CJ, Naughton MT, Barter CE *et al*. The prevalence of OSA in hypertensives. *Am J Respir Crit Care Med* 1998; **157**: 111–15.

67. Neito FJ, Young TB, Lind BK. Association of sleep-disordered breathing, sleep apnea, and hypertension in a large community-based study. *J Am Med Assoc* 2000; **283**: 1829–36.

68. Peppard PE, Young T, Palta M, Skatrud J. Prospective study of the association between sleep-disordered breathing and hypertension. *N Engl J Med* 2000; **342**: 1378–84.

●69. Brooks D, Horner RL, Kozar LF *et al*. OSA as a cause of systemic hypertension. Evidence from a canine model. *J Clin Invest* 1997; **99**: 106–9.

70. Carlson JT, Hedner J, Elam M *et al*. Augmented resting sympathetic activity in awake patients with and without OSA. *Chest* 1993; **103**: 1763–8.

71. Kato M, Roberts-Thompson P, Phillips BG *et al*. Impairment of resistance vessels in OSA. *Circulation* 2000; **102**: 2607–10.

72. Pepperell JC, Ramdassingh-Dow S *et al*. Ambulatory blood pressure following therapeutic and sub-therapeutic nasal CPAP for OSA: a randomised controlled parallel trial. *Lancet* 2002; **359**: 204–10.

73. Faccenda JF, Mackay TW, Boon NA *et al*. Randomised controlled trial of CPAP therapy for the sleep apnoea/hypopnoea syndrome. *Am J Respir Crit Care Med* 2001; **163**: 344–8.

●74. Becker HF, Jerrentrup A, Ploch T *et al*. Effect of nasal CPAP treatment on blood pressure in patients with OSA. *Circulation* 2003; **107**: 68–73.

◆75. NHLBI. *The Seventh Report of the Joint National Committee on Prevention, Detection, Evaluation and Treatment of High Blood Pressure* (JNC 7). NIH Publication No. 03-5233. Bethesda, MD: NHLBI, 2003. (Online: http://www.nhbli.nih.gov).

76. Levy D, Kenchaiah S, Larson MG *et al*. Long-term trends in the incidence of and survival with heart failure. *N Engl J Med* 2002; **347**: 1397–1402.

77. Kenchaiah S, Evans JC, Levy D *et al*. Obesity and the risk of heart failure. *N Engl J Med* 2002; **347**: 305–13.

78. Dougherty AH, Naccarelli GV, Gray EL *et al*. CHF with normal systolic function. *Am J Cardiol* 1984; **54**: 778–82.

79. Clarkson P, Wheeldon NM, Macdonald TM. Left ventricular diastolic dysfunction. *Quart J Med* 1994; **87**: 143–8.

80. Serizawa T, Vogel WM, Apstein CS, Grossman W. Comparison of acute alterations in left ventricular relaxation and diastolic chamber stiffness induced by hypoxia and ischemia. Role of

myocardial oxygen supply-demand imbalance. *J Clin Invest* 1981; **68**: 91–102.

81. Laaban JP, Pascal-Sebaoun S, Bloch E *et al.* Left ventricular systolic dysfunction in patients with OSA syndrome. *Chest* 2002; **122**: 1133–38.

82. Amin RS, Kimball TR, Bean JA *et al.* Left ventricular hypertrophy and abnormal ventricular geometry in children and adolescents with OSA. *Am Respir Crit Care Med* 2002; **165**: 1395–9.

83. Chan J, Sanderson J, Chan W *et al.* Prevalence of sleep-disordered breathing in diastolic heart failure. *Chest* 1997; **111**: 1488–93.

84. Shahar E, Whitney CW, Redline S *et al.* Sleep disordered breathing and cardiovascular disease. Cross sectional results of the sleep heart health study. *Am J Respir Crit Care Med* 2001; **163**: 19–25.

85. Morgan BJ, Denahan T, Ebert TJ. Neurocirculatory consequences of negative intrathoracic pressure vs asphyxia during voluntary apnea. *J Appl Physiol* 1993; **74**: 2969–75.

86. Mansfield D, Gollogly NC, Bergin P *et al.* Congestive heart failure and obstructive sleep apnea trial of continuous positive airway pressure. *Am J Respir Cit Care Med* 2004; **169**: 361–6.

●87. Kaneko Y, Floras JS, Usui K *et al.* Cardiovascular effects of CPAP in patients with CHF and OSA. *N Engl J Med* 2003; **348**: 1233–41.

88. Wessendorf TE, Wang YM, Thilmann AF *et al.* Treatment of OSA with nasal CPAP in stroke. *Eur Respir J* 2001; **18**: 623–9.

89. Peker Y, Kraiczi H, Hedner L *et al.* An independent association between OSA and coronary heart disease. *Eur Respir J* 1999; **13**: 179–84.

90. Hanly P, Sasson Z, Zuberi N, Lunn K. ST-segment depression during sleep in OSA. *Am J Cardiol* 1993; **71**: 1341–5.

91. Hung J, Whitford EG, Parsons RW *et al.* Association of sleep apnoea with myocardial infarction in men. *Lancet* 1990; **336**: 261–4.

●92. Franklin KA, Nilsson JB, Sahlin C, Naslund U. Sleep apnoea in nocturnal angina. *Lancet* 1995; **345**: 1085–7.

93. Mooe T, Franklin KA, Wiklund U *et al.* Sleep-disordered breathing and myocardial ischemia in patients with coronary artery disease. *Chest* 2000; **117**: 1597–1602.

94. Peker Y, Hedner J, Norum J *et al.* Increased incidence of cardiovascular disease in middle-aged men with OSA: a 7-year follow-up. *Am J Respir Crit Care Med* 2002; **166**: 159–65.

95. Freidlander AH, Friedlander IK, Yueh R, Littner MR. The prevalence of carotid atheromas seen on panoramic radiographs of patients with OSA and their relation to risk factors for atherosclerosis. *J Oral Maxillofac Surg* 1999; **57**: 516–22.

96. Chin K, Ohi M, Kita H *et al.* Effects of CPAP therapy on fibrinogen levels in OSA. *Am J Respir Crit Care Med* 1996; **153**: 1972–6.

●97. Bassetti C, Aldrich MS. Sleep apnea in acute cerebrovascular diseases:final report on 128 patients. *Sleep* 1999; **22**: 217–23.

98. Milanova A, Pfaffli B, Gugger M, Bassetti C. Sleep apnea in acute stroke: diagnosis, treatment and follow-up in 100 patients. *Sleep Res Online* 1999; **2**: 405.

99. Good DC, Henkle JQ, Gelber D *et al.* Sleep-disordered breathing and poor functional outcome after stroke. *Stroke* 1996; **27**: 252–9.

100. Sandberg O, Franklin KA, Bucht G *et al.* Nasal CPAP in stroke patients with sleep apnea: a randomised treatment study. *Eur Respir J* 2001; **18**: 630–4.

●101. Bradley TD, McNicholas WT, Rutherford R *et al.* Clinical and physiological heterogeneity of the central sleep apnea syndrome. *Am Rev Respir Dis* 1986; **134**: 217–21.

102. Stevenson TW and Perloff JK. The limited reliability of physical signs for estimating hemodynamics in chronic heart failure. *J Am Med Assoc* 1989; **261**: 884–8.

103. Xie A, Skatrud JB, Puleo DS *et al.* Apnea-hypopnea threshold for CO_2 in patients with congestive heart failure. *Am J Respir Crit Care Med* 2002; **165**: 1245–50.

104. Naughton MT, Benard DC, Liu PP *et al.* Effects of nasal CPAP on sympathetic activity in patients with heart failure and central sleep apnea. *Am J Respir Crit Care Med* 1995; **152**: 473–9.

105. Sun SY, Wang W, Zucker IH, Schultz HD. Enhanced peripheral chemoreceptor function in conscious rabbits with pacing induced heart failure. *J Appl Physiol* 1999; **86**: 1264–72.

106. Teichtahl H, Prodromidis A, Miller B *et al.* Sleep-disordered breathing in stable methadone programme patients: a pilot study. *Addiction* 2001; **96**: 395–403.

107. Wilkinson MH, Berger PJ, Blanch N *et al.* Paradoxical effect of oxygen administration on breathing stability following post hyperventilation apnoea in lambs. *J Physiol* 1997; **504**: 199–209.

108. Berger PJ, Skuza EM, Brodecky V *et al.* Unusual response to oxygen in an infant with repetitive cyanotic episodes. *Am J Respir Crit Care* 2000; **161**: 2107–11.

109. Mansfield D, Kaye DM, Brunner LaRocca H *et al.* Raised sympathetic nerve activity in heart failure and central sleep apnea is due to heart failure severity. *Circulation* 2003; **107**: 1396–400.

110. Solin P, Kaye DM, Little PJ *et al.* Impact of sleep apnea on sympathetic nervous system activity in heart failure. *Chest* 2003; **123**: 1119–26.

111. Lanfranchi PA, Braghiroli A, Bosimini E *et al.* Prognostic value of nocturnal Cheyne-Stokes respiration in chronic heart failure. *Circulation* 1999; **99**: 1435–40.

112. Solin P, Roebuck T, Swieca J *et al.* Effects of cardiac dysfunction on non-hypercapnic central sleep apnea. *Chest* 1998; **113**: 104–10.

113. Solin P, Roebuck T, Johns DP *et al.* Peripheral and central ventilatory responses in central sleep apnea with and without congestive heart failure. *Am J Respir Crit Care Med* 2000; **162**: 2194–200.

●114. Solin P, Bergin P, Richardson M *et al.* Influence of pulmonary capillary wedge pressure on central apnea in heart failure. *Circulation* 1999; **99**: 1574–9.

115. Roberston CH, Pagel MA, Johnson RL. The distribution of blood flow, oxygen consumption and work output among the respiratory muscles during unobstructed hyperventilation. *J Clin Invest* 1977; **59**: 43–50.

116. Levine M, Cleave JP, Dodds C. Can periodic breathing have advantages for oxygenation? *J. Theor Biol* 1995; **172**: 355–68.

117. Maze SS, Kotler MN, Parry WR. Doppler evaluation of changing cardiac dynamics during Cheyne-Stokes respiration. *Chest* 1989; **95**: 525–9.

118. Naughton MT, Floras JS, Rahman MA *et al.* Respiratory correlates of muscle sympathetic nerve activity in heart failure. *Clin Sci* 1998; **95**: 277–85.

119. DeBacker WA, Verbraeken J, Wilemen M *et al.* Central apnea index decreases after prolonged treatment with acetazolamide. *Am J Respir Crit Care Med* 1995; **151**: 87–91.

120. Haque WA, Boehmer J, Clemson BS, *et al.* Hemodynamic effects of supplemental oxygen administration in CHF. *J Am Coll Cardiol* 1996; **27**: 353–7.

121. Mansfield D, Solin P, Naughton MT. Central sleep apnea following successful heart transplant and attenuation of sympathetic activity. *Chest* 2003; **124**: 1675–81.

●122. Bersten AD, Holt AW, Vedig A *et al.* Treatment of severe cardiogenic pulmonary edema with CPAP delivered by a face mask. *N Engl J Med* 1991; **325**: 1825–30.

●123. Naughton MT, Liu PP, Benard DC *et al.* Treatment of congestive heart failure and Cheyne-Stokes respiration during sleep by CPAP. *Am J Respir Crit Care Med* 1995; **151**: 92–7.

124. Kaye DM, Mansfield D, Aggarwal A *et al.* Acute effects of CPAP on cardiac sympathetic tone in CHF. *Circulation* 2001; **103**: 2336–8.

125. Teschler H, Dohring J, Wang YM, Berthon-Jones M. Adaptive pressure support servo-ventilation. A novel treatment for Cheyne-Stokes respiration in heart failure. *Am J Respir Crit Care Med* 2001; **164**: 614–19.

126. Franklin KA, Eriksson P, Sahlin C *et al.* Reversal of central sleep apnoea with oxygen. *Chest* 1997; **111**: 163–9.

127. Mak S, Azevedo ER, Liu PP, Newton GE. Effect of hyperoxia on left ventricular function and filling pressures in patients with and without CHF. *Chest* 2001; **120**: 467–3.

128. Clark THJ and Hetzel MR. Diurnal variation of asthma. *Br J Dis Chest* 1977; **71**: 87–92.

129. Chan CS, Woolcock AJ, Sullivan CE. Nocturnal asthma: role of snoring and OSA. *Am Rev Respir Dis* 1988; **137**: 1502–4.

◆130. McNicholas WT. Impact of sleep in respiratory failure. *Eur Resp J* 1997; **10**: 920–33.

131. Breslin E, Van der Schans, Breubink S *et al.* Perception of fatigue and quality of life in patients with COPD. *Chest* 1998; **114**: 958–64.

132. Chan CS, Bye PTP, Woolcock AJ *et al.* Eucapnia and hypercapnia in patients with chronic airflow limitation: the role of the upper airway. *Am Rev Respir Dis* 1990; **141**: 861–5.

133. Fletcher EC, Donner CF, Midgren B *et al.* Survival in COPD patients with a daytime $PaO_2 > 60$ mmHg with and without nocturnal oxyhemoglobin desaturation. *Chest* 1992; **101**: 649–55.

134. Flick MR, Block AJ. Nocturnal vs diurnal arrhythmias in patients with chronic obstructive pulmonary disease. *Chest* 1989; **95**: 757–66.

135. Heijdra YF, Dekhuijzen PNR, van Herwaarden CLA, Folgering HThM. Nocturnal saturation and respiratory muscle function in patients with chronic obstructive pulmonary disease. *Thorax* 1995; **50**: 610–12.

136. Sanders MH, Newman AB, Haggerty CL *et al.* Sleep and sleep-disordered breathing in adults with predominately mild obstructive airay disease. *Am J Respir Crit Care Med* 2003; **167**: 7–14.

137. McEvoy RD, Mykytyn I, Sajkov D *et al.* Sleep apnoea in patients with quadriplegia. *Thorax* 1995; **50**: 613–19.

138. Sawicka EH Branthwaite MA. Respiration during sleep in kyphoscoliosis. *Thorax* 1987; **42**: 801–8.

139. Ellis ER, Grunstein RR, Chan S *et al.* Non-invasive ventilatory support during sleep improves respiratory failure in kyphoscoliosis. *Chest* 1988; **94**: 811–15.

140. Bourke SC, Shaw PJ, Gibson GJ. Respiratory function vs sleep-disordered breathing as predictors of QOL in ALS. *Neurology* 2001; **57**: 2040–4.

141. Kleopa KA, Shernman M, Neal B *et al.* BiPAP improves survival and rate of pulmonary function decline in patients with ALS. *J Neurol Sci* 1999; **164**: 82–8.

12

Pathophysiology of exercise and exercise assessment

LUCA BIANCHI, JOSEP ROCA

INTRODUCTION

Patients suffering from chronic lung disease frequently experience exercise intolerance, as a result of an imbalance between the load placed on their cardiorespiratory and muscle-metabolic system and their capacity to accomplish the task. Each compartment, in particular, has its own task.

The muscle's task involves utilization of the energy of stored substrates of ingested food. Utilization of these substrates within the muscles requires that oxygen be properly carried from its atmospheric source to the site of its utilization (i.e. the cellular mitochondria). Subsequently the by-products of energy transformation (heat and CO_2) must be cleared, respectively, through the skin and the lungs. Thus, the lungs appear to be the crucial beginning and terminus of gas exchange, which makes them the critical point in determining the individual's tolerance to exercise.

Chronic lung diseases encompass a group of nosological entities characterized by diverse constraints of exercise capacity (disability). As a result, exercise intolerance increases, a process long recognized as representative of the 'dyspnoea spiral' or, more properly, an 'incapacity spiral'. Exercise intolerance is therefore a hallmark of chronic pulmonary diseases. It is commonly associated with reduced quality of life and increased mortality (handicap) (1–3).

The physiological basis of exercise limitation is multifactorial (4). Ventilatory impairment, sensation of dyspnoea, cardiopulmonary interactions, skeletal and respiratory muscle dysfunction, and general systemic illness may all contribute in certain patients. An understanding of contributors to diminished exercise capacity is important for improvements in pulmonary rehabilitation programmes and for the development of new therapeutic strategies that may enhance physical performance.

Chronic obstructive pulmonary disease (COPD) has been extensively studied and therefore most of the current concepts of pathophysiology of exercise pertain to this disease. The aims of this chapter are to provide a basic understanding of the factors limiting exercise in patients with pulmonary disease and to indicate the best test to be performed in various settings.

FACTORS LIMITING EXERCISE RESPONSE IN HEALTHY SUBJECTS

The physiology of exercise in the healthy individual gives an important frame of reference for understanding the constraints of exercising for those with lung disease. Factors limiting maximal exercise in normal untrained subjects are the unpleasant perceptions of muscular fatigue and/or breathlessness, due to an O_2 demand that exceeds the maximal O_2 transport capability. Energy for muscular work derives from both aerobic (oxygen taken up from the inspired air and from the body's stores) and anaerobic (depletion of creatine phosphate stores and production of lactate and H^+) stores.

Submaximal muscle oxygen uptake ($\dot{V}_{O_2}$) in response to a ramp-type incremental exercise is controlled by the turnover of the high energy phosphate pool, at least for moderate exercise (5). $\dot{V}_{O_2}$ response during a ramp-type incremental test increases in a monophase linear fashion (c. 10 mL/min per W). This linearity has been shown to be maintained only up to lactate threshold (LT). Above LT, the slope is less for high increments of work and greater for low increments of work.

At moderate-intensity exercise, until LT is reached (c. 50 per cent of maximal $\dot{V}_{O_2}$), pulmonary CO_2 output is relatively linear with work rate, and it reflects oxidation of substrate mixture but is underestimated by increased tissue CO_2 storage (6).

At this moderate-intensity exercise, ventilation ($\dot{V}_E$) increases proportionally with $\dot{V}CO_2$: arterial pH and partial pressure of CO_2 (P_aCO_2) are regulated close to resting levels.

At higher work rate, resulting in sustained metabolic acidaemia (above LT), $\dot{V}CO_2$ profile steepens both with respect to work rate and $\dot{V}O_2$. This results from increased CO_2 from the bicarbonate (HCO_3^-) buffering of lactic acid in muscles and blood. $\dot{V}_E$ must therefore increase as a compensatory mechanism of increased $\dot{V}CO_2$ (7).

As a result of the above-described metabolic and gas exchange mechanisms, the $\dot{V}CO_2$–$\dot{V}O_2$ relationship during incremental exercise is characterized by a fairly linear trend during moderate exercise. The slope of this relationship immediately before LT steepens, following a similar linear trend thereafter. The intersection of the two slopes identifies a point which has been shown to estimate closely the increase in the blood concentration of lactates (V-slope method for non-invasive estimation of lactate threshold) (Fig. 12.1) (8).

Most healthy, untrained subjects have significant ventilatory reserve at maximum exercise: this means that $\dot{V}_E$ reached at maximum effort ($\dot{V}_{E,max}$) is usually less than the maximum voluntary ventilation (MVV). Only elite athletes can actually achieve airflows during part of the expiration equivalent to that achieved with maximum volitional effort (9).

Increase in $\dot{V}_E$ during exercise is highly variable in different subjects and may be the result of increase in respiratory frequency (f_R) tidal volume (V_T) or both. Most characteristically during moderate-intensity exercise, increase in $\dot{V}_E$ is determined by an increase in V_T, whereas during heavier exercise hyperpnoea is achieved mainly by increasing f_R. This strategy optimizes the work of breathing, limiting further increase in the elastic work of breathing, at high lung volumes. These mechanisms explain the importance of knowing slow and fast dynamic vital capacity and inspiratory capacity in predicting the breathing pattern response to exercise in different lung diseases: in restrictive diseases, for example, increase in f_R plays a more dominant role, thus resulting in a V_T approaching or even reaching the subject's resting inspiratory capacity and a f_R in excess of 50 breaths/min (10).

Arterial hypoxaemia is uncommon at sea level even during maximum exercise effort, but it may occur in some elite, highly fit athletes during high-intensity exercise (11). Inefficiency of pulmonary gas exchange as showed by widening of alveolar to arterial P_O_2 difference, is normal during exercise, becoming more evident during heavier exercise. This probably results from some ventilation/perfusion mismatching and diffusion impairment (11, 12).

Cardiac output ($\dot{Q}$), which is a determinant of muscle blood flow, has not been found to be significantly different between fit and unfit normal subjects at a given work rate; but as a consequence of higher stroke volume in trained subjects, higher work rates can be reached prior to maximum cardiac frequency being attained, thus resulting in higher achievable levels of $\dot{Q}$.

In summary, the causes and mechanisms of exercise limitation in healthy subjects are difficult to establish because of the difficulty in establishing the relative importance of each of the contributing factors to maximal exercise limitation. At maximal exercise there is significant ventilatory reserve (9). Oxygen saturation and content remain close to baseline values, despite some widening of the alveolar-to-arterial oxygen difference. As oxygen delivery to the skeletal muscles is increased, exercise performance is increased.

Therefore, in healthy subjects, maximal exercise appears to be limited by O_2 delivery, the product of cardiac output and arterial O_2 content. As arterial O_2 content is maintained, even at peak exercise, cardiac output is likely to be the limiting link. In fact, adding other exercising muscles to the two-legged exercise does not increase maximal $\dot{V}O_2$, suggesting that O_2 blood flow (cardiac output) has reached its maximal capacity.

EXERCISE RESPONSE IN LUNG DISEASE

The overall response to exercise in patients with lung disease is not substantially different from that of normal subjects. During exercise, O_2 uptake, CO_2 production, ventilation and cardiac output increase. However, the peak levels attained in disease become lower as lung impairment increases. The response to exercise depends upon the nature and severity of the underlying pulmonary disease. The influence of anthropometric values on exercise outcomes should also be accounted for (13–15).

For the sake of simplicity, the characteristics of exercise response in the two main categories of chronic lung diseases will be described in this chapter: obstructive diseases, as best represented by COPD, and restrictive diseases.

Obstructive lung diseases: mechanisms by which COPD affects exercise tolerance

Patients with COPD experience exertional dyspnoea but demonstrate widely variable exercise capacities. The ventilatory constraint, associated with reduced airflow, is the most important contributor to exercise intolerance in COPD

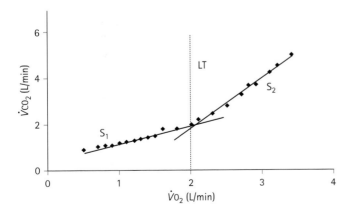

Figure 12.1 *Lactic threshold (LT) detection by the 'V-slope' method (see text for further explanations). The intercept of the slopes of the two linear phases (S_1 and S_2) is the LT.*

patients. Nonetheless, dyspnoea is not the only factor limiting exercise performance, suggesting that abnormal pulmonary gas exchange, pulmonary hypertension, reduced cardiac output and peripheral muscle dysfunction play important roles (16, 17).

VENTILATORY RESPONSE

The inspiratory muscle pump is excessively loaded during exercise in COPD, as a consequence of expiratory airflow limitation (Box 12.1). Patients with COPD have to generate increased minute ventilation to maintain blood gas homeostasis, because the destruction of lung tissue generates ventilation/perfusion mismatching (18) and because physiological dead space is increased. Even at rest, the load to the muscle pump is increased, as demonstrated by the increased transdiaphragmatic pressure generation, increased firing rates in motor units of the diaphragm and extradiaphragmatic inspiratory muscles (19–21).

During exercise, $\dot{V}_E$ increases and its relationship with work rate, in patients with COPD, has a slope similar to that of healthy individuals. But, as it happens at rest, $\dot{V}_E$ is somewhat higher than in normal subjects at the same workload. The increase in $\dot{V}_E$ may be obtained by two complementary mechanisms. The first option is to actively increase tidal volume by increasing lung volume into a region where maximum available airflow is higher (unlike normal subjects who breathe at a lower end-expiratory lung volume [EELV]) without necessarily reducing timing (T_I/T_{TOT}). The second option is to actively increase f_R, by reducing T_I/T_{TOT} in order to reduce the required expiratory flow at a given ventilation. The former requires tonic activation of inspiratory muscles and is

energetically costly. The latter requires a deliberate reduction of T_I/T_{TOT} from its naturally selected value. Although energetically superior, this approach might result in less breathlessness. It is possible that patients with strong inspiratory muscles choose the first option, whereas those with weaker muscles are driven to follow the second course. The impact of T_I/T_{TOT} on inspiratory muscle function is not so definite. Although, at a given $\dot{V}_E$, a shorter T_I/T_{TOT} translates into a greater inspiratory flow, the inspiratory muscles need to generate more pressure during inspiration. However, they contract for a shorter fraction of cycle time, which tends to reduce the tension-time index (22).

This scenario would offer a plausible explanation for much of the variability in maximum exercise performance in COPD, which would depend upon differences in ventilatory response to exercise (13) and in the subject's susceptibility to dynamic hyperinflation. This latter, in particular, has been shown to be an important influence on the patient's ability to generate higher flow rates during expiration (23).

GAS EXCHANGE

The homeostasis of arterial P_{CO_2} in healthy subjects and in patients with COPD is guaranteed by chemoreceptor sensitivity, the capacity of the respiratory pump to increase $\dot{V}_E$, and the linear shape of the dissociation curve for carbon dioxide (CO_2). These mechanisms compensate for increased levels of P_aCO_2 as a consequence of ventilation/perfusion mismatching, even if at a higher $\dot{V}_E$ and cost of breathing than normal. Nonetheless, in some COPD patients, the balance between the need for increased ventilation and the cost of breathing is struck and this results in a small increase in P_aCO_2. Some possible explanations exist for this phenomenon. The first is that even in the presence of a higher $\dot{V}_E$, reduced clearance of CO_2 from the blood persists, as a consequence of slow CO_2 output kinetics in the presence of increased physiological dead space (24). The second possibility is the development of worsening of $\dot{V}_A/\dot{Q}$ relationships during exercise in COPD. Whereas studies using the multiple inert gas elimination technique have shown that alteration of the ventilation/perfusion relationship, as well as shunts and diffusion alterations, do not occur on exercise in COPD patients (25), it has been reported that clinically stable COPD patients who developed hypercapnia during a hyperoxic breathing test were more likely to develop significant CO_2 retention during exercise (26). If hyperoxia, through suppression of the hypoxic vasoconstriction, represents an indirect measure of the extent of $\dot{V}/\dot{Q}$ inequalities at rest, patients who show more compromised gas exchange capabilities at rest may be more prone to develop hypercapnia during exercise, when challenged with increased $\dot{V}_{CO_2}$ and progressive mechanical restriction.

Most patients with severe COPD show decreased P_aO_2 at rest. The role of O_2 diffusion limitation due to alterations of the alveolar-capillary membrane appears to be negligible in these patients, unlike those with interstitial lung diseases (see below). Arterial P_{O_2} during exercise usually falls, but may sometimes even increase.

Box 12.1 Mechanisms by which respiratory system load is increased in chronic obstructive pulmonary disease patients

Resting

- Need to increase tidal volume (due to ventilation/perfusion ratio mismatch and/or increased alveolar dead space)
- Increase in chest wall elastance (breathing in the higher portion of the pressure/volume curve)
- Increased resistance of airways

During exercise

- Increase in inspiratory flow rate (as a consequence of increase in respiratory frequency and reduction of inspiratory phase of duty cycle)
- Development of dynamic hyperinflation from reduced airflow, resulting in breathing at higher lung volumes where lung compliance is reduced
- Increased CO_2 production from anaerobic metabolism in the limb muscles

HAEMODYNAMICS

The cardiac output response to exercise increases as the metabolic rate increases, but at peak exercise it is about 50 per cent of that achieved by a healthy age-matched subject. The cardiac output during exercise in lung disease may be limited to matching the intensity of exercise and $\dot{V}O_2$ attainable, depending upon the severity of the underlying disease. Breathlessness could exert some protective effect on the cardiovascular system, thus hiding underlying cardiovascular disorders (27), which would only be disclosed when factors limiting exercise performance in COPD are reduced, for instance, by adding inspiratory pressure support (27).

Pulmonary hypertension is a common complication of COPD (28). It is associated with shorter survival rates, worse clinical outcomes and increased use of health resources (29, 30). In COPD, pulmonary hypertension is considered to be present when the mean pressure of the pulmonary artery (P_{pa}) exceeds 20 mmHg (2.66 kPa). At rest the P_{pa} rarely exceeds 40 mmHg (5.32 kPa). A variety of causes may contribute to the development and maintenance of pulmonary hypertension in COPD, the most important of which are remodelling of pulmonary vessels and hypoxic vasoconstriction. The initial event in the natural history of pulmonary hypertension could develop in the pulmonary endothelium from cigarette smoke-induced downregulation of endothelial nitric oxide synthase (eNOS) expression and impairment of endothelial function (31, 32). At this stage, the reactivity of pulmonary arteries to hypoxia might also be altered in some patients with mild COPD (33–35), hence contributing to ventilation/perfusion mismatching and promoting the development of arterial hypoxaemia.

Patients prone to pulmonary hypertension may show an abnormal increase in P_{pa} during exercise, years before pulmonary hypertension is evident at rest (36). Possible causes of a further increase of P_{pa} during exercise in COPD include hypoxic vasoconstriction, reduction of the capillary bed by emphysema, extramural compression by increased alveolar pressure or impaired release of endothelium-derived relaxing factors. Since pulmonary hypertension may develop at moderate levels of exercise, it has been suggested that repeated episodes of pulmonary hypertension during daily activities, e.g. climbing stairs or even walking, could contribute to the development of right ventricular hypertrophy (36).

MUSCLES

Multiple factors combine to limit exercise performance in COPD. Peripheral muscle dysfunction is also an important contributing factor (37, 38). A detailed review of the peripheral muscles is found in Chapter 9. There is a recognized association between reduced muscle mass and survival in COPD, independent of the reduction in FEV_1 (39). Inactivity, acidosis, hypoxaemia, chronic inflammation, malnutrition, coexisting heart disease, severe deconditioning and medications, especially corticosteroids, have all been proposed as contributors to skeletal muscle dysfunction in COPD patients.

Studies on muscle function in COPD are limited by the relatively small number of subjects enrolled in randomized controlled trials, the lack of age-matched controls and methodological differences in work rates and patient selection criteria. Immobility-associated quadriceps weakness is greater than that of other muscle groups (40). However, malnutrition, androgen deficiency and inflammatory processes might all contribute to muscle weakness (41).

Biopsy of the quadriceps of patients with COPD has shown a loss of aerobic type I fibres (42) and a reduction in oxidative enzymes (43), suggesting a switch to anaerobic metabolism at a lower level of exercise than control subjects (44). Given that anaerobic metabolism produces lactate as an end-product, the increased lactate, buffered by bicarbonate with the consequent release of CO_2, imposes an additional ventilatory load on the respiratory muscles. Anaerobic metabolism also makes the muscle more susceptible to fatigue (44). It has been recently postulated that quadriceps muscles have a significant metabolic reserve, as isolated limb muscle performance can be improved by improving oxygen delivery (45); this would mean that anaerobic limb muscle metabolism would represent a significant additional load for exercising COPD patients.

In summary, in COPD, ventilatory, haemodynamic and peripheral muscle factors combine to limit exercise capacity. Therapies such as bronchodilators, oxygen, exercise training for specific skeletal muscle groups, nutritional intervention and anabolic hormones should be considered in the approach to disease management.

Determinants of exercise limitation in interstitial lung diseases

Beyond morphological, anatomical and histological differences among diseases that encompass the nosological entity of interstitial lung diseases (ILDs), these latter have in common some clinical, radiological and physiological characteristics. Restriction of the lung volumes, increased elastic recoil and low transfer factor of the lung for carbon monoxide are almost always present. Exertional dyspnoea and exercise intolerance represent very common complaints by ILD patients.

The mechanisms of exertional dyspnoea are multifactorial. Exertional dyspnoea in ILD may be aggravated by hypoxaemia (46) or by concomitant expiratory flow limitation (47). Abnormalities in ventilatory mechanics, gas exchange and circulatory impairment appear to contribute to exercise intolerance in these patients.

VENTILATORY RESPONSE

Hyperventilation at rest is a frequent finding in patients with ILD. It is unlikely to be caused by hypoxic stimulation of the peripheral chemoceptors, as it persists, even with a relatively normal arterial P_aO. One explanation is that hyperopnoea is consequent upon activation of J-receptors following the derangement of alveolar architecture (48).

The relationship between ventilation and work rate or $\dot{V}O_2$ in ILD patients has a similar slope to that in healthy patients, but during both rest and exercise, $\dot{V}_E$ is higher for any given workload. Reduced lung compliance requires more inspiratory muscle effort, which increases the work of breathing. During steady-state conditions, $\dot{V}_{O_2}$ increases as power output increases, as in healthy subjects.

The response of the respiratory system in ILD is restricted. Inspiratory capacity (IC) is reduced, tidal volume (V_T) expansion is constrained and must 'cycle' close to total lung capacity (TLC) on the upper non-linear extreme of the contracted pressure–volume (P–V) relationship of the respiratory system. As a consequence, f_R increases, reaching a higher level for a given $\dot{V}_E$ (49). There is no change in EELV, as dynamic hyperinflation does not contribute to exercise limitation (50). Reduced efficiency of gas exchange and, to some extent, circulatory impairment limit maximal exercise performance in ILD (51, 52).

HAEMODYNAMICS

At peak exercise, cardiac output is lower than in healthy subjects even if it seems to increase normally during exercise in patients with ILD. Pulmonary hypertension, not always evident at rest, increases significantly during exercise, especially when ILD is advanced, in keeping with the altered interstitium which interferes with vascular recruitment during exercise (53). The increase in pulmonary artery pressure occurs more frequently in those patients with a reduced resting T_LCO (lung transfer factor for CO) (53). In fact, T_LCO, rather than other measurements of lung function at rest, better predicts exercise performance in ILD patients, reflecting the predominant role of an altered lung capillary bed in exercise limitation (51).

GAS–EXCHANGE RESPONSE

Homeostasis of gas exchange is usually preserved at rest, but hypoxaemia is evident as the disease advances, whereas hypercapnia is seldom observed in ILD. Typically $P_{a}O_2$ falls, even dramatically, during exercise, due to $\dot{V}_A/\dot{Q}$ mismatch or shunt and especially due to the limitation of the O_2 transfer by the alveolar-capillary membrane. The abnormalities are further enhanced by a reduction of the capillary transit time and of $P_{v}O_2$ (53).

EXERCISE ASSESSMENT

Exercise testing has become a versatile tool for diagnosis, risk stratification for surgery, measuring disability and evaluating response to interventions such as exercise training. Resting pulmonary and cardiac function do not predict exercise capacity (54–56), and exertional symptoms correlate poorly with resting cardiopulmonary measurements (16, 57, 58). Although exertional dyspnoea is a common symptom in patients with respiratory disease, exercise limitations also include leg discomfort, chest pain and fatigue (16, 55).

Exercise capacity can be assessed by both simple and sophisticated tests. The global assessment from a cardiopulmonary exercise test (CPET) permits an objective determination of the factors limiting exercise, such as the respiratory vs. the cardiac contribution to exercise limitation. CPET is also useful for monitoring disease progression and treatment response (59). In contrast, the 6-min walking test (6-MWT) requires only a hallway. The latter has been standardized and has gained in popularity (60–63), such that both the 6-MWT and CPET are used for exercise assessment, the choice being determined by the question to be answered.

Cardiopulmonary exercise test

The cardiopulmonary exercise test provides a global assessment of the integrative exercise response involving the pulmonary, cardiovascular, haematopoietic, neuropsychological and skeletal muscle systems that is not adequately reflected through the measurement of resting function (59). The main clinical applications of CPET include the evaluation of exercise-induced symptoms and the determination of functional capacity. CPET can be used in diagnosis, assessment of severity, prognosis and response to treatment. Box 12.2 lists the indications for CPET.

CPET is particularly useful for monitoring the efficacy of interventions directed at reducing breathlessness by improving breathing strategy and dynamic hyperinflation in COPD

Box 12.2   Main indications for CPET

Evaluation of exercise tolerance

- Determination of functional impairment or capacity ($\dot{V}_{O_2,peak}$)
- Determination of exercise-limiting factors and pathophysiological mechanisms

Evaluation of undiagnosed exercise intolerance

- Assessing contribution of cardiac and pulmonary aetiology in coexisting disease
- Symptoms disproportionate to resting pulmonary and cardiac tests
- Unexplained dyspnoea when initial cardiopulmonary testing is non-diagnostic

Evaluation of patients with cardiovascular disease

- Functional evaluation and prognosis in patients with heart failure
- Selection for cardiac transplantation
- Exercise prescription and monitoring response to exercise training for cardiac rehabilitation

Evaluation of patients with respiratory disease

- Functional impairment assessment
- In COPD:
  - establishing exercise limitation(s) and assessing other potential contributing factors, especially occult heart disease (ischaemia)

- determination of magnitude of hypoxaemia and for O_2 prescription
- when objective determination of therapeutic intervention is necessary and not adequately addressed by standard pulmonary function testing
- Interstitial lung diseases
  - detection of early (occult) gas exchange abnormalities
  - overall assessment/monitoring of pulmonary gas exchange
  - determination of magnitude of hypoxaemia and for O_2 prescription
  - determination of potential exercise-limiting factors
  - documentation of therapeutic response to potentially toxic therapy
- Pulmonary vascular disease (careful risk–benefit analysis required)
- Cystic fibrosis
- Exercise-induced bronchospasm

Specific clinical applications

- Preoperative evaluation
  - lung resectional surgery
  - elderly patients undergoing major abdominal surgery
  - lung volume resectional surgery for emphysema (currently investigational)
- Exercise evaluation and prescription for pulmonary rehabilitation
- Evaluation for impairment/disability
- Evaluation for lung, heart–lung transplantation

> **Box 12.3**   Main contraindications of cardiopulmonary exercise testing
>
> **Absolute**
>
> - Recent acute myocardial infarction (3–5 days)
> - Unstable angina
> - Symptomatic and uncontrolled arrhythmias causing instability of haemodynamics
> - Acute endocarditis, myocarditis or pericarditis
> - Symptomatic severe aortic stenosis
> - Acute cardiac failure
> - Acute pulmonary thromboembolism or pulmonary infarction
> - Acute disorders potentially affecting exercising or worsened by exercise (infection, renal failure)
>
> **Relative**
>
> - Left main coronary stenosis or equivalent
> - Moderate stenotic valvular cardiac disease
> - Severe hypertension (systolic >200 mmHg and diastolic >120 mmHg)
> - Electrolyte abnormalities
> - Significant pulmonary hypertension
> - Arrhythmias
> - Hypertrophic cardiomyopathy
> - Atrioventricular block of high degree
> - Thrombotic disease of lower limbs
> - Inability to cooperate

---

patients. These include exercise rehabilitation training (64), non-invasive ventilation (65), bronchodilators (66), lung volume reduction surgery (67) and skeletal muscle dysfunction (43). The preoperative measurement of oxygen uptake ($\dot{V}O_2$) has been shown to predict postoperative complications accurately (68, 69). A $\dot{V}O_{2,peak}$ <50–60 per cent of predicted is associated with a higher morbidity and mortality after lung resection (68–70). The use of an algorithm for the functional assessment of patients being considered for lung resection reduced morbidity and mortality by half without unnecessarily excluding patients from surgery (71).

Exercise training is a key part of pulmonary rehabilitation (64, 72–75). The CPET provides information before training, to determine safety and to optimize training intensity. After training it is used to document improvement and refine training levels. Physiological training can be accomplished even in severe COPD and even without achieving lactic acidosis. Improved ventilatory efficiency and improved skeletal muscle bioenergetics have been suggested as physiological explanations (74). A training-induced reduction in skeletal muscle redox status has been demonstrated in patients with COPD (76, 77). The optimal training regimens, such as the combination of strength and endurance training, remain the subject of clinical trials (78).

Box 12.3 summarizes the main contraindications for exercise assessment. Absolute contraindications are often obvious, but relative contraindications must be carefully weighed against the potential gains from the test.

CPET commonly employs two modes of exercise, treadmill walking and stationary cycling (Table 12.1), each with its own advantages. Whatever the test modality, the same exercise modality for testing should be used as for the exercise training prescription. Treadmill exercise closely resembles daily living activities. Its main disadvantage is in accurately quantifying the external work rate. The relationship between treadmill speed and elevation and the metabolic cost ($\dot{V}O_2$) of performing work is only an estimate (79), influenced by the weight of the subject as well as the pacing strategy. Weight has much less influence on cycle ergometry, which provides a more accurate estimate of external work.

Exercise testing includes incremental protocols and constant-work rate protocols (59). Incremental cycle ergometry measures the integrated responses to the tolerable range of work rates (80). As work increases, the variables of interest, such as $\dot{V}_E$, $\dot{V}CO_2$ and $\dot{V}O_2$, will change. A standard incremental cycle ergometry test consists of 3 min of rest, followed by 3 min of unloaded pedalling and then an incremental phase of loaded cycling every minute until the patient is limited by symptoms or the test is interrupted by the physician (Table 12.1). The increment size (5–25 W/min) should be decided

Table 12.1 *Advantages and disadvantages of treadmill and cycle ergometry*

	Cycle	Treadmill
$\dot{V}_{O_2,max}$	Lower	Higher
Work rate measurement	More accurate	Less accurate
Noise and artifacts	Less	More
Blood gas sampling	Easier	More difficult
Safety	Safer	Less safe
Weight-bearing in obese	Less	More
Degree of leg muscle training	Less	More

according to the characteristics of the patient in order to obtain approximately 10 min of loaded exercise. Exercise tests in which the incremental phase lasts 8–12 min are efficient and provide useful diagnostic information (59, 81). If a treadmill is used, the incremental protocol is similar. The Balke's protocol is simple and feasible even in patients with moderate to severe pulmonary disease: the speed of the treadmill is kept constant at 3.3 mph and the elevation is increased by 1 per cent every minute (82).

Constant-work rate exercise may yield a steady-state response provided that the work rate is of moderate intensity. Such protocols are increasingly used to monitor treatment responses to cardiopulmonary rehabilitation, bronchodilators, surgery and medical devices (64–67). Oxygen requirements during exercise are easily attainable at work rates that simulate daily activity. Inspiratory capacity measurements are used to identify dynamic hyperinflation (4). A constant-work rate test should be performed after an incremental test in order to use 50–70 per cent of the maximal work rate. At least 6 min of continuous exercise is the minimum duration of this test. A constant-work rate test for 5–10 min often achieves 70–90 per cent of $\dot{V}_{O_2,max}$ achieved during an incremental test (59).

CPET involves the measurement of respiratory gas exchange: oxygen uptake ($\dot{V}_{O_2}$), carbon dioxide output ($\dot{V}_{CO_2}$), and minute ventilation ($\dot{V}_E$), in addition to monitoring electrocardiography, blood pressure and oxygen saturation by pulse oximetry. When appropriate, arterial sampling provides more detailed information about pulmonary gas exchange (59).

Not infrequently, patients with cardiopulmonary disorders performing a CPET are symptom-limited rather than physiologically limited. Therefore, symptom assessment of effort is helpful. The availability of reliable measurement tools, and the clear relationship between symptoms and physiological variables, have made it possible to characterize and quantify symptoms during exercise (16, 83–87). Patients with respiratory disease usually report that breathlessness and/or leg discomfort are the major symptoms that 'limit' exercise (88). The Visual Analogue Scale (VAS) (89, 90) and the Category Ratio (CR)-10 Scale developed by Borg (91) are the major instruments used to quantify symptoms during an exercise test. There are several theoretical advantages of the CR-10 Scale:

- A numeric descriptor on the CR-10 Scale is easier to use as a dyspnoea target than the length in millimetres on the VAS.

- The CR-10 Scale is open-ended, so that the patient can select a number greater than 10. In contrast, the VAS has a ceiling, as the highest possible rating is 100 mm.
- Descriptors on the CR-10 Scale enable direct comparisons between individuals at a specific rating (e.g. 3 or moderate breathlessness). Comparison of VAS dyspnoea ratings between individuals is problematic because the only anchors are no breathlessness or maximal breathlessness, which may be distinct for each person.

In general, most subjects discontinue exercise at ratings of 5–8 on the CR-10 Scale or 50–80 on the VAS, with few subjects rating dyspnoea or leg effort as maximal (10 on the modified Borg Scale) at the time of cessation (90–92).

INTERPRETATION STRATEGIES

Exercise limitation in a healthy person is generally due to limitation of cardiac output (9). Precise exercise responses during CPET, for various clinical entities, are difficult to predict as there is wide overlap and often several factors contribute to exercise limitation. However, some patterns of change do occur (Table 12.2 and Fig. 12.2).

In obesity, $\dot{V}_{O_2,peak}$ may be reduced when it is expressed per kilogram of actual body weight, or normal when it is expressed per kilogram of ideal body weight. The excessive metabolic requirement for a given amount of work reflects the high cost of moving the weight of the legs. Obese individuals, in performing daily activities while 'loaded' with a greater body mass, do show a sort of training effect, which is reflected by usually normal $\dot{V}_{O_2,peak}$, peak O_2 pulse and anaerobic threshold (AT). As a result of the increased metabolic requirement, $\dot{V}_E$ at a given external work rate is higher in obese than in lean subjects. Expiratory flow limitation also occurs in obese patients as a consequence of their breathing at low lung volumes and their inability to increase EELV sufficiently during exercise, presumably secondary to the increased inspiratory load (93, 94). The increased elastic load of excess adipose tissue is the primary cause of the increased work of breathing. The typical breathing pattern in obesity, characterized by increased respiratory rate and reduced tidal volume compared with normal subjects, might be an attempt to reduce work of breathing (95). Abnormal resting $P_{a}O_2$ and $P_{(A-a)}O_2$ may result from the decrease in chest wall and lung compliance as well as segmental atelectasis (96). These abnormalities may improve as the tidal volume increases during exercise and the overall $\dot{V}/\dot{Q}$ relationships improve. Diastolic dysfunction, a subclinical form of cardiomyopathy, also occurs even in asymptomatic, morbidly obese patients (97, 98).

In psychogenic disorders, exertional dyspnoea, chest pain and light-headedness are presenting complaints. These symptoms are seen in anxiety reactions, hysteria, panic disorders and obsessional behaviour (99–101). Hyperventilation, as evident from abnormal increases in $\dot{V}_E$, $\dot{V}_E/\dot{V}_{CO_2}$ and respiratory rate, are the main CPET response characteristics of these patients, with consequent respiratory alkalosis (101, 102). A normal or near-normal $\dot{V}_{O_2,peak}$ and work rate, together with a careful history, will provide a correct diagnosis.

Table 12.2 *Pattern of cardiopulmonary response*

Measurement	COPD	ILD	Obesity	Deconditioning	Malingering
$\dot{V}O_{2,max}$ or $\dot{V}O_{2,peak}$	↓	↓	↓ or =	↓	↓
AT	↓ = or ND	= or ↓	=	= or ↓	ND
Peak HR	↑ or = in mild	↓	= or ↓	= or ↓	↓
O_2 pulse	= or ↓	= or ↓	=	↓	↓
$\dot{V}_E/MVV$ (%)	↑	= or ↑	=	=	↑ or =
$\dot{V}_E/\dot{V}CO_2$ (at AT)	↑	↑	=	=	↑ or =
V_D/V_T	↑	↑	=	=	=
P_aO_2	↑↓=	↓	= or ↓	=	=
$P_{(A-a)}O_2$	↑↓=	↑	= or ↓	=	=

COPD, chronic obstructive pulmonary disease; ILD, interstitial lung disease; AT, anaerobic threshold; $\dot{V}O_2$, oxygen uptake; HR, heart rate; $\dot{V}_E/MVV$, ventilatory reserve; $\dot{V}_E/\dot{V}CO_2$, ventilatory equivalent for CO_2; V_D/V_T, physiological dead space to tidal volume ratio; P_aO_2, partial arterial oxygen pressure; $P_{(A-a)}O_2$, alveolar–arterial difference for oxygen pressure.

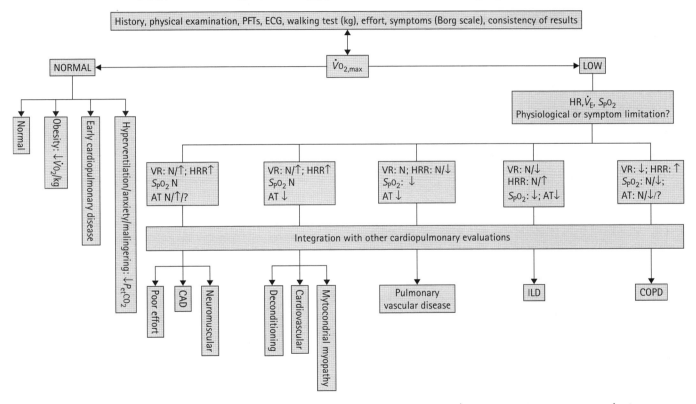

Figure 12.2 *Algorithm for interpretation of exercise response. PFT, pulmonary function tests; $\dot{V}O_{2,max}$, maximal oxygen uptake; $\dot{V}O_2/kg$, oxygen uptake per kg; HR, heart rate; $\dot{V}_E$, minute ventilation; S_pO_2, oxygen saturation by pulse oximetry; $P_{et}CO_2$, end-tidal CO_2; VR, $\dot{V}_E/MVV \times 100$, ventilatory reserve; HRR, heart rate reserve; AT, anaerobic threshold; CAD, coronary artery disease; ILD, interstitial lung disease; COPD, chronic obstructive pulmonary disease.*

Deliberately inadequate effort may be hard to identify unless there is knowledge of the secondary gain. Poor effort is characterized by early cessation of exercise and a reduced $\dot{V}O_{2,peak}$, normal or unattained AT, a low R-value at exercise cessation, and substantial heart rate as well as ventilatory reserve with no readily apparent peripheral abnormality. Erratic breathing patterns, intermittent hyperventilation and hypoventilation, irregular respiratory rates and fluctuation in $P_{et}CO_2$ and P_aCO_2 unrelated to work rate are signs of an uncooperative subject. Symptom scores may be totally disproportionate to the level of effort.

In summary, CPET interpretation involves an understanding of the integrative approach to the physiology of exercise limitation in which the specific patterns of exercise response can be associated with various clinical entities (Fig. 12.2).

Walking tests

Timed-walking tests are increasingly being used in clinical practice to assess exercise tolerance in patients affected with chronic respiratory conditions (60–62, 103, 104).

The 6-MWT is a simple and practical test, used to evaluate walking (63). It does not provide specific information on each of the systems involved with exercise but it reflects functional capacity (63). The 6-MWT has good reliability, validity and interpretability as a measure of functional capacity (60–62). Its utility has been enhanced by the availability of normative tables (105–107). The product of body weight and walking distance accounts for differences in body weight and thereby estimates both work and energy expenditure as force distance (108). In some clinical situations, the 6-MWT is a better index of ability to perform daily activities than peak oxygen uptake, as it correlates better with measures of quality of life (109). Changes in 6-MWT after therapeutic interventions correlate with subjective improvements in dyspnoea (110, 111). The 6-MWT is also sensitive in detecting exercise-induced desaturation in patients with COPD (112).

In summary, the 6-MWT is useful and complementary to the CPET in the comprehensive evaluation of patients with respiratory disease. In severe COPD the 6-min walk distance predicts mortality better than other traditional markers of disease severity such as body mass index (BMI) or degree of co-morbidity (113).

The shuttle-walking test uses an audio signal from a tape cassette to direct the walking pace of the patient back and forth on a 10 m course (114–117). The walking speed is increased every minute, and the test ends when the patient cannot reach the turnaround point within the required time. The exercise performed is similar to a symptom-limited, maximal, incremental treadmill test. An advantage of the shuttle-walking test is that it has a better correlation with peak oxygen uptake than the 6-MWT. Disadvantages include less validation, less widespread use and more potential for cardiovascular problems.

Key points

● Pathophysiology of exercise in the healthy subject.
● Factors limiting exercise performance in chronic obstructive pulmonary disease and interstitial lung diseases.
● Assessment of exercise tolerance in chronic lung diseases by cardiopulmonary exercise testing and by walking tests.
● Interpretation of exercise response in chronic pulmonary diseases.

REFERENCES

◆1. American Thoracic Society. Standards for the diagnosis and care of patients with chronic obstructive pulmonary disease (COPD) and asthma. *Am J Respir Crit Care Med* 1995; **152**: S77–121.
2. Ries AL, Kaplan RM, Limberg TM, Prewitt LM. Effects of pulmonary rehabilitation on physiological and psychosocial outcomes in patients with chronic obstructive pulmonary disease. *Ann Intern Med* 1995; **122**: 823–32.
3. Gerardi DA, Lovett L, Benoit-Connors ML *et al.* Variables related to increased mortality following out-patient pulmonary rehabilitation. *Eur Respir J* 1996; **9**: 431–5.
●4. O'Donnell DE, Revill SM, Webb KA. Dynamic hyperinflation and exercise intolerance in chronic obstructive pulmonary disease. *Am J Respir Crit Care Med* 2001; **164**: 770–7.
5. Kushmerick MJ, Meyer RA, Brown TR. Regulation of oxygen consumption in fast- and slow-twitch muscle. *Am J Physiol* 1992; **263**: C598–606.
●6. Whipp BJ. The bioenergetic and gas-exchange basis for exercise testing. *Clin Chest Med* 1994; **15**: 173–92.
7. Douglas CG. Co-ordination of the respiration and circulation with variations in bodily activity. *Lancet* 1927; **2**: 213–18.
●8. Beaver WL, Wassermann K, Whipp BJ. A new method for detecting the anaerobic threshold by gas exchange. *J Appl Physiol* 1986; **60**: 2020–7.
9. Johnson BD, Dempsey JA. Demand vs capacity in the aging pulmonary system. *Ex Sports Sci Rev* 1991; **19**: 171–210.
◆10. Jones NL, Killian KJ, Stubbing DG. The thorax in exercise. In: Roussos CH, Macklem PT, eds. *The Thorax. Lung Biology in Health and Disease*, Vol. 29. New York: Marcel Dekker, 1988; 627–62.
11. Wagner PD, Gale GE, Moon RE, Torre-Bueno J, Stolp BW, Saltzman HA. Pulmonary gas exchange in humans exercising at sea levels and stimulated altitude. *J Appl Physiol* 1986; **60**: 260–70.
12. Powers SK, Lawler J, Dempsey JA, Dodd S, Landry G. Effects of incomplete pulmonary gas exchange on VO$_2$max. *J Appl Physiol* 1986; **66**: 2491–5.
13. Bauerle O, Younes M. Role of ventilatory response to exercise in determining exercise capacity in COPD. *J Appl Physiol* 1995; **79**: 1870–7.
14. Riddle W, Younes M, Remmers J. Graphical analysis of patient performance in the pulmonary function laboratory. *Fourth Annual Symposium on Computer Applications in Medical Care, November 2–5.* Washington, DC: IEEE, 1980; 282–290.
◆15. Younes M. Interpretation of clinical exercise testing in respiratory disease. *Clin Chest Med* 1980; **5**: 189–206.
●16. Killian KJ, Leblanc P, Martin DH *et al.* Exercise capacity and ventilatory, circulatory, and symptom limitation in patients with chronic airflow limitation. *Am Rev Respir Dis* 1992; **146**: 935–40.
◆17. Polkey MI. Muscle metabolism and exercise tolerance in COPD. *Chest* 2002; **121**: 131–5S.
18. Wagner PD, Dantzker DR, Dueck R *et al.* Ventilation-perfusion inequality in chronic obstructive pulmonary disease. *J Clin Invest* 1977; **59**: 203–16.
19. Bellemare F, Grassino A. Force reserve of the diaphragm in patients with chronic obstructive pulmonary disease. *J Appl Physiol* 1983; **55**: 8–15.
20. De Troyer A, Leeper JB, McKenzie DK *et al.* Neural drive of the diaphragm in patients with severe COPD. *Am J Respir Crit Care Med* 1997; **155**: 1335–40.
21. Gandevia SC, Leeper JB, McKenzie DK *et al.* Discharge frequencies of parasternal intercostal and scalene motor units during breathing in normal and COPD subjects. *Am J Respir Crit Care Med* 1996; **153**: 622–8.
●22. Bellemare F, Grassino A. Effect of pressure and timing of contraction on human diaphragm fatigue. *J Appl Physiol* 1982; **53**: 1190–5.
23. Bauerle O, Chrusch CA, Younes M. Mechanisms by which COPD affects exercise tolerance. *Am J Respir Crit Care Med* 1998; **157**: 57–68.
24. Diaz O, Villafranca C, Ghezzo H *et al.* Breathing pattern and gas exchange at peak exercise in COPD patients with and without tidal flow limitation at rest. *Eur Respir J* 2001; **17**: 1120–7.

25. Dantzker DR, D'Alonzo GE. The effect of exercise on pulmonary gas-exchange in patients with severe chronic obstructive pulmonary disease. *Am Rev Respir Dis* 1986; **134**: 1135–9.

26. O'Donnel DE, D'Arsigny C, Fitzpatrick M, Webb KA. Exercise hypercapnia in advanced chronic obstructive pulmonary disease. *Am J Respir Crit Care Med* 2002; **166**: 663–8.

27. Bianchi L, Foglio K, Porta R et al. Lack of additional effect of adjunct of assisted ventilation to pulmonary rehabilitation in mild COPD patients. *Respir Med* 2002; **96**: 359–67.

28. Scharf SM, Iqbal M, Keller C et al. Hemodynamic characterization of patients with severe emphysema. *Am J Respir Crit Care Med* 2002; **166**: 314–22.

29. Burrows B, Kettel L J, Niden AH et al. Patterns of cardiovascular dysfunction in chronic obstructive lung disease. *N Engl J Med* 1972; **286**: 912–18.

30. Weitzenblum E, Hirth C, Ducolone A et al. Prognostic value of pulmonary artery pressure in chronic obstructive pulmonary disease. *Thorax* 1981; **36**: 752–758.

31. Dinh-Xuan AT, Higenbottam TW, Clelland CA et al. Impairment of endothelium-dependent pulmonary-artery relaxation in chronic obstructive lung disease. *N Engl J Med* 1991; **324**: 1539–47.

32. Clini E, Cremona G, Campana M et al. Production of endogenous nitric oxide in chronic obstructive pulmonary disease and patients with cor pulmonale: correlates with echo-Doppler assessment. *Am J Respir Crit Care Med* 2000; **162**: 446–50.

33. Wright JL, Petty T, Thurlbeck WM. Analysis of the structure of the muscular pulmonary arteries in patients with pulmonary hypertension and COPD. National Institutes of Health Nocturnal Oxygen Therapy Trial. *Lung* 1992; **170**: 109–24.

34. Ashutosh K, Mead G, Dunsky M. Early effects of oxygen administration and prognosis in chronic obstructive pulmonary disease and cor pulmonale. *Am Rev Respir Dis* 1983; **127**: 399–404.

35. Peinado VI, Santos S, Ramirez J et al. Response to hypoxia of pulmonary arteries in COPD. an in vitro study. *Eur Respir J* 2002; **20**: 332–8.

36. Kessler R, Faller M, Weitzenblum E et al. 'Natural history' of pulmonary hypertension in a series of 131 patients with chronic obstructive lung disease. *Am J Respir Crit Care Med* 2001; **164**: 219–24.

37. Casaburi R. Limitation to exercise tolerance in chronic obstructive pulmonary disease. Look to the muscles of deambulation. *Am J Respir Crit Care Med* 2003; **168**: 409–10.

38. Saey D, Debigaré R, Leblanc P et al. Contractile leg fatigue after cycle exercise a factor limiting exercise in patients with chronic obstructive pulmonary disease. *Am J Respir Crit Care Med* 2003; **168**: 425–30.

◆39. Marquis K, Debigaré R, Lacasse Y et al. Midthigh muscle cross-sectional area is better predictor of mortality than body mass index in patients with chronic obstructive pulmonary disease. *Am J Respir Crit Care Med* 2002; **166**: 809–13.

◆40. Bernard S, Leblanc P, Whittom F et al. Peripheral muscle weakness in patients with chronic obstructive pulmonary disease. *Am J Respir Crit Care Med* 1998; **158**: 629–34.

41. Schols AM, Buurman WA. Staal van den Brekel AJ et al. Evidence for a relation between metabolic derangements and increased levels of inflammatory mediators in a subgroup of patients with chronic obstructive pulmonary disease. *Thorax* 1996; **51**: 819–24.

42. Jakobsson P, Jorfeldt L, Brundin A. Skeletal muscle metabolites and fibre types in patients with advanced chronic obstructive

pulmonary disease, with and without chronic respiratory failure. *Eur Respir J* 1990; **3**: 192–6.

43. Maltais F, Simard A-A, Simard C et al. Oxidative capacity of the skeletal muscle and lactic acid kinetics during exercise in normal subjects and in patients with COPD. *Am J Respir Crit Care Med* 1996; **153**: 288–93.

44. Mador MJ, Kufel TJ, Pineda L. Quadriceps fatigue after cycle exercise in patients with chronic obstructive pulmonary disease. *Am J Respir Crit Care Med* 2000; **161**: 447–53.

45. Richardson RS, Sheldon J, Poole DC et al. Evidence of skeletal muscle metabolic reserve during whole body exercise in patients with chronic obstructive pulmonary disease. *Am J Respir Crit Care Med* 1999; **159**: 881–5.

46. Bye PTB, Anderson SD, Woodcock AJ et al. Bicycle endurance performance of patients with interstitial lung disease breathing air and oxygen. *Am Rev Respir Dis* 1982; **126**: 1005–12.

47. Marciniuk DD, Sridhar G, Clemens RE et al. Lung volumes and expiratory flow limitation during exercise in interstitial lung disease. *J Appl Physiol* 1994; **77**: 963–73.

48. Paintal AS. Vagal sensory receptors and their reflex effects. *Physiol Rev* 1973; **53**: 159–227.

49. Younes M. *Determinants of Thoracic Excursions During Exercise.* In: Whipp BJ, Wasserman K, eds. *Exercise, Pulmonary Physiology and Pathophysiology*, Vol. 52. (Lung Biol. Health Dis. Ser.). New York: Dekker, 1991; 1–65.

50. Marciniuk DD, Sridhar G, Clemens RE, Zintel TA, Gallagher CG. Lung volumes and expiratory flow limitation during exercise in interstitial lung disease. *J Appl Physiol* 1994; **77**: 963–73.

51. Harris-Eze AO, Sridhar G, Clemens RE et al. Role of hypoxemia and pulmonary mechanics in exercise limitation in interstitial lung disease. *Am J Respir Crit Care Med* 1996; **154**: 994–1001.

52. Hansen JE, Wasserman K. Pathophysiology of activity limitation in patients with interstitial lung disease. *Chest* 1996; **109**: 1566–76.

53. Agusti AG, Roca J, Gea J et al. Mechanisms of gas-exchange impairment in ideopathic pulmonary fibrosis. *Am Rev Respir Dis* 1991; **143**: 219–25.

54. Wasserman K, Hansen JE, Sue DY et al. *Principles of Exercise Testing and Interpretation: Including Pathophysiology and Clinical Applications*, 3rd edn. Philadelphia: Lippincott Williams & Wilkins, 1999; 15.

55. Hamilton AL, Killian KJ, Summers E, Jones NL. Muscle strength, symptom intensity, and exercise capacity in patients with cardiorespiratory disorders. *Am J Respir Crit Care Med* 1995; **152**: 2021–31.

56. Weisman IM, Zeballos RJ. Clinical exercise testing. *Clin Chest Med* 2001; **22**: 679–701.

57. Franciosa JA, Park M, Levine TB. Lack of correlation between exercise capacity and indexes of resting left ventricular performance in heart failure. *Am J Cardiol* 1981; **47**: 33–9.

58. Weber KT, Janicki JS. *Cardiopulmonary Exercise Testing: Physiologic Principles and Clinical Applications.* Philadelphia: WB Saunders, 1986; 16.

◆59. American Thoracic Society/American College of Chest Physicians. ATS/ACCP statement on cardiopulmonary exercise testing. *Am J Respir Crit Care Med* 2003; **167**: 211–77.

60. Guyatt GH, Sullivan MJ, Thompson PJ et al. The six-minute walk test: a new measure of exercise capacity in patients with chronic heart failure. *Can Med Assoc J* 1985; **132**: 919–23.

61. Butland RJA, Pang J, Gross ER et al. Two-, six-, and 12-minute walking tests in respiratory disease. *Br Med J* 1982; **284**: 1607–8.

62. Solway S, Brooks D, Lacasse Y, Thomas S. A qualitative systematic overview of the measurement properties of functional walk tests used in the cardiorespiratory domain. *Chest* 2001; **119**: 256–70.

◆63. ATS Statement. Guidelines for the six-minute walk test. *Am J Respir Crit Care Med* 2002; **166**: 111–17.

◆64. American Thoracic Society. Pulmonary rehabilitation – 1999. *Am J Respir Crit Care Med* 1999; **159**: 1666–82.

◆65. van't Hul A, Kwakkel G, Gosselink R. The acute effects of noninvasive ventilatory support during exercise on exercise endurance and dyspnea in patients with chronic obstructive pulmonary disease. A systematic review. *J Cardiopulm Rehab* 2002; **22**: 290–7.

◆66. Liesker JJW, Wijkstra PJ, Ten Hacken NHT *et al.* A systematic review of the effects of bronchodilators on exercise capacity in patients with COPD. *Chest* 2002; **121**: 597–608.

67. American Thoracic Society. Lung volume reduction surgery: official statement of the American Thoracic Society. *Am J Respir Crit Care Med* 1996; **154**: 1151–2.

68. Bolliger CT, Jordan P, Soler M *et al.* Exercise capacity as a predictor of postoperative complications in lung resection candidates. *Am J Respir Crit Care Med* 1995; **151**: 1472–80.

69. Bolliger CT, Perruchoud AP. Functional evaluation of the lung resection candidate. *Eur Respir J* 1998; **11**: 198–212.

70. Morice RC, Peters EJ, Ryan MB *et al.* Redefining the lowest exercise peak oxygen consumption acceptable for lung resection of high risk patients. *Chest* 1996; **110**: 161S.

71. Wyser C, Stulz P, Soler M *et al.* Prospective evaluation of an algorithm for the functional assessment of lung resection candidates. *Am J Respir Crit Care Med* 1999; **159**: 1450–6.

◆72. American Association of Cardiovascular and Pulmonary Rehabilitation. Pulmonary rehabilitation: joint ACCP/AACVPR evidence-based guidelines. ACCP/AACVPR Pulmonary Rehabilitation Guidelines Panel. *Chest* 1997; **112**: 1363–96.

73. Maltais F, Leblanc P, Jobin J *et al.* Intensity of training and physiologic adaptation in patients with chronic obstructive pulmonary disease. *Am J Respir Crit Care Med* 1997; **155**: 555–61.

74. Casaburi R, Porszasz J, Burns MR *et al.* Physiologic benefits of exercise training in rehabilitation of patients with severe chronic obstructive pulmonary disease. *Am J Respir Crit Care Medical* 1997; **155**: 1541–51.

75. Sala E, Roca J, Marrades RM *et al.* Effects of endurance training on skeletal muscle bioenergetics in chronic obstructive pulmonary disease. *Am J Respir Crit Care Med* 1999; **159**: 1726–34.

76. Rabinovich RA, Ardite E, Troosters T *et al.* Reduced muscle redox capacity after endurance training in patients with chronic obstructive pulmonary disease. *Am J Respir Crit Care Med* 2001; **164**: 1114–18.

77. Reid MB. COPD as a muscle disease. *Am J Respir Crit Care Med* 2001; **164**: 1101–2.

◆78. Ortega F, Toral J, Cejudo P *et al.* Comparison of effects of strength and endurance training in patients with chronic obstructive pulmnary disease. *Am J Respir Crit Care Med* 2002; **166**: 669–74.

79. Committee on Exercise Testing. ACC/AHA guidelines for exercise testing: a report of the American College of Cardiology/American Heart Association Task Force on Practice Guidelines. *J Am Coll Cardiol* 1997; **30**: 260–311.

80. Whipp BJ, Davis JA, Torres F, Wasserman K. A test to determine parameters of aerobic function during exercise. *J Appl Physiol* 1981; **50**: 217–21.

81. Buchfuhrer MJ, Hansen JE, Robinson TE *et al.* Optimizing the exercise protocol for cardiopulmonary assessment. *J Appl Physiol* 1983; **55**: 1558–64.

82. Nagle FJ, Balke B, Naughton JP. Gradational step tests for assessing work capacity. *J Appl Physiol* 1965; **20**: 745–8.

83. Mahler DA. The measurement of dyspnea during exercise in patients with lung disease. *Chest* 1992; **101**(Suppl.): 242–7S.

84. Mahler DA, Guyatt GH, Jones PW. Clinical measurement of dyspnea. In: Mahler DA, ed. *Lung Biology in Health and Disease*, Vol. III. *Dyspnea*. New York: Marcel Dekker, 1998; 149–98.

85. Mejia R, Ward J, Lentine T, Mahler DA. Target dyspnea ratings predict expected oxygen consumption as well as target heart rate values. *Am J Respir Crit Care Med* 1999; **159**: 1485–9.

86. O'Donnell DE, Webb KA. Exertional breathlessness in patients with chronic airflow limitation: the role of lung hyperinflation. *Am Rev Respir Dis* 1993; **148**: 1351–7.

87. Mahler DA, Mejia-Alfaro R, Ward R, Baird C. Continuous measurement of breathlessness during exercise. Validity, reliability, and responsiveness. *J Appl Physiol* 2001; **90**: 2188–96.

●88. Jones NL, Killian KJ. Exercise limitation in health and disease. *N Engl J Med* 2000; **343**: 632–41.

89. Aitken RC. Measurement of feelings using visual analogue scales. *Proc R Soc Med* 1969; **62**: 989–93.

90. Gift AG. Visual analogue scales: measurement of subjective phenomena. *Nurs Res* 1989; **38**: 286–8.

91. Borg GA. Psychophysical bases of perceived exertion. *Med Sci Sports Exerc* 1982; **14**: 377–81.

92. Mahler DA, Horowitz MB. Clinical evaluation of exertional dyspnea. *Clin Chest Med* 1994; **15**: 259–69.

93. Johnson BD, Weisman IM, Zeballos RJ, Beck KC. Emerging concepts in the evaluation of ventilatory limitation during exercise: the exercise tidal flow–volume loop. *Chest* 1999; **116**: 488–503.

94. Babb TG, Buskirk ER, Hodgson JL. Exercise end-expiratory lung volume in lean and moderately obese women. *Int J Obes* 1989; **13**: 11–9.

95. Sakamoto S, Ishikawa K, Senda S *et al.* The effect of obesity on ventilatory response and anaerobic threshold during exercise. *J Med Syst* 1993; **17**: 227–31.

96. Ray CS, Sue DY, Bray G *et al.* Effects of obesity on respiratory function. *Am Rev Respir Dis* 1983; **128**: 501–6.

97. Salvadori A, Fanari P, Fontana M *et al.* Oxygen uptake and cardiac performance in obese and normal subjects during exercise. *Respiration* 1999; **66**: 25–33.

98. Zarich SW, Kowalchuk GJ, McGuire MP *et al.* Left ventricular filling abnormalities in asymptomatic morbid obesity. *Am J Cardiol* 1991; **68**: 377–81.

99. Magarian GJ. Hyperventilation syndromes: infrequently recognized common expressions of anxiety and stress. *Medicine (Baltimore)* 1982; **61**: 219–36.

100. Gardner WN. The pathophysiology of hyperventilation disorders. *Chest* 1996: **109**: 516–34.

101. Gardner WN, Meah MS, Bass C. Controlled study of respiratory responses during prolonged measurement in patients with chronic hyperventilation. *Lancet* 1986; **2**: 826–30.

102. Kinnula VL, Sovijarvi AR. Elevated ventilatory equivalents during exercise in patients with hyperventilation syndrome. *Respiration* 1993; **60**: 273–8.

103. Lipkin DP, Scrivin AJ, Crake T, Poole-Wilson PA. Six minute walking test for assessing exercise capacity in chronic heart failure. *Br Med J* 1986; **292**: 653–5.

104. Troosters T, Gosselink R, Decramer M. Six minute walking distance in healthy elderly subjects. *Eur Respir J* 1999; **14**: 270–4.

105. Guyatt GH, Townsend M, Keller J *et al.* Measuring functional status in chronic lung disease: conclusions from a random control trial. *Respir Med* 1991; **85**(Suppl. B): 17–21.

●106. Gibbons WJ, Fruchter N, Sloan S *et al.* Reference values for multiple repetition 6-minute walk test in healthy adults older than 20 years. *J Cardiopulm Rehabil* 2001; **21**: 87–93.

●107. Enright PL, Sherrill DL. Reference equations for the six-minute walk in healthy adults. *Am J Respir Crit Care Med* 1998; **158**: 1384–7.

108. Chuang ML, Lin IF, Wasserman K. The body weight-walking distance product as related to lung function, anaerobic threshold and peak VO_2 in COPD patients. *Respir Med* 2001; **95**: 618–26.

109. Carter R, Holiday DB, Nwasuruba C *et al.* 6-minute walk work for assessment of functional capacity in patients with COPD. *Chest* 2003; **123**: 1408–15.

110. Niederman MS, Clemente PH, Fein AM *etal.* Benefits of a multidisciplinary pulmonary rehabilitation program: improvements are independent of lung function. *Chest* 1991; **99**: 798–804.

111. Noseda A, Carpiaux J, Prigogine T, Schmerber J. Lung function, maximum and submaximum exercise testing in COPD patients: reproducibility over a long interval. *Lung* 1989; **167**: 247–57.

112. Poulain M, Durand F, Palomba B *et al.* 6-Minute walk testing is more sensitive than maximal incremental cycle testing for detecting oxygen desaturation in patients with COPD. *Chest* 2003; **123**: 1401–7.

113. Pinto-Plata VM, Cote C, Cabral H *et al.* The 6-min walk distance: change over time and value as a predictor of survival in severe COPD. *Eur Respir J* 2004; **23**: 28–33.

114. Singh SJ, Morgan MDL, Scott S *et al.* Development of a shuttle walking test of disability in patients with chronic airways obstruction. *Thorax* 1992; **47**: 1019–24.

115. Revill SM, Morgan MDL, Singh SJ *et al.* The endurance shuttle walk: a new field test for the assessment of endurance capacity in chronic obstructive pulmonary disease. *Thorax* 1999; **54**: 213–22.

116. Singh SJ, Morgan MDL, Hardman AE *et al.* Comparison of oxygen uptake during a conventional treadmill test and the shuttle walking test in chronic airflow limitation. *Eur Respir J* 1994; **7**: 2016–20.

117. Morales FJ, Martinez A, Mendez M *et al.* A shuttle walk test for assessment of functional capacity in chronic heart failure. *Am Heart J* 1999; **138**: 292–8.

13

Physiological basis of dyspnoea

NHA VODUC, KATHERINE WEBB, DENIS O'DONNELL

DEFINITION

Dyspnoea is the most common symptom in patients suffering from chronic respiratory diseases and leads to a curtailment of physical activity and a diminished quality of life. Dyspnoea has been defined as 'difficult, labored, uncomfortable breathing' (1). However, this definition does not do justice to the broad range of sensations that are encompassed by the symptom. A multitude of distinct sensory processes ultimately shape the individual's perception of respiratory discomfort. The breathing discomfort reported by a healthy subject during heavy exercise has a different aetiology and quality to that experienced by a patient suffering from an acute exacerbation of chronic obstructive pulmonary disease (COPD). The American Thoracic Society consensus committee on dyspnoea attempted to recognize this diversity with their comprehensive, albeit unwieldy, definition (2):

> ...a term used to characterize a subjective experience of breathing discomfort that consists of qualitatively distinct sensations that vary in intensity. The experience derives from interactions among multiple physiological, psychological, social and environmental factors, and may induce secondary physiological and behavioral responses.

This statement acknowledges that the symptom of dyspnoea not only has a measurable intensity, but also has a range of discrete qualitative dimensions, which may vary depending on the individual, the disease process and numerous other circumstances.

With this definition in mind, we briefly review what is currently known about the neurosensory underpinnings of dyspnoea, examine the pathophysiological basis of dyspnoea in the clinical arena and, finally, discuss a physiological rationale for alleviation of dyspnoea following common therapeutic interventions. Since the majority of clinical studies on dyspnoea have been conducted in patients with COPD, this is the main focus of this review.

NEUROPHYSIOLOGICAL BASIS OF DYSPNOEA (SEE BOX 13.1)

Chemoreceptors

Peripheral and centrally located chemoreceptors are capable of sensing changes in arterial oxygen (Po_2), carbon dioxide (Pco_2) and pH (Fig. 13.1). These receptors play an important role in the control of breathing and ensure that alveolar ventilation is closely matched to the prevailing metabolic needs under diverse physical and environmental conditions. Given that oxygen uptake and elimination of carbon dioxide are

---

Box 13.1 Neurophysiological mechanisms of dyspnoea in COPD

Central (corollary discharge)

- ↑ Motor drive (inspiratory effort) – cortical
- ↑ Reflexic drive (chemical, neural) – medullary

Peripheral (afferent activity)

- Altered vagal afferent activity (stretch, A-fibres)
- Altered chest wall afferent activity (muscle spindles, Golgi tendon organs, joint receptors)

Integrated central–peripheral

- Neuromechanical dissociation

among the most important functions of the respiratory system, it would not be unreasonable to assume that dyspnoea is the result of increased chemoreceptor activity in the setting of arterial hypoxia or hypercarbia. Indeed, this assumption has prevailed since the nineteenth century. At that time, dyspnoea was believed to be the result of one of two processes: 'want of oxygen' and 'carbon dioxide retention' (3). Haldane and Priestley (4) demonstrated that in healthy humans small increases in CO_2 (~3 per cent) produced dyspnoea and hyperventilation, whereas a reduction of O_2 in the order of 14 per cent of the baseline value was required to induce the same effect (4).

Numerous studies have demonstrated that dyspnoea is reported by healthy subjects when hypercapnia is experimentally produced (5, 6). Many of these studies did not control for the increased ventilation (and respiratory muscle work) that occurs as a consequence of hypercapnia. When ventilatory activity is controlled for, the results of research in this area are somewhat contradictory. Campbell *et al.* (7) observed that subjects paralysed with curare did not complain of air hunger after the inhalation of CO_2. On the other hand, Banzett *et al.* (8) found that patients with high-level quadriplegia (and almost total respiratory muscle paralysis) reported 'air hunger' with increasing levels of carbon dioxide, in the absence of any increase in ventilation. Most recently, Gandevia *et al.* (9) demonstrated that healthy subjects who were completely paralysed with high doses of atracurium would still report severe dyspnoea in response to relatively mild hypercapnia (a change of 4.0 mmHg). There is no satisfactory explanation for the disparity in results between these most recent studies and the older study by Campbell *et al.* but nevertheless it would seem that the sum of existing evidence favours a role for CO_2 in the pathogenesis of dyspnoea and, in particular, the perception of air hunger.

The effects of arterial hypoxia on dyspnoea are more complex and less well understood (10). The response to induced

hypoxaemia in health is quite variable, and the response to supplemental O_2 in patients with pulmonary diseases is unpredictable, even in patients with severe resting hypoxaemia (11). The effects of hypoxia are multifactorial: critical arterial hypoxia (<60 mmHg) acutely stimulates peripheral chemoreceptors, whose afferent activity may directly reach consciousness. Additionally, the resultant ventilatory stimulation with increased central motor output and respiratory muscle activation may contribute to breathing discomfort. Hypoxic effects on the cardiac pump and the pulmonary vasculature may have negative sensory consequences, but these are poorly understood.

In the exercising subject, the sensory effects of hypoxia are even more complex. Low arterial oxygenation will alter the metabolic milieu and the level of sympathetic activation at the peripheral muscle level and, consequently, influence ventilatory and sensory responses during exercise (12, 13). In elderly healthy individuals and in patients with expiratory airflow limitation, hypoxic hyperventilation will result in air-trapping and dynamic lung overinflation, which may, of itself, contribute to dyspnoea. Hypoxia may cause ventilatory muscle fatigue, which would require greater motor activation and effort for a given muscle contraction. This increased perceived effort may contribute to respiratory discomfort. The relative contribution of all of the multiple sensory inputs that arise as a consequence of hypoxia is difficult to determine with any precision.

Pulmonary receptors

Three different classes of sensory receptors have been identified in the lung (14). Slowly adapting stretch receptors are located principally in large airways, and respond to increases in lung volume (15). Rapidly adapting receptors (RARs), also known as irritant receptors, are present in the airway epithelium. They respond to a wide range of stimuli, including particulate irritants, direct stimulation of the airways and pulmonary congestion. Juxtapulmonary (J) receptors (also known as pulmonary c-fibres) are non-myelinated fibres that are located throughout the lung near pulmonary capillaries and in the bronchial and laryngeal mucosa. These fibres (similar to RARs) are stimulated by a variety of mechanical and chemical stimuli. C-fibre stimulation results in apnoea, a rapid shallow breathing pattern, bronchoconstriction, and mucous hypersecretion (16, 17). There have been several attempts to implicate pulmonary receptors, particularly c-fibres, in the sensation of dyspnoea (Fig. 13.1). For example, inhaled lidocaine has been shown to reduce breathlessness associated with bronchoconstriction, but not breathlessness caused by external loading (18). Raj *et al.* (19) injected lobeline (a J-receptor stimulant) into 26 normal subjects, 12 of whom consequently reported a sensation similar to dyspnoea.

Almost all of the afferent signals from pulmonary receptors are ultimately carried to the central nervous system via the vagus nerve. Several studies have examined the effects of vagal nerve block or vagotomy on respiratory sensation. Guz *et al.* (20) found that the dyspnoea associated with breath-holding was decreased following injection of lidocaine around both vagus

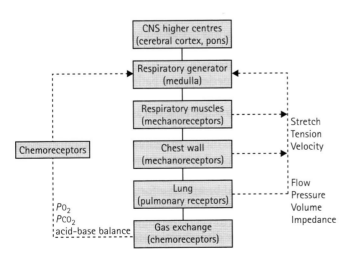

Figure 13.1 *Neurophysiological basis of dyspnoea. Events in the lung and chest wall stimulate receptors in the airways, lung parenchyma and respiratory muscles which then provide sensory feedback via vagal, phrenic and intercostal nerves to the spinal cord, medulla and higher centres.*

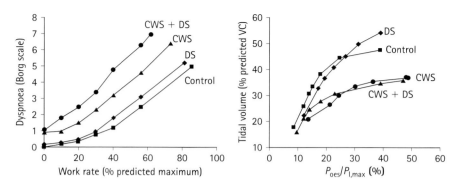

Figure 13.2 *Compared with control, dyspnoea intensity was increased significantly by chest wall strapping (CWS) and dead-space loading (DS), alone or in combination, during exercise in 12 healthy young men (left panel). Dyspnoea increased progressively as greater mechanical constraints on tidal volume expansion were imposed, shown relative to inspiratory effort ($P_{oes}/P_{I,max}$) (right panel). During CWS, vital capacity (VC) was reduced to approximately 60 per cent of the baseline value; during DS, 0.6 L was added to the dead space of the breathing circuit. Adapted from O'Donnell et al. (43).*

validation of scales, such as the Borg and visual analogue scales to measure dyspnoea intensity (44, 45); and second, Leblanc *et al.* (46) pioneered the use of stepwise multiple regression analysis to explore dyspnoea in the clinical setting. The use of Borg ratings of dyspnoea intensity as the dependent variable vs. a number of relevant independent physiological variables permitted the identification of major contributing factors to respiratory discomfort during exercise in patients with cardiopulmonary diseases. Extending this type of analysis, it also became possible to evaluate mechanisms of improvement in dyspnoea following a number of therapeutic interventions, thus gaining new insights into its source. Here, the change in dyspnoea ratings at a standardized stimulus (i.e. work rate, $\dot{V}O_2$, ventilation) was used as the dependent variable vs. simultaneous change in potential contributory physiological variables.

The majority of studies examining dyspnoea have focused on COPD. Expiratory flow limitation is the pathophysiological hallmark of COPD. This arises because of intrinsic airway factors that increase resistance (i.e. mucosal inflammation/oedema, airway remodelling and secretions), and extrinsic airway factors (i.e. reduced airway tethering from emphysema and regional extraluminal compression by adjacent overinflated alveolar units). Emphysematous destruction also reduces elastic lung recoil and, thus, the driving pressure for expiratory flow, further compounding flow limitation. Expiratory flow limitation with dynamic collapse of the small airways compromises the ability of patients to expel air during forced and quiet expiration; thus, alveolar air retention and lung overinflation occur.

Reduced lung recoil in emphysema alters the balance of forces between the lung and chest wall to a higher end-expiratory lung volume (EELV). Moreover, EELV is a continuous dynamic variable in flow-limited patients with COPD: inspiration begins before tidal expiration is complete and lung hyperinflation results. When breathing rate acutely increases (and expiratory time diminishes), as for example during exercise or hyperventilation, there is further 'dynamic' lung hyperinflation (DH) as a result of air trapping, which has serious mechanical and sensory consequences (Fig. 13.3). The pattern and magnitude of DH during exercise are highly variable and depend on the extent of expiratory flow limitation, the ventilatory demand and the level of resting lung hyperinflation (47). Serial inspiratory capacity (IC) measurements can be used to track dynamic changes in EELV since total lung capacity is unaltered with exercise (48, 49). The resting IC represents the true operating limits for tidal volume (V_T) expansion during exercise: the smaller the IC, the greater the constraints on V_T expansion during exercise (47). Faced with this mechanical restriction, patients rely on an increasing breathing frequency to increase ventilation, but this rebounds to cause even further DH in a vicious cycle. In patients with severely compromised gas exchange capabilities (with high physiological dead space), reduced IC and poor V_T expansion during exercise contribute importantly to exercise hypercapnia (50).

The mechanical consequences of acute-on-chronic hyperinflation are well described. DH results in increased elastic and inspiratory threshold loading of inspiratory muscles already burdened with increased resistive work. Moreover, acute-on-chronic hyperinflation compromises the ability of the ventilatory muscles, particularly the diaphragm, to increase pressure generation in response to the increased drive to breathe during exercise.

Dynamic hyperinflation and dyspnoea

Several studies have shown a close correlation between hyperinflation (the reduction of IC) during exercise and the intensity of exertional dyspnoea (41, 42). The relationship between dyspnoea and lung hyperinflation is complex. The slope of the relationship between IC and Borg dyspnoea ratings is alinear in COPD: when the IC (and inspiratory reserve volume [IRV]) reaches a critically reduced level, dyspnoea rises steeply to intolerable levels. Thus, with increasing exercise, V_T expands maximally to reach a minimal IRV of approximately of 0.5 L; thereafter, dyspnoea rises rapidly as a function of the increasing chemical drive to breathe (47). Close intercorrelations have been found between the intensity of exertional dyspnoea, the

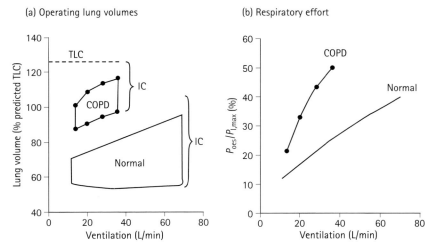

Figure 13.3   *Behaviour of operating lung volumes (a) and respiratory effort ($P_{oes}/P_{I,max}$) (b) as ventilation increases during exercise in COPD and in age-matched normal subjects. In COPD, tidal volume takes up a larger proportion of the reduced IC at any given ventilation – mechanical constraints on tidal volume expansion are further compounded because of dynamic hyperinflation during exercise. As a result of functionally weakened inspiratory muscles and increased mechanical loading, tidal inspiratory pressures represent a much higher fraction of their maximal force-generating capacity in COPD than in health. Adapted from O'Donnell et al. (47).*

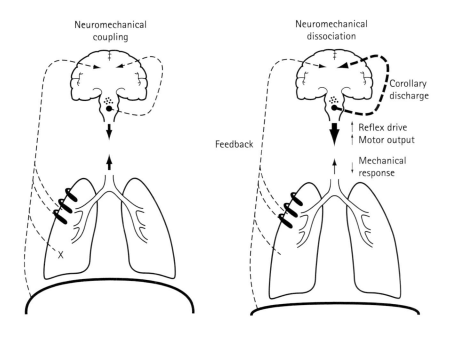

Figure 13.4   *In health during exercise, there is a harmonious matching of motor output (via corollary discharge) to the mechanical response of the respiratory system (via afferent peripheral feedback from multiple mechanoreceptors), i.e. neuromechanical coupling. In COPD, there is a mismatch between inspiratory effort and the mechanical response of the system, i.e. neuromechanical dissociation. This disparity gives rise to sensations of respiratory discomfort such as 'unsatisfied inspiratory effort'.*

reduction in IC and the increased ratio of effort (tidal oesophageal pressure relative to maximum) to tidal volume during exercise (42). This increased effort:displacement ratio is a crude measure of neuromechanical uncoupling of the respiratory system in COPD. As already mentioned, the inability to expand tidal volume appropriately in response to the increased central drive to breathe appears to contribute importantly to the intensity and quality of dyspnoea in COPD. Interestingly, in contrast to healthy subjects who report a perception of increased effort/work at the end of exhaustive exercise, patients with COPD invariably select descriptors which allude to inspiratory difficulty and unsatisfied inspiration (i.e. 'can't get enough air in') (42). Neuromechanical dissociation

may form the basis for these discrete qualitative dimensions of dyspnoea.

The neuromechanical dissociation hypothesis implies that dyspnoea not only is a function of the amplitude of central motor output, but is also importantly modulated by peripheral feedback from a variety of mechanoreceptors throughout the respiratory system (51–54) (Fig. 13.4). The psychophysical basis of neuromechanical dissociation is likely to reside in the complex central processing and integration of signals that mediate: (i) central motor command output (via central corollary discharge) (31, 55); and (ii) sensory feedback from a variety of mechanoreceptors that provide precise, instantaneous proprioceptive information about muscle displacement (muscle spindles and joint receptors), tension development (Golgi tendon organs), and change in respired volume or flow (lung and airway mechanoreceptors) (8, 56–62).

Dyspnoea and reduced diffusion capacity

A common clinical observation is that patients with COPD who have a reduced diffusion capacity for carbon monoxide (D_LCO), signifying a reduced surface area for gas exchange, often experience more severe dyspnoea and disability than those with a preserved D_LCO. In one study in patients with a similar FEV_1 (forced expiratory volume in 1 s), those with a reduced D_LCO (<50 per cent predicted) experienced greater exertional dyspnoea than those with a more preserved D_LCO (47). During exercise, patients with a reduced D_LCO have a higher physiological dead space, greater arterial hypoxaemia, and higher submaximal ventilation levels throughout exercise. Patients with clinical and physiological characteristics of emphysema therefore appear to have greater expiratory flow limitation (reduced lung recoil and tethering) and greater ventilatory demand (increased ventilation/perfusion mismatching), which together would predispose them to greater acute-on-chronic hyperinflation. In this regard, it was recently determined that, among patients with an identical FEV_1, those with the lower D_LCO had a more rapid rate of rise of DH early in exercise, with greater mechanical constraints on ventilation (reduced peak ventilation) and, consequently, greater exertional dyspnoea and lower symptom-limited $\dot{V}O_2$ compared with patients with a better preserved D_LCO (47). This latter group had similar rest-to-peak changes in DH during exercise, but hyperinflation occurred at a more constant rate as ventilation increased.

MECHANISMS OF DYSPNOEA: LESSONS FROM THERAPEUTIC INTERVENTIONS (TABLE 13.1)

Bronchodilators

Bronchodilator therapy is the first step in the management of dyspnoea in COPD. Several studies have shown that important improvements in dyspnoea can occur after bronchodilators with minimal or no changes in the FEV_1 (63–65).

Bronchodilators improve airway conductance during a forced expiratory manoeuvre, thus facilitating lung emptying as reflected by the increased vital capacity and the reduced residual volume (66, 67). Improvements in volume-corrected maximal expiratory flows over the operating range in the order of 40–60 per cent are frequently seen after bronchodilators in severe COPD (64, 67, 68). These improvements in flow are clinically relevant in flow-limited patients and indicate that greater expiratory flows are now available during tidal breathing (Fig. 13.5). Thus, bronchodilators improve dynamic expiratory flow rates, facilitating lung emptying with each tidal expiration. When this is integrated over time, the dynamically determined EELV is reduced to a volume closer to the respiratory system's relaxation volume. This reduction in EELV is reflected by an increased resting IC. Bronchodilators therefore allow patients to meet their alveolar ventilation requirements at a lower lung volume and at a lower oxygen cost of breathing.

During exercise, this pharmacological volume reduction (increased resting IC) allows for greater tidal volume expansion (65, 67). In other words, the increased resting IC delays the mechanical limitation of ventilation, allowing greater exercise

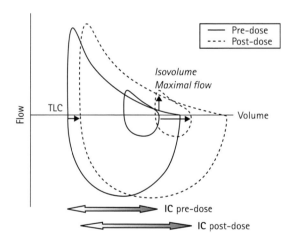

Figure 13.5 *Effect of a bronchodilator on maximal and tidal flow–volume curves in COPD. Improvements in isovolume maximal expiratory flows allow greater lung emptying with each tidal expiration. As dynamic EELV is reduced, resting IC and IRV are increased. Total lung capacity (TLC) either remains unchanged or is minimally reduced in response to bronchodilators.*

Table 13.1 *Putative mechanisms of dyspnoea relief with various interventions*

	Reduced ventilation	Reduced mechanical loading	Ventilatory muscle strengthening	Altered perceptual response
Bronchodilators	+	+	−	−
Exercise training	+	−	+	+
Oxygen therapy	+	+	−	+
Volume reduction surgery	−	+	+	−

+, present; −, absent.

performance (Fig. 13.6) and significantly delaying the onset of intolerable dyspnoea (69). In some patients, greater V_T expansion can also contribute to more effective CO_2 elimination and possibly to decreased chemical drive to breathe during exercise. Thus, bronchodilators may reduce exertional dyspnoea in COPD by both delaying the onset of mechanical limitation caused by dynamic hyperinflation and by decreasing respiratory drive. In patients with advanced disease and lung hyperinflation, small improvements in resting IC in the order of 0.3 L (i.e. 10 per cent predicted) appear to be clinically meaningful.

Exercise training

The relief of dyspnoea after pulmonary rehabilitation has been shown to result from exercise training (EXT) rather than the educational component per se (70). Several studies have shown important improvements in dyspnoea, which contribute to improved health status in individuals with COPD (71–73). Symptom improvement is multifactorial, and not fully understood. Potential mechanisms include reduced central motor drive related to decreased metabolic acidosis (74) that accompanies the improved oxidative capacity following muscle training (75). Alterations in the metabolic milieu at the peripheral muscle level may also affect sympathetic activation and, in turn, reduce central drive and ventilation. The magnitude of decrease in submaximal ventilation at a standardized time during exercise varies from 3 to 5 L/min, and correlates well with reduced Borg ratings (76, 77).

In one study, the resting IC improved significantly after exercise training by 0.3 L compared with control (76). The mechanisms of increased IC are unclear, but may reflect resting breathing pattern alterations, particularly reduced frequency and increased expiratory time, which promotes lung deflation. Improved static inspiratory muscle strength at rest, as a result of exercise training, may also favourably alter the IC. Following EXT, several studies have shown that the breathing pattern changes to a slower deeper pattern (76–79). Reduced breathing frequency would be expected to contribute to reduced DH during exercise, which has been demonstrated in one study (78). Global exercise training improves the strength of both the inspiratory and expiratory muscles and increases inspiratory muscle endurance by threefold, on average (77). Improved functional strength means less electrical activation (or drive) for a given force generation by the muscle, which should translate into reduced perceived effort.

After EXT, breathlessness also diminishes at any given ventilation (76, 78) (Fig. 13.7), suggesting a reduction in the mechanical load (i.e. hyperinflation) or increased tolerance or desensitization to the symptom. During pulmonary rehabilitation, patients can overcome their fear of dyspnoea and may learn to tolerate higher levels of discomfort. In other words, consistent attention in a secure health care environment will provide psychosocial support, which may alter the affective responses to dyspnoea. This effect has been difficult to quantify with any precision, but is undoubtedly important.

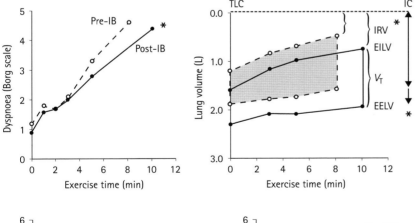

Figure 13.6   *In response to a bronchodilator (nebulized ipratropium bromide [IB], 500 μg), exertional dyspnoea decreased significantly (*P < 0.05) during constant-load cycle exercise. Operating lung volumes also improved, i.e. mechanical constraints on V_T expansion were reduced as IC and IRV increased significantly (*P < 0.05). EELV, end-expiratory lung volume; EILV, end-inspiratory lung volume; TLC, total lung capacity. Modified from O'Donnell and Webb (64).*

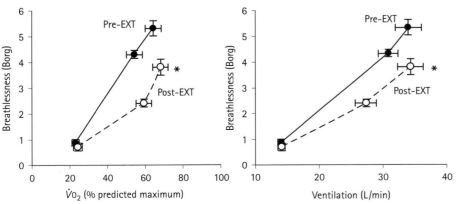

Figure 13.7   *Slopes of exertional dyspnoea intensity (Borg ratings) relative to oxygen uptake ($\dot{V}O_2$) and ventilation decreased significantly (*P < 0.05) after a supervised EXT in 30 patients with COPD. Modified from O'Donnell (76).*

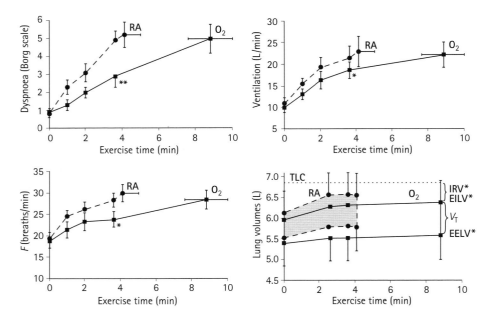

Figure 13.8 *Dyspnoea, ventilation, breathing frequency (F) and operating lung volumes are plotted against time during constant-load exercise during room air (RA) and 60 per cent oxygen (O₂). While breathing oxygen, there were significant decreases in dyspnoea ventilation, F, EELV; i.e. increased inspiratory capacity and end-inspiratory lung volume (EILV; i.e. increased inspiratory reserve volume [IRV]) at isotime during exercise (*P < 0.05, **P < 0.01). TLC, total lung capacity; V_T, tidal volume. Adapted from O'Donnell et al. (80).*

Oxygen therapy

The effect of oxygen on dyspnoea in a given individual with symptomatic COPD is unpredictable. Potential mechanisms of improvement include reduced ventilatory drive and ventilation. These reductions may be secondary to a combination of diminished hypoxic drive from peripheral chemoreceptors and reduced metabolic acidosis (blood lactate) during exercise. However, in some studies, the reduction of dyspnoea during oxygen appears disproportionate for the small changes in ventilation that were induced. Possible explanations for this include the following:

- reduced respiratory muscle impedance as a result of reduced airways resistance
- reduced dynamic lung hyperinflation (secondary to decreased breathing frequency and increased expiratory time)
- a delay in the inspiratory muscle fatigue because of increased oxygen-rich blood perfusion to the muscles
- altered central perception of dyspnoeogenic stimuli as the result of the effects of oxygen
- a decrease in afferent inputs from the pulmonary vasculature and right heart secondary to acute decreases in pulmonary artery pressures.

The relative importance of these various factors is difficult, if not impossible, to quantify, and is likely to vary between individuals.

Three recent studies in COPD provided evidence that improvement in dyspnoea and exercise endurance during oxygen may also be related to reduced DH as a consequence of the reduced ventilation (13, 80, 81). As in the case of bronchodilators, reduced operating volumes delay critical mechanical limitation of ventilation and improve exercise endurance (Fig. 13.8). Even in normoxic COPD patients, improvements

in operating lung volumes and endurance time have been shown to increase in a dose-dependent manner with the fractional concentration of oxygen until reaching a plateau at a value of 0.5 (13). Improvements following oxygen therapy relate mainly to increased dynamic IRV during exercise: V_T remains constant and the reduction in ventilation is mainly due to reduced breathing frequencies. The net effect of added oxygen is therefore to reduce the drive to breathe while at the same time reducing restrictive ventilatory mechanics (i.e. enhanced neuromechanical coupling).

SUMMARY

After reviewing the available literature on dyspnoea, it becomes apparent that this ubiquitous symptom is complex and not fully understood. However, despite our incomplete understanding of the mechanisms, our ability to measure and characterize the subjective experience of dyspnoea accurately has advanced significantly. New insights into the pathophysiological basis of dyspnoea during exercise in COPD have laid the foundation for the development of effective combined management strategies for this distressing symptom.

Key points

- Dyspnoea is the subjective experience of breathing discomfort that consists of qualitatively distinct sensations that vary in intensity.
- The mechanisms of dyspnoea are complex and multifactorial – there is no unique central or peripheral source of this symptom.

- Increased chemoreceptor activation in response to hypercapnia leads to the perception of air hunger. Sensory responses to hypoxia are less consistent.
- The sense of heightened inspiratory effort is an integral component of exertional dyspnoea and is pervasive across health and disease.
- The neuromechanical dissociation (NMD) theory of dyspnoea states that the symptom arises when there is a disparity between the central reflexic drive to breathe (efferent discharge) and the simultaneous afferent feedback from a multitude of peripheral sensory receptors throughout the respiratory system. This feedback system provides information about the extent and appropriateness of the mechanical response to central drive.
- In COPD, the intensity and quality of dyspnoea during activity correlates with the magnitude of lung hyperinflation which, in turn, results in severe NMD.
- Therapeutic interventions that reduce the mechanical load on the inspiratory muscles, increase inspiratory muscle strength and reduce ventilatory demand, either singly or in combination, effectively alleviate dyspnoea.

REFERENCES

1. Comroe JH. Some theories of the mechanism of dyspnea. In: Howell JB, Campbell EJM, eds. *Breathlessness*. Boston: Blackwell Scientific Publications, 1966; 1–7.
◆2. American Thoracic Society. Dyspnea. Mechanisms, assessment and management: a consensus statement. *Am J Respir Crit Care Med* 1999; **159**: 321–40.
3. Meakins J. The cause and treatment of dyspnoea in cardiovascular disease. *Br Med J* 1923; 1043–5.
●4. Haldane JS, Priestley JG. The regulation of lung-ventilation. *J Physiol* 1905; **32**: 225–66.
5. Haldane JS, Smith JL. The physiological effects of air vitiated by respiration. *J Path Bacteriol* 1892; **1**: 168.
6. Hill L, Flack F. The effect of excess of carbon dioxide and of want of oxygen upon the respiration and the circulation. *J Physiol* 1908; **37**: 77–111.
7. Campbell EJM, Godfrey S, Clark TJH *et al.* The effect of muscular paralysis induced by tubocurarine on the duration and sensation of breath-holding during hypercapnia. *Clin Sci* 1969; **36**: 323–8.
8. Banzett RB, Lansing RW, Reid MB, Brown R. 'Air Hunger' arising from increasing PCO_2 in mechanically ventilated quadriplegics. *Respir Physiol* 1989; **76**: 53–68.
●9. Gandevia SC, Killian K, McKenzie DK *et al.* Respiratory sensations, cardiovascular control, kinaesthesia and transcranial stimulation during paralysis in humans. *J Physiol* 1993; **470**: 85–107.
10. Lane R, Cockcroft A, Adams L, Guz A. Arterial oxygen saturation and breathlessness in patients with chronic obstructive airways disease. *Clin Sci* 1987; **72**: 693–8.
●11. Mak VHF, Bugler JR, Roberts CM, Spiro SG. Effect of arterial oxygen desaturation on six-minute walk distance, perceived effort and perceived breathlessness in patients with airflow limitation. *Thorax* 1993; **48**: 33–48.
12. O'Donnell DE, Bain DJ, Webb KA. Factors contributing to relief of exertional breathlessness during hyperoxia in chronic airflow limitation. *Am J Respir Crit Care Med* 1997; **155**: 530–5.
●13. Somfay A, Porszasz J, Lee SM, Casaburi R. Dose–response effect of oxygen on hyperinflation and exercise endurance in nonhypoxaemic COPD patients. *Eur Respir J* 2001; **18**: 77–84.
◆14. Coleridge HM, Coleridge JCG. Reflexes evoked from tracheobronchial tree and lungs. In. *Handbook of Physiology, Section 3: the Respiratory System, Vol. 2: Control of Breathing, Part 1*. Bethesda, MD: American Physiological Society, 1986; 395–429.
◆15. Bradley GW. Control of breathing pattern. In: Widdicombe JG, ed. *Respiratory Physiology II, Vol. 14*. Baltimore, MD: University Park, 1977; 185–217.
16. Paintal AS. Mechanism of stimulation of type J pulmonary receptors. *J Physiol* 1969; **203**: 511–32.
17. Green JF, Schmidt ND, Schultz HD *et al.* Pulmonary C-fibers evoke both apnea and tachypnea of pulmonary chemoreflex. *J Appl Physiol* 1984; **57**: 562–7.
18. Taguchi O, Kikuchi Y, Hida W *et al.* Effects of bronchoconstriction and external resistive loading on the sensation of dyspnea. *J Appl Physiol* 1991; **71**: 2183–90.
19. Raj H, Singh VK, Anand A, Paintal AS. Sensory origin of lobeline-induced sensations: a correlative study in man and cat. *J Physiol* 1995; **482**: 235–46.
●20. Guz A, Noble MIM, Widdicombe JG *et al.* The role of vagal and glossopharyngeal afferent nerves in respiratory sensation, control of breathing and arterial pressure regulation in concious man. *Clin Sci* 1966; **30**: 161–70.
21. Bradley GW, Hale T, Pimble J *et al.* Effect of vagotomy on the breathing pattern and exercise ability in emphysematous patients. *Clin Sci* 1982; **62**: 311–19.
●22. Winning AJ, Hamilton RD, Guz A. Ventilation and breathlessness on maximal exercise in patients with interstitial lung disease after local anesthetic aerosol inhalation. *Clin Sci* 1988; **74**: 275–81.
23. Kimoff RJ, Cheong TH, Cosio MG *et al.* Pulmonary denervation in humans: Effects on dyspnea and ventilatory pattern during exercise. *Am Rev Respir Dis* 1990; **142**: 1034–40.
24. Lougheed MD, Flannery J, Webb KA, O'Donnell DE. Respiratory sensation and ventilatory mechanics during induced bronchoconstriction in spontaneously breathing low cervical quadriplegia. *Am J Respir Crit Care Med* 2002; **166**: 370–6.
◆25. Shannon R. Reflexes from respiratory muscles and costovertebral joints. In: Cherniak NS, Widdcombe JG, eds. *Handbook of Physiology, section 3: The Respiratory System, Vol. 2: Control of Breathing, Part 1*. Bethesda, MD: American Physiological Society, 1986; 431–47.
26. Mithoefer JC, Stevens CD, Ryder HW, McGuire J. Lung volume restriction, hypoxia and hypercapnia as interrelated respiratory stimuli in normal man. *J Appl Physiol* 1953; **5**: 797–802.
27. Fowler WS. Breaking point of breath-holding. *J Appl Physiol* 1954; **6**: 539–45.
28. Sibuya M, Yamada M, Kanamaru A *et al.* Effect of chest wall vibration on dyspnea in patients with chronic respiratory disease. *Am J Respir Crit Care Med* 1994; **149**: 1235–40.
29. Chonan T, Mulholland MB, Cherniak NS, Altose MD. Effects of voluntary constraining of thoracic displacement during hypercapnia. *J Appl Physiol* 1987; **63**: 1822–8.
◆30. McCloskey DI. Corollary discharges: motor commands and perception. In: Brookahrt JM, Mountcastle VB, eds. *Handbook of Physiology Section 1: The Nervous System*, Vol. 2. Bethesda, MD: American Physiological Society, 1981; 1415–47.

31. Chen Z, Eldridge FL, Wagner PG. Respiratory-associated firing of midbrain neurones in cats: relation to level of respiratory drive. *J Physiol* 1991; **437**: 305–25.

32. Redline S, Gottfried SB, Altose MD. Effect of changes in inspiratory muscle strength on the sensation of respiratory force. *J Appl Physiol* 1991; **70**: 240–5.

33. Killian KJ, Gandevia SC, Summers E, Campbell EJM. Effect of increased lung volume on perception of breathlessness, effort and tension. *J Appl Physiol* 1984; **57**: 686–91.

34. El-Manshawi A, Killian KJ, Summers E, Jones NL. Breathlessness and exercise with and without resistive loading. *J Appl Physiol* 1986; **61**: 896–905.

35. Gandevia SC, Killian KJ, Campbell EJM. The effect of respiratory muscle fatigue on respiratory sensations. *Clin Sci* 1981; **60**: 463–6.

●36. Hamilton AL, Killian KJ, Summers E, Jones NL. Muscle strength, symptom intensity, and exercise capacity in patients with cardiorespiratory disorders. *Am J Respir Crit Care Med* 1995; **152**: 2021–31.

37. Campbell EJM, Freedman S, Smith PS, Taylor ME. The ability of man to detect added elastic loads to breathing. *Clin Sci* 1961; **20**: 223–31 (and Wylie RL, Zechman FW. Perception of added airflow resistance in humans. *Respir Physiol* 1966; **2**: 73–87).

38. Lougheed MD, Webb KA, O'Donnell DE. Breathlessness during induced lung hyperinflation in asthma: the role of the inspiratory threshold load. *Am J Respir Crit Care Med* 1995; **152**: 911–20.

39. Campbell EJM, Howell JBL. The sensation of breathlessness. *Br Med Bull* 1963; **18**: 36–40.

●40. Schwartzstein RM, Simon PM, Weiss JW *et al.* Breathlessness induced by dissociation between ventilation and chemical drive. *Am Rev Respir Dis* 1989; **139**: 1231–7.

●41. O'Donnell DE, Webb KA. Exertional breathlessness in patients with chronic airflow limitation: the role of hyperinflation. *Am Rev Respir Dis* 1993; **148**: 1351–7.

●42. O'Donnell DE, Bertley JC, Chau LKL, Webb KA. Qualitative aspects of exertional breathlessness in chronic airflow limitation: pathophysiologic mechanisms. *Am J Respir Crit Care Med* 1997; **155**: 109–15.

43. O'Donnell DE, Hong HH, Webb KA. Respiratory sensation during chest wall restriction and dead space loading in exercising men. *J Appl Physio* 2000; **88**: 1859–69.

●44. Mahler DA, Weinberg DH, Wells CK, Feinstein AR. The measurement of dyspnea: contents, interobserver agreement, and physiologic correlates of two new clinical indexes. *Chest* 1984; **85**: 751–8.

45. Borg GAV. Psychophysical basis of perceived exertion. *Med Sci Sports Exerc* 1982; **14**: 377–81.

●46. Leblanc P, Bowie DM, Summers E *et al.* Breathlessness and exercise in patients with cardio-respiratory disease. *Am Rev Respir Dis* 1986; **133**: 21–5.

●47. O'Donnell DE, Revill SM, Webb KA. Dynamic hyperinflation and exercise intolerance in COPD. *Am J Respir Crit Care Med* 2001; **164**: 770–7.

48. Stubbing DG, Pengelly LD, Morse C, Jones NL. Pulmonary mechanics during exercise in normal males. *J Appl Physiol* 1908; **49**: 506–10.

49. Stubbing DG, Pengelly LD, Morse C, Jones NL. Pulmonary mechanics during exercise in subjects with chronic airflow obstruction. *J Appl Physiol* 1908; **49**: 511–15.

50. O'Donnell DE, D'Arsigny C, Fitzpatrick M, Webb KA. Exercise hypercapnia in advanced COPD. the role of lung hyperinflation. *Am J Respir Crit Care Med* 2002; **166**: 663–8.

◆51. Meek PM, Schwartzstein RMS, Adams L *et al.* Dyspnea mechanisms, assessment and management: a consensus statement (American Thoracic Society). *Am J Respir Crit Care Med* 1999; **159**: 321–40.

◆52. O'Donnell DE. Exertional breathlessness in chronic respiratory disease. In: Mahler DA, ed. *Lung Biology in Health and Disease, Vol. III: Dyspnea.* New York: Marcel Dekker, 1998; 97–147.

◆53. Killian KJ, Campbell EJM. Dyspnea. In. Roussos C, Macklem PT, eds. *Lung Biology in Health and Disease, Vol. 29 (Part B): The Thorax.* New York: Marcel Dekker, 1985; 787–828.

54. Altose M, Cherniack N, Fishman AP. Respiratory sensations and dyspnea: perspectives. *J Appl Physiol* 1985; **58**: 1051–4.

55. Davenport PW, Friedman WA, Thompson FJ, Franzen O. Respiratory-related cortical potentials evoked by inspiratory occlusion in humans. *J Appl Physiol* 1986; **60**: 1843–8.

56. Gandevia SC, Macefield G. Projection of low threshold afferents from human intercostal muscles to the cerebral cortex. *Respir Physiol* 1989; **77**: 203–14.

57. Homma I, Kanamara A, Sibuya M. Proprioceptive chest wall afferents and the effect on respiratory sensation. In: Von Euler C, Katz-Salamon M, eds. *Respiratory Psychophysiology.* New York: Stockton Press, 1988; 161–6.

58. Altose MD, Syed I, Shoos L. Effects of chest wall vibration on the intensity of dyspnea during constrained breathing. *Proc Int Union Physiol Sci* 1989; **17**: 288.

59. Matthews PBC. Where does Sherrington's 'muscular sense' originate: muscles, joints, corollary discharge? *Ann Rev Neurosci* 1982; **5**: 189–218.

60. Roland PE, Ladegaard-Pederson HA. A quantitative analysis of sensation of tension and kinaesthesia in man. Evidence for peripherally originating muscular sense and a sense of effort. *Brain* 1977; **100**: 671–92.

61. Noble MIM, Eisele JH, Trenchard D, Guz A. Effect of selective peripheral nerve blocks on respiratory sensations. In: Porter R, ed. *Breathing: Hering-Breyer Symposium.* London: Churchill, 1970; 233–46.

◆62. Zechman FR Jr, Wiley RL. Afferent inputs to breathing: respiratory sensation. In: Fishman AP, eds. *Handbook of Physiology, Section 3, Vol. II Part 2: The Respiratory System.* Bethesda, MD: American Physiology Society, 1986; 449–74.

◆63. Liesker JJW, Wijkstra PJ, Ten Hacken NHT *et al.* A systematic review of the effects of bronchodilators on exercise capacity in patients with COPD. *Chest* 2002; **121**: 597–608.

64. O'Donnell DE, Lam M, Webb KA. Spirometric correlates of improvement in exercise performance after anticholinergic therapy in chronic obstructive pulmonary disease. *Am J Respir Crit Care Med* 1999; **160**: 542–9.

●65. O'Donnell DE, Lam M, Webb KA. Measurement of exertional symptoms, dynamic hyperinflation and exercise endurance in COPD: reproducibility and responsiveness *Am J Resp Crit Care Med* 1998; **158**: 1557–65.

●66. O'Donnell DE, Forkert L, Webb KA. Evaluation of bronchodilator responses in patients with 'irreversible' emphysema. *Eur Respir J* 2001; **18**: 914–20.

67. O'Donnell DE, Magnussen H, Gerken F *et al.* Mechanisms of improved exercise tolerance in COPD in response to tiotropium [abstract]. *Eur Respir J* 2002; **20**.

68. Tantucci C, Duguet A, Similowski T *et al.* Effect of salbutamol on dynamic hyperinflation in chronic obstructive pulmonary disease patients. *Eur Respir J* 1998; **12**: 799–804.

69. O'Donnell DE, Webb KA. Pharmacological volume reduction delays the threshold for intolerable dyspnea during acute hyperinflation in COPD [abstract]. *Am J Respir Crit Care Med* 2003, 167.

●70. Ries AL, Kaplan RM, Limberg TM, Prewitt LM. Effects of pulmonary rehabilitation on physiologic and psychosocial outcomes in patients with chronic obstructive pulmonary disease. *Ann Intern Med* 1995; **122**: 823–32.

◆71. Lacasse T, Wong E, Guyatt GH *et al.* Meta-analysis of respiratory rehabilitation in chronic obstructive lung disease. *Lancet* 1996; **348**: 1115–19.

◆72. American Thoracic Society. Pulmonary rehabilitation – 1999. *Am J Respir Crit Care Med* 1999; **159**: 1666–82.

73. Goldstein RS, Gort EH, Stubbing D *et al.* Randomised controlled trial of respiratory rehabilitation. *Lancet* 1994; **344**: 1394–7.

74. Casaburi P, Patessio A, Ioli F *et al.* Reductions in exercise lactic acidosis and ventilation as a result of exercise training in patients with obstructive lung disease. *Am Rev Respir Dis* 1991; **143**: 9–18.

75. Maltais F, Leblanc P, Simard C *et al.* Skeletal muscle adaptation to endurance training in patients with chronic obstructive pulmonary disease. *Am J Respir Crit Care Med* 1996; **154**: 442–7.

76. O'Donnell DE, McGuire M, Samis L, Webb KA. The impact of exercise reconditioning on breathlessness in severe chronic airflow limitation. *Am J Respir Crit Care Med* 1995; **152**: 2005–13.

77. O'Donnell DE, McGuire M, Samis L, Webb KA. General exercise training improves ventilatory and peripheral muscle strength and endurance in chronic airflow limitation. *Am J Respir Crit Care Med* 1998; **157**: 1489–97.

78. Gigliotti F, Coli C, Bianchi R *et al.* Exercise training improves exertional dyspnea in patients with COPD: evidence of the role of mechanical factors. *Chest* 2003; **123**: 1794–802.

●79. Casaburi R, Porszasz J, Burns MR *et al.* Physiologic benefits of exercise training in rehabilitation of patients with severe chronic obstructive pulmonary disease. *Am J Respir Crit Care Med* 1997; **155**: 1541–51.

●80. O'Donnell DE, D'Arsigny C, Webb KA. Effects of hyperoxia on ventilatory limitation during exercise in advanced chronic obstructive pulmonary disease. *Am J Respir Crit Care Med* 2001; **163**: 892–8.

81. Alvisi V, Mirkovic T, Nesme P *et al.* Acute effects of hyperoxia on dyspnea in hypoxemia patients with chronic airway obstruction at rest. *Chest* 2003; **123**: 1038–46.

14

Measurement of dyspnoea

DONALD A. MAHLER

INTRODUCTION

The two major purposes for measuring dyspnoea are: (i) to differentiate between people who have less dyspnoea and those who have more dyspnoea; and (ii) to determine how dyspnoea changes in response to a medical intervention. Although dyspnoea is a subjective sensation, the principles of psychophysics (the study of the relationship between a stimulus and the response) can be applied in order to quantify the severity of breathing difficulty (1). To illustrate this approach, in 1946 Stevens (2) stated: 'Measurement is defined as the assignment of numerals to objects or events according to rules.'

Accordingly, dyspnoea can be measured by examining the stimulus–response relationship. To measure or grade the severity of dyspnoea, both the presumed stimulus and the available instruments used to quantify the response need to be considered.

WHAT IS THE STIMULUS FOR DYSPNOEA DURING EXERCISE?

At the present time the exact mechanisms and precise stimuli for exertional breathlessness have not been completely identified. Nevertheless, two different approaches are used as probable stimuli for quantifying dyspnoea (Box 14.1). For example, patients with chronic respiratory disease typically report that activities of daily living provoke breathlessness and are an important reason that they seek medical attention. Thus, activities of daily living have a direct impact on an individual's ability to work and perform tasks. Consideration of

---

Box 14.1   Presumed stimuli for measuring the intensity of dyspnoea and instruments used to measure the response

Activities of daily living

- Baseline and Transition Dyspnoea Indexes

or

- Dyspnoea component of the CRQ

or

- UCSD Shortness of Breath questionnaire

Exercise test

- 0–10 category-ratio (CR-10) scale

or

- Visual analogue scale (VAS)

CRQ, chronic respiratory questionnaire; UCSD, University of California San Diego; VAS, visual analogue scale.

---

activities of daily living as a stimulus depends on a person's recall and description of daily tasks, ability to function, time and effort to complete an activity, etc. (3).

A second approach uses exercise testing on the cycle ergometer or a treadmill as a direct stimulus to elicit both physiological and perceptual responses (3). During a cardiopulmonary exercise test, the subject performs work which can be considered as a stimulus for perceptual responses such as dyspnoea and leg discomfort. Presently, variables such as power production (watts) or oxygen consumption ($\dot{V}O_2$ in mL/kg per min) are used as putative stimuli for causing dyspnoea during exertion (3, 4).

TYPES OF INSTRUMENTS AND MEASUREMENT CRITERIA

A discriminative instrument used to quantify dyspnoea can differentiate between people who have less dyspnoea and those who have more dyspnoea, whereas an evaluative instrument can determine how much dyspnoea has changed (3, 5).

Validity, reliability (for a discriminative instrument), responsiveness (for an evaluative instrument) and interpretability are important measurement criteria (Box 14.2). Validity concerns whether an instrument measures what it is intended to measure. For a discriminative instrument, validity is strengthened if different measures of dyspnoea categorize patients in a similar manner and should correlate highly with one another. For an evaluative instrument, validity is supported if changes in dyspnoea scores correlate with expected changes in other parameters (e.g. exercise performance) consistent with expectations.

Moreover, a satisfactory instrument should have a high signal-to-noise ratio. For a discriminative instrument, reliability is the method for quantifying the signal to noise. An instrument is considered reliable if the variability in scores between patients (the signal) is considerably greater than the variability within subjects (the noise). For an evaluative instrument, responsiveness is the method for determining the signal-to-noise ratio. Physicians and/or investigators want to be confident that they can detect an important difference in dyspnoea even if it is small. Responsiveness is related to the magnitude of the differences in scores in patients who have improved or deteriorated (the signal) compared with the extent to which patients who have not changed have more or less the same scores (the noise).

Box 14.2   Criteria to assess instruments used to measure dyspnoea (adapted from Mahler *et al.* [3])

Discriminative instrument (differentiates between people who have less dyspnoea and those who have more dyspnoea)

- Reliability – stable patients should have only small changes in dyspnoea scores with repeated testing when compared with differences in dyspnoea scores between patients
- Validity – a dyspnoea score from one instrument should correlate with the dyspnoea score from another instrument

Evaluative instrument (determines how much dyspnoea has changed)

- Responsiveness – ability to detect change if it has occurred
- Construct validity – changes in dyspnoea scores should correlate with expected changes in other variables, such as lung function or exercise performance, as a result of an intervention

---

Interpretability is another important criterion when considering a particular score or rating. For an evaluative instrument, a specific change in the score could represent a trivial, small but important, moderate or large improvement or deterioration in dyspnoea. Furthermore, a threshold level has been established for some instruments that represents a 'minimal important difference' (MID) that is considered as clinically meaningful (6).

INSTRUMENTS USED TO MEASURE DYSPNOEA

Clinical dyspnoea ratings

Since 1959 the Medical Research Council (MRC) scale (7) has been used extensively as a discriminative instrument based on a single dimension (i.e. magnitude of task) that provokes dyspnoea. In 1982, the American Thoracic Society (8) published a dyspnoea scale that was nearly identical to the MRC scale. Although these scales are appropriate discriminative instruments, they are limited by two factors. Both scales focus only on one dimension that affects breathlessness; and the grades are quite broad so that it may be difficult to detect small but important changes with particular interventions (3).

To enhance the ability to measure changes in dyspnoea, multidimensional instruments were developed that considered additional factors that influenced the sensation of dyspnoea experienced by patients. The Baseline (BDI) and Transition (TDI) Dyspnoea Indexes were published in 1984 and included two components – functional impairment and magnitude of effort – in addition to magnitude of task that provoked breathing difficulty (9). The BDI was developed as a discriminative instrument to measure dyspnoea at a single point in time, whereas the TDI was developed as an evaluative instrument to measure changes in dyspnoea from the baseline state. Ratings or scores for dyspnoea are obtained from an interviewer (physician, nurse or pulmonary function technician) as part of taking a medical history relating to respiratory disease; the interviewer selects a score for each of the three components based on the patient's answers using the specific criteria for the grades as described for the instruments.

An interview approach was used rather than a self-administered questionnaire for two specific reasons. First, dyspnoea could be graded as part of obtaining a standard medical history of a patient with respiratory disease; and second, the questions posed by the interviewer could uncover subtleties relating to dyspnoea that might be missed by the patient simply checking a box to indicate a grade. More recently, a self-administered computerized version of the BDI has been shown to provide comparable scores as obtained by two different interviewers (10).

In 1987 the Chronic Respiratory Questionnaire (CRQ) was described and included dyspnoea as one of four components of a quality of life instrument in patients with respiratory disease (11). The individual patient is asked to select the five most important activities that caused breathlessness over the past 2 weeks by recall and by then reading from a list of

26 activities. The severity of dyspnoea is graded by the patient selecting a score on a scale (range, 1–7) for each of the five activities. The overall score can then be divided by the number of activities (usually five) selected by the patient. The CRQ was developed as an evaluative instrument. Williams *et al.* (12) developed a self-administered CRQ and observed a significant difference in the dyspnoea scores between the interviewer and the self-report versions, although the differences were less than the MID for the dyspnoea dimension. Schunemann *et al.* (13) have standardized the five activities that otherwise were selected by each patient as part of the dyspnoea dimension of the CRQ.

Other multidimensional questionnaires include the UCSD Shortness of Breath Questionnaire (14) and the Pulmonary Functional Status and Dyspnoea Questionnaire (15). The UCSD questionnaire asks patients to indicate how frequently they experience shortness of breath on a seven-point scale during 21 activities of daily living. There are three additional questions about limitations due to shortness of breath, fear of harm from over-exertion, and fear of shortness of breath for a total of 24 items. Although the St George's Respiratory Questionnaire includes questions about dyspnoea as part of the symptoms component for measuring health status, there is no specific score or grade for dyspnoea (16).

In 1995 Eakin *et al.* (17) reported that the BDI/TDI and the UCSD Shortness of Breath questionnaire demonstrated the highest levels of reliability and validity among six different measures of dyspnoea (including the American Thoracic Society dyspnoea scale, oxygen cost diagram, visual analogue scale, and the 0–10 Borg scale). In this cross-sectional study the BDI exhibited consistently higher correlations with the 6-min walking distance, quality of well-being score, lung function, depression score and anxiety score compared with the UCSD questionnaire (17).

In 1995 the Outcomes Committee of the American Association of Cardiovascular and Pulmonary Rehabilitation reviewed the available clinical instruments to measure dyspnoea and stated that, 'The recommended measure of overall dyspnoea is the Baseline Dyspnoea Index (BDI)/Transition Dyspnoea Index (TDI)', for assessment of clinical outcomes in rehabilitation programmes (18).

Ratings during exercise

During an exercise test the individual can provide ratings of dyspnoea using a visual analogue scale (VAS) or a category-ratio scale (3). In addition to rating the intensity of breathlessness, subjects can also be instructed to rate leg discomfort or chest pain if it is a predominant complaint.

The VAS is a continuous scale that is typically a vertical line, usually 100 mm in length, with or without descriptors positioned as anchors (19). As an example, descriptors may be 'no breathlessness' and 'greatest breathlessness' at the two extremes. The subject places a mark on the VAS with a pen or can adjust a linear potentiometer (or the cursor on a computer screen) to indicate his/her level of dyspnoea on the VAS displayed on a monitor.

However, the most widely used scale for enabling individuals to rate dyspnoea during exercise testing is the 0–10 category-ratio scale (CR-10) developed by Borg (20). This scale consists of a vertical line labelled 0–10 with non-linear spacing of verbal descriptors of severity corresponding to specific numbers that can be chosen by the subject to reflect presumed ratio properties of sensation or symptom intensity.

Investigators have shown that the VAS and the CR-10 scale provide similar scores during incremental cardiopulmonary exercise testing in healthy subjects (21) and in patients with COPD (22). However, the CR-10 scale has at least two advantages for measuring dyspnoea during exercise. First, the descriptors on the CR-10 scale permit comparisons between or among individuals based on the assumption that the verbal descriptors on the scale describe the same intensity for different subjects. For example, two subjects may have different levels of cardiorespiratory fitness, but nonetheless both may select the number '8' on the CR-10 scale as the proper indication of their subjective maximum breathlessness. Second, a numerical value or descriptor on the CR-10 scale may be used as a dyspnoea 'target' (as opposed to a measured length in mm on the VAS) for prescribing and monitoring exercise training (23, 24).

Initially, investigators were interested in peak values of dyspnoea on the VAS or the CR-10 scale during exercise testing. Although a wide range of values have been reported, both healthy individuals and patients with cardiorespiratory disease usually stop exercise on the cycle ergometer at submaximal (at ratings between 5 and 8 on the CR-10 scale) intensities of dyspnoea and/or leg discomfort. For example, Killian *et al.* (25) reported that 320 healthy subjects (63 ± 4 years) had a median dyspnoea intensity of 6 at peak exertion, while the 25–75th percentile values were 5–9. Patients with varying severity of COPD had similar ratings for peak values for dyspnoea. However, as expected, the peak power output on the cycle ergometer was almost twice as high in the healthy subjects as it was in the patients with COPD.

Although data on peak values of symptoms may be useful, there are clearly limits to the use of such information, particularly when evaluating the effect of an intervention such as pulmonary rehabilitation. The next step in the development process for obtaining breathlessness ratings was to instruct patients to give ratings at specific times or workloads during the exercise test (3). The most frequently used exercise protocols incorporated an increase in power output on the cycle ergometer each minute. Accordingly, the subject was instructed to provide ratings at each increment (typically at 1-min intervals) 'on cue' during the exercise test. A series of discrete dyspnoea ratings can be obtained over the course of 1-min intervals of time. Based on these data the slope and intercept of the stimulus–response relationship can be calculated over a range of stimulus values (3, 4, 25, 26). In general, the slope of the regression between power production and dyspnoea is higher in patients with respiratory disease than in healthy individuals (3, 26, 27).

In 1993 Harty *et al.* (28) described the methodology and results of the continuous measurement (subjects adjusted a potentiometer to give ratings on a VAS displayed on a monitor) of breathlessness during exercise. In 2001 Mahler *et al.* (29) reported on a continuous method in which subjects moved a computer mouse that controlled the length of a vertical bar adjacent to values along the CR-10 scale to represent the current level of perceived dyspnoea throughout exercise. This method enabled subjects to provide spontaneous and continuous ratings while exercising without waiting for a cue or request from the physician or exercise specialist. In addition, the continuous method provides more ratings of dyspnoea throughout the course of exercise than are obtained with the discrete method (29, 30). For example, 24 patients with COPD (aged 66 ± 10 years) gave significantly more ratings (11 ± 4) with the continuous method than with the discrete method (5 ± 1) during an incremental exercise test (31).

The advantages of the continuous method for measuring dyspnoea include the following (28–31):

- dyspnoea ratings are spontaneous rather than 'on cue' each minute with the discrete method
- more dyspnoea ratings are obtained, which can then be used for statistical analyses
- it has the ability to calculate an absolute threshold for breathlessness.

MINIMAL IMPORTANT DIFFERENCE

Although an experienced physician may be confident in interpreting changes in lung function or infiltrates on chest radiographs, the change in a score for breathlessness is not intuitively obvious. Accordingly, the concept of a MID has been used to provide an estimate as to the clinical importance of the magnitude of the treatment effect. Moreover, regulatory agencies have been interested in understanding whether a change in dyspnoea not only is statistically significant, but also represents a clinically meaningful response. Jaeschke *et al.* (32) defined the MID as: 'The smallest difference in score in the domain of interest which patients perceive as beneficial and would mandate, in the absence of troublesome side-effects and excessive cost, a change in the patient's management.'

Both an anchor approach and standard statistical methods have been used to determine the MID for dyspnoea and health status instruments (6, 33).

For the TDI focal score, a change of at least one unit re-presents the MID (9, 34, 35). First, a change of one unit or more in the TDI is inherent in the instrument itself as representing meaningful change (improvement or deterioration) (9). Second, Witek and Mahler (34, 35) used the physician's global evaluation (PGE) score (range 1–8) of individual patients with COPD as an anchor to demonstrate that a change of one unit in the TDI focal score corresponded to a minimal improvement or decline in the PGE. Furthermore, those TDI responders (≥1 unit improvement) in a randomized controlled trial evaluating a long-acting inhaled bronchodilator, tiotropium, used less supplemental albuterol, had better health status and fewer exacerbations (34, 35). The

responses in these clinical outcomes provide additional support for one unit as the MID for the TDI.

For example, a one unit change in the TDI represents:

+1 Able to return to work at reduced pace or has resumed some customary activities with more vigour than previously, due to improvement in shortness of breath (for the component functional impairment).

or

+1 If a patient was short of breath with light activities such as walking on the level or washing, and now becomes short of breath with moderate or average tasks such as walking up a gradual hill or carrying a light load on the level (for the component magnitude of task).

or

+1 Able to do things with distinctly greater effort without shortness of breath. May be able to carry out tasks somewhat more rapidly than previously (for the component magnitude of effort).

If the individual patient achieved improvement in all three components as described above, the TDI focal score would be +3!

For the dyspnoea component of the CRQ, Redelmeier *et al.* (6) 'found that scores, on average, needed to differ by about 0.5 per question for patients to stop rating themselves as "about the same" and start rating themselves as either "a little bit better" or "a little bit worse" '. Therefore, as there are five questions or activities related to dyspnoea as part of the CRQ, the MID for the composite dyspnoea score would be 0.5 (a total summation score of at least 2.5 divided by five activities) (6).

At the present time, a minimal important difference has not been determined for ratings of dyspnoea during exercise testing.

CLINICAL APPLICATIONS IN PULMONARY REHABILITATION

Clinical dyspnoea ratings

The majority of studies evaluating the benefits of pulmonary rehabilitation have used the TDI and/or the dyspnoea component of the CRQ to measure the relief of dyspnoea related to activities of daily living. The changes in dyspnoea after pulmonary rehabilitation in randomized trials are summarized in Table 14.1. In these selected studies, the improvements in breathlessness with pulmonary rehabilitation are highly consistent (36–48). Furthermore, the magnitude of the changes in the TDI and/or in the dyspnoea component of the CRQ exceed the respective MIDs and are generally greater than the responses observed with inhaled bronchodilator therapy (49).

In a study of 37 patients with COPD, de Torres *et al.* (50) evaluated the responsiveness of various outcome measures and found clinically significant changes for the MRC

Table 14.1   *Changes in dyspnoea as measured by the TDI and/or by the dyspnoea component of CRQ in patients with chronic obstructive pulmonary disease after pulmonary rehabilitation*

Author	No. of subjects	Months of study	TDI	Dyspnoea–CRQ[a]
Carrieri-Kohlman	24 (coached)	3	2.4 ± 2.2	1.2 ± 0.3
Berry	16, 36 and 99	3		0.7, 0.5, 0.5
Foglio	26	2	5.6 ± 2.2	
Foy	118	3		0.7 ± 0.1
Goldstein	89	2	2.7 (0.8–4.6)	0.6 (0.1–1.1)
O'Donnell	60	1.5	2.8 ± 0.3	
O'Donnell	20	1.5	3.2 ± 0.3	
Reardon	20	1.5	2.1	
Guell	30	24		1.0 (0.2–1.7)
Behnke	30	6	7.2	0.5
Ortega	17 (strength)	3		0.8
	16 (endurance)			0.9
	14 (combined)			0.9
Wijkstra	58	3		0.9
Ries[b]	164	2	2.7 ± 2.3	0.9

Scores for Transition Dyspnoea Index (TDI) and/or dyspnoea component of the Chronic Respiratory Questionnaire (CRQ) are differences between pre- and post-rehabilitation values. Values in parenthesis represent ranges.
[a]Total scores for the changes in the dyspnoea component of the CRQ are divided by five for the number of activities selected.
[b]Change in the UCSD Shortness of Breath questionnaire was –10.0 after pulmonary rehabilitation in this study (47).

dyspnoea scale in 29 per cent of patients, for the VAS at peak exercise in 48 per cent of patients, and for the TDI and the CRQ in >50 per cent of patients after pulmonary rehabilitation. The authors concluded that the VAS peak exercise, BDI/TDI and the CRQ 'adequately reflect the beneficial effects of pulmonary rehabilitation' (50).

In addition, Ries *et al.* (48, 51) showed a significant reduction in dyspnoea on the UCSD Shortness of Breath questionnaire and/or TDI after 2 months of pulmonary rehabilitation compared with an education group or with a standard care control group.

Ratings during exercise

Various studies have demonstrated that exercise training, as part of a comprehensive pulmonary rehabilitation programme reduces dyspnoea ratings during exercise (38, 41, 42, 45, 48, 51–54). For example, Ries *et al.* (51) showed that breathlessness ratings on the CR-10 scale were significantly lower during endurance treadmill exercise in those with COPD who did exercise training than in those who received only education. O'Donnell *et al.* (41) reported that the slope of the oxygen consumption–breathlessness curve fell significantly ($P < 0.01$) in patients who performed 2.5 h of exercise training three times per week for 6 weeks compared with a control group. Similarly, Ramirez-Venegas *et al.* (52) demonstrated a reduction in the slope of the power (watts)–dyspnoea relationship (pre: 0.12; post: 0.09; $P < 0.05$) during incremental exercise testing after training in 44 patients with COPD. These reports illustrate the beneficial effects of pulmonary rehabilitation on relieving exertional breathlessness as measured during standard exercise testing.

RECOMMENDATION

The severity of dyspnoea should be routinely measured in all patients at the start and upon completion of their participation in a pulmonary rehabilitation programme (3, 18, 55). Established instruments are available to measure the intensity of breathlessness based on activities of daily living or during exercise testing. Numerous studies performed in Europe and in North America (Table 14.1) have demonstrated consistent and substantial improvements in dyspnoea in patients with COPD as a result of pulmonary rehabilitation (3, 4, 17, 30, 55).

Key points

- The reduction of dyspnoea is an important objective of pulmonary rehabilitation.
- Valid, reliable and responsive instruments are available to measure the severity of breathlessness in patients with respiratory disease.
- Both activities of daily living and exercise testing can be used as stimuli to assess the dyspnoea response.
- Numerous randomized controlled trials of pulmonary rehabilitation have demonstrated the consistent benefits for relief of breathlessness.
- The severity of dyspnoea should be measured routinely as a standard outcome measure to evaluate the efficacy of all pulmonary rehabilitation programmes.

REFERENCES

1. Baird JC, Noma E. *Fundamentals of Scaling and Psychophysics.* New York: Wiley Interscience, 1978.

2. Stevens SS. On the theory of scales of measurement. *Science* 1946; **103**: 677–80.

◆3. Mahler DA, Jones PW, Guyatt GH. Clinical measurement of dyspnea. In: Mahler DA, ed. *Dyspnea.* New York: Marcel Dekker, Inc. 1998, 149–98.

4. Killian KJ. The objective measurement of dyspnea. *Chest* 1985; **85**(Suppl.): 84S–90S.

5. Guyatt GH, Feeny DH, Patrick DL. Measuring health-related quality of life. *Ann Intern Med* 1993; **118**: 622–19.

6. Redelmeier D, Guyatt GH, Goldstein RS. Assessing the minimal important difference in symptoms: a comparison of two techniques. *J Clin Epidemiol* 1996; **49**: 1215–19.

7. Fletcher CM, Elmes PC, Wood CH. The significance of respiratory symptoms and the diagnosis of chronic bronchitis in a working population. *Br Med J* 1959; **1**: 257–66.

8. Brooks SM (chairman). Task group on surveillance for respiratory hazards in the occupational setting. *ATS News* 1982; **8**: 12–16.

●9. Mahler DA, Weinberg DH, Wells CK, Feinstein AR. The measurement of dyspnea: contents, interobserver agreement, and physiologic correlates of two new clinical indexes. *Chest* 1984; **85**: 751–8.

10. Mahler DA, Ward J, Baird JC. Validity of a self-administered computerized (SAC) baseline dyspnea index. *Am J Respir Crit Care Med* 2003; **167**: A312 (abstract).

●11. Guyatt GH, Berman LB, Townshend M *et al.* A measure of quality of life for clinical trials in chronic lung disease. *Thorax* 1987; **42**: 773–8.

12. Williams JEA, Singh SJ, Sewell L *et al.* Development of a self-reported Chronic Respiratory Questionnaire (CRQ-SR). *Thorax* 2001; **56**: 954–9.

13. Schunemann HJ, Griffith L, Goldstein R *et al.* A comparison of the original Chronic Respiratory Questionnaire (CRQ) with a standardized version. *Am J Respir Crit Care Med* 2003; **167**: A226 (abstract).

14. Eakin EG, Resnikoff PM, Prewitt LM *et al.* Validation of a new dyspnea measure: the UCSD shortness of breath questionnaire. *Chest* 1998; **113**: 619–24.

15. Lareau SC, Carrieri-Kohlman V, Janson-Bjerklie Ross PJ. Development and testing of the pulmonary functional status and dyspnea questionnaire. *Heart Lung* 1994; **23**: 242–50.

16. Jones PW, Quirk FH, Baveystock CM, Littlejohns P. A self-complete measure of health status for chronic airflow limitation. The St George's Respiratory Questionnaire. *Am Rev Respir Dis* 1992; **145**: 1321–7.

17. Eakin EG, Sassi-Dambron DE, Ries AL, Kaplan RM. Reliability and validity of dyspnea measures in patients with obstructive lung disease. *Int J Behav Med* 1995; **2**: 118–34.

◆18. AACVPR outcomes committee. Outcome measurement in cardiac and pulmonary rehabilitation. *J Cardiopulm Rehab* 1995; **15**: 394–405.

19. Gift AG. Visual analogue scales: measurement of subjective phenomena. *Nurs Res* 1989; **38**: 286–8.

20. Borg GAV. Psychological bases of perceived exertion. *Med Sci Sport Exer* 1982; **14**: 377–81.

21. Wilson RC, Jones PW. A comparison of the visual analogue scale and modified Borg scale for the measurement of dyspnea during exercise. *Clin Sci* 1989; **76**: 277–82.

22. Muza SR, Silverman MT, Gilmore GC *et al.* Comparison of scales used to quantitate the sense of effort to breathe in patients with chronic obstructive pulmonary disease. *Am Rev Respir Dis* 1990; **141**: 909–13.

23. Mejia R, Ward J, Lentine T, Mahler DA. Target dyspnea ratings predict expected oxygen consumption as well as target heart rate values. *Am J Respir Crit Care Med* 1999; **159**: 1485–9.

24. Mahler DA, Ward J, Mejia-Alfaro R. Stability of dyspnea ratings after exercise training in patients with COPD. *Med Sci Sports Exerc* 2003; **35**: 1083–7.

25. Killian KJ, Leblanc P, Martin DH *et al.* Exercise capacity and ventilatory, circulatory, and symptom limitation in patients with chronic airflow limitation. *Am Rev Respir Dis* 1992; **146**: 935–40.

26. Hamilton AL, Killian KJ, Summers E, Jones NL. Symptom intensity and subjective limitation to exercise in patients with cardiorespiratory disorders. *Chest* 1996; **110**: 1255–63.

27. O'Donnell DE, Chau LKL, Webb KA. Qualitative aspects of exertional dyspnea in patients with interstitial lung disease. *J Appl Physiol* 1998; **84**: 2000–9.

28. Harty HR, Heywood P, Adams L. Comparison between continuous and discrete measurements of breathlessness during exercise in normal subjects using a visual anlogue scale. *Clin Sci* 1993; **85**: 229–36.

29. Mahler DA, Mejia-Alfaro R, Ward J, Baird JC. Continuous measurement of breathlessness during exercise: validity, reliability, and responsiveness. *J Appl Physiol* 2001; **90**: 2188–96.

30. Mahler DA, Fierro-Carrion G, Baird JC. Mechanisms and measurement of exertional dyspnea. In: Weisman IM, Zeballos RJ, eds. *Clinical Exercise Testing.* Basel: Karger, 2002; 72–80.

31. Fierro-Carrion G, Mahler DA, Ward J, Baird JC. Comparison of continuous and discrete measurements of dyspnea during exercise in patients with COPD and normals. *Chest* 2004; **125**: 77–84.

32. Jaeschke R, Singer J, Guyatt GH. Measurement of health status. Ascertaining the minimal clinically important difference. *Control Clin Trials* 1989; **10**: 407–15.

33. Wyrwich KW, Tierney WM, Wolinsky FD. Further evidence supporting an SEM-based criterion for identifying meaningful intra-individual changes in health-related quality of life. *J Clin Epidemiol* 1999; **52**: 861–73.

34. Witek TJ Jr, Mahler DA. Meaningful effect size and patterns of response of the transition dyspnea index. *J Clin Epidemiol* 2003; **56**: 248–55.

35. Witek TJ Jr, Mahler DA. Minimal important difference of the transition dyspnea index in a multi-national clinical trial. *Eur Respir J* 2003; **21**: 267–72.

36. Carrieri-Kohlman V, Gormley JM, Douglas MK *et al.* Exercise training decreases dyspnea and the distress and anxiety associated with it. *Chest* 1996; **110**: 1526–35.

37. Berry MJ, Rejeski WJ, Adair NE, Zaccaro D. Exercise rehabilitation and chronic obstructive pulmonary disease stage. *Am J Respir Crit Care Med* 1999; **160**: 1248–53.

38. Foglio K, Bianchi L, Bruletti G *et al.* Long-term effectiveness of pulmonary rehabilitation in patients with chronic airway obstruction. *Eur Respir J* 1999; **13**: 125–32.

39. Foy CG, Rejeski WJ, Berry MJ *et al.* Gender moderates the effects of exercise therapy on health-related quality of life among COPD patients. *Chest* 2001; **119**: 70–6.

●40. Goldstein RS, Gort EH, Stubbing D *et al.* Randomised controlled trial of respiratory rehabilitation. *Lancet* 1994; **344**: 1394–7.

●41. O'Donnell DE, McGuire MA, Samis L, Webb KA. The impact of exercise reconditioning on breathlessness in severe chronic airflow limitation. *Am J Respir Crit Care Med* 1995; **152**: 2005–13.

42. O'Donnell DE, McGuire M, Samis L, Webb KA. General exercise training improves ventilatory and peripheral muscle strength and endurance in chronic airflow limitation. *Am J Respir Crit Care Med* 1998; **157**: 1489–97.

43. Readon J, Awad E, Normandin E *et al.* The effect of comprehensive outpatient pulmonary rehabilitation on dyspnea. *Chest* 1994; **105**: 1046–52.

44. Guell R, Casan P, Belda J *et al.* Long-term effects of outpatient rehabilitation of COPD. *Chest* 2000; **117**: 976–83.

45. Behnke M, Taube C, Kirsten D *et al.* Home-based exercise is capable of preserving hospital-based improvements in severe chronic obstructive pulmonary disease. *Respir Med* 2000; **94**: 1184–91.

46. Ortega F, Toral J, Cejudo P *et al.* Comparison of effects of strength and endurance training in patients with chronic obstructive pulmonary disease. *Am J Respir Crit Care Med* 2002; **166**: 669–74.

47. Wijkstra PJ, van Altena R, Kraan J *et al.* Quality of life in patients with chronic obstructive pulmonary disease improves after rehabilitation at home. *Eur Respir J* 1994; **7**: 269–73.

●48. Ries AL, Kaplan RM, Myers R, Prewitt LM. Maintenance after pulmonary rehabilitation in chronic lung disease. *Am J Respir Crit Care Med* 2003; **167**: 880–8.

49. Mahler DA. Dyspnea. In: Celli BR, ed. *Pharmacotherapy of COPD*. New York: Marcel Dekker, Inc, 2003.

50. de Torres JP, Pinto-Plata V, Ingenito E *et al.* Power of outcome measurements to detect clinically significant changes in pulmonary rehabilitation of patients with COPD. *Chest* 2002; **121**: 1092–8.

●51. Ries AL, Kaplan RM, Limberg TM, Prewitt LM. Effects of pulmonary rehabilitation on physiologic and psychosocial outcomes in patients with chronic obstructive pulmonary disease. *Ann Intern Med* 1995; **122**: 823–32.

52. Ramirez-Venegas A, Ward JL, Olmstead EM *et al.* Effect of exercise training on dyspnea measures in patients with chronic obstructive pulmonary disease. *J Cardiopulm Rehab* 1997; **17**: 103–9.

53. Strijbos JH, Postma DS, van Altena R *et al.* A comparison between an outpatient hospital-based pulmonary rehabilitation program and a home-care pulmonary rehabilitation program in patients with COPD. *Chest* 1996; **109**: 366–72.

54. Wijkstra PJ, van der Mark TW, Kraan J *et al.* Effects of home rehabilitation on physical performance in patients with chronic obstructive pulmonary disease (COPD). *Eur Respir J* 1996; **9**: 104–10.

◆55. Mahler DA, Harver A. Dyspnea. In: Fishman AP, ed. *Pulmonary Rehabilitation*. New York: Marcel Dekker, Inc., 1996; 97–116.

15

Impact of health status ('quality of life') issues in chronic lung disease

MAURO CARONE, PAUL W. JONES

Chronic respiratory diseases affect the lungs, but also have effects in other organs. These secondary effects must be addressed if the patient's quality of life (QoL) is to be improved. This applies especially when the disease interferes with daily activities such as washing, dressing and cooking. There are several ways in which respiratory disease may impair the QoL of patients with chronic obstructive pulmonary disease (COPD) (Fig. 15.1). Although cough and sputum production are troublesome, especially at night, dyspnoea and fatigue are the dominant symptoms which lead to exercise limitation, physical disability and the capacity to perform routine daily activities. Disuse-induced muscle wasting and the influence of the subject's personality may constitute self-reinforcing feedback loops that may lead to a vicious cycle that inevitably leads to progressive worsening of the patient's state. Over and above the pathophysiological elements, the personality of individual subjects, their mood, hopes and fears, and expectations from life are important, as they represent the subjective aspect of the impaired health, which varies from patient to patient. From the patients' perspective, interference with their health, as reflected in their symptoms and the disturbance to daily life, is more important than variables such as pulmonary function tests or arterial blood gas analysis (1, 2).

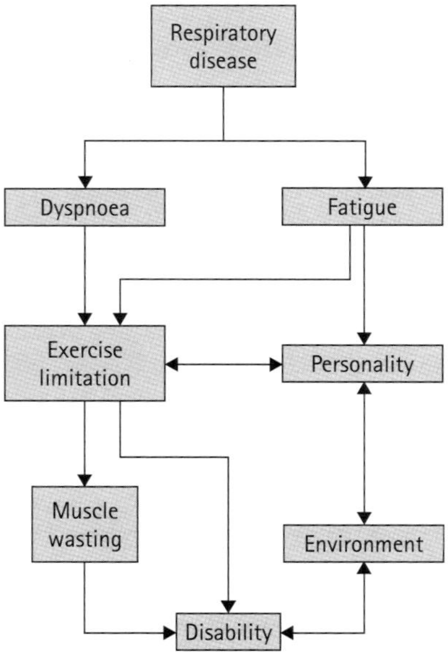

COPD is the commonest cause of respiratory-induced disability. Like most chronic respiratory causes, it is incurable, but unlike them it is also usually progressive. Therapy and rehabilitation are directed towards a reduction of exacerbations, minimization of symptom severity, and improvement, or at least maintenance, of the patients' health. In view of the multiplicity of pathways or mechanisms that lead to impaired health, it is clear that a comprehensive approach is required for the management of these patients. Pulmonary rehabilitation is a multidisciplinary therapeutic intervention that incorporates a number of modalities discussed elsewhere in this book. A typical programme will contain many components that produce a range of benefits. The relative contribution of each component will vary between programmes and patients. Whilst each component may have a more or less specific effect, measurable using appropriate instruments, the outcome of greatest interest is the overall effect on health. However,

Figure 15.1 *Pathways linking lung disease to disability.*

health states should be measured directly using appropriate instruments, since the level of health impairment cannot be inferred reliably by measurement of one of the components that contribute to impaired health. Most physiological measurements correlate relatively poorly with patient-reported impairment of physical function or overall health status, although exercise performance, especially as measured using the 6-min walk test, is a much better correlate than the FEV_1 (forced expiratory volume in 1 s) (3). In practice, the only method that can provide an overall estimate of the patient's health is the use of suitably designed questionnaires.

QUALITY OF LIFE, HEALTH–RELATED QUALITY OF LIFE AND HEALTH STATUS MEASUREMENTS

A number of different terms are applied to the measurements used to quantify the impact of COPD on a patient's daily life and well-being. For instance, the terms 'quality of life' and 'health status measurement' are too often used interchangeably. This can lead to confusion through overlap and differences of interpretation and definition between authors. A further problem arises in the tension generated between theoreticians who wish to analyse and define the concept of ill health due to disease, and those who wish to develop valid and practical methods for measuring ill health.

Quality of life is a general term that applies to all individuals, whether diseased or healthy. QoL can be broadly defined as the gap between what is desired in life and the degree to which this desire is achieved, i.e. between wishes and achievements. It can be influenced by many factors, including financial status, housing conditions, spirituality, family and social support, and health.

Within the context of medicine, the focus is more upon the effects of disease. For this reason, the term 'health-related quality of life' (HRQL) has been proposed to signify the effect of disease on the gap between desires and the degree to which they are achievable. Both QoL and HRQL should be thought of as indicators of how individuals rate their lives.

Measurement requires standardization, so questionnaires designed to measure HRQL must be applicable to each patient with the disease. In other words, they treat each patient as if he or she were a typical patient. They rarely permit any indiviuality. For this reason we prefer to draw a distinction between HRQL that applies to individuals and health status that applies to populations. Health status questionnaires are made up of a set of items that are appropriate and common to all subjects with the disease in question. Inevitably this means that they tend to address essential activities and functions of daily living specifically, and examine social and recreational matters in a more general manner. Whilst this might seem to be a limitation, standardization does permit health status scores to be used in the same way as any other standardized measure, e.g. spirometry. An easy-to-understand definition of health status measurement may be: 'quantification of the impact of disease on daily life and well-being in a formal and standardised manner' (4).

HEALTH STATUS (QUALITY OF LIFE) MEASUREMENTS IN COPD

Health status–QoL measurements are designed to:

- define the health of groups of patients
- measure changes over time in health of groups of patients
- predict future health events and resource use
- assess the impact of disease and treatment on an individual basis.

Health status questionnaires used in COPD fall into two main classes: generic questionnaires, such as the Medical Outcomes Study Short-Form Health Survey (SF36) (5, 6), Sickness Impact Profile (SIP) (7), EuroQoL (8), and disease-specific questionnaires; among the latter are the Chronic Respiratory Questionnaire (CRQ) (9), Maugeri Respiratory Failure Questionnaire (MRF-28) (10), Quality-of-Life for Respiratory Illness Questionnaire (QOL-RIQ) (11) and St George's Respiratory Questionnaire (SGRQ) (12). These all meet criteria for validity, reliability and responsiveness. The disease-specific questionnaires have both discriminative properties (i.e. ability to detect differences in health status among patients at a given moment), and evaluative properties (i.e. ability to detect changes in health status within the same group), but only the MRF-28 and SGRQ were designed specifically to have both discriminative and evaluative properties. It was necessary for these two questionnaires to have good performance in both of these functions, because they were intended for long-term studies over years as well as over much shorter time periods. All of the questionnaires listed above are complex and relatively time-consuming. Another much shorter and simpler questionnaire, the AQ20, has been developed and validated for use in COPD (13, 14), but there are fewer studies reporting data with instrument, as yet.

Currently, the most used application of health status measurement is to assess the effectiveness of different treatments in COPD, and improvement in health status has become a goal of new management strategies, as recommended in numerous management guidelines (15–18). For example, the Global Initiative for Chronic Obstructive Lung Disease (GOLD) outlines the importance of health status and symptom relief as goals for effective COPD management (18). In addition, the European Agency for the Evaluation of Medicinal Products recommends the inclusion of measures of symptomatic benefit such as the SGRQ along with FEV_1 measurement as co-primary end-points in studies of new medicinal products for the treatment of COPD (19).

IMPACT OF LONG–TERM OXYGEN THERAPY ON HEALTH STATUS

There has been much interest in the effect of chronic hypoxaemia on health status, particularly cognitive function, but it is still not possible to draw a final conclusion on the efficacy of long-term oxygen therapy (LTOT) on cognitive function, mood state or overall health status of patients with chronic respiratory failure.

Unfortunately the large NOTT study (20) and the related IPPB study (21) used the SIP – a generic questionnaire. Okubadejo *et al.* (22) showed that the SGRQ was correlated with arterial Po_2, suggesting that it was a valid instrument for use in COPD (22). These authors then used this instrument to assess the impact of LTOT on patients' health status (23). They were unable to carry out a randomized controlled trial of the effect of LTOT for ethical reasons, so used a control group of COPD patients with a similar level of FEV_1, but with severe hypoxia. They found no apparent benefit in the use of LTOT delivered by a concentrator after 6 months and concluded that LTOT did not improve health status. This result is open to some re-interpretation in the light of the more recent observation that health status in COPD declines at a measurable rate (24). Okubadejo *et al.* (23) noted that the health of the control patients deteriorated a little, but that of the LTOT patients did not. This suggests that LTOT might preserve health status, at least for a while. To date there has been no randomized trial of ambulatory oxygen, but this might improve QoL and health status, since it may permit more activities outside the home.

IMPACT OF CHRONIC MECHANICAL VENTILATION ON HEALTH STATUS

A number of studies have investigated the health status impact of non-invasive positive pressure ventilation (NIPPV). For example, using the SF36, it was shown that hypoxaemic COPD patients on NIPPV have better health status score in comparison with hypoxaemic COPD patients who, for one reason or another, used neither LTOT nor NIPPV (25). There have also been some intervention studies. In a crossover study in severely hypoxic patients on LTOT, the patients had better SGRQ scores when they were in the NIPPV limb of the study than when they were on LTOT alone (26). The reason for this is not clear since the greatest benefit was seen in the 'symptoms' component of the SGRQ rather than the 'activity' component or the 'impacts' component, which includes factors such as sleep and mood. Another study (27) utilized the SGRQ and demonstrated that, after 6 months of treatment, health status improved significantly, both statistically and clinically, when judged in terms of the size of change in the SGRQ score (Fig. 15.2). This improvement was more than double the threshold for clinical significance, being –9 units for 'impact' and –10 units for total score.

Even more interesting are the data from a 2-year multicentre Italian study, which compared NIPPV plus LTOT with LTOT alone in 122 COPD patients (28). In that study, the SGRQ did not show any difference between the two groups, but the MRF-28 appeared to be more specific and sensitive. At the end of the 2 years' follow-up, patients on LTOT alone showed slightly worsened health status scores, measured using the MRF-28, whereas patients who received LTOT and NIPPV had improved scores (Fig. 15.3). This study is important

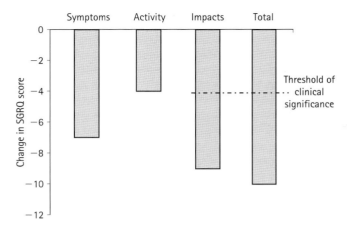

Figure 15.2   *Change in St George's Respiratory Questionnaire score (SGRQ) following 6 months of non-invasive positive pressure ventilation. Negative values indicate health status improvements. The 4-unit value for the threshold for clinical significance applies only to the impacts and total score.*

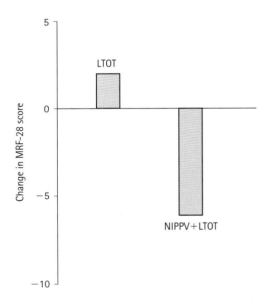

Figure 15.3   *Change in MRF-28 score following 2 years of non-invasive positive pressure ventilation (NIPPV). Negative values indicate improved health. LTOT, long-term oxygen therapy.*

because it suggests that for the most severe patients with respiratory failure, a condition-specific questionnaire such as the MRF-28 (developed specifically for use in such patients) may be more appropriate than a disease-specific questionnaire such as the SGRQ.

IMPACT OF REHABILITATION PROGRAMMES ON PATIENTS' HEALTH STATUS

Numerous studies have contributed to the body of evidence that shows very clearly that rehabilitation improves HRQL

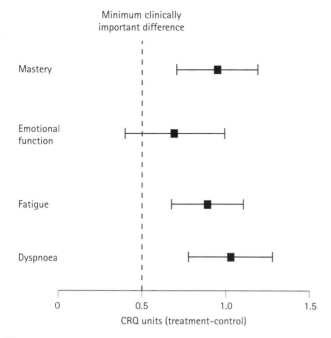

Figure 15.4 *Weighted mean difference in Chronic Respiratory Questionnaire (CRQ) component scores for difference between rehabilitation and control groups from a meta-analysis of randomized trials of rehabilitation in COPD. The error bars are 99 per cent confidence intervals. Data from (29).*

and health status in COPD patients (30–33). These benefits have been shown principally using the CRQ and SGRQ, but the 'physical function' component of the SF-36 has also been shown to be responsive (33). A recent meta-analysis of eight randomized controlled trials has summarized the health status gains assessed using the CRQ (34). This showed that there was a statistically significant improvement in all components of the SGRQ (Fig. 15.4). Furthermore, for three components – fatigue, mastery and dyspnoea – the lower 99 per cent confidence interval was greater than the minimum clinically important difference for this questionnaire.

Similar evidence is available for the SGRQ. In a study performed on 60 patients randomized to enter a 6-week rehabilitation programme or a control group, the SGRQ score was the same in the two subgroups at baseline (32). At the third and sixth months following rehabilitation, there had been a significant improvement in the patients in the rehabilitation arm that exceeded the 4-unit improvement needed with this questionnaire to be clinically significant. In another very large study, 182 COPD patients were randomized either to enter ($n = 93$) or not to enter ($n = 89$) a 6-week, three half days/week, 2 h/day rehabilitation programme (33). As in the previous study, at the end of the programme the improvement in health status was present only in the rehabilitated group but not in the control group. This improvement was both statistically and clinically significant (improvement in SGRQ score = 9 units). Perhaps more importantly, the improvement in SGRQ score was still significant after 1 year

(SGRQ improvement = 5 units). The CRQ also showed a clinically significant improvement at the end of the study, but this was not sustained to 1 year. It is not clear why that difference was seen between these two questionnaires, but it may be related to the psychometric properties of the SGRQ and the fact that it was designed for use in long-term studies.

One of the most useful properties of health status questionnaires is that they permit comparisons of the size of the treatment effect between very different therapeutic modalities. The large improvements in SGRQ score seen with rehabilitation should be contrasted with the size of improvement seen with modern pharmacological therapy, where the improvements are typically of the order of 4 units (35–38). This constitutes powerful evidence that rehabilitation is a very important component of COPD management.

IMPACT OF EDUCATIONAL PROGRAMMES ON PATIENTS' HEALTH STATUS

The efficacy of educational programmes on chronic asthma has been established, but the efficacy of such programmes in COPD on health outcomes has not been completely assessed, even though guidelines stress the fact that education must be a key point of any therapeutic strategy (39).

PREDICTING OUTCOME AND HEALTH STATUS

There is much evidence that health status questionnaires have concurrent validity, i.e. they relate to other measures of disease severity made in the patients at the same time (3). It has already been shown that health status can predict the risk of subsequent hospitalizations (40) and exacerbations of COPD (41). More recently there is evidence that they can predict mortality in COPD, independent of factors such as age, FEV_1 and body mass index (BMI) (42). Two studies, one in Spain (42) and the other in Japan (43), have shown that a 4-unit difference in SGRQ between patients with moderately severe COPD is associated with a 12 per cent difference in mortality at 3 years. In more severe patients with respiratory failure, interim data from the Quality of Life Evaluation and Survival Study (QuESS) (44) suggest that health status assessment provides a better predictor of mortality than functional parameters such as FEV_1 and exercise performance (45).

HEALTH STATUS MEASUREMENTS IN ROUTINE PRACTICE

Health status questionnaires were developed as research tools and are quite complex to administer or score. Self-administered versions of the CRQ are becoming available, as are computer programmes for the SGRQ, which allow keyboard data entry by patient or clinician coupled with automated scoring. In routine practice, there may be a role for using simpler questionnaires, such as the AQ20, for the routine assessment of patients, since this takes only 3 min to complete and score (46, 13). Pulmonary rehabilitation programmes are required to produce evidence of the efficacy of their programme for reimbursement processes, quite unlike other aspects of respiratory therapy. The CRQ and the SGRQ have been used widely for this purpose, as have two functional performance instruments, the Pulmonary Functional Status and Dyspnoea Questionnaire (PFSDQ-M) (2) and the Pulmonary Functional Status Scale (PFSS) (47). All of these can be used to monitor the effects of changes to the programme. The much simpler AQ20 could serve in the same way.

The major limitation with all of these questionnaires is that they treat each patient as if they were 'typical'. This means that whilst they are very useful for assessing change in groups of patients, they are not really suitable for monitoring changes in individual patients. However, they can complement spirometric measurements very usefully for the assessment of individual patients, because the correlation between the FEV_1 and health status scores is weak. Many patients can have poor health status, yet only mild disease when assessed in terms of their degree of airway obstruction. Routine use of health status questionnaires will identify patients who might otherwise be judged ineligible based upon their lung function assessment.

Key points

- Chronic respiratory diseases affect the lungs, but also have effects in other organs.
- Respiratory disease may impair the quality of life of patients with COPD.
- From the patients' perspective, interference with their health is more important than variables such as pulmonary function tests or arterial blood gas analysis.
- Therapy and rehabilitation are directed towards a reduction of exacerbations, minimization of symptom severity, and improvement, or at least maintenance, of patients' health.
- Health states should be measured directly using appropriate instruments, since the level of health impairment cannot be inferred reliably by measurement of one of the components that contribute to impaired health.
- Health status questionnaires used in COPD fall into two main classes: generic questionnaires and disease-specific questionnaires.
- The disease-specific questionnaires have both discriminative properties (i.e. ability to detect differences in health status among patients at a given moment) and evaluative properties (i.e. ability to detect changes in health status within the same group), but only the MRF-28 and SGRQ were designed specifically to have both discriminative and evaluative properties.
- Currently, the most used application of health status measurement is to assess the effectiveness of different treatments in COPD, and improvement in health status has become a goal of new management strategies.
- There has been much interest in the effect of chronic hypoxaemia on health status, particularly cognitive function, but it is still not possible to draw a final conclusion on the efficacy of LTOT on cognitive function, mood state or overall health status of patients with chronic respiratory failure.
- A number of studies have investigated the health status impact of NIPPV, and showed that it improves patients' health.
- Numerous studies have contributed to the body of evidence that shows very clearly that rehabilitation improves quality of life and health status in COPD patients.
- The efficacy of educational programmes in COPD on health outcomes has not been completely assessed, even though guidelines stress the fact that education must be a key point of any therapeutic strategy.
- The major limitation with all of these questionnaires is that they treat all patients as if they were 'typical'. This means that whilst they are very useful for assessing change in groups of patients, they are not really suitable for monitoring changes in individual patients. However, they can complement spirometric measurements very usefully for the assessment of individual patients.

REFERENCES

1. Mahler DA. How should health-related quality of life be assessed in patients with COPD? *Chest* 2000; **117**(2 Suppl.): 54S–7.
2. Lareau SC, Breslin EH, Meek PM. Functional status instruments: outcome measure in the evaluation of patients with chronic obstructive pulmonary disease. *Heart Lung* 1996; **25**: 212–24.
◆3. Jones PW. Health status measurement in chronic obstructive pulmonary disease. *Thorax* 2001; **56**: 880–7.
◆4. Jones PW, Quirk FH, Baveystock CM. Why quality of life measures should be used in the treatment of patients with respiratory illness. *Monaldi Arch Chest Dis* 1994; **49**: 79–82.
5. Stewart AL, Hays RD, Ware JE. The MOS Short Form General Health Survey: reliability and validity in a patient population. *Med Care* 1988; **26**: 724–32.
●6. Mahler DA, Mackowiak JI. Evaluation of the short-form 36-item questionnaire to measure health-related quality of life in patients with COPD. *Chest* 1995; **107**: 1585–9.

●7. Bergner M, Bobbit RA, Carter WB, Gilson BS. The Sickness Impact Profile: development and final revision of a health status measure. *Med Care* 1981; **19**: 787–805.

8. The Euroqol Group. EuroQol – a new facility for the measurement of health-related quality of life. *Health Policy* 1992; **20**: 321–8.

●9. Guyatt GH, Berman LB, Townsend M *et al.* A measure of quality of life for clinical trials in chronic lung disease. *Thorax* 1987; **42**: 773–8.

●10. Carone M, Bertolotti G, Anchisi F *et al.* Analysis of factors that characterize health impairment in patients with chronic respiratory failure. Quality of Life in Chronic Respiratory Failure Group. *Eur Respir J* 1999; **13**: 1293–300.

11. Maille AR, Koning CJ, Zwinderman AH *et al.* The development of the 'Quality-of-life for Respiratory Illness Questionnaire (QOL-RIQ) ': a disease-specific quality-of-life questionnaire for patients with mild to moderate chronic non-specific lung disease. *Respir Med* 1997; **91**: 297–309.

●12. Jones PW, Quirk FH, Baveystock CM, Littlejohns P. A self-complete measure for chronic airflow limitation – the St George's Respiratory Questionnaire. *Am Rev Respir Dis* 1992; **145**: 1321–7.

13. Hajiro T, Nishimura K, Jones PW *et al.* A novel, short and simple questionnaire to measure health-related quality of life in patients with chronic obstructive pulmonary disease. *Am J Respir Crit Care Med* 1999; **159**: 1874–8.

14. Alemayehu B, Aubert RE, Feifer RA, Paul LD. Comparative analysis of two quality-of-life instruments for patients with chronic obstructive pulmonary disease. *Value Health* 2002; **5**: 436–41.

15. American Thoracic Society. Standards for the diagnosis and care of patients with chronic obstructive pulmonary disease. *Am J Respir Crit Care Med* 1995; **152**: s1–s121.

16. Siafakas NM, Vermeire P, Pride NB *et al.* Optimal assessment and management of chronic obstructive pulmonary disease (COPD). The European Respiratory Society Task Force. *Eur Respir J* 1995; **8**: 1398–420.

17. The COPD Guidelines Group of the Standards of Care Committee of the BTS. BTS guidelines for the management of chronic obstructive pulmonary disease. *Thorax* 1997; **52**: s1–28.

18. Pauwels RA, Buist AS, Calverley PM et al. Global strategy for the diagnosis, management, and prevention of chronic obstructive pulmonary disease. NHLBI/WHO Global Initiative for Chronic Obstructive Lung Disease (GOLD) Workshop summary. *Am J Respir Crit Care Med* 2001; **163**: 1256–76.

19. European Agency for the Evaluation of Medicinal Products. Committee for Proprietary Medicinal Products (CPMP). Efficacy Working Party (EWP). Points to consider on clinical investigation of medicinal products in the chronic treatment of patients with chronic obstructive pulmonary disease (COPD). CPMP/EWP/562/98 ed. Luxembourg: Office for Official Publications of the European Communities, 1999.

20. Nocturnal Oxygen Therapy Trial Group. Continuous or nocturnal oxygen therapy in hypoxemic chronic obstructive lung disease. *Ann Intern Med* 1980; **93**: 391–8.

21. Intermittent Positive Pressure Trial Group. Intermittent positive pressure breathing therapy of chronic obstructive pulmonary disease. *Ann Int Med* 1983; **99**: 612–20.

●22. Okubadejo AA, Jones PW, Wedzicha JA. Quality of life in patients with chronic obstructive pulmonary disease and severe hypoxaemia. *Thorax* 1996; **51**: 44–7.

23. Okubadejo AA, Paul EA, Jones PW, Wedzicha JA. Does long-term oxygen therapy affect quality of life in patients with chronic obstructive pulmonary disease and severe hypoxaemia? *Eur Respir J* 1996; **9**: 2335–9.

24. Spencer S, Calverley PMA, Burge PS, Jones PW. Health status deterioration in patients with chronic obstructive pulmonary disease. *Am J Respir Crit Care Med* 2001; **163**: 122–8.

25. Crockett AJ, Cranston JM, Moss JR, Alpers JH. The MOS SF-36 health survey questionnaire in severe chronic airflow limitation: comparison with the Nottingham Health Profile. *Qual Life Res* 1996; **5**: 330–8.

26. Meecham Jones DJ, Paul EA, Jones PW, Wedzicha JA. Nasal pressure support ventilation plus oxygen compared with oxygen therapy alone in hypercapnic COPD. *Am J Respir Crit Care Med* 1995; **152**: 538–44.

27. Perrin C, El Far Y, Vandenbos F *et al.* Domiciliary nasal intermittent positive pressure ventilation in severe COPD. Effects on lung function and quality of life. *Eur Respir J* 1997; **10**: 2835–9.

●28. Clini E, Sturani C, Rossi A *et al.* The Italian multicentre study on noninvasive ventilation in chronic obstructive pulmonary disease patients. *Eur Respir J* 2002; **20**: 529–38.

29. Lacasse Y, Wong E, Guyatt GH *et al.* Meta-analysis of respiratory rehabilitation in chronic obstructive pulmonary disease. *Lancet* 1996; **348**: 1115–19.

30. Wijkstra PJ, Tenvergert EM, Van Altena R *et al.* Reliability and validity of the chronic respiratory questionnaire (CRQ). *Thorax* 1994; **49**: 465–7.

31. Guell R, Casan P, Belda J *et al.* Long-term effects of outpatient rehabilitation of COPD. A randomized trial. *Chest* 2000; **117**: 976–83.

32. Finnerty JP, Keeping I, Bullough I, Jones J. The effectiveness of outpatient pulmonary rehabilitation in chronic lung disease: a randomized controlled trial. *Chest* 2001; **119**: 1705–10.

●33. Griffiths TL, Burr ML, Campbell IA *et al.* Results at 1 year of outpatient multidisciplinary pulmonary rehabilitation: a randomised controlled trial. *Lancet* 2000, 2003; **29**: 362–8.

◆34. Lacasse Y, Brosseau L, Milne S *et al.* Pulmonary rehabilitation for chronic obstructive pulmonary disease (Cochrane Review). In: *The Cochrane Library, Issue 4,* Chichester, UK: John Wiley.

35. Dahl R, Greefhorst LAPM, Nowak D *et al.* Inhaled formoterol dry powder versus ipratropium bromide in chronic obstructive pulmonary disease. *Am J Respir Crit Care Med* 2001; **164**: 778–84.

36. Casaburi R, Mahler DA, Jones PW *et al.* A long-term evaluation of once daily inhaled tiotropium in chronic obstructive pulmonary disease. *Eur Respir J* 2002; **19**: 209–16.

37. Szafranski W, Cukier A, Ramirez A *et al.* Efficacy and safety of budesonide/formoterol in the management of chronic obstructive pulmonary disease. *Eur Respir J* 2003; **21**: 74–81.

38. Calverley PMA, Pauwels R, Vestbo J *et al.* Combined salmeterol and fluticasone in the treatment of chronic obstructive pulmonary disease. *Lancet* 2003; **361**: 449.

39. Global Initiative for Chronic Obstructive Lung Disease (GOLD). Global strategy for the diagnosis, management, and prevention of chronic obstructive pulmonary disease. NHLBI/WHO, workshop report. Bethesda, MD: National Heart, Lung, and Blood Institute, 2001.

40. Osman L, Silverman M. Measuring quality of life for young children with asthma and their families. *Eur Respir J Suppl* 1996; **21**: 35s–41s.

41. Seemungal TA, Donaldson GC, Paul EA *et al.* Effect of exacerbation on quality of life in patients with chronic obstructive pulmonary disease. *Am J Respir Crit Care Med* 1998; **157**(5 Part 1): 1418–22.

42. Domingo-Salvany A, Lamarca R, Ferrer M *et al.* Health-related quality of life and mortality in male patients with chronic obstructive pulmonary disease. *Am J Respir Crit Care Med* 2002; **166**: 680–5.

43. Oga T, Nishimura K, Tsukino M, Sato S, Hajiro T. Analysis of the factors related to mortality in chronic obstructive pulmonary disease: role of exercise capacity and health status. *Am J Respir Crit Care Med* 2003; **167**: 544–9.

●44. Carone M, Jones PW, on behalf of the QuESS Group. Quality of Life Evaluation and Survival Study: a 3-year prospective multinational study on patients with chronic respiratory failure. *Monaldi Arch Chest Dis* 2001; **56**: 17–22.

45. Carone M, Bertolotti G, Donner CF, Jones PW, on behalf of the QuESS Group. Mortality in chronic respiratory failure is detected better by health status (QoL) than by functional parameters. *Am J Respir Crit Care Med* 2001; **163**: A13.

46. Barley EA, Quirk FH, Jones PW. Asthma health status measurement in clinical practice: validity of a new short and simple instrument. *Respir Med* 1998; **92**: 1207–14.

47. Weaver TE, Narsavage GL, Guilfoyle MJ. The development and psychometric evaluation of the Pulmonary Functional Status Scale: an instrument to assess functional status in pulmonary disease. *J Cardiopulm Rehab* 1998; **18**: 105–11.

16

Evaluation of impairment and disability and outcome measures for rehabilitation

HOLGER J. SCHÜNEMANN, RICHARD ZUWALLACK

INTRODUCTION

Assessment of patients' impairment, disability and handicap has become a focus of investigation, specifically in the evaluation of effects of pulmonary rehabilitation. The World Health Organization (WHO) defined impairment as 'abnormalities of body structure, appearance, organ or system function resulting from any cause'; disability as a 'restriction or lack of ability to perform an activity in a manner or within the range considered normal for a human being'; and handicap as a 'disadvantage for a given individual resulting from an impairment or a disability, that limits or prevents fulfilment of a role that is normal for that individual' (1). The WHO has recently moved away from these definitions in its International Classification of Functioning Disability and Health (ICF) (2).

The WHO classification developed from being 'consequences of disease' (1) to emphasizing the 'components of health' (2). It now utilizes the terms (i) body functions and structures, and (ii) activities and participation. Thus, the focus has shifted to what a person with a disease or disorder does do or can do. Functioning encompasses all body functions, activities and participation. Disability now serves as an umbrella term for impairments, activity limitations or participation restrictions. These terms, which replace the formerly used terms 'impairment', 'disability' and 'handicap', allow the description and evaluation of positive experiences. In that sense, the new WHO classification merges with the aim of pulmonary rehabilitation, which is to provide positive experience and yield (at least temporary) improvement in functioning, activities and participation.

RATIONALE FOR OUTCOME ASSESSMENT IN PULMONARY REHABILITATION

Outcome assessment in pulmonary rehabilitation goes far beyond assessment of physiological variables. Comprehensive pulmonary rehabilitation results in improvements in multiple outcome areas in individuals with chronic respiratory disease (3). These positive results are often of sufficient magnitude to be meaningful to the patient. Outcome assessment in pulmonary rehabilitation is used to quantify these varied beneficial effects.

Outcome assessment can focus on immediate goals, such as being able to walk up a flight of stairs, or long-term goals, such as mastering the social consequences of respiratory disease, including the mastery of respiratory symptoms such as coughing or shortness of breath.

Since pulmonary rehabilitation represents the collaboration of efforts of the patient and a multidisciplinary team of professionals in the setting of a health care system, outcome assessment can have differing perspectives and goals. Thus, for a patient, the perceived needs and achievement of success in meeting those needs might differ from those of the pulmonary rehabilitation staff or third party payers. Although there are a number of outcomes that can be measured, there is little doubt that quantifying the benefits of rehabilitation is important for patients, clinicians and third party payers. However, as with any health care intervention, benefits have to be balanced against the adverse effects, burden and cost of the intervention. Therefore, the downsides of pulmonary rehabilitation should be considered in deciding to participate in a pulmonary rehabilitation programme (patient perspective), maintain or start a pulmonary rehabilitation programme (clinician perspective) and reimburse for a rehabilitation programme (society's and payer's perspective). Balancing downsides against benefits from each of these perspectives is a challenging task and in the early stages of evaluation. Box 16.1 presents the rationale for assessing outcomes in pulmonary rehabilitation.

Patient perspective

Patients increasingly want to become involved in medical decision-making (4). Active patient involvement in the process of health care delivery may improve outcomes such as quality of life and, possibly, reduce health care expenditures (5). Defined outcomes can help patients to set goals for their rehabilitation programme. Monitoring progress or disease impact can provide patients with feedback on specific gains from rehabilitation. Care providers may have different views and expectations of patients. Setting goals and monitoring progress can help to communicate these goals and expectations.

In order to help people make specific and deliberative choices among options, investigators and clinicians have developed decision aids for a variety of chronic diseases (6). These aids provide (at a minimum) information on the alternatives, benefits and downsides pertaining to the patients' clinical condition. No decision aids exist that help patients make decisions regarding whether they should participate in pulmonary rehabilitation. Another reason to involve patients in the assessment of outcomes is that patients and clinicians differ in their evaluation of the magnitude of the effects of the intervention on functioning and disability. In a study of patients undergoing pulmonary rehabilitation, there was little agreement between physicians and patients on whether rehabilitation was beneficial, and, in addition, physicians systematically overestimated the impact of rehabilitation on the patients' health-related quality of life (HRQL) (7).

Pulmonary rehabilitation programme perspective

From the clinicians' perspective, assessment of outcomes is important to satisfy their desire to provide care and to maintain quality improvement programmes (Box 16.1). Systematic outcome assessment provides ongoing information on the effectiveness of the various components of the rehabilitation programme which may be used for the purposes of continuous quality improvement. Documentation of the overall success of the intervention increases staff morale. Since patients beginning pulmonary rehabilitation differ widely in their response to treatment, measuring their response will help identify those who require more intensive interventions. Because objective measures of lung function, such as the forced expiratory volume in 1 s (FEV_1), do not change with pulmonary rehabilitation, they cannot be used as surrogate markers for improvements in dyspnoea or heath status. Finally, from a programme perspective, outcome assessment may facilitate evaluation of the rehabilitation team.

Box 16.1   The rationale for outcome assessment in pulmonary rehabilitation: differing perspectives

Patient perspective

- May help with patient goal-setting and decision-making.
- Direct positive feedback to the patient on specific gains made during the rehabilitation intervention may increase morale, improve motivation and enhance adherence to the pulmonary rehabilitation process.
- May help to compare treatment effects patients experience with those of providers.

Pulmonary rehabilitation programme perspective

- Evaluation of outcomes in several areas provides ongoing information to personnel on the effectiveness of the various components of the pulmonary rehabilitation programme that may be used for continuous quality improvement purposes.
- Documentation of the overall success of the intervention in outcome areas serves to increase staff morale.
- Patients beginning pulmonary rehabilitation differ widely in their response to rehabilitation.
- Objective measures of lung function, such as the FEV_1, do not change with pulmonary rehabilitation and therefore cannot be used as surrogate markers for improvement in areas of importance to the patient, such as relief of dyspnoea or improvement in heath status.
- Comparison of different interventions and effectiveness (performance) of rehabilitation staff.

Third party payer perspective

- Objective assessment of health care utilization outcomes provides information on the cost effectiveness of pulmonary rehabilitation.
- Assessment of pre- to post-rehabilitation outcomes of importance to the patient can provide useful information on the success of the individual pulmonary rehabilitation programme.
- National and international comparison of rehabilitation programmes.
- Incentives for rehabilitation programmes.

Third party payer perspective

For third party payers and society as a whole, costs drive resource allocation. Standardized outcome measures that permit economic evaluation are indispensable in making economic comparisons between alternative health care interventions. Third party payers are interested in comparing rehabilitation programmes on a national and international level. Finally, in

---

Box 16.2   Outcome areas for pulmonary rehabilitation

- Symptoms
- Exercise ability
- Respiratory muscle strength
- Functional status
- Nutritional status
- The individual patient's knowledge of the disease and its treatment
- Psychological status
- Health care utilization
- Survival
- Health-related quality of life (HRQL)

---

an incentive-driven market, outcome assessment can become a basis for providing incentives to rehabilitation programmes.

TYPES OF OUTCOME

A patient with severe chronic obstructive pulmonary disease (COPD) is usually limited by exertional dyspnoea (impairment and activity limitation) attributable to the underlying lung disease. Peripheral muscle dysfunction (associated morbidity with impact on body structure) may aggravate the sensation of dyspnoea. Coexisting cardiac disease (co-morbidity) may also play a role in the patient's breathlessness. Pulmonary rehabilitation attempts to reduce the impact of the disease on disability and thereby improve functioning.

Since many factors influence the health of individuals with chronic lung disease, multiple outcomes can be used to assess the effectiveness of pulmonary rehabilitation. Potential outcomes for pulmonary rehabilitation are listed in Box 16.2. There is no widely accepted definition of quality of life so that we use the term health-related quality of life (HRQL) as it excludes widely valued aspects of quality of life such as income, freedom and the environment (8).

Investigators and clinicians often use health status, functional status and quality of life interchangeably to describe the same domain of health. These terms include physical functioning assessment (ability to carry out activities of daily living such as walking around), psychological functioning (emotional well-being) and social functioning (relationships with others and participation in social activities), and overall satisfaction with life (9).

In this chapter we will discuss the effects of pulmonary rehabilitation on key outcomes.

Design of outcome analyses in pulmonary rehabilitation

Several pulmonary rehabilitation outcome assessments have used parallel group designs, with randomization of patients to

rehabilitation treatment or control groups. Since withholding rehabilitation from control subjects is no longer an option, pre- to post-rehabilitation changes in selected outcome areas are sufficient to document programme effectiveness and individual patient responses. An alternative is to compare a new intervention with an established one, using as controls the group receiving 'usual care'.

Rehabilitation patients cannot be blinded to their treatment. Moreover, effort-dependent outcomes such as timed walks can be influenced by subject motivation (10). Subjective assessments of health status can be biased by the patient's 'need to please' bias. However, in a recent randomized controlled trial comparing the effects of informing patients about their pre-treatment responses to two commonly used HRQL questionnaires, the Chronic Respiratory Questionnaire (CRQ) and the St George's Respiratory Questionnaire (SGRQ), there were no systematic between-group differences in HRQL changes after 2 months of pulmonary rehabilitation, i.e. informed patients did not report greater improvement (11).

The demonstration of rehabilitation resulting in a statistically significant improvement raises the issue of the thresholds representing a minimal important difference (MID) to the patient. The need for assessing the MID is discussed later in this chapter.

Assessment post-rehabilitation should follow a period of living in the community to enable patients to experience the effects of rehabilitation in their usual environment. Although it is easier to measure outcomes before and shortly after rehabilitation, documentation of longer-term benefit is essential as many of the benefits diminish with time (12–14). Monitoring longer-term outcomes will allow for innovations in rehabilitation designed to counter this diminution of benefit.

DYSPNOEA

Dyspnoea is the 'subjective experience of breathing discomfort that consists of qualitatively distinct sensations that vary in intensity'. (15) Dyspnoea is the predominant symptom in COPD and has the most important influence on HRQL (16, 17). Although dyspnoea is broadly related to airways obstruction, psychological, social and environmental factors influence this sensation (15). Box 16.3 lists several dyspnoea measures that are commonly used in outcome assessment for pulmonary rehabilitation.

Exertional dyspnoea

Dyspnoea during exercise testing is usually measured using a Borg Category Scale (18) or a visual analogue scale (VAS). Assessment of dyspnoea is further discussed in detail in Chapter 14.

Examples of pulmonary rehabilitation studies that report a reduction in exertional dyspnoea are summarized in Table 16.1 (13, 19, 20, 21).

Dyspnoea during daily activities

Dyspnoea can be measured using a category scale, such as the modified Medical Research Council (MRC) dyspnoea scale. The Baseline and Transitional Dyspnoea Indexes (BDI and TDI) (22), the University of California, San Diego Shortness of Breath Questionnaire (SOBQ) (23) and the dyspnoea domain of the CRQ (24, 25) are also commonly used to rate dyspnoea associated with daily activities. The BDI rates dyspnoea in three areas – functional impairment, magnitude of task and magnitude of effort – with each score ranging from 4 (no

impairment) to 0 (severe). The focal score, which sums the three areas, ranges from zero (most dyspnoea) to 12 (no dyspnoea). The TDI rates change over time in each of the above three areas. The BDI focal score correlates well with other measures of dyspnoea, while the TDI has proven very responsive to therapeutic intervention (21).

The SOBQ is a 24-item self-complete questionnaire that measures breathlessness during a variety of activities of daily living. Dyspnoea with each activity is rated on a six-point scale, from 0 (not at all) to 5 (maximal, or unable to do because of breathlessness). The 24 responses are summed to give a total score, which can range from 0 to 120. The usefulness of this questionnaire as an outcome measure was demonstrated by the controlled trial of pulmonary rehabilitation by Ries et al. (13). Comprehensive outpatient pulmonary rehabilitation led to a 7-unit decrease in dyspnoea shortly following its completion, equivalent to nearly a 20 per cent improvement over baseline.

The CRQ (24, 25) is a 20-item questionnaire that measures HRQL in patients with chronic airflow limitation. One of its four domains, the dyspnoea domain, has five items on which respondents rate the level of breathlessness on a seven-point scale ranging from 1 (maximum impairment) to 7 (no impairment). The version including the original individualized dyspnoea domain lets patients choose five activities that are most important to them in their daily lives. Patients then rate the degree of dyspnoea on these self-selected activities during subsequent administrations of the CRQ. A new standardized version includes standardized dyspnoea questions

---

Box 16.3 Some instruments for rating dyspnoea

Exertional dyspnoea

- The Borg category scale (1–10)
- The linear visual analogue scale

Dyspnoea with daily activities

- The Medical Research Council (MRC) questionnaire
- The Baseline and Transitional Dyspnoea Indexes (BDI and TDI)
- The University of California, San Diego, Shortness of Breath Questionnaire (SOBQ)
- The dyspnoea domain of the Chronic Respiratory Questionnaire (CRQ)

Table 16.1 *Pulmonary rehabilitation and exertional dyspnoea*

Reference	Total number	Active intervention(s)	Dyspnoea measure	Outcome
Reardon *et al.* (21)	20	6 weeks OPR vs. standard rx	200 mm VAS; incremental ET	Dyspnoea at peak exercise improved significantly post-OPR, from 74 to 51% of VAS line length; this effect became apparent by the second minute of exercise testing
Ries *et al.* (13)	119	8 weeks OPR	10-unit category scale; submaximal ET	Perceived breathlessness during submaximal ET decreased; this effect persisted for 24 months
O'Donnell *et al.* (19)	20	6 weeks endurance exercise training	10-unit category scale; incremental and submaximal ET	Reduction in exertional dyspnoea (Borg-time and Borg-$\dot{V}o_{2n}$ slopes) during incremental exercise testing and dyspnoea at isotime during endurance testing. Dyspnoea relief correlated with a reduction in breathing of frequency post-exercise training
Normandin *et al.* (20)	40	High-intensity training vs. classroom calisthenics	200 mm VAS at 50% and 80% of peak $\dot{V}o_2$ during incremental ET	Higher-intensity training on the treadmill and cycle ergometer led to significant reductions in exertional dyspnoea compared with lower-intensity classroom calisthenics training

ET, exercise test; OPR, outpatient pulmonary rehabilitation; VAS, visual analogue scale.

that ask patients to rate their dyspnoea on the same five activities (26):

- feeling emotional such as angry or upset
- taking care of your basic needs (bathing, showering, eating or dressing)
- walking
- performing chores (such as housework, shopping, groceries)
- participating in social activities.

The individualized version of the dyspnoea domain shows slightly greater responsiveness to therapy, but reduces comparability between patients and across settings. The CRQ is now available as a self-administered standardized instrument (27). Table 16.2 summarizes several studies showing the effect of comprehensive pulmonary rehabilitation on dyspnoea (13, 14, 19, 21, 28, 29).

EXERCISE

Exercise training is a necessary component of pulmonary rehabilitation, and improvement in exercise performance is an important and frequently measured outcome of this therapy. Exercise tests can vary from simple to complex. For the purposes of this chapter, commonly used exercise tests have been categorized into laboratory tests, which include incremental cardiopulmonary exercise testing and constant-workload endurance testing, and field tests, which include the timed-walk test and the shuttle-walk test.

Incremental exercise tests in pulmonary rehabilitation

Cardiopulmonary exercise testing on a stationary cycle ergometer or treadmill, with gradual increases in work rate to a peak effort, is the 'gold standard' of exercise performance evaluation. Exercise is terminated when the patient's heart rate approaches the predicted maximum or, more commonly in patients with advanced lung disease, when severe breathlessness or leg fatigue limits further exertion. Physiological variables are measured at regular intervals during testing, including blood pressure, heart rate, respiratory rate, electrocardiogram and oxygen saturation. Breath-by-breath analysis of expired gas permits the determination of important physiological variables such as tidal volume and minute ventilation, oxygen consumption, carbon dioxide production, respiratory ratio, anaerobic threshold and oxygen pulse.

Incremental exercise testing to maximal tolerance allows for the determination of not only work rate and oxygen consumption ($\dot{V}O_2$) at peak work rate, but also normal and abnormal physiological changes occurring up to this maximum. Useful information is often provided on mechanisms for exercise limitation, the presence of co-morbidity (especially cardiac disease), and whether a true physiological training effect took place following exercise training. This testing requires relatively expensive equipment and trained personnel;

Table 16.2 *Pulmonary rehabilitation and dyspnoea during daily activities*

Reference	Total number	Active intervention(s)	Dyspnoea measure	Outcome
Goldstein et al. (28)	89	8 weeks OPR, then 16 weeks supervision	CRQ dyspnoea, BDI/TDI	Significant improvement in both dyspnoea measures. CRQ dyspnoea improvement >MCID, the TDI increase was +2.7 units
Reardon et al. (21)	20	6 weeks OPR	BDI/TDI	The TDI focal score of the treatment group was +2.3 units, which was significantly greater than the +0.2 increase in the control
Ries et al. (13)	119	8 weeks OPR	UCSD SOBQ	Significant improvement in the SOBQ; effect lasted 6 months
O'Donnell et al. (19)		6 weeks endurance training	BDI/TDI, OCD	The TDI focal score increased by +3.2 units following exercise training and the OCD increased by approximately 7 mm
Güell et al. (29)	60	6 months OPR plus EM	10 cm VAS[a], MRC CRQ dyspnoea	Dyspnoea improved in all three measures in the treatment group
Griffiths et al. (14)	200	6 weeks OPR	CRQ dyspnoea	Significant improvement in CRQ dyspnoea at 8 weeks and 1 year. Treatment effect >MCID at 8 weeks

[a] Stratified by MRC dyspnoea level (MRC 3/4 (*n* = 66) treated in a facility; MRC 5 (*n* = 60) treated at home).
BDI/TDI, Baseline and Transitional Dyspnoea Indexes; CRQ, Chronic Respiratory Disease Questionnaire; EM, exercise maintenance; ET, exercise test; MCID, minimal clinically important difference; MRC, Medical Research Council dyspnoea scale; OCD, Oxygen Cost Diagram; OPR, outpatient pulmonary rehabilitation; UCSD SOBQ, University of California San Diego Shortness of Breath Questionnaire; VAS, visual analogue scale (rating dyspnoea associated with daily activities).

Table 16.3 *Pulmonary rehabilitation and maximal exercise capacity*

Reference	Total number	Active intervention(s)	Exercise test	Outcome
Casaburi *et al.* (75)	19	8 weeks exercise training programme; high vs. moderate intensity	Incremental cycle ergometry	Exercise led to a physiological training effect which was enhanced with higher intensity training
Ries *et al.* (13)	119	8 weeks OPR vs. education only	Incremental treadmill walking exercise	Maximal oxygen consumption increased by 0.11 L/min after OPR. However, there was no treatment-control difference in this variable at 1 year
Clark *et al.* (76)	48	Low-intensity peripheral muscle training vs. control	Incremental cycle ergometry	No significant difference between treatment and control in maximal exercise capacity variables
Wijkstra *et al.* (77)	43	12 weeks home-based pulmonary rehabilitation vs. control	Incremental cycle ergometry	Peak work rate increased by 8 watts and maximal oxygen consumption by 0.1 L/min over baseline in the rehabilitation group. The change in maximal oxygen consumption was greater than control
Maltais *et al.* (78)	42	12 weeks of high-intensity exercise training; comparison to baseline	Incremental cycle ergometry	An 11% increase in peak $\dot{V}O_2$, and a 16% increase in peak work rate, accompanied by a 6% decrease in minute ventilation and a 17% decrease in lactate concentration
Bernard *et al.* (79)	45	12 weeks: aerobic training vs. aerobic + strength training	Incremental cycle ergometry	No significant change in peak oxygen consumption, $\dot{V}_E$, or lactate levels. At isotime during testing, significant reductions were observed in $\dot{V}_e$, heart rate, and lactate production in both groups
Coppoolse *et al.* (80)	21	8 weeks: interval vs. continuous exercise training	Incremental cycle ergometry	Continuous training resulted in a 17% increase in peak oxygen consumption, and decreased $\dot{V}_E/\dot{V}O_2$ and $\dot{V}_E/\dot{V}CO_2$ at peak exercise. No changes in these measures were observed following interval training
Spruit *et al.* (81)	48	Resistance vs. endurance training	Incremental cycle ergometry	Peak work rate increased by 15 watts following resistance training and 14 watts following endurance training; only endurance training resulted in increased oxygen consumption: +89 mL/min

OPR, outpatient pulmonary rehabilitation; $\dot{V}_E$, minute ventilation; $\dot{V}CO_2$, carbon dioxide production; $\dot{V}O_2$, oxygen consumption.

therefore it is not available to many pulmonary rehabilitation centres.

Pulmonary rehabilitation has been demonstrated to result in significant improvement in maximal exercise capacity, either in the form of increased work rate, such as peak watts, or as increased peak $\dot{V}O_2$. However, in general, the degree of improvement in maximal exercise capacity has been lower than that of submaximal endurance testing or field tests of exercise ability. Casaburi *et al.* (75) compared high-intensity and moderate-intensity exercise training in patients with COPD. Although the authors maintained the total amount of work at equal levels in the two groups, the patients who completed the programme involving higher levels of training had lower lactate production and lower minute ventilation at equal work rates and were therefore able to achieve a physiological training effect. Examples of studies reporting incremental testing in pulmonary rehabilitation are given in Table 16.3.

Submaximal endurance exercise in pulmonary rehabilitation

Stationary cycle or treadmill exercise testing at a constant work rate, such as at 80 per cent of maximal, is a common measure

Table 16.4   *Pulmonary rehabilitation and endurance exercise*

Reference	Total number	Active intervention(s)	Exercise test	Outcome
Goldstein *et al.* (18)	89	8 weeks OPR, then 16 weeks supervision vs. control	Submaximal cycle time at 60% of maximum	Highly significant increase in submaximal cycle time (4.7 min[a]) in the treatment group
Ries *et al.* (13)	119	8 weeks OPR vs. education only	Treadmill endurance	Significant improvement in treadmill endurance time
Clark *et al.* (76)	48	Low-intensity peripheral muscle training vs. control	Endurance walk test on a treadmill at a speed 1.5–3.5 km/h	The treatment group that did low-intensity exercise had a highly significant increase in endurance work (J) compared with control group
O'Donnell *et al.* (19)	20	6 weeks multimodality endurance training	Cycle ergometry and treadmill, at 75% of maximal work rate; arm ergometry at 60 rpm	Significant improvements in endurance time in all those outcome areas
Coppoolse *et al.* (80)	21	8 weeks: interval vs. continuous exercise training	Cycle ergometry at 90% of maximal work rate	Lactate production at submaximal work rates was decreased in both groups following exercise training, indicating a physiological training effect. Leg discomfort was less after interval training
Normandin *et al.* (20)	40	High-intensity training vs. classroom calisthenics	Treadmill endurance at 85% of maximal workrate	Treadmill endurance time increased significantly only in the high-intensity training group: +8.4 min. Endurance time was significantly greater than that of the low-intensity group

[a] Treatment effect.

Derby Hospitals NHS Foundation Trust
Library and Knowledge Service

of exercise endurance for pulmonary rehabilitation. Usually, duration of exercise at this work rate is measured. Physiological variables, pulmonary function tests such as inspiratory capacity, and exertional dyspnoea can also be measured.

Submaximal endurance testing is very responsive to pulmonary rehabilitation, probably reflecting its emphasis on lower extremity training. It is not unusual to observe increases in endurance time of greater than 50 per cent following exercise-training programmes. Physiological measurements before and after the intervention at isotime or at constant work rate allow for the evaluation of cardiopulmonary responses to that intervention. Examples of endurance testing studies of pulmonary rehabilitation or exercise training are given in Table 16.4.

Field tests of exercise ability

The timed-walk test is undoubtedly the most frequently used outcome measure of exercise ability in pulmonary rehabilitation. For this test of functional exercise capacity, the patient must walk as far as possible in a hallway, corridor, large room or auditorium during the allotted period of time. Self-pacing is required, and patients are allowed to stop and rest as often as necessary, although additional time is not allotted for rests. Although the 12-min walk test was more common in earlier pulmonary rehabilitation assessments (30), the 6-min test has become the standard in the past few years.

The popularity of this outcome measure probably stems from its ease of administration, its relevance to daily activities, and its responsiveness to the pulmonary rehabilitation intervention. The walk test is simple to perform, requires no extra equipment, and is usually well tolerated. The intensity, duration and type of exercise required for the timed-walk test are similar to those required for many activities of daily living, making this a reasonable test of functional ability (31). This is reflected by a strong correlation between the walk distance and questionnaire-measured functional performance (32). The 6-min walk distance appears to be a separate construct from dyspnoea measures and health status measures, thereby making it desirable as an outcome measure for pulmonary rehabilitation. In patients completing pulmonary rehabilitation, this measure of functional exercise ability was even found to be a stronger predictor of survival than the FEV_1 (33).

Potential drawbacks of the timed-walk test are its intrinsic variability, a not insignificant learning effect from successive walk tests, and the potential effects of encouragement and motivation on performance. In a recent study of successive 12-min walk tests (34), a 7 per cent improvement was seen between walk one and two, a 4 per cent improvement between walk two and three, but only a 2 per cent improvement between walk three and four. Because of this, it is advisable to perform one or more practice walk tests initially before the actual measurement. Rests of at least 15 min between tests are necessary. Simple encouragement of the effort-dependent 6-min walk test can increase the distance by approximately 30 m, which is similar in magnitude to the effect of pulmonary rehabilitation in some trials (35). Even the awareness of walk test duration can affect performance, since walk distance in a 6-min walk test is longer than that in the first half of a 12-min walk test. Despite these potentially confounding influences, the timed-walk test has been poorly standardized among pulmonary rehabilitation programmes (36). Therefore, strict standardization of walk test administration should be a requirement, and guidelines for its administration have become available to this purpose (37).

Performance on the 6- and 12-min walk tests correlate reasonably well with each other (38), although their comparability as an outcome measure for pulmonary rehabilitation has received relatively little attention. Since performing two or three 6-min walks in succession is simpler than doing 12-min walks, the shorter test has risen to the top of the list of field tests of functional exercise capacity.

As mentioned above, a major reason for the popularity of the timed-walk test is its remarkable responsiveness to the pulmonary rehabilitation intervention. This probably reflects the emphasis on lower extremity training and pacing instructions in pulmonary rehabilitation. High levels of functional impairment do not preclude a successful outcome in walk distance following pulmonary rehabilitation, providing the patient can participate in the exercise training (39, 40). The estimated threshold of clinical importance for changes in the 6-min walk distance (the minimal clinically important difference) is 54 m (41).

A listing of results from selected published series is given in Table 16.5.

The incremental and endurance shuttle–walk tests

The 10 m shuttle-walk test developed by Singh *et al.* (42) is an externally paced incremental measure of exercise capacity for COPD. It entails walking up and down a 10 m course in a corridor at gradually increasing speeds. Marker cones are placed 0.5 m from either end for ease in turning. Instructions are given to walk at a steady pace with a goal of reaching the opposite marker cone at the next beeping signal from the cassette player. The initial speed (set by the interval between beeps) is 0.5 m/s, but this is increased after every minute by shortening the time between successive beeps. The test endpoint is determined when the patient becomes too breathless to keep up with the pace and is unable to complete the shuttle in the time allowed. The total distance walked is calculated and recorded as the result.

This field test of exercise ability differs considerably from the 6-min walk test. First, it involves incrementally increased work and therefore is more closely a measure of exercise capacity. Second, the pace is set by the external signal, not the patient. The shuttle test is reproducible (43) and, not unexpectedly, correlates well with peak oxygen consumption measured during cardiopulmonary testing on a treadmill (44). An

estimate of a threshold for a clinically meaningful change in this exercise test is not available.

A newer variation of the shuttle-walk test is the endurance shuttle-walk test. Pulmonary rehabilitation leads to significant increases in the shuttle-walk distance. A listing of results from selected published series is given in Table 16.5.

HEALTH–RELATED QUALITY OF LIFE INSTRUMENTS

Generic instruments

There are two types of HRQL instrument: generic and disease-specific. Generic instruments are broad (Fig. 16.1) and can be used to assess HRQL across a wide area of diseases and populations.

HEALTH PROFILES

Among the generic HRQL instruments we distinguish health profiles and preference (utility) instruments. An example of a generic HRQL instrument used in pulmonary rehabilitation is the Medical Outcomes Short-Form 36 (SF-36) (45). The SF-36 has demonstrated validity (i.e. it measures what it is intended to measure) and responsiveness (i.e. it is able to detect true changes in HRQL over time) in patients undergoing respiratory rehabilitation (46). Another health profile is the Sickness Impact Profile (SIP) (47). The SIP includes a physical domain (ambulation, mobility and body care and movement), a psychosocial domain (social interaction, alertness behaviour, communication and emotional behaviour) and five additional independent categories (eating, work, home management, sleep and rest, and recreations). The SIP has been used in several studies assessing HRQL in pulmonary rehabilitation, but has not consistently been shown to be responsive to changes in HRQL (11, 46). Health profiles allow for comparisons of the relative impact of various health care programmes. For example, one could compare the impact on HRQL of pulmonary rehabilitation with that of cardiac rehabilitation programmes.

PREFERENCE INSTRUMENTS

Another class of generic HRQL instruments are preference-based instruments. There are two approaches to measuring preferences. One is to use a multi-attribute utility measure in which patients describe their health state, and the preference for that health state is calculated using a published formula representing preferences of the general population (48). The Euroquol (49), Quality of Well-Being Index (50), and the Health Utilities Index (HUI) (51) are examples of this approach. These instruments have been used in respiratory rehabilitation (11, 46, 52, 53); the HUI and the rating scale of the EQ-5D have demonstrated responsiveness (26, 53). However, the limitation of these instruments lies in their low responsiveness. Health profiles and multi-attribute utility tools may

Table 16.5 *Pulmonary rehabilitation and field tests of exercise ability*

Reference	Total number	Active intervention(s)	Exercise test	Outcome
Goldstein *et al.* (28)	89	8 weeks OPR, then 16 weeks supervision vs. control	6-min walk distance	Walk distance increased by 37.9 m (treatment effect). This was statistically significant, although somewhat less than the suggested MCID of 54 m
Wijkstra *et al.* (77)	43	12 weeks home-based pulmonary rehabilitation vs. control	6-min walk distance	At 12 weeks, the 6-min walk distance in the rehabilitation group increased from 438 to 447 m. This was statistically significant, although far less than the suggested MCID of 54 m
Wedzicha *et al.* (82)	126	OPR or home-based rehabilitation vs. control	Incremental shuttle-walk test	In the group given OPR, the shuttle-walk distance increased significantly, by 191 m. Home-based rehabilitation did not lead to improvement in exercise performance
Bernard *et al.* (79)	45	12 weeks: aerobic training vs. aerobic + strength training	6-min walk distance	A 66 m increase in the 6-min walk distance in the aerobic-only group and an 88 m increase in the combined aerobic-strength group. These both surpassed of the MCID
Berry *et al.* (83)	151	12 weeks: upper and lower extremity training, stratification by disease severity	6-min walk distance	Significant increases in the 6-min walk distances in patients of mild or moderate severity (61 and 73 m, respectively, which surpass the MCID). No significant improvement in the severe group
Griffiths *et al.* (14)	200	6 weeks multidisciplinary OPR vs. control	Incremental shuttle-walk test	The shuttle-walk distance increased by 75.9 m following OPR, and by 28.1 m at 1 year following the intervention (treatment effects)
Hernandez *et al.* (84)	37	12 weeks of home-based pulmonary rehabilitation vs. control	Incremental and endurance shuttle-walk test (70% of max. speed over 20 m course)	No significant improvement in the incremental shuttle-walk distance; significant increase in submaximal walk test distance, from 1247 to 2650 m
Green *et al.* (85)	44	7 weeks vs. 4 weeks OPR	Incremental shuttle-walk test	There was a trend for greater increase in the shuttle-walk distance in group given 7 weeks' rehabilitation
Spruit *et al.* (81)	48	Resistance vs. endurance training	6-min walk distance	Both resistance training and endurance training led to significant increase in 6-min walk distance: 38 and 41% improvements over baseline, respectively

MCID, minimal clinically important difference; OPR, outpatient pulmonary rehabilitation.

detect changes in domains that disease-specific instruments do not include. Similar to other generic tools, they allow comparison across diseases.

An alternative approach to measuring utilities is the use of direct preference measures (54–56). Using this approach, patients place a value or utility score on their current health state, typically on a 0–1.0 scale, where 0 equals dead and 1.0 is full health. Direct preference measures include the standard gamble (SG), time-trade off (TTO) and the feeling thermometer (FT) (54). Patients completing the SG choose between two options, continuing in their current health state or a gamble. Typically, choosing the gamble results in a probability p of returning to full health, and a probability of $(1 - p)$ of immediate death. The value of p at which patients are indifferent between continuing in their current health state and the gamble represents their preference for their current health state on a utility scale where dead is 0.0 and full health is 1.0.

The SG meets theoretical criteria for utility measurement best (54), but requires administration by an interviewer. It may be conceptually challenging for the patient, and although

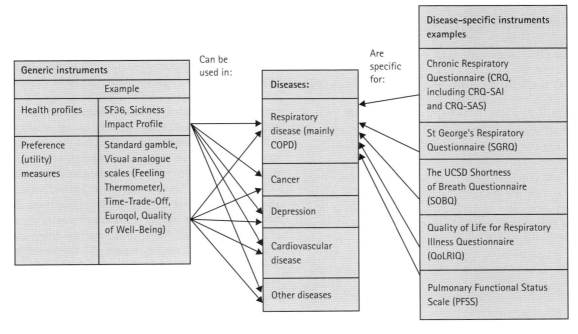

Figure 16.1 *Health-related quality of life (HRQL) instruments*

investigators used the SG in respiratory rehabilitation studies and found that it is valid, it may be unresponsive to small but important changes in HRQL (46, 53). The FT is a visual analogue scale presented in the form of a thermometer. Patients choose the score on the thermometer that represents the value they place on their health state.

The FT is far simpler and has shown surprisingly good responsiveness and validity in respiratory rehabilitation. In a study of 85 patients undergoing respiratory rehabilitation, Schünemann *et al.* (53) found a mean increase of 0.11 (SD = 0.20) from a baseline of 0.57 (0.21) on the scale ranging from 0 to 1.0. Corresponding mean changes on the CRQ in these patients were 1.42 (1.22) on the dyspnoea, 1.13 (1.34) on the fatigue, 0.89 (1.20) on the mastery and 1.12 (1.20) on the emotional function domain. On the SGRQ the mean change scores were 4.2 (14.9) on the symptoms domain, 8.4 (16.3) on the activity domain, 9.0 (12.9) on the impacts domain, and 8.1 (20.4) for the total score. The FT showed slightly greater responsiveness when patients first rated three clinical marker states. The rationale for use of disease-specific marker states in patients with COPD is that patients become oriented to the task and more thoughtful about their rating. The FT administered with and without marker states also showed good cross-sectional and longitudinal construct validity when compared with the CRQ and SGRQ. Thus, there is evidence that simple preference instruments are useful for the evaluation of treatment response to pulmonary rehabilitation.

Preference instruments, in particular the standard gamble, may allow for cost-utility analysis and expression of benefits in terms of quality-adjusted life-years (QALYs). However, as we described above, these instruments may fail to detect important changes in HRQL that patients experience as part of

pulmonary rehabilitation programmes. For use in cost analysis, one would require a preference instrument to fulfil the following four criteria:

- it should be usable in any population (to allow comparison between alternate health interventions
- it should be tied to full health and death (correspond to a 0–1 scale)
- it should be valid
- it should be responsive to change in quality of life.

If the first two are fulfilled, one should choose the instrument that performs best in terms of validity and responsiveness (the third and fourth criteria). The FT fulfils these criteria in respiratory rehabilitation.

Disease-specific instruments

Disease-specific HRQL instruments offer a significant advantage over generic instruments. The two most frequently used instruments to measure HRQL in patients suitable for pulmonary rehabilitation are the CRQ and the SGRQ.

As described above, the CRQ includes 20 questions divided into four domains: dyspnoea (five questions), fatigue (four questions), emotional functioning (seven questions) and mastery (four questions) (26, 27). The results are expressed as the mean score for each domain and the mean overall score. The psychometric properties, including responsiveness, cross-sectional and longitudinal construct validity and interpretability, have been extensively studied (11, 26, 46, 57). The questionnaire takes approximately 8 (self-administered standardized version) to 20 min (interviewer-administered individualized version during the first administration) to complete (27). In addition to application in patients with COPD, investigators have used the CRQ in patients with pulmonary fibrosis and cystic fibrosis (58, 59).

The SGRQ is a self-administered instrument designed to measure the impact of respiratory disease on HRQL and well-being (60). The responses to its 76 items can be aggregated into an overall score and three subscores for the domains symptoms, activity and impact. The number of response options per question varies from two (yes/no responses on the activity and impacts domain) to a Likert-type five-point scale for the symptoms domain. Patients' scores are calculated by weighting each item and dividing the summed weights by the maximum possible weight derived by the developer and expressing the result as a percentage. Zero per cent represents the best possible score and 100 per cent the worst. The self-administered SGRQ is valid, responsive and reliable in patients with COPD, asthma and pulmonary fibrosis (58, 60).

We described the UCSD SOBQ on page 154 (23). This instrument focuses on the assessment of dyspnoea and has three additional questions that ask about fear of harm from over-exertion, limitations and fear caused by shortness of breath. An interesting feature of this instrument is that patients are asked to estimate their shortness of breath on activities that they do not routinely perform. Internal consistency, reliability and validity of the SOBQ have been found to have excellent internal consistency, reliability and moderate-to-strong correlations with measures of exercise tolerance, disease severity, depression and perceived breathlessness ratings following a 6-min walk test (6-MWT).

The Quality-of-Life for Respiratory Illness Questionnaire (QoLRIQ) (61) includes 55 questions across seven domains: breathing problems (nine items); physical problems (nine items); emotions (nine items); situations triggering or enhancing breathing problems (seven items); daily and domestic activities (10 items); social activities, relationships and sexuality (seven items) and general activities (four items). A recent study suggested that the QoLRIQ is responsive to change and valid (62).

The Pulmonary Functional Status Scale (PFSS) (63) is a 53-item questionnaire, that includes the three domains: daily activities/social functioning, psychological functioning and sexual functioning. This instrument has demonstrated content validity and concurrent validity (63, 64). In addition, it showed discriminant validity after pulmonary rehabilitation (65).

The COPD Self-Efficacy Scale (CSES) is a self-reported, COPD-specific measure that contains 34 items describing situations or activities that cause shortness of breath in patients with COPD (66). It contains five domains: negative affect, intense emotional arousal, weather/environment, physical exertion and behavioural risk factors. Respondents rate how confident they are, on a five-point Likert-type scale, that they could manage breathing difficulty or avoid breathing difficulty on each of the 34 items. The measurement properties of this instrument have not been extensively investigated.

MINIMAL IMPORTANT DIFFERENCE OF DIFFERENT OUTCOME MEASURES

Interpreting changes in HRQL remains a challenge for clinicians, patients and investigators. One way of describing and interpreting changes in HRQL is through the MID, the smallest difference in score in the outcome of interest that informed patients or informed proxies perceive as important, either beneficial or harmful, and which would lead the patient or clinician to consider a change in the management. Approaches to establishing the MID include distribution-based methods (statistical methods), reliance on experts (opinion-based methods), and approaches that depend on sequential hypothesis formation and testing (predictive or data-driven) (67). An example of the last approach (also called anchor-based methods) for evaluating the MID relies on examining the associations between scores on the instrument that is under investigation and an anchor, typically an independent measure of HRQL that clinicians can easily interpret.

Among all disease-specific HRQL questionnaires, the CRQ and the SGRQ have been most widely evaluated, in particular using anchor-based approaches. A substantial body of evidence suggests that the MID of the CRQ is approximately 0.5 on the seven-point scale. Changes of 1.0 and 1.5 correspond, respectively, to moderate and large improvement or deterioration (68). Jones et al. (69) suggested score changes of 4, 8 and 12 on the SGRQ for minimal, moderate and large changes. A change of 1 unit on the TDI can be considered important (70), while the MID for the FT ranges from 0.04 to 0.08 (71). Further reports will help clinicians understand how best to interpret changes for outcome measures used to assess patients undergoing rehabilitation (68).

SPECIFIC RECOMMENDATIONS FOR THE INDIVIDUAL PROGRAMME

Outcome assessment is part of pulmonary rehabilitation (72). The individual pulmonary rehabilitation programme must balance the time required for measurement against the value of any particular measure. A good choice will include a few measures that are valid, responsive, interpretable and easy to administer.

The three general areas are exercise ability, dyspnoea and HRQL, with assessments at baseline and at set times subsequent to the intervention. The 6-min walk test, with one or two practice trials, is a valid, responsive, relatively easy to administer test of functional exercise ability. An alternative might be the shuttle-walk test, which is less open to bias by practice or motivation, yet is also responsive to detecting change from the therapeutic intervention. BDI and TDI are easy to administer, are established measures of overall dyspnoea and show good responsiveness to rehabilitation. An alternative might be the modified Medical Research Council dyspnoea questionnaire. The CRQ and SGRQ are both valid and responsive health status instruments for pulmonary rehabilitation, with established thresholds for clinically meaningful change. A few studies indicate that the CRQ is probably more responsive to changes resulting from intervention than the SGRQ (73, 74). The new self-administered standardized CRQ does not require interviewer administration and individualized elicitation of activities. The total time spent in supervising the 6-min walk test, assessing the patient for the BDI/TDI, and scoring the self-administered CRQ would be less than an hour. Information gained from these assessments should make this time spent well worthwhile.

Key points

- Assessment of patients' impairment, disability and handicap has become a focus of clinical investigation.
- Since many factors influence the health of individuals with chronic lung disease, measuring outcomes in several areas may be needed to assess fully the effectiveness of pulmonary rehabilitation.
- Comprehensive pulmonary rehabilitation results in improvements in multiple outcome areas of importance to individuals with chronic respiratory disease.
- The effectiveness of pulmonary rehabilitation can be assessed from several perspectives, including those of the patient, the pulmonary rehabilitation team, and third party payers.
- Common outcome areas in pulmonary rehabilitation include dyspnoea, exercise performance and HRQL.
- Disease-specific measures of HRQL are more responsive to measuring change in HRQL associated with an intervention; the minimal important difference facilitates interpretation of changes in HRQL.

REFERENCES

1. World Health Organization. *International Classification of Impairment, Disabilities and Handicaps.* Geneva: World Health Organization, 1980.
◆2. World Health Organization. *International Classification of Functioning, Disability and Health.* Online. http://www3.who.int/icf/icftemplate.cfm (accessed 15 November 2004).
3. Pulmonary rehabilitation. Joint ACCP/AACVPR evidence-based guidelines. *J Cardiopulm Rehabil* 1997; **17**: 371–405.
4. Guyatt G, Devereaux PJ, Montori V *et al.* Putting the patient first. In our practice, and in our use of language. *ACP J Club,* 2004; **140**: A11.
5. Stewart MA. Effective physician-patient communication and health outcomes: a review. *Can Med Assoc J* 1995; **152**: 1423–33.
6. O'Connor AM, Legare F, Stacey D. Risk communication in practice: the contribution of decision aids. *Br Med J,* 2003; **327**: 736–40.
7. Puhan MA, Behnke M, Devereaux PJ *et al.* Does patients' evaluation of their response to therapy differ from that of their doctors? A prospective study. *Respir Med* 2004, in press.

◆8. Guyatt GH, Feeny DH, Patrick DL. Measuring Health-related Quality of Life. *Ann Intern Med* 1993; **118**: 622–9.
9. Sanders C, Egger M, Donovan J *et al.* Reporting on quality of life in randomised controlled trials: bibliographic study. *Br Med J* 1998; **317**: 1191–4.
10. Guyatt GH, Pugsley O, Sullivan MJ *et al.* Effect of encouragement on walking test performance. *Thorax* 1984; **39**: 818–22.
11. Schünemann HJ, Guyatt GH, Griffith L *et al.* A randomized controlled trial to evaluate the effect of informing patients about their pretreatment responses to two respiratory questionnaires. *Chest* 2002; **122**: 1701–8.
●12. Vale F, Reardon JZ, Zuwallack RL. The long-term benefits of outpatient pulmonary rehabilitation on exercise endurance and quality of life. *Chest* 1993; **103**: 42–5.
●13. Ries AL, Kaplan RM, Limberg TM, Prewitt LM. Effects of pulmonary rehabilitation on physiologic and psychosocial outcomes in patients with chronic obstructive pulmonary disease. *Ann Intern Med* 1995; **122**: 823–32.
◆14. Griffiths TL, Burr ML, Campbell IA *et al.* Results at 1 year of outpatient multidisciplinary pulmonary rehabilitation: a randomised controlled trial. *Lancet* 2000; **355**: 362–8.
15. American Thoracic Society. Dyspnea. Mechanisms, assessment, and management: a consensus statement. *Am J Respir Crit Care Med* 1999; **159**: 321–40.
16. Shoup R, Dalsky G, Warner S *et al.* Body composition and health-related quality of life in patients with chronic obstructive airways disease. *Eur Respir J* 1997; **10**: 1576–80.
17. Siafakas NM, Schiza S, Xirouhaki N, Bouros D. Is dyspnoea the main determinant of quality of life in the failing lung? A review. *Eur Respir Rev* 1997; **7**: 53–6.
18. Borg GAV. Psychophysical bases of perceived exertion. *Med Sci Sports Exer* 1982; **14**: 377–81.
◆19. O'Donnell DE, McGuire M, Samis L, Webb KA. General exercise training improves ventilatory and peripheral muscle strength and endurance in chronic airflow limitation. *Am J Respir Crit Care Med* 1998; **157**: 1489–97.
20. Normandin EA, McCusker C, Connors ML *et al.* An evaluation of two approaches to exercise conditioning in pulmonary rehabilitation. *Chest* 2002; **121**: 1085–91.
◆21. Reardon J, Awad E, Normandin E *et al.* The effect of comprehensive outpatient pulmonary rehabilitation on dyspnea. *Chest* 1994; **105**: 1046–52.
◆22. Mahler DA, Weinberg DH, Wells CK *et al.* The measurement of dyspnea: contents, interobserver agreement, and physiologic correlations of two new clinical indexes. *Chest* 1984; **85**: 751–8.
23. Eakin EG, Resnikoff PM, Prewitt LM *et al.* Validation of a new dyspnea measure. The UCSD shortness of breath questionnaire. *Chest* 1998; **113**: 619–24.
24. Guyatt GH, Berman LB, Townsend M *et al.* A measure of quality of life for clinical trials in chronic lung disease. *Thorax* 1987; **42**: 773–8.
25. Schünemann HJ, Guyatt GH, Ståhl E *et al.* Validation of a new version of the chronic respiratory questionnaire (CRQ): the self-administered standardized CRQ. *Eur Respir J* 2002; **20**: 156S.
26. Schünemann HJ, Griffith L, Jaeschke R *et al.* A comparison of the original chronic respiratory questionnaire with a standardized version. *Chest* 2003; **124**: 1421–9.
27. Puhan MA, Behnke M, Laschke M *et al.* Self-administration and standardisation of the chronic respiratory questionnaire: A randomized trial in three German-speaking countries. *Respir Med* 2004; **98**: 342–50.
●28. Goldstein RS, Gort EH, Stubbing D *et al.* Randomised controlled trial of respiratory rehabilitation. *Lancet* 1994; **344**: 1394–7.

29. Güell R, Casan P, Belda J et al. Long-term effects of outpatient rehabilitation of COPD. Chest 2000; 117: 976–83.

30. McGavin CR, Gupta SP, McHardy GJR. Twelve-minute walking test for assessing disability in chronic bronchitis. Br Med J 1976: 822–3.

31. Larson JL, Covey MK, Vitalo CA et al. Reliability and validity of the 12-minute distance walk in patients with chronic obstructive pulmonary disease. Nursing Res 1996; 45: 203–10.

32. Bowen JB, Votto JJ, Thrall RS et al. Functional status and survival following pulmonary rehabilitation Chest 2000; 118: 697–703.

●33. Gerardi DA, Lovett L, Benoit-Connors ML et al. Variables related to increased mortality following out-patient pulmonary rehabilitation. Eur Respir J 1996; 9: 431–5.

34. Larson JLMK, Covey CA, Vitalo C et al. Reliability and validity of the 12-minute distance walk in patients with chronic obstructive pulmonary disease. Nursing Res 1996; 45: 203–10.

35. Guyatt GH, Pugsley O, Sullivan MJ et al. Effect of encouragement on walking test performance. Thorax 1984; 39: 818–22.

36. Elpern EH, Stevens D, Kesten S. Variability in performance of the timed walk tests in pulmonary rehabilitation programs. Chest 2000; 118: 98–105.

37. Steele B. Timed walking tests of exercise capacity in chronic cardiopulmonary disease. J Cardiopulm Rehabil 1996; 16: 25–33.

38. Butland RJA, Pang J, Gross ER et al. Two-, six-, and 12-minute walking tests in respiratory disease. Br Med J 1982; 284: 1607–8.

39. Zuwallack RL, Patel K, Reardon JZ et al. Predictors of improvement in the 12-minute walking distance following a six-week outpatient pulmonary rehabilitation program. Chest 1991; 99: 805–8.

40. Votto J, Bowen J, Scalise P et al. Short-stay comprehensive inpatient pulmonary rehabilitation for advanced chronic obstructive pulmonary disease. Arch Phy Med Rehabil 1996; 77: 1115–18.

◆41. Redelmeier DA, Bayoumi AM, Goldstein RS, Guyatt GH. Interpreting small differences in functional status: the six minute walk test in chronic lung disease patients. Am J Respir Crit Care Med 1997; 155: 1278–82.

42. Singh SJ, Morgan MDL, Scott S et al. Development of a shuttle walking test of disability in patients with chronic airways obstruction. Thorax 1992; 47: 1019–24.

43. Hernandez MTE, Guerra JF, Marin JT et al. Reproducibilidad de un test de paseo de carga progresiva (shuttle walking test) en pacientes con enfermedad pulmonar obstructiva cronica. Arch Bronconeumol 1997; 33: 64–8.

44. Singh SJ, Morgan MDL, Hardman AE et al. Comparison of oxygen uptake during a conventional treadmill test and the shuttle walking test in chronic airflow limitation. Eur Respir J 1994; 7: 2016–20.

45. Ware JE, Snow KK, Kosinski MA. SF-36 Health Survey Manual and Interpretation Guide. Boston, Massachusetts: New England Medical Centre, 1993.

●46. Guyatt GH, King DR, Feeny DH et al. Generic and specific measurement of health-related quality of life in a clinical trial of respiratory rehabilitation. J Clin Epidemiol 1999; 52: 187–92.

47. Bergner M, Bobbitt RA, Carter WB et al. The Sickness Impact Profile: development and final revision of a health status measure. Med Care 1981: 787–805.

48. Feeny DH, Furlong W, Boyle M, Torrance GW. Multiattribute health status classification system. Health Utilities Index. Pharmacoeconomics 1995; 6: 490–502.

49. Euroqol Group. EuroQol – a new facility for the measurement of health-related quality of life. Health Pol 1990; 16: 199–208.

50. Kaplan RM, Bush JW, Berry CC. Health status. Types validity index well-being. Health Services Res 1976; 11: 478–507.

51. Torrance GW, Furlong W, Feeny DH, Boyle M. Multiattribute preferences functions. Health Utilities Index. Pharmacoeconomics 1995; 6: 503–20.

52. Harper R, Brazier JE, Waterhouse JC et al. Comparison of outcome measures for patients with chronic obstructive pulmonary disease (COPD) in an outpatient setting. Thorax 1997; 52: 879–87.

53. Schünemann H, Griffith L, Stubbing D et al. A clinical trial to evaluate the responsiveness and validity of two direct health state preference instruments administered with and without hypothetical marker states in chronic respiratory disease. Med Decis Making 2003; 23: 140–9.

54. Bennet KJ, Torrance GW. Measuring health state preferences and utilities: rating scale, time trade-off, and standard gamble techniques. In: Spilker B. Quality of Life and Pharmacoeconomics in Clinical Trials, 2nd edn. Philadelphia: Lippincott-Raven, 1996; 259.

55. Brazier J, Deverill M, Green C. The use of health status measures in economic evaluation. In: Stevens A, Abrams K, Brazier J, Fitzpatrick R, Lilford R, eds. The Advanced Handbook of Methods in Evidence Based Healthcare. London: Sage Publications, 2000; 195–214.

56. Neumann PJ, Goldie SJ, Weinstein MC. Preference-based measures in economic evaluation in health care. Annu Rev Public Health 2000; 21: 587–611.

57. Wijkstra PJ, Ten Vergert EM, Van Altena R et al. Reliability and validity of the chronic respiratory questionnaire (CRQ). Thorax 1994; 49: 465–7.

58. Chang JA, Curtis JR, Patrick DL, Raghu G. Assessment of health-related quality of life in patients with interstitial lung disease. Chest 1999; 116: 1175–82.

59. Bradley J, Dempster M, Wallace E, Elborn S. The adaptations of a quality of life questionnaire for routine use in clinical practice: the Chronic Respiratory Disease Questionnaire in cystic fibrosis. Qual Life Res 1999; 8: 65–71.

◆60. Jones PW, Quirk FH, Baveystock CM, Littlejohns P. A self-complete measure of health status for chronic airflow limitation. The St George's Respiratory Questionnaire. Am Rev Respir Dis 1992; 145: 1321–72.

61. Maille AR, Koning CJM, Zwinderman AH et al. The development of the 'Quality-of-Life for Respiratory Illness Questionnaire (QOL-RIQ)': a disease-specific quality-of-life questionnaire for patients with mild to moderate chronic non-specific lung disease. Respir Med 1997; 91: 297–309.

62. van Stel HF, Maille AR, Colland VT, Everaerd W. Interpretation of change and longitudinal validity of the quality of life for respiratory illness questionnaire (QoLRIQ) in inpatient pulmonary rehabilitation. Quality Life Res 2003; 12: 133–45.

63. Weaver TW, Narsavage GL, Guilfoyle MJ. The development and psychometric evaluation of the Pulmonary Functional Status Scale (PFSS): An instrument to assess functional status in pulmonary disease. J Cardiopulmon Rehabil 1998; 18: 105–11.

64. Stockdale-Woolley R, Zuwallack R, Haggerty MC. Correlations among various measurements used to evaluate the effects of pulmonary rehabilitation. Am J Crit Care Med 1995; 151: A686.

65. Votto J, Bowen J, Scalise P et al. Short-stay comprehensive in-patient pulmonary rehabilitation for advanced chronic obstructive pulmonary disease. Arch Phys Med Rehabil 1996; 77: 1115–18.

66. Wigal JK, Creer TL, Kostes H. The COPD Self-Efficacy Scale. Chest 1991; 99: 1193–6.

67. Lassere MN, van der Heijde D, Johnson KR. Foundations of the minimal clinically important difference for imaging. *J Rheumatol* 2001; **28**: 890–1.

◆68. Schünemann H, Goldstein R, Jaeschke R *et al*. The minimum important difference of the Chronic Respiratory Questionnaire. *J Chron Obstruct Pulm Dis* 2004, in press.

69. Jones PW, Quirk FH, Baveystock CM, Littlejohns P. A self-complete measure of health status for chronic airflow limitation. The St George's Respiratory Questionnaire. *Am Rev Respir Dis* 1992; **145**: 1321–72.

70. Witek TJ Jr, Mahler DA. Minimal important difference of the transition dyspnoea index in a multinational clinical trial. *Eur Respir J* 2003; **21**: 267–72.

71. Schünemann HJ, Griffith L, Jaeschke R *et al*. Evaluation of the minimal important difference for the feeling thermometer and St. Georges Respiratory Questionnaire in patients with chronic airflow limitation. *J Clin Epidemiol* 2003; **56**: 1170–6.

◆72. Pulmonary rehabilitation. Official statement of the American Thoracic Society. *Am J Respir Crit Care Med* 1999; **159**: 1666–82.

73. Singh SJ, Sodergren SC, Hyland ME *et al*. A comparison of three disease-specific and two generic health-status measures to evaluate the outcome of pulmonary rehabilitation in COPD. *Respir Med* 2001; **95**: 71–7.

74. de Torres JP, Pinto-Plata V, Ingenito E *et al*. Power of outcome measurements to detect clinically significant changes in pulmonary rehabilitation of patients with COPD. *Chest* 2002; **121**: 1092–8.

75. Casaburi R, Patessio A, Ioli F *et al*. Reductions in lactic acidosis and ventilation as a result of exercise training in patient with obstructive lung disease. *Am Rev Respir Dis* 1991; **143**: 9–18.

76. Clark CJ, Cochrane L, Mackay E. Low intensity peripheral muscle conditioning improves exercise tolerance and breathlessness in COPD. *Eur Respir J* 1996; **9**: 2590–6.

77. Wijkstra PJ, van der Mark TW, Kraan J *et al*. Effects of home rehabilitation on physical performance in patients with chronic obstructive pulmonary disease (COPD). *Eur Respir J* 1996; **9**: 104–10.

78. Maltais F, LeBlanc P, Jobin J *et al*. Intensity of training and physiologic adaptation in patients with chronic obstructive pulmonary disease. *Am J Respir Crit Care Med* 1997; **155**: 555–61.

79. Bernard S, Whitom F, LeBlanc P *et al*. Aerobic and strength training in patients with chronic obstructive pulmonary disease. *Am J Respir Crit Care Med* 1999; **159**: 896–901.

80. Coppoolse R, Schols AMWJ, Baarends EM *et al*. Interval versus continuous training in patients with severe COPD: a randomized clinical trial. *Eur Respir J* 1999; **14**: 258–63.

81. Spruit MA, Gosselink R, Troosters T *et al*. Resistance versus endurance training in patients with COPD and peripheral muscle weakness. *Eur Respir J* 2002; **19**: 1072–8.

82. Wedzicha JA, Bestall JC, Garrod R *et al*. Randomized controlled trial of pulmonary rehabilitation in severe chronic obstructive pulmonary disease patients, stratified with the MRC dyspnoea scale. *Eur Respir J* 1998; **12**: 363–9.

83. Berry MJ, Rejeski J, Adair NE, Zaccaro D. Exercise rehabilitation and chronic obstructive pulmonary disease stage. *Am J Respir Crit Care Med* 1999; **160**: 1248–53.

84. Hernandez MTE, Rubio TM, Ruiz FO *et al*. Results of a home-based training program for patients with COPD. *Chest* 2000; **118**: 106–14.

85. Green RH, Singh SJ, Williams J, Morgan MDL. A randomised controlled trial of four weeks versus seven weeks of pulmonary rehabilitation in chronic obstructive pulmonary disease. *Thorax* 2001; **56**: 143–5.

17

The economics of pulmonary rehabilitation and self-management education for patients with chronic obstructive pulmonary disease

T. L. GRIFFITHS, J. BOURBEAU

INTRODUCTION

The clinical effectiveness of pulmonary rehabilitation and supported self-management education is now well established, and supported by evidence provided by randomized controlled trials (RCTs) and, in the case of pulmonary rehabilitation, meta-analysis (1, 2). The use of multidisciplinary pulmonary rehabilitation in the management of patients with chronic obstructive pulmonary disease (COPD) is now being widely adopted. Supported self-management education programmes are gaining wider acceptance as they reduce the use of hospital resources and may improve aspects of patient well-being (3). In addition to the clinical effectiveness of a service, those who allocate resources will wish to know the cost of service provision; the financial return made on the investment and the downstream changes in overall resource utilization. As a result, in considering the best disease management strategies for COPD, there is considerable interest in the economic evaluation of the various management approaches.

The effect of changing patterns of care for acute exacerbations of COPD is particularly important as the cost saving associated with reduced admissions to hospital or a reduced length of stay is the prime driver of its overall cost or cost–benefit. As changes in acute care reduce the average bed occupancy incurred by exacerbations, strategies for chronic disease management may become apparently less cost-beneficial. When comparing economic analyses originating in different health care systems, the results of studies undertaken in one health care system should only be generalized to other health care systems with extreme caution.

This chapter reviews predominantly RCTs of pulmonary rehabilitation and supported self-management education that report outcomes related to clinical effectiveness but which also report outcomes of economic relevance such as the cost of providing the intervention, the impact on medication cost, primary and secondary health care usage or a fuller cost–benefit or cost-effectiveness analysis. The review covers in-patient, outpatient and community-based rehabilitation, as well as supported self-management education, as isolated entities. However, these modalities are not mutually exclusive and the health economic outcomes of these individual interventions would change if modalities of chronic care were combined or models of delivery of acute care were to evolve, as they seem likely to do, with more emphasis being placed on management of exacerbations in the community.

ECONOMIC EVALUATION

Economic evaluation compares alternative interventions in terms of both costs and consequences. It provides important additional information to assist decision-makers to arrive at appropriate choices about effective and efficient resource allocation.

It is standard practice in health economic evaluation to provide not only a point estimate of cost or cost-effectiveness but also an estimate of the precision of this figure or a sensitivity analysis indicating realistic best- and worst-case scenarios. However, many studies of rehabilitation fail to provide full costing of the intervention and subsequent health costs. They also neglect to provide an indication of the precision of this figure. In a number of studies, downstream cost effects are implied from observations of hospital admission rates or (the more economically meaningful) bed usage. RCTs reporting both the cost and effect of adding multidisciplinary pulmonary rehabilitation or supported self-management education to standard care have been published in the last 7 years with appropriate indications of the precision of their cost-effectiveness estimates. However, difficulties remain comparing the cost-effectiveness of different rehabilitation programmes that vary in their content, delivery and the patient-centred outcomes recorded.

The kinds of analysis employed in the trials described in this review are of the following types:

- *Analysis of the direct costs of providing the intervention.* This is considered to be a partial economic analysis as it is restricted to the cost of the intervention. The analysis is usually done taking a provider's perspective of the costs of running the service per patient included. Occasionally a wider perspective is taken to include costs to patients and their carers, such as transport and lost income.
- *Cost–benefit analysis.* In this kind of analysis, both the costs and the outcome are measured in monetary units. The information on the cost of caring for patients, including the use of the service, is compared with the cost of caring for patients in a comparator fashion (most often usual care). Cost–benefit analysis is used to assess the overall effect on cost to the health service of adding a given intervention to patients' care. The outcome of this kind of analysis may vary with the duration of follow-up of 'downstream' effects and the comprehensiveness of the costs that are taken into account. Many studies have reported the effect of rehabilitation on health service usage, e.g. post-rehabilitation hospital admissions, but few have analysed simultaneously both the cost of intervention and the cost of subsequent care from a health service perspective. In none of the studies in pulmonary rehabilitation has a full societal perspective on cost–benefit analysis been taken.
- *Cost-effectiveness analysis.* In this mode of analysis, the cost of intervention is related to the clinical benefits obtained. Cost-effectiveness analysis is a method designed to assess the comparative impacts of expenditures on different health interventions. It is critical to the understanding of this kind of analysis to know whether the costs referred to are simply those of providing the intervention, or whether later modulations of overall cost are being taken into account. Whereas incremental cost–benefit analysis balances the cost of adding the intervention with any cost reductions that might ensue, incremental cost-effectiveness analysis relates the overall

cost of adding the intervention to standard care to the incremental clinical benefit gained. Thus the cost per unit of benefit can be determined. To carry out this kind of analysis, a RCT design is needed, making appropriate estimates of cost and clinical outcome.

- *Cost–utility analysis.* In this variant of cost-effectiveness analysis, the value placed on the health outcomes of the intervention by patients forms a key element of the effectiveness measure. In studies where mortality or survival are also recorded, the duration of life as well as its patient-determined value may become a utility measure. The benefits may then be expressed in quality-adjusted life-years (QALYs) or 'well years'.

As yet no prospective economic analysis comparing in-patient, outpatient and community-based rehabilitation has been reported and so rehabilitation in different settings will be discussed separately.

IN-PATIENT PULMONARY REHABILITATION

Direct cost of programme provision

In 1994, Goldstein *et al.* (4) reported the clinical outcomes of a Canadian rehabilitation programme incorporating an initial 2-month multidisciplinary in-patient period followed by a home exercise programme with scaling down of professional contact over the subsequent 4 months. This highly effective intervention was then subjected to a detailed costing which estimated the average cost of providing in-patient rehabilitation per patient to be Canadian \$10 228 (~£4600) (5). Figure 17.1

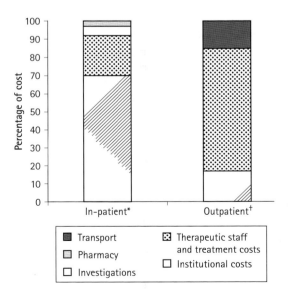

Figure 17.1 *Percentage contributions to costs of pulmonary rehabilitation in in-patient and outpatient settings. *8-week in-patient programme Goldstein* et al. *(4, 5);* †*6-week outpatient programme Griffiths* et al. *(14, 15).*

shows in percentage terms the relative contributions to the overall cost of the programme made by medical investigations and drugs, hospital overheads, staff, transport and (the largest component) the cost of providing 'hotel' services. The need to provide accommodation to patients is clearly a major driver of cost and is what makes in-patient programmes more expensive to run than outpatient or community programmes.

Cost–benefit

Set beside their detailed costing of service provision, Goldstein *et al.* (4, 5) undertook to analyse the cost–benefits of in-patient rehabilitation. The cost of care for patients over 6 months was found to be greater in their rehabilitation than in their standard care group despite the costs of prescribed drugs and community services being less in the rehabilitated group. When all costs had been taken into account, adding in-patient pulmonary rehabilitation to standard care increased the overall health service bill by Can$11 597 per patient.

Cost–effectiveness

As part of their economic evaluation of in-patient-based pulmonary rehabilitation, Goldstein *et al.* (4, 5), also reported an estimate of the number needed to treat (NNT) to obtain one more patient with the minimum clinically important benefit in the rehabilitation group as compared with control. The number needed to treat is given by:

$$NNT = 1/(P_I - P_C)$$

where P_I and P_C are the proportions gaining a minimum clinically important benefit in the intervention and control groups, respectively.

The NNT provides a measure of the effectiveness of health care interventions in terms of the proportion of patients who would be expected to derive a specified level of benefit as a result of applying the intervention to a population of subjects. More effective interventions will have smaller NNTs. If the average incremental cost of rehabilitation per patient is multiplied by the NNT, the product is the programme's cost to provide one patient with a minimal clinically important benefit – an index of cost-effectiveness. In this study (4, 5), disease-specific health status was measured using the Chronic Respiratory Disease Questionnaire (6). An average change in response score of 0.5 points in each of its domains of dyspnoea, fatigue, emotion and mastery was accepted as the minimum clinically important change. This level of change was used as the threshold of clinical effectiveness in the NNT calculations. The NNT estimates for this study were as follows: dyspnoea, 4.1; fatigue, 4.4; emotion, 3.3; and mastery, 4.4. The incremental cost of achieving one patient with the minimum clinically important benefit was: for dyspnoea, Can$47 548; for fatigue, Can$51 027; for emotion, Can$38 272; and for mastery, Can$28 993.

OUTPATIENT REHABILITATION

Direct cost of programme provision

There are now a number of reports in the literature, addressing the cost of providing pulmonary rehabilitation programmes in an outpatient setting.

An analysis of a rehabilitation programme mixing outpatient and in-patient components was reported by Burton *et al.* (7) and Dunham *et al.* (8) from California in 1982. The costs of all aspects of this multidisciplinary programme were accounted for, but because the programme was individually tailored, the number of sessions patients received was variable. However, when the total cost of programme provision was divided by the total number of graduates, an average cost of $452 (US$ unless otherwise stated) per patient per year was calculated. An exclusively outpatient programme of once-weekly exercise, respiratory muscle and breathing training for 6 weeks was reported from Seattle in 1988 (9). The cost of this intervention, which improved exercise capacity, was reported to be $600–800 per patient. A 10-week programme of once per week multidisciplinary intervention supplemented by a domiciliary exercise and respiratory muscle training was reported from Newark, New Jersey (10). Programme graduates showed significant improvements in exercise tolerance and breathlessness with an estimated programme cost of $650 per patient. More recent reports from the UK have estimated the cost per patient of providing effective outpatient rehabilitation to be £422 per patient for a 7-week, 14-session multidisciplinary programme in Leicester (11) and £400 for a 6-week, 12-session, multidisciplinary programme in Bristol (12). A recent Belgian study of a thrice-weekly 6-month outpatient strength and endurance training programme (13) estimated that the direct cost of providing the programme, from Belgian National Health Insurance reimbursement, expressed as the average cost per patient, was $2615 (SD, $625).

In 2000, a RCT of an 18-session, 6-week, multidisciplinary rehabilitation programme was reported by Griffiths *et al.* (14) from Wales accompanied by a health economic analysis (15). The programme included exercise reconditioning, education, dietetic support, stress management and relaxation training. The proportionate contributions of staff, equipment and consumables, travel and institutional overhead costs are shown in Fig. 17.1. A conservative cost analysis of the programme was made as if the programme were run at 85 per cent capacity of its maximum 20 patients every 6 weeks, to reflect the fact that all programmes lose participants over time. The programme showed important functional and health status benefits at an estimated cost of £725 per patient. From Fig. 17.1, it is clear that staff costs form the largest single component of the cost of providing outpatient pulmonary rehabilitation with considerably less hospital-related cost than is seen for in-patient rehabilitation.

Cost–benefit

In 1969, Petty *et al.* (16) reported a non-randomized study of 182 patients with moderate to severe COPD who had undergone a programme of exercise with the option of in-patient care for those undergoing clinical deterioration. Hospital admissions for the year prior to entering the programme were compared with the year after. A 48 per cent reduction in days spent in hospital was observed. The longer-term requirement for hospitalization for respiratory problems in graduates of this programme was subsequently reported (17). Using recall data from 113 patients, the number of days patients spent in hospital in each of the 4 years after entering the programme was compared with their experience in the year before entering the programme. Major reductions in hospital usage following rehabilitation were reported. The authors considered that the effect on hospital usage was likely to be of economic importance.

A retrospective analysis of the influence of rehabilitation on subsequent hospital usage was reported from Loma Linda (7, 8). Eighty patients were noted to have spent a mean of 17.41 days in hospital in the year before rehabilitation and 7.78, 4.91, 2.74, 2.22 and 3.26 days in each of the 5 years after rehabilitation. The estimated per-capita cost of rehabilitation was $452. With a day spent in hospital being allocated a notional cost of $400, the average cost–benefit per patient could be estimated at $3852 in the first year. Although this report lacked statistical detail and did not include a control group, it seemed to indicate that pulmonary rehabilitation might be cost-beneficial.

Now that a *prime facie* case had been established for the cost benefits of pulmonary rehabilitation in uncontrolled studies, the scene was set for the important RCT reported from San Diego by Ries *et al.* (18) that would avoid recruitment bias and changes in patients' condition with time alone. In this large study, subjects were randomized to receive either multidisciplinary pulmonary rehabilitation or a purely educational programme. Rehabilitation was delivered in 12 sessions over 8 weeks with monthly follow-up over a year. Interestingly, the dramatic effects reported in the non-randomized studies were not replicated. While rehabilitated patients tended to take up fewer hospital bed-days, the difference was not statistically different from that seen in the education group. The questions remained, therefore: had the earlier studies suffered from recruitment bias and regression to the mean effects, or had the management of COPD exacerbation perhaps changed? Finally, could outpatient rehabilitation reduce subsequent health service utilisation or not?

The study of Griffiths *et al.* (14, 15) was designed to address the effect of outpatient pulmonary rehabilitation on health service usage and costs. The authors estimated the cost of providing care over 1 year of follow-up in a group of 200 patients randomized to receive either 6 weeks of multidisciplinary, outpatient, pulmonary rehabilitation or standard care. The difference in average patient costs reflected the incremental cost of adding rehabilitation to standard care. Rehabilitation was not associated with a reduction in the number of patients needing at least one hospital admission during the follow-up year. Despite this, overall, the number of days spent in hospital and the number of admissions were both significantly reduced in those who were admitted in the

rehabilitated group compared with controls. The findings represented a halving of hospital usage from 8 to 4 days when averaged across the entire group. Significant effects were also observed in the pattern of primary care utilization, with rehabilitated patients seeking consultation in their general practitioners' premises more frequently and in their own homes less frequently than those in the control group. Taking into account primary and secondary care utilization and drug costs, the annual mean per-capita cost of standard care was £1826 (SD 3295) and that for care including rehabilitation was £1674 (SD 1588). The £150 difference in the cost of care was not statistically significant. These findings strongly support the contention that multidisciplinary pulmonary rehabilitation does indeed reduce subsequent health service utilization to the extent that the cost of providing the rehabilitation is balanced by later cost reductions.

A recent, innovative study from nine collaborating rehabilitation groups in California described the effect of rehabilitation on health state and health care utilization in 'real life' practice (19). All the centres provided exercise training, education and psychosocial support, but the programmes were not uniform in content, referral pattern or setting. Outcomes from 521 graduates confirmed important benefits in health status as well as reductions in health service usage. Compared with the 3-month period prior to entering rehabilitation, days spent in hospital, urgent care visits, phone calls to medical attendants and physician visits were all significantly reduced over the subsequent 18 months. Results were relatively homogeneous across rehabilitation centres, confirming the general applicability and effectiveness of the intervention.

There is now a body of evidence in support of outpatient pulmonary rehabilitation being at least cost-neutral and reducing subsequent health care utilization. Studies allowing direct comparison between the cost–benefits of in-patient, outpatient and home rehabilitation in a single health delivery system are needed.

Cost–effectiveness

As part of their RCT and allied economic analysis, Griffiths *et al.* (14, 15) undertook an NNT analysis similar to that described by Goldstein *et al.* (4, 5). Using a change of 0.5 points in responses to the dyspnoea, fatigue, emotion and mastery domains of the CRQ, they found that after their 18-session, 6-week outpatient programme the NNT was as follows: for dyspnoea, 2.3; for fatigue, 2.5; for emotion, 2.2; and for mastery, 2.5. The corresponding cost of providing rehabilitation to obtain one subject with the minimum clinically important change over and above standard care was: for dyspnoea, £1730; for fatigue, £1880; for emotion, £1654; and for mastery, £1880. Direct comparison between outcomes of this study and that of Goldstein *et al.* and other studies is not possible due to differences in patient characteristics, health services and timing of outcome measurement. However, it is clear that whilst both in-patient and outpatient rehabilitation programmes are effective in achieving improvements of health state, the inclusion of an in-patient component to the programme does increase the cost. In order to quantify differences in cost-effectiveness between different programme formats, further randomized trials addressing the question would be needed.

Cost–utility

Cost–utility analysis is a method of applying cost-effectiveness analysis in such a way as to enable comparisons to be made between different interventions in different conditions. This form of analysis was undertaken by Griffiths et al. (14, 15). One of the outcome measures in this study was the SF-36 generic health status questionnaire. Subject responses to this questionnaire were mapped onto the much more concise SF-6D (20). The states of health described by the possible 'responses' to the SF-6D carry a preference value placed upon them by a reference population. The SF-6D thus provides a preference-based indication of the 'value' placed on the health state described for each individual from 0 (the least valued health state) to 1 (the most valued heath state). As survival was also recorded in this study, the measure of utility could be further refined to determine the length of life as well as the value placed on that life. The resulting unit, the QALY, was the product of the SF-6D utility score and duration of life for each subject in the study.

For the purpose of their cost–utility analysis, the difference in the mean cost in monetary units for providing care for the rehabilitation and control groups was determined as the mean incremental cost. Similarly the difference in the mean utility in QALYs for the rehabilitation and control groups was determined as the incremental utility. The point estimate of incremental cost was –£152 (95 per cent confidence interval [CI] = –880–577) and the point estimate for incremental utility gain was 0.03 (0.002–0.058). The ratio of these two values forms the cost–utility ratio and, in this study, it indicated that there was a negative cost per QALY gained by rehabilitation.

The cost–utility ratio is unlikely to be a normally distributed variable and so non-parametric methods are appropriate to determine its statistical precision. The authors did this using statistical modelling known as the 'bootstrap' technique (21). They concluded that the probability that the true cost–utility ratio fell below £0 per QALY was 0.64. The probability that the true cost per QALY was less than £3000 was 0.74, and the probability the cost per QALY was below £10 000 was 0.9.

Griffiths et al. (15) compared cost per QALY ratios for their rehabilitation programme with published cost per QALY ratios for some well-accepted interventions in other areas of medicine such as hip replacement surgery (£1180 per QALY), coronary artery bypass graft (£2090 per QALY), hospital haemodialysis (£21 970 per QALY) and treating hypertension with beta-blockade in middle-aged men and women (£26 796 and £67 678 per QALY, respectively). With this level of cost–utility, outpatient pulmonary rehabilitation

is becoming increasingly available in a variety of health care systems.

COMMUNITY-BASED REHABILITATION

Direct cost of programme provision

A community or primary care setting for pulmonary rehabilitation places rehabilitation closer to patients' homes and avoids the overheads associated with hospital-based rehabilitation. Few community-based rehabilitation programmes have been evaluated economically. Depending of the programme's location, associated costs would be expected to be quite variable. For example, the need for individual or small group participation may increase the staff costs, but the community setting may reduce transport costs. A Dutch study reported in 1996 by Wijkstra et al. (22, 23) analysed outcomes of a community-based rehabilitation programme. Subjects were randomized to a control group or to receive either 3 months of twice-weekly rehabilitation based in a community setting followed by a weekly or monthly physiotherapist visit for the next 18 months. In this study, once per month maintenance appeared to be more effective than a weekly maintenance programme when compared with the control group, but the two maintenance strategies were not shown to be significantly different from each other. Subsequently, the authors estimated the cost of their programme in a community location with weekly maintenance home visits to be $2300 per patient (24). They also estimated the cost of a programme of similar intensity, undertaken in a hospital facility, and arrived at a figure of $4250 per patient. The main cost difference between community and hospital settings was the cost of patient transport to and from sessions. However, their calculations may have neglected the fact that hospital-based rehabilitation can be offered to groups of patients together, thus introducing economies of staff time. These methodological issues highlight the need for appropriate randomized trials to compare cost and cost-effectiveness between rehabilitation settings.

Cost–benefit

There are no RCTs addressing the cost–benefit of community-based pulmonary rehabilitation. However, the cost and health service utilization effects of a community support programme were reported in 1982 by Roselle and D'Amico (25). Their intervention took the form of comprehensive home respiratory therapist support for up to 1 year. When compared with the year before entry into the programme, there were significant reductions in both hospital admission rates and the number of days spent in hospital – a reduction in secondary care usage of 66 per cent. With the proviso that this study has all the problems inherent in studies lacking an appropriate control group, the authors estimated a cost reduction of $2625 per patient in the first year of follow-up. Another, retrospective analysis of a home care programme has been reported from Connecticut (26). Again this compared periods before and after entering a home care. A reduction in the monthly cost of care for patients undergoing the programme of $328 was indicated. More comprehensive, prospective studies are needed before the cost–benefits of community rehabilitation programmes become clear.

Cost-effectiveness

The cost-effectiveness of community-based rehabilitation programmes has not been systematically studied or reported.

SUPPORTED SELF-MANAGEMENT EDUCATION

A relatively new concept in chronic disease management for patients with COPD is to offer a supported self-management plan with the goal of improving health state and of reducing the impact of acute exacerbations on the patient and health care system. The first aim of these self-management programmes is to educate patients and their family, empowering them to make therapeutic, behavioural and environmental adjustments in accordance with recommendations given to them in advance. These education programmes offer a combination of one or more of the following modalities delivered to individuals in the community as a package:

- skill-orientated education in chronic and acute disease management
- an exercise programme
- ongoing attention from and communication with a case manager who supervises the programme individually
- rapid access to care services for assessment and treatment of acute exacerbations.

In 2003, a systematic review of self-management education programmes for patients with COPD was published (27). The conclusion of this review was that self-management had no effect on hospital admissions, emergency room visits, days lost from work or lung function. Variable effects were seen on health status and use of primary care services. Self-management education has now become more directed towards inducing behavioural change than simply imparting information to patients. A number of recent RCTs have reported the effectiveness and cost-effectiveness of supported self-management in the community (Table 17.1).

A Norwegian trial of an education programme was reported in 2000 (28). Sixty-two patients with COPD were randomized to standard care or two 2-h group sessions and one to two 40-min individual sessions with a specialist nurse or physiotherapist. The self-management was a multi-component education programme and included a written action plan to deal with acute exacerbation. This plan involved a prescription of doubling inhaled corticosteroids or prednisone for self-administration. The subjects in their study had a mean FEV_1 of 56–59 per cent of predicted. The usual care group accrued an average of 2.5 hospital bed-days in the year of follow-up. The intervention did not have a significant effect on this low level of hospital usage but GP visits were significantly reduced from 3.4 per patient to 0.5 in the intervention group. In the accompanying economic analysis taken from a societal perspective (29), it was found that the cost of providing the educational intervention was 1600 Norwegian kroner (NOK). The overall average per-capita cost of a year's care for the control group was NOK 19 900 and that for educated the educated group was NOK 10 600. This revealed a clear cost benefit from this type of intervention resulting from reductions in primary and secondary care usage.

These results contrast with a recent study of a self-management programme (30) reported as a randomized trial in which 248 patients with moderate COPD (mean FEV_1

Table 17.1 *Comparison of self-management programme effectiveness, direct cost and cost–benefit per patient per year*[a]

	Gallefoss and Bakke (28, 29)	Monninkhof et al. (30, 31)	Farrero et al. (32)	Bourbeau et al. (3), Bourbeau (33)[b]
Country	Norway	Netherlands	Spain	Canada
COPD patients	62	248	94	191
FEV_1 predicted	56–59%	57%		40%
Long-term oxygen	Unknown	Unknown	100%	12–15%
Effectiveness	Emergency visits	Days with limitation post-exacerbation	Emergency visits and hospital admissions	Emergency visits and hospital admissions Health-related quality of life
Cost of the programme	$1600	$664	$832	$1056 (50:1), $808 (70:1)
Ratio cost–benefit	1:4.8	1:0.45	1:2.2	1:1.8–2.6

[a]The ratio cost–benefit of 1:1 means that for every $1 put into patient self-management education, there is a saving of $1; ratio cost–benefit of 1:0.5 means that education costs twice as much as usual care.

[b]The number in parenthesis represents the patient caseload per case manager: a 50-patient caseload in the setting of a nursing home practice, and a 70-patient caseload per case manager in the setting of an outpatient clinic.

approximately 57 per cent of predicted) were randomized to usual care or a 4-month programme of five 2-h group, self-management, educational sessions together with one or two group exercise sessions per week supported by a booklet. The multi-component education programme highlighted chronic and acute disease self-management, exercise, communication and social relationships. The self-management programme included an action plan for exacerbations with a short course of oral corticosteroids and antibiotic and a near-home fitness programme that was under the guidance of a physiotherapist. The intervention could be characterized as a low-intensity outpatient, community rehabilitation programme. Both control and intervention groups had standard pharmacological treatment and could report to the study staff in the case of exacerbation for advice. In this study, no benefit was seen in in-patient health status or exacerbation rates. More exacerbations requiring oral corticosteroids were reported in the intervention group, but early recognition and treatment of exacerbations were goals of the educational component. This resulted in a reduction in doctor consultations per patient compared with the usual care group. A recent paper (31) reported that the programme applied to patients with moderate COPD and relatively good health status was twice as expensive as usual care and had no measurable beneficial effects on QALYs.

A different approach has been reported from Spain. Farrero *et al.* (32) described a home-care programme for patients with severe COPD receiving long-term oxygen therapy. Ninety-four patients completed 1-year follow-up. The programme combined scheduled home support by a respiratory nurse specialist and a chest physician with a weekly phone call and a 3-monthly home visit. The team was also available to meet the patients' needs 'on demand' with a 'usually immediate' response to requests for help. This service offered home-care support with rapid, easy access to hospital facilities. In the intervention group, emergency department visits were significantly reduced by 70 per cent, and hospital admissions and days spent in hospital were reduced by 60 per cent. The authors attributed much of the success to the fact that the same clinical team were managing home and acute care with ready access to the means of investigation and treatment of exacerbations. In this study, the estimated cost of providing home-care was $832 per patient. There was an average per-capita cost saving in the intervention group compared with the control group of $1850 due to the reduction in use of secondary care in-patient facilities. Although no estimate of the precision of these point estimates of cost was given, the statistically significant reduction in secondary care use suggests that this kind of approach is likely to be cost-beneficial, although no improvement in health status or mortality was found.

An important study of combined supported home self-management education and access to specialist secondary care staff was reported from Canada by Bourbeau *et al.* (3) in 2003. This multi-centre RCT enrolled 191 patients with COPD (mean FEV_1 approximately 1.0 L or 40 per cent of predicted) and a history of hospital admission in the previous year. Patients were randomized to receive standard care or a modular,

disease-specific self-management programme based on a skill-orientated workbook *Living Well with COPD* designed by health educators. Modules of self-care were covered in a weekly home visit by a trained health care professional over 2 months. A home exercise programme and an exacerbation plan with a short course of oral corticosteroids and antibiotic were advised and a case manager was allocated to make telephone contact each month and to advise at other times on management if symptoms became worse despite the home management plan. The intervention group did not show statistically significant reductions in the number of symptomatic exacerbations. However, there was a statistically significant 60 per cent reduction in the number of emergency room visits and 40 per cent admissions for COPD exacerbations and associated bed-days used in the intervention group compared with standard care. The average number of days spent in hospital per capita was 12.5 in the usual care group, and 7.2 in the intervention group. Economic analysis suggested that this programme, applied to patients with severe COPD, reduced health status and previous hospitalization, is likely to be cost-beneficial (33). However, to be cost-beneficial, the case manager needs to have a caseload of 50 patients or more to follow in a year (Table 17.1). In a real-life situation where a case manager will usually follow 50 patients or more, a self-management programme would save over Can$1700 per patient per year.

Thus, there is growing evidence in favour of supported self-management programmes. Further studies will be needed to establish its cost–benefit and cost-effectiveness in populations of varying COPD severity and delivery settings.

CONCLUSION

Multidisciplinary pulmonary rehabilitation now has an established place in the management of patients disabled by chronic lung disease. The evidence upon which this is based includes not only data on clinical effectiveness but also accumulating information on health resource utilization. The health economic data suggest that the costs of providing rehabilitation will depend on the content and setting of the programme. Outpatient programmes are less expensive than in-patient programmes, although they may be appropriate for different patient groups. In addition to being cost-beneficial, outpatient rehabilitation generates patient benefit at costs that would generally be accepted as cost-effective. Thus, investment in pulmonary rehabilitation is clinically and economically justified.

Supported self-management education programmes have a developing evidence base, suggesting that this form of management used as an integral component of patient care may reduce primary and secondary health service usage and be cost-beneficial when applied to patients with severe COPD, especially those with reduced quality of life who use hospital in-patient services. The cost-effectiveness of supported self-management education in terms of clinical outcome and utility remain to be determined.

Key points

● The economic evaluation of pulmonary rehabilitation and self-management education programmes is a developing area of interest that will inform the development and general application of these services.

● Data on cost, cost–benefit, cost-effectiveness and cost–utility are available for pulmonary rehabilitation and the evidence base for supported self-management is growing.

● Pulmonary rehabilitation is a cost-effective intervention that reduces subsequent health service usage.

● Rehabilitation programmes with an in-patient component are more costly to implement than outpatient programmes.

● Outpatient rehabilitation is likely to be cost-neutral to the health service at the same time as improving patient well-being.

● Supported self-management education programmes can reduce primary and secondary care usage and are likely to provide a cost-effective modality of chronic disease management in patients with more severe COPD or a history of hospital admission.

● Care should be exercised in generalizing the results of health economic analyses from one health care system to another.

REFERENCES

◆1. Lacasse Y, Wong E, Guyatt GH et al. Meta-analysis of respiratory rehabilitation in chronic obstructive pulmonary disease. Lancet 1996; 348: 1115–19.

◆2. Lacasse Y, Brosseau L, Milne S et al. Pulmonary rehabilitation for chronic obstructive pulmonary disease (Cochrane Review). The Cochrane Library, issue 4. Chichester, UK: John Wiley, 2004.

●3. Bourbeau J, Julien M, Maltais F et al. Reduction of hospitalization in patients with chronic obstructive pulmonary disease. Arch Intern Med 2003; 163: 585–91.

●4. Goldstein RS, Gort EH, Stubbing D et al. Randomised controlled trial of respiratory rehabilitation. Lancet 1994; 344: 1394–7.

●5. Goldstein RS, Gort EH, Guyatt GH, Feeny D. Economic analysis of respiratory rehabilitation. Chest 1997; 112: 370–9.

6. Guyatt GH, Berman LB, Townsend M et al. A measure of quality of life for clinical trials in chronic lung disease. Thorax 1987; 42: 773–8.

7. Burton GG, Gee G, Hodgkin JE, Dunham JL. Cost effectiveness studies in respiratory care. On overview and some possible early solutions. Hospitals 1975; 49: 61–71.

8. Dunham JL, Hodgkin JE, Nicol J, Burton GG. Cost effectiveness of pulmonary rehabilitation programs. In: Connors GL, ed. Pulmonary Rehabilitation: Guidelines to Success. Boston: Butterworth, 1984; 389–402.

9. Holle RHO, Williams DV, Vandree JC et al. Increased muscle efficiency and sustained benefits in an outpatient community hospital-based pulmonary rehabilitation program. Chest 1988; 94: 1161–8.

10. Reina-Rosenbaum R, Bach JR, Penek J. The costs/benefits of outpatient-based pulmonary rehabilitation. Arch Phys Med Rehabil 1997; 78: 240–4.

11. Singh SJ, Smith DL, Hyland ME, Morgan MD. A short outpatient rehabilitation programme: immediate and longer-term effects on exercise performance and quality of life. Resp Med 1998; 92: 1146–54.

12. White RJ, Rudkin ST, Ashley J et al. Outpatient pulmonary rehabilitation in severe chronic obstructive pulmonary disease. J R Coll Phys 1997; 31: 541–5.

13. Troosters T, Gosselink R, Decramer M. Short- and long-term effects of outpatient rehabilitation in patients with chronic obstructive pulmonary disease: a randomised controlled trial. Am J Med 2000; 109: 207–12.

●14. Griffiths TL, Burr ML, Campbell IA et al. Results at 1 year of outpatient multidisciplinary pulmonary rehabilitation: a randomised controlled trial. Lancet 2000; 355: 362–8.

●15. Griffiths TL, Phillips CJ, Davies S et al. Cost effectiveness of an outpatient multidisciplinary pulmonary rehabilitation programme. Thorax 2001; 56: 779–84.

16. Petty TL, Nett LM, Finigan MM et al. A comprehensive care program for chronic airway obstruction: methods and preliminary evaluation of symptomatic and functional improvement. Ann Intern Med 1969; 70: 1109–20.

17. Hudson LD, Tyler ML, Petty TL. Hospitalization needs during an outpatient rehabilitation program for severe chronic airway obstruction. Chest 1976; 70: 606–10.

●18. Ries AL, Kaplan RM, Limberg TM, Prewitt L. Effects of pulmonary rehabilitation on physiologic and psychosocial outcomes in patients with chronic obstructive pulmonary disease. Ann Intern Med 1995; 122: 823–32.

19. Ries AL. Effects of pulmonary rehabilitation on dyspnoea, quality of life, and healthcare costs in California. J Cardiopulm Rehab 2004; 24: 52–62.

20. Brazier JE, Harper R, Thomas K et al. Deriving a preference-based single index measure from the SF-36. J Clin Epidemiol 1998; 51: 1115–29.

21. Briggs A, Wonderling D, Mooney C. Pulling cost-effectiveness analysis up by its bootstraps: a non-parametric approach to confidence interval estimation. Health Econ 1997; 6: 327–40.

22. Wijkstra PJ, Ten Vergert EM, van Altena R et al. Long term benefits of rehabilitation at home on quality of life and exercise tolerance in patients with chronic obstructive pulmonary disease. Thorax 1995; 50: 824–8.

23. Wijkstra PJ, van der Mark TW, Kraan J et al. Long-term effects of home rehabilitation on physical performance in chronic obstructive pulmonary disease. Am J Respir Crit Care Med 1996; 153: 1234–41.

◆24. Wijkstra PJ, Strijbos JH, Koeter GH. Home-based rehabilitation for patients with COPD. Organization, effects and financial implications. Monaldi Arch Chest Dis 2000; 55: 130–4.

25. Roselle S, D'Amico FJ. The effect of home respiratory therapy on hospital readmission rates of patients with chronic obstructive pulmonary disease. Respir Care 1982; 27: 1194–9.

26. Campbell Haggerty M, Stockdale-Woolley R, Nair S. Respi-care. An innovative home care program for the patient with chronic obstructive pulmonary disease. Chest 1991; 100: 607–12.

◆27. Monnikhof M, Valk Pvd, Palen JVD et al. Self-management education for patients with chronic obstructive pulmonary disease: a systematic review. Thorax 2003; 58: 394–8.

● 28. Gallefoss F, Bakke PS. Impact of patient education and self-management on morbidity in asthmatics and patients with chronic obstructive pulmonary disease. *Respir Med* 2000; **94**: 279–87.

● 29. Gallefoss F, Bakke P. Cost-benefit and cost-effectiveness analysis of self-management in patients with COPD. A 1-year follow-up randomized, controlled trial. *Respir Med* 2002; **96**: 424–31.

● 30. Monninkhof E, van der Valk P, van der Palen J *et al.* Effects of a comprehensive self-management programme in patients with chronic obstructive pulmonary disease. *Eur Respir J* 2003; **22**: 815–20.

● 31. Monninkhof E, Valk PVD, Schermer T *et al.* Economic evaluation of a comprehensive self-management programme in patients with COPD. *Chron Respir Dis* 2004, **1**: 7–16.

● 32. Farrero E, Escarrabill J, Prats E *et al.* Impact of a hospital-based home-care program on the management of COPD patients receiving long-term oxygen therapy. *Chest* 2001; **119**: 364–9.

◆ 33. Bourbeau J. Self-management interventions to improve outcomes in patients suffering from COPD. *Expert Rev Pharmacoeconomics Outcomes Res* 2004; **4**: 71–7.

PART 3

Delivering pulmonary rehabilitation: general aspects

Table 18.1   *Major papers (from Cochrane Review) programme duration*

Setting	Authors	Year	Sample no.	Duration (weeks)
In-patient	Cockcroft et al. (14)	1981	24	6
	Goldstein et al. (17)	1994	79	8
	Vallet et al. (30)	1994	20	8
Hospital outpatients	Lake et al. (19)	1990	14	8
	Weiner et al. (100)	1992	24	26
	Reardon et al. (25)	1994	20	6
	Güell et al. (26)	2000	56	26
	Bendstrup et al. (9)	1997	32	12
	Emery et al. (15)	1998	50	10
	Engstrom et al. (16)	1999	50	52
	Gosselink et al. (48)	2000	70	24
	Griffiths et al. (29)	2000	184	6
	Ringbaek et al. (21)	2000	36	8
Community	Wijkstra et al. (101)	1994	43	12
	Cambach et al. (12)	1997	23	12
Home-based	McGavin et al. (20)	1977	24	15 (approx.)
	Booker (10)	1984	69	9
	Jones et al. (18)	1985	14	10
	Busch and McClements (11)	1988	12	18
	Clark et al. (13)	1996	48	12
	Strijbos et al. (24)	1996	45	12
	Hernandez et al. (27)	2000	37	12

Table 18.2   *Rehabilitation settings*

	Advantages	Disadvantages
In-patient	Intensive	Cost
	Residential	Exclusion of relatives
	No safety issues	
Hospital outpatient	Economy	Daily travel
	Safety	
Community	Close to home	Availability of staff
	Potential volume	Quality of supervision
Home	Domestic relevance	Cost
	No travel	No group effect

location in papers from the Cochrane review of rehabilitation are shown in Table 18.1 and the major features of the various locations are summarised in Table 18.2 (9–29).

In-patient rehabilitation

Patients may be admitted for planned in-patient rehabilitation, or rehabilitation may be implemented during an admission for an acute exacerbation. The earlier reports of successful rehabilitation were from planned in-patient programmes (14, 17, 30). In one of these randomized controlled trials, patients with chronic obstructive pulmonary disease (COPD) achieved the now familiar benefits in exercise performance and health status after an 8-week in-patient programme followed by 4 months of less intensive outpatient care (17). The results were highly significant at the time but comparable improvements have since been achieved in much less expensive outpatient programmes. There is an argument

in favour of providing in-patient rehabilitation for people with particularly severe disease, multiple co-morbidities or where geographical preferences apply.

Recently, there has been some interest in short-duration in-patient rehabilitation either to precondition patients for lung volume reduction surgery or to reduce the impact of the admission for acute exacerbation. A very short intensive in-patient physical training may produce some rapid improvements in physical performance and health status (31–33). However, all of the short-term in-patient studies that have been reported so far are uncontrolled and therefore difficult to compare to the main bulk of evidence. Prospective trials in this area would be welcome.

There is considerable interest in in-patient rehabilitation immediately following hospital admission for exacerbation. Unfortunately there is little published evidence to support the practice. Studies in this area are difficult to conduct but would be valuable. Peripheral muscle deconditioning occurs rapidly following admission (34) and there is evidence that transcutaneous electrical neuromuscular stimulation may reverse this process (35), although further prospective trials are required.

Hospital outpatient rehabilitation

Most programmes are carried out on an outpatient basis, as reflected in the Cochrane review of rehabilitation and other successful descriptions (36). Some in-patient programmes are followed by outpatient attendance. Advantages of hospital-based services include the convenience of transport links, the availability of trained personnel, the security of safety facilities and the economy of scale. From the health care providers' perspective, they are the most efficient and cost-effective option. Disadvantages include accessibility and saturation of service provision as the demand for services increases.

Community and home-based rehabilitation

Most pulmonary rehabilitation could be conducted at a community centre close to the patient's home (community-based) or at home. Some trials described as 'home-based' were actually home care community studies (37) or a mixture of local physiotherapy practice and home training (38). Several studies have demonstrated benefit from unsupervised and supervised home training (20, 27, 39). One major home study failed to show benefit when restricted to severely disabled patients (40). Rehabilitation may be provided directly from the primary care centres without referral to a specialist centre. Two pilot studies have noted the same short-term benefits as conventional hospital-based programmes (41–42).

Comparisons between settings

Similar benefits in exercise performance and health status have been described in all the settings. The content of a rehabilitation programme appears to be more important in determining success than the setting. Two studies have made direct comparisons between settings. In the first, hospital outpatient rehabilitation was compared with home rehabilitation and a control group (24). Somewhat surprisingly, the home-based group had more prolonged benefit in exercise performance. The authors argued that home-based training might, in context, have a more enduring effect. In another study, more disabled patients with COPD were offered home training while the less disabled patients had hospital outpatient therapy (40). In this case, the home-based treatment was ineffective compared with the hospital rehabilitation, but this was not a true comparison of settings. So far the literature has failed to demonstrate conclusively the benefits of one setting over another. For the present, the cost-effectiveness of outpatient or community-based rehabilitation is likely to make them the most attractive options.

PATIENT SELECTION, ASSESSMENT AND EXERCISE PRESCRIPTION

Selection

The success of a rehabilitation programme depends, at least in part, upon the selection of patients. Most patients have an established diagnosis of chronic respiratory disease, usually but not exclusively, COPD. The American and British Thoracic Society statements suggest that individuals should be considered for rehabilitation when they are adversely effected by their lung disease (2, 4). This is most frequently judged to be a perceived reduction in exercise capacity, as might be reflected in their Medical Research Council Dyspnoea score (43). The

aims of rehabilitation extend beyond improving exercise tolerance and so it may be important to consider other factors such as depression, coping skills and individual health status. Inclusion criteria for rehabilitation are quite broad. Exclusion criteria are significant orthopaedic or neurological problems that reduce mobility, poorly controlled coexisting medical problems, such as cardiovascular or psychiatric conditions, and recent events such as myocardial infarction. Some centres disqualify current smokers. Age is not an exclusion factor (44) but poorly motivated patients do not do so well. The timing of rehabilitation for maximum impact may be important to secure the agreement of the patient. However, there is little scientific exploration of this area.

Pre-rehabilitation assessment

The assessment of patients should broadly follow measures of impairment, activity limitation and activity participation.

ASSESSMENT OF IMPAIRMENT

Spirometry
Simple spirometry is largely irrelevant as a selection mechanism, except to define the population and, in some countries, to categorize severity (45). Recently there has been interest in the measurement of dynamic hyperinflation (46, 47) to identify patients with ventilatory limitation who may require a different approach to exercise retraining.

Secondary measures of impairment
Nutritional status and peripheral muscle function are useful outcome measures. Reduced muscle strength has been repeatedly identified in patients with COPD (48). Preserved peripheral muscle strength may indicate a reduced likelihood of a positive benefit following exercise training (49). Body mass index (BMI) is a basic measure of nutritional status; more complex measures include fat-free mass. Nutritionally depleted patients can be referred to a dietician for support. Rehabilitation seems to be effective even in those with a low BMI (50).

ASSESSMENT OF ACTIVITY LIMITATION

The gold standard measure of disability is the laboratory-based incremental or constant workload exercise test. Less technically demanding tests include the 6-min walk test (6-MWT) (51), the incremental and endurance shuttle-walk test (52, 53) and treadmill-based walking tests (54).

The 6-MWT is simple to perform (55) in a corridor or on a treadmill. During both tests, patients choose their own speed of walking and can stop or slow down. Alternatives to self-paced tests are the shuttle-walk tests. Both the incremental and endurance shuttle-walk tests are conducted around an elliptical 10 m course, with the speed of walking dictated by pre-recorded signals. The incremental shuttle-walk test requires the patient to walk at increasing speeds, whilst the endurance speed is a constant work rate test; the load (speed) is set by performance on the incremental test. The 6-MWT, incremental and endurance shuttle-walk tests have been shown to be sensitive to change after a course of rehabilitation (28, 29, 53). The incremental shuttle-walk test appears to induce a similar response to the symptom-limited laboratory-based exercise test (56). There are no suggested upper or lower levels of performance that would exclude the individuals from rehabilitation and a wide rage of values for both tests has been reported in the literature.

Adjuncts to field walking tests include measures of heart rate (usually by a short-range telemetry device), oxygen saturation (simple pulse oximeter) and subjective evaluation of breathlessness. Self-reported measures of breathlessness could be made at rest and at the end of exercise. A recent national statement on rehabilitation suggested that patients on grades 3–5 of the MRC Dyspnoea Scale are most appropriate for rehabilitation (57). Measures of breathlessness during or immediately after an exercise test need to be quick and simple to administer. The two most commonly employed are a visual analogue scale and the Borg Breathlessness scale (58).

ASSESSMENT OF HEALTH STATUS

Assessment of health status should be included in all rehabilitation programmes. Generic questionnaires such as the Short Form 36 (SF-36; 59) are often used. Disease-specific questionnaires focus on domains specific to a particular disease that will influence health status. The St George's Respiratory Questionnaire (SGRQ) (60) and the Chronic Respiratory Questionnaire (CRQ) are valid and sensitive to change (61). The SGRQ is self-administered. Until recently the CRQ was available only as an interviewer-administered questionnaire but a self-reported CRQ has now been validated and its sensitivity to rehabilitation established (62, 63). Both the SGRQ and the CRQ are interpretable, with their minimum clinically important difference (MCID) defined. Although measurements of depression are embedded in the generic and disease-specific questionnaires, many centres include additional measures such as the Hospital Depression and Anxiety Scale as well as the Psychosocial Adjustment to Illness Scale – Self Report (64). Evidence supports a reduction of anxiety and depression post-rehabilitation (29).

ACTIVITIES OF DAILY LIVING

Completion of domestic activities can be assessed by questionnaire, although some questionnaires have their origins in health care of the elderly and they frequently have a ceiling effect such that they may be insensitive to change for patients with COPD. Like the health status measures, components of activities may be assessed in segments of questionnaires that reflect the impact of symptoms on activities. Choices include the Pulmonary Functional Status and Dyspnoea Questionnaire (65), the London Chest Activities of Daily Living scale (66) and the Canadian Occupational Performance Measure (67). Activity monitors have also been used to describe domestic physical activity (68). Additional outcomes could include measures of cognitive function and motivation.

IDENTIFYING A CLINICALLY IMPORTANT DIFFERENCE

Statistically significant improvements in a particular outcome do not necessarily reflect a clinically important improvement. Redelmeier et al. (69) identified the MCID for the 6-MWT to be 54 m. Interestingly, a recent meta-analysis showed that the weighted mean difference was lower than the identified important difference at 49 m for the 23 randomized controlled trials included (8). The MCID has also been identified for the SGRQ and the CRQ. Troosters et al. (49) also nominated a 10-point improvement in the CRQ and a 25 per cent improvement in the 6-MWT as arbitrary indicators of success. This latter study suggested that patients with a ventilatory limit and higher measures of peripheral muscle strength were less likely to benefit from rehabilitation. However, while minimum important differences can be calculated for aggregate data, it is not known how the MCID can be interpreted for individual improvement.

Exercise prescription

Lower limb aerobic exercise is mandatory for patients with COPD in order to improve exercise capacity and health status. For healthy individuals, the exercise prescription is based on the relationship between external work and heart rate. For patients with COPD, as this relationship is not linear, the prescription is based upon exercise testing, to identify a training load that corresponds to 60–80 per cent of peak oxygen consumption. Exercise can be on a cycle ergometer, a treadmill or simply by free walking. The optimum profile of the training programme is less clear, with both continuous exercise and interval training being used. Training should be performed at least five times per week for 30 min (including home exercise), in sessions that are supervised and unsupervised, although entirely unsupervised exercise may be less effective than a supervised programme (7).

UPPER LIMB TRAINING

Although it is generally assumed that upper limb training is important for improving the functional abilities of patients with COPD, this has been difficult to establish in the literature. Upper limb function may be relatively well preserved in patients with COPD (70). Upper limb training is usually delivered as a functional activity, e.g. raising and lowering a pole for a set period of time, strength training, using weights to improve peripheral muscle strength, or as an endurance activity using an upper limb cycle ergometer.

RESPIRATORY MUSCLE TRAINING

Inspiratory muscle function may be reduced in COPD, although in many centres measurements beyond inspiratory muscle strength are not routinely included at initial assessment. A recent meta-analysis concluded that respiratory muscle training improved respiratory muscle strength and endurance but failed to have significant benefits on functional exercise capacity (71). There may be an important role for this type of training in pre-selected patients who have demonstrable reductions in respiratory muscle strength. Further research is required to clarify the role of this form of training.

STRENGTH TRAINING

This directly addresses peripheral muscle weakness, which is believed to be an important factor in the disability associated with the disease. Strength training requires the identification of an appropriate training load and graduated training programme. Recently, successful regimes have been described in the literature (72, 73). Equipment employed can range from sophisticated multigyms to simple free weights.

EDUCATION

The educational content of a comprehensive pulmonary rehabilitation programme is designed around the individualized needs of the patient, with patients having differing educational, functional, nutritional and psychological requirements. Education can be complex as it also involves addressing co-morbidities, including issues such as memory, that require strategies to help patients remember what is learned. Staff must be skilled in communicating with patients with complex pathology and varying learning needs. The programme length allows for frequent observations of patients and many opportunities to understand the needs of both patients and their families.

Learning theories

Teaching strategies used in pulmonary rehabilitation (74) should consider cultural, educational, emotional, cognitive and physical characteristics of the patient population. Whilst the benefits of education appear obvious, patients with chronic conditions require self-care skills to deal with their ongoing problems. Recent evidence has noted that self-management skills can reduce hospital admissions for exacerbations, hospital admissions for other health problems as well as emergency room and unscheduled health care provider visits (75). Changes in behaviour require an understanding of the diversity of patients' learning styles. Whereas education alone does not ensure a change in behaviour, it does help patients make appropriate decisions about their health. The education process also provides a supportive bonding environment (76).

Educational topics

The educational opportunities provided in programmes are both formal and informal. The educational components of rehabilitation programmes generally contain the topics identified in Box 18.1. The major purpose of education in pulmonary rehabilitation is to foster self-management. Patients who integrate the educational information can assume more responsibility for their health care and communicate important changes in their condition to their health care provider in a more timely fashion.

Box 18.1   Education topics for a pulmonary rehabilitation programme

- Anatomy and normal function of the lung
- Pathophysiology of lung disease
- Medications
- Oxygen
- Prevention and control of respiratory infections
- Breathing strategies
- Bronchial hygiene
- Role and benefits of exercise
- Energy conservation
- Symptom management, dyspnoea, fatigue
- Nutrition
- Coping with chronic lung disease
- End-of-life planning
- Panic control
- Travel
- Sexuality
- Staying healthy

Anatomy and normal function of the lung
This is necessary for patients to understand their condition. Being aware of the role of mucus production and ciliary clearance helps patients to understand why sputum colour and characteristics such as quantity and viscosity are used to monitor for infection.

Pathophysiology of lung disease
An explanation of the pathophysiology of bronchitis, emphysema and asthma is helpful, especially the role of smoking in the development of COPD. Misconceptions about the lack of benefit of smoking cessation after COPD has developed can be discouraging.

Medication
Rehabilitation sessions offer multiple opportunities to observe the technique and frequency of medication use. Discussions regarding the common categories of medications, their actions and side-effects, as well as how to select the best delivery system, provide opportunities to clarify misconceptions and enhance medication effectiveness.

Oxygen is discussed as a therapeutic modality with emphasis on the indications for supplemental oxygen, how to accommodate the equipment and how to maintain an active lifestyle while receiving oxygen therapy. Given the variety of oxygen systems and equipment (liquid oxygen, oxygen-conserving devices, etc.) the rehabilitation staff should be well versed in which oxygen delivery systems are available in their area.

Exacerbation management
Exacerbation management can be optimized if the patients know when to seek help. Learning to communicate with their provider is critical to successful prevention. Encouraging patients to recognize the presence of infection (yellow or green sputum production, increase in sputum production, etc.) is important. Some patients are unable to make decisions about

their condition, in which case very specific, but simple, instructions are provided.

Breathing strategies

Breathing strategies such as pursed lip breathing and diaphragmatic breathing are thought to relieve breathlessness, although the clinical evidence of the effectiveness of diaphragmatic breathing remains to be shown (77). In one review, only six out of 42 reports on diaphragmatic breathing noted symptom benefit (78) and only 10 identified physiological changes. Many patients spontaneously breathe with pursed lips. Breathing retraining has recently been shown to be effective in asthmatic patients with dysfunctional breathing (79). Other approaches to reduce breathlessness on exertion include the use of a wheeled walking aid (80). Breathing strategies are incorporated into panic control, demonstrating how slow, controlled breathing can allow patients to be 'in control' of their breathing.

Bronchial hygiene

Bronchial hygiene usually refers to facilitating mobilization of sputum. Increasing fluid intake, medications, cough manoeuvres, cough-enhancing devices, or postural drainage, percussion and vibration can enhance mobilization. Not all patients with COPD require assistance with expectoration.

Role and benefits of physical exercise

Exercise is essential but this is not always obvious to the dyspnoeic patient who elects to limit activities to avoid dyspnoea. Understanding the importance of continuing to exercise after the intensive phase of the programme is important. Many facilities provide a less intense, once or twice a week, maintenance programme.

Energy conservation

Energy conservation techniques apply breathing strategies and ergonomics to activities of daily living. Such strategies reduce rushing and breath-holding as well as encouraging planned activities.

Nutrition

A dietician or nutritionist familiar with the needs of pulmonary patients can provide nutritional content. Strategies take into account the energy demands of breathing in pulmonary patients and the best approaches to healthy nutrition. Within any group there will be patients who are obese and also those with nutritional depletion. Each patient will require individual advice.

Coping with chronic lung disease

Coping is important for patients and care providers, being best taught by individuals with skills in psychology and social work.

End-of-life planning

Pulmonary rehabilitation is an ideal setting for the discussion of advance directives. Both patients and health care providers appreciate discussing end-of-life decision-making and communicating specific directives to their primary care provider (81).

Travel

Emphasis is placed on ways of adapting travel plans and anticipating events, to avoid patients' fear of becoming ill away from their provider as well as self-imposed isolation and anxiety. Patients often do not realize that travelling with oxygen is possible. The goal is to support patients in maximizing their travel patterns. Written advice is available from several sources (82, 83).

Sexuality

The rehabilitation programme can offer education about the impact of lung disease on sexual performance and ways to decrease dyspnoea during sexual activity. Recommendations can include using an inhaled bronchodilator prior to sex, using oxygen during sex (if oxygen is indicated during exercise), assuming non-dominant positions, or even a water bed (84).

PROGRAMME DURATION

The objective of a pulmonary rehabilitation programme is to produce an improvement in disability that is sustained by a lasting change in lifestyle. Rehabilitation is a relatively expensive therapy that is still not widely available, so it is important for the process to be as efficient and cost-effective as possible. The duration of the programme is an important determination of cost and capacity. Obviously the length of a programme has to be sufficient to achieve a lasting training effect and deliver the educational programme. Successful outpatient programmes have been described with durations varying from 4 to 78 weeks, with few comparisons of programme durations or the rate of improvement during the programme. Since published trials have similar short- and long-term results, it appears that once a minimum threshold has been achieved, the total duration of the programme may not be critical. Training programmes that build up gradually will obviously take longer to have an effect. In one report, improvements continued beyond 12 weeks (28), and in others, lengthened programmes did not provide additional benefit (85). The issue of cost-effectiveness is important to any consideration of longer programmes (86).

Improvements in exercise performance and health status may not occur concurrently (87), with the gains in exercise performance preceding the improvements in health status. Therefore current recommendations suggest that an intensive outpatient programme in excess of 6 weeks is associated with significant sustainable benefits. The optimum duration may even turn out to be less than this.

STAFFING AND REIMBURSEMENT

A programme of pulmonary rehabilitation is delivered by a multidisciplinary team. Minimum staff requirements include a medical director, programme coordinator and a pulmonary rehabilitation specialist, with the last two roles being combined in some instances. The medical director should be a licensed physician able to assume responsibility for all medical aspects of the programme, to develop and evaluate the treatment plan

16. Engstrom CP, Persson LO, Larsson S, Sullivan M. Long-term effects of a pulmonary rehabilitation programme in outpatients with chronic obstructive pulmonary disease: a randomized controlled study. *Scand J Rehab Med* 1999; **31**: 207–13.

●17. Goldstein RS, Gort EH, Stubbing D *et al*. Randomised controlled trial of respiratory rehabilitation. *Lancet* 1994; **344**: 1394–7.

18. Jones DT, Thomson RJ, Sears MR. Physical exercise and resistive breathing training in severe chronic airways obstruction – are they effective? *Eur J Respir Dis* 1985; **67**: 159–66.

19. Lake FR, Henderson K, Briffa T *et al*. Upper-limb and lower-limb exercise training in patients with chronic airflow obstruction. *Chest* 1990; **97**: 1077–82.

20. McGavin CR, Gupta SP, Lloyd EL, McHardy GJ. Physical rehabilitation for the chronic bronchitic: results of a controlled trial of exercises in the home. *Thorax* 1977; **32**: 307–11.

21. Ringbaek TJ, Broendum E, Hemmingsen L *et al*. Rehabilitation of patients with chronic obstructive pulmonary disease. Exercise twice a week is not sufficient! *Respir Med* 2000; **94**: 150–4.

22. Simpson K, Killian K, McCartney N *et al*. Randomised controlled trial of weightlifting exercise in patients with chronic airflow limitation. *Thorax* 1992; **47**: 70–5.

23. Strijbos JH, Koeter GH, Meinesz AF. Home care rehabilitation and perception of dyspnea in chronic obstructive pulmonary disease (COPD) patients. *Chest* 1990; **97**: 109S–110S.

24. Strijbos JH, Postma DS, van Altena R *et al*. A comparison between an outpatient hospital-based pulmonary rehabilitation program and a home-care pulmonary rehabilitation program in patients with COPD. A follow-up of 18 months. *Chest* 1996; **109**: 366–72.

25. Reardon J, Awad E, Normandin E *et al*. The effect of comprehensive outpatient pulmonary rehabilitation on dyspnea. *Chest* 1994; **105**: 1046–52.

26. Güell R, Casan P, Belda J *et al*. Long-term effects of outpatient rehabilitation of COPD. A randomized trial. *Chest* 2000; **117**: 976–83.

27. Hernandez MT, Rubio TM, Ruiz FO *et al*. Results of a home-based training program for patients with COPD. *Chest* 2000; **118**: 106–14.

28. Troosters T, Gosselink R, Decramer M. Short- and long-term effects of outpatient rehabilitation in patients with chronic obstructive pulmonary disease: a randomized trial. *Am J Med* 2000; **109**: 207–12.

●29. Griffiths TL, Burr ML, Campbell IA *et al*. Results at 1 year of outpatient multidisciplinary pulmonary rehabilitation: a randomised controlled trial. *Lancet* 2000; **355**: 362–8.

30. Vallet G, Ahmaidi S, Serres I *et al*. Comparison of two training programmes in chronic airway limitation patients: standardized versus individualized protocols. *Eur Respir J* 1997; **10**: 114–22.

31. Clini E, Foglio K, Bianchi L *et al*. In-hospital short-term training program for patients with chronic airway obstruction. *Chest* 2001; **120**: 1500–5.

32. Fuchs-Climent D, Le Gallais D, Varray A *et al*. Quality of life and exercise tolerance in chronic obstructive pulmonary disease: effects of a short and intensive inpatient rehabilitation program. *Am J Phys Med Rehab* 1999; **78**: 330–5.

33. Stewart DG, Drake DF, Robertson C *et al*. Benefits of an inpatient pulmonary rehabilitation program: a prospective analysis. *Arch Phys Med Rehabil* 2001; **82**: 347–52.

34. Spruit MA, Gosselink R, Troosters T *et al*. Muscle force during an acute exacerbation in hospitalised patients with COPD and its relationship with CXCL8 and IGF-I. *Thorax* 2003; **58**: 752–6.

●35. Bourjeily-Habr G, Rochester CL, Palermo F *et al*. Randomised controlled trial of transcutaneous electrical muscle stimulation of the lower extremities in patients with chronic obstructive pulmonary disease. *Thorax* 2002; **57**: 1045–9.

36. Finnerty JP, Keeping I, Bullough I, Jones J. The effectiveness of outpatient pulmonary rehabilitation in chronic lung disease: a randomized controlled trial. *Chest* 2001; **119**: 1705–10.

37. Cambach W, Chadwick-Straver RV, Wagenaar RC *et al*. The effects of a community-based pulmonary rehabilitation programme on exercise tolerance and quality of life: a randomized controlled trial. *Eur Respir J* 1997; **10**: 104–13.

38. Wijkstra PJ, van der Mark TW, Kraan J *et al*. Effects of home rehabilitation on physical performance in patients with chronic obstructive pulmonary disease (COPD). *Eur Respir J* 1996; **9**: 104–10.

39. Strijbos JH, Postma DS, van Altena R *et al*. Feasibility and effects of a home-care rehabilitation program in patients with chronic obstructive pulmonary disease. *J Cardiopulm Rehabil* 1996; **16**: 386–93.

●40. Wedzicha JA, Bestall JC, Garrod R *et al*. Randomized controlled trial of pulmonary rehabilitation in severe chronic obstructive pulmonary disease patients, stratified with the MRC dyspnoea scale. *Eur Respir J* 1998; **12**: 363–9.

41. Jones RC, Copper S, Riley O, Dobbs F. A pilot study of pulmonary rehabilitation in primary care. *Br J Gen Pract* 2002; **52**: 567–8.

42. Ward JA, Akers G, Ward DG *et al*. Feasibility and effectiveness of a pulmonary rehabilitation programme in a community hospital setting. *Br J Gen Pract* 2002; **52**: 539–42.

43. Cotes JE. Medical Research Council questionnaire on respiratory symptoms (1986). *Lancet* 1987; **2**: 1028.

44. Yohannes AM. Pulmonary rehabilitation and outcome measures in elderly patients with chronic obstructive pulmonary disease. *Gerontology* 2001; **47**: 241–5.

45. Pauwels RA, Buist AS, Ma P *et al*. Global strategy for the diagnosis, management, and prevention of chronic obstructive pulmonary disease: National Heart, Lung, and Blood Institute and World Health Organization Global Initiative for Chronic Obstructive Lung Disease (GOLD): executive summary. *Respir Care* 2001; **46**: 798–825.

46. Saey D, Debigare R, Leblanc P *et al*. Contractile leg fatigue after cycle exercise: a factor limiting exercise in patients with chronic obstructive pulmonary disease. *Am J Respir Crit Care Med* 2003; **168**: 425–30.

●47. O'Donnell DE, Revill SM, Webb KA. Dynamic hyperinflation and exercise intolerance in chronic obstructive pulmonary disease. *Am J Respir Crit Care Med* 2001; **164**: 770–7.

48. Gosselink R, Troosters T, Decramer M. Distribution of muscle weakness in patients with stable chronic obstructive pulmonary disease. *J Cardiopulm Rehabil* 2000; **20**: 353–60.

49. Troosters T, Gosselink R, Decramer M. Exercise training in COPD: how to distinguish responders from nonresponders. *J Cardiopulm Rehabil* 2001; **21**: 10–17.

50. Steiner MC, Barton RL, Singh SJ, Morgan MD. Nutritional enhancement of exercise performance in chronic obstructive pulmonary disease: a randomised controlled trial. *Thorax* 2003; **58**: 745–51.

51. Butland RJ, Pang J, Gross ER *et al*. Two-, six-, and 12-minute walking tests in respiratory disease. *Br Med J (Clin Res Ed)* 1982; **284**: 1607–8.

52. Singh SJ, Morgan MD, Scott S *et al*. Development of a shuttle walking test of disability in patients with chronic airways obstruction. *Thorax* 1992; **47**: 1019–24.

53. Revill SM, Morgan MD, Singh SJ *et al*. The endurance shuttle walk. A new field test for the assessment of endurance capacity in chronic obstructive pulmonary disease. *Thorax* 1999; **54**: 213–22.

54. Stevens D, Elpern E, Sharma K et al. Comparison of hallway and treadmill six-minute walk tests. Am J Respir Crit Care Med 1999; **160**: 1540–3.

◆55. ATS Statement. Guidelines for the six-minute walk test. Am J Respir Crit Care Med 2002; **166**: 111–17.

56. Onorati P, Antonucci R, Valli G et al. Non-invasive evaluation of gas exchange during a shuttle walking test vs. a 6-min walking test to assess exercise tolerance in COPD patients. Eur J Appl Physiol 2003; **89**: 331–6.

57. BTS Standards of Care Subcommittee on Pulmonary Rehabilitation. Pulmonary rehabilitation. Thorax 2001; **56**: 827–34.

58. Borg GA. Psychophysical bases of perceived exertion. Med Sci Sports Exerc 1982; **14**: 377–81.

59. Ware JE Jr, Sherbourne CD. The MOS 36-item short-form health survey (SF-36). I. Conceptual framework and item selection. Med Care 1992; **30**: 473–83.

60. Jones PW, Quirk FH, Baveystock CM, Littlejohns P. A self-complete measure of health status for chronic airflow limitation. The St George's Respiratory Questionnaire. Am Rev Respir Dis 1992; **145**: 1321–7.

61. Guyatt GH, Berman LB, Townsend M et al. A measure of quality of life for clinical trials in chronic lung disease. Thorax 1987; **42**: 773–8.

62. Williams JE, Singh SJ, Sewell L et al. Development of a self-reported Chronic Respiratory Questionnaire (CRQ-SR). Thorax 2001; **56**: 954–9.

63. Williams JE, Singh SJ, Sewell L, Morgan MD. Health status measurement: sensitivity of the self-reported Chronic Respiratory Questionnaire (CRQ-SR) in pulmonary rehabilitation. Thorax 2003; **58**: 515–18.

64. Morrow GR, Chiarello RJ, Derogatis LR. A new scale for assessing patients' psychosocial adjustment to medical illness. Psychol Med 1978; **8**: 605–10.

65. Lareau SC, Meek PM, Roos PJ. Development and testing of the modified version of the pulmonary functional status and dyspnea questionnaire (PFSDQ-M). Heart Lung 1998; **27**: 159–68.

66. Garrod R, Paul EA, Wedzicha JA. An evaluation of the reliability and sensitivity of the London Chest Activity of Daily Living Scale (LCADL). Respir Med 2002; **96**: 725–30.

67. Sewell 1 Singh SJ. The Canadian Occupational Performance Measure. Is it a reliable measure in clients with COPD? Br J Occup Ther 2001; **64**: 305–10.

68. Singh S, Morgan MD. Activity monitors can detect brisk walking in patients with chronic obstructive pulmonary disease. J Cardiopulm Rehabil 2001; **21**: 143–8.

69. Redelmeier DA, Bayoumi AM, Goldstein RS, Guyatt GH. Interpreting small differences in functional status: the six minute walk test in chronic lung disease patients. Am J Respir Crit Care Med 1997; **155**: 1278–82.

70. Franssen FM, Wouters EF, Baarends EM et al. Arm mechanical efficiency and arm exercise capacity are relatively preserved in chronic obstructive pulmonary disease. Med Sci Sports Exerc 2002; **34**: 1570–6.

71. Lotters F, van Tol B, Kwakkel G, Gosselink R. Effects of controlled inspiratory muscle training in patients with COPD. A meta-analysis. Eur Respir J 2002; **20**: 570–6.

72. Spruit MA, Gosselin R, Troosters T et al. Resistance versus endurance training in patients with COPD and peripheral muscle weakness. Eur Respir J 2002; **19**: 1072–8.

73. Ortega F, Toral J, Cejudo P et al. Comparison of effects of strength and endurance training in patients with chronic obstructive pulmonary disease. Am J Respir Crit Care Med 2002; **166**: 669–74.

74. Lareau SC, Insel KC. Education of patient and family. In: Hodgkin JE, Celli BR, Connors GL, eds. Pulmonary Rehabilitation. Philadelphia: Lippincott, Williams & Wilkins, 2000.

●75. Bourbeau J, Julien M, Maltais F et al. Reduction of hospital utilization in patients with chronic obstructive pulmonary disease: a disease-specific self-management intervention. Arch Intern Med 2003; **163**: 585–91.

76. Sassi-Dambron DE, Eakin EG, Ries AL, Kaplan RM. Treatment of dyspnea in COPD. A controlled clinical trial of dyspnea management strategies. Chest 1995; **107**: 724–9.

77. Gosselink RA, Wagenaar RC, Rijswijk H et al. Diaphragmatic breathing reduces efficiency of breathing in patients with chronic obstructive pulmonary disease. Am J Respir Crit Care Med 1995; **151**: 1136–42.

78. Cahalin LP, Braga M, Matsuo Y, Hernandez ED. Efficacy of diaphragmatic breathing in persons with chronic obstructive pulmonary disease: a review of the literature. J Cardiopulm Rehabil 2002; **22**: 7–21.

79. Thomas M, McKinley RK, Freeman E et al. Breathing retraining for dysfunctional breathing in asthma: a randomised controlled trial. Thorax 2003; **58**: 110–15.

80. Solway S, Brooks D, Lau L, Goldstein R. The short-term effect of a rollator on functional exercise capacity among individuals with severe COPD. Chest 2002; **122**: 56–65.

81. Heffner JE, Fahy B, Hilling L, Barbieri C. Attitudes regarding advance directives among patients in pulmonary rehabilitation. Am J Respir Crit Care Med 1996; **154**: 1735–40.

82. Breathin' Easy Travel Guide. Breathin' Easy: A Guide for Travellers with Pulmonary Disabilities. Online. http://www.oxygen4travel.com. Napa, CA: Breathin' Easy Travel Guide.

83. British Thoracic Society. Managing passengers with respiratory disease planning air travel: British Thoracic Society recommendations. Thorax 2002; **57**: 289–304.

84. Law C. Sexual health and the respiratory patient. Nurs Times 2001; **97**: XI–XII.

85. Criner GJ, Cordova FC, Furukawa S et al. Prospective randomized trial comparing bilateral lung volume reduction surgery to pulmonary rehabilitation in severe chronic obstructive pulmonary disease. Am J Respir Crit Care Med 1999; **160**: 2018–27.

●86. Griffiths TL, Phillips CJ, Davies S et al. Cost effectiveness of an outpatient multidisciplinary pulmonary rehabilitation programme. Thorax 2001; **56**: 779–84.

87. Green RH, Singh SJ, Williams J, Morgan MD. A randomised controlled trial of four weeks versus seven weeks of pulmonary rehabilitation in chronic obstructive pulmonary disease. Thorax 2001; **56**: 143–5.

88. American Association of Cardiovascular and Pulmonary Rehabilitation. Appendix B: Clinical Competency Guidelines for Pulmonary Rehabilitation. Guidelines for Pulmonary Rehabilitation Programs. Champaign, IL: AACPR, 2003.

89. Hoberty PD, Chiu CY, Hoberty RJ. Staffing exercise sessions in pulmonary rehabilitation. Respir Care 2001; **46**: 694–7.

90. Foglio K, Bianchi L, Bruletti G et al. Long-term effectiveness of pulmonary rehabilitation in patients with chronic airway obstruction. Eur Respir J 1999; **13**: 125–32.

91. Foglio K, Bianchi L, Ambrosino N. Is it really useful to repeat outpatient pulmonary rehabilitation programs in patients with chronic airway obstruction? A 2-year controlled study. Chest 2001; **119**: 1696–704.

92. Berry MJ, Rejeski WJ, Adair NE et al. A randomized, controlled trial comparing long-term and short-term exercise in patients with

chronic obstructive pulmonary disease. *J Cardiopulm Rehabil* 2003; **23**: 60–8.

93. Bowen JB, Votto JJ, Thrall RS *et al.* Functional status and survival following pulmonary rehabilitation. *Chest* 2000; **118**: 697–703.

◆94. American College of Sports Medicine. *Guidelines for Exercise Testing and Prescription*, 6th edn. Philidelphia: Lippincott, Williams & Wilkins, 2000.

95. Spence DP, Hay JG, Carter J *et al.* Oxygen desaturation and breathlessness during corridor walking in chronic obstructive pulmonary disease: effect of oxitropium bromide. *Thorax* 1993; **48**: 1145–50.

96. Garrod R, Paul EA, Wedzicha JA. Supplemental oxygen during pulmonary rehabilitation in patients with COPD with exercise hypoxaemia. *Thorax* 2000; **55**: 539–43.

97. Rooyackers JM, Dekhuijzen PN, van Herwaarden CL *et al.* Training with supplemental oxygen in patients with COPD and hypoxaemia at peak exercise. *Eur Respir J* 1997; **10**: 1278–84.

98. AACVPR Program Certification Committee. *Program Certification*. Online. http://www.aacvpr.org/certification/2002pulmonary.doc. Chicago, IL: AACVPR, 2003.

99. AACVPR. *Program Certification*. Online. http://www.aacvpr.org/certification/program_cert_action.cfm. Chicago, IL: AACVPR, 2003.

100. Weiner P, Azgad Y, Ganam R. Inspiratory muscle training combined with general exercise reconditioning in patients with COPD. *Chest* 1992; **102**: 1351–6.

101. Wijkstra PJ, van Altena R, Kraan J *et al.* Quality of life in patients with chronic obstructive pulmonary disease improves after rehabilitation at home. *Eur Respir J* 1994; **7**: 269–73.

19

Respiratory physiotherapy

RIK GOSSELINK

INTRODUCTION

Respiratory physiotherapy is relevant to the treatment of patients with acute and chronic lung disease, but also effective in patients with advanced neuromuscular disorders, or in patients admitted to major surgery and patients on the intensive care unit. Physiotherapy contributes to assessment and treatment of various aspects of respiratory disorders, such as airflow obstruction, alterations in ventilatory pump function and impaired exercise performance. In addition, physiotherapy aims to alleviate dyspnoea and improve quality of life. Since lack of compliance with treatment is a well-known problem in the prescription of techniques for airway clearance and the maintenance of the effects of exercise training after rehabilitation, physiotherapy also includes patient education. In this chapter, airway clearance techniques, breathing retraining, exercise training, and peripheral and respiratory muscle training in a variety of conditions affecting the respiratory system are discussed.

TECHNIQUES FOR AIRWAY CLEARANCE AND LUNG INFLATION

Hypersecretion and impaired mucociliary transport are important pathophysiological features of obstructive lung diseases like cystic fibrosis (CF) and chronic bronchitis as well as in patients with acute lung disease, i.e. atelectasis and pneumonia. Hypersecretion is associated with an increased rate of decline of pulmonary function and excess mortality in patients with chronic obstructive pulmonary disease (COPD) (1). In patients with more advanced neuromuscular disease, mucus retention and pulmonary complications significantly contribute to morbidity and mortality (2). Although a cause–effect relationship has not been proven in these conditions, improvement of

airway clearance is considered to be an important aim of treatment of these patients.

Mucus retention results from excessive mucus production or abnormal rheological properties, on the one hand, or impaired mucociliary function or cough clearance on the other. Pharmaceutical interventions and physical therapy are effective to enhance mucus transport by improving rheological properties of the mucus layer, stimulating ciliary action or utilization of compensatory physical mechanisms such as gravity, two-phase gas–liquid interaction, vibration, oscillation or airway compression. In a recent meta-analysis in patients with CF (3), it was concluded that the combined standard treatment of postural drainage, percussion and vibration resulted in significantly greater sputum expectoration compared with no treatment. No differences were observed between standard treatment and other treatment modalities. In patients with COPD and bronchiectasis, it was concluded in a recent Cochrane library review (4) that the combination of postural drainage, percussion and forced expiration improved airway clearance but not pulmonary function. There is certainly a need for further research to support or refute the use of physiotherapy aimed at improving bronchial hygiene.

Forced expiration

The concept of therapeutic forced expiratory manoeuvres is to enhance mucus transport with high airflow velocities. A higher airflow velocity makes mucus move to the central airways due to the interaction and energy transfer between the air stream and the mucus layer (two-phase gas–liquid interaction). The effectiveness of this transmission, and hence of mucus transport, depends on the thickness of the mucus layer and airflow velocity. A thicker mucus layer is easier to move as more kinetic energy is transmitted to it (5). Huffing and coughing and also, though to a lesser extent, ventilation at rest or during exercise induce higher airflow velocities which stimulate mucus transport significantly (6, 7). High expiratory flow rate and dynamic airway compression during forced expiratory manoeuvres accelerate the air stream velocity considerably. The combination of high expiratory force and low lung volume may cause extensive narrowing of the airways, up to the fourth generation, and thus high expiratory airflow velocities to expel mucus into the central airways. However, in patients with airway instability (pulmonary emphysema), forced expiratory manoeuvres may result in airway collapse and impair mucus transport. Patients with neuromuscular disorders often experience expiratory muscle weakness, and hence forced expiratory manoeuvres will be ineffective.

Forced expiratory manoeuvres, huffing and coughing are considered the cornerstone of airway clearance techniques and thus an essential part in every combination of treatment modalities. Although it is generally believed that mucus clearance techniques are only effective in patients with excessive hypersecretion, forced expiratory manoeuvres were also found to be effective in patients with unproductive coughing (7).

Huffing and coughing consist of a deep inspiration followed by a forced expiration, without and with glottis closure, respectively. During huffing, lower pleural pressures and peak flow rates were generated compared with coughing (8). However, both techniques have been shown to increase mucus clearance from central and intermediate lung zones (6–8). No differences were observed in overall mucus transport (6, 8), or in peripheral mucus clearance between huffing and coughing. The forced expiration technique (FET) combines huffing, coughing and diaphragmatic breathing and was recently expanded with deep breathing retraining and renamed to active cycle of breathing technique (ACBT). The autogenic drainage (AD) aims to enhance mucus transport in peripheral airways by forced expirations at low lung volumes. Expiratory force is significantly lower in AD than in ACBT and FET to prevent airway collapse, but none of these techniques has been shown to be superior. Airway collapse is a major risk during forced expiration in patients with airway instability and reduces mucus transport significantly. Indeed, manual chest wall compression during forced expiration decreased peak cough flow rate in patients with severe COPD (9). This was probably due to premature airway closure. Therefore, forced expiratory manoeuvres should be carefully adapted to altered pulmonary mechanics in patients with more severe airflow obstruction. The lack of association between tracheobronchial clearance and peak flow achieved during cough and FET implies that excessive attempts to achieve the highest flow rates are not necessary (7). Indeed, forced expirations also contribute to alterations in viscoelastic properties of the mucus layer. Repetitive strain on the mucus by repeated huffing or coughing reduces viscosity and promotes mucus transport.

In neuromuscular disease, the reduced expiratory muscle strength limits effective huffing and coughing. Manual assistance with chest wall compression enhances peak cough flow rate in patients with neuromuscular disease without scoliosis, but was not beneficial in patients with chest wall deformities (9). Mechanical insufflation and exsufflation and manually

assisted coughing are effective and safe to facilitate clearance of airway secretions (10). In addition, deep lung insufflation increases maximum insufflation capacity and peak cough flow in patients with progressive neuromuscular disease (9). Glossopharyngeal breathing (GPB) is also used to improve the efficacy of coughing in patients with neuromuscular disease and intact upper airway function. It has been shown that this technique increases vital capacity and thereby improves expiratory flow rates. Recently, GPB has once again been receiving attention as a treatment option in patients with high spinal cord injury (11).

Chest expansion and lung inflation

Mechanically ventilated patients are often, due to lack of consciousness, unable to perform forced expiratory manoeuvres effectively. Manual hyperinflation combined with chest wall compression during expiration ('bag squeezing') are frequently applied in clinical practice. However, controversy exists regarding the safety and effectiveness of the approach. In particular, the detrimental cardiovascular effects must be taken into consideration when applying manual hyperinflation (12). Its effectiveness in preventing pulmonary complications and pneumonia was questioned, but recent data provide some evidence that physiotherapy might indeed add to the prevention of ventilator-associated pneumonia (13).

Postoperative pulmonary complications after thoracic and abdominal surgery remain a major cause of morbidity and mortality. Prolonged hospitalization and intensive care stay may result. Evidence for the effectiveness of physiotherapy in preventing postoperative pulmonary complications after abdominal surgery is provided in randomized controlled trials (14). In addition, absence of preoperative physiotherapy was an independent factor associated with a higher risk on postoperative pulmonary complications in patients with lung resection (15). A meta-analysis confirmed the beneficial effect of physiotherapy on prevention of complications after abdominal surgery (16).

In addition to deep breathing retraining, coughing and early mobilization, positive expiratory pressure (PEP) mask breathing and incentive spirometry (IS) are provided to patients with the aim of reducing pulmonary complications. Although IS is widely used in clinical practice, it has not been shown to be of additional value after major abdominal, lung and cardiac surgery (17). After abdominal surgery, Hall et al. (18) concluded that IS was as effective as chest physiotherapy in both low- and high-risk patients. In thoracic surgery for lung or oesophageal resection, IS had no additional effect on recovery of pulmonary function, pulmonary complications and hospital stay (19).

Exercise

During exercise, increased ventilation and release of mediators in the airways may be effective in enhancing mucus transport (20). Indeed, increased mucus transport has been observed during exercise in healthy subjects and patients with chronic bronchitis (21), but it was less effective than conventional physiotherapy in patients with CF (22). During exercise combined with physiotherapy, significantly more sputum volume was expectorated than during physiotherapy alone (23).

Postural drainage and body position

During postural drainage, the major bronchi are positioned in a more vertical position to allow gravitational forces to promote mucus transport to the central airways. Postural drainage is usually combined with other treatment modalities. Studies investigating the efficacy of postural drainage and using radio-aerosol tracer assessment showed no additional improvement in mucus transport after postural drainage (24), but in patients with bronchiectasis and excessive mucus production, postural drainage alone enhanced mucus transport and expectoration (25).

Body position has also been shown to affect oxygenation. This effect has not always been acknowledged in clinical care. In patients with unilateral lung disease, the lateral decubitus position with the unaffected side down in general improves oxygenation (26). In patients with acute respiratory distress syndrome, the prone position increased arterial P_{O_2}. Alterations in ventilation/perfusion inequality have been suggested as the main reason for improved oxygenation in these body positions (27).

Percussion and vibration

Manual or mechanical percussion and vibration are based on the assumption of transmission of oscillatory forces to the bronchi. Although such oscillations are observed during bronchoscopy in the central airways, it is believed that absorption of the forces by air and lung parenchyma prevents transmission to smaller and intermediate airways. This probably explains the lack of additional effects on mucus transport of adding chest percussion and vibration to breathing retraining, postural drainage and coughing (28). Another explanation might be the frequency dependence of the effects of vibration and oscillation. The optimal frequency enhancing mucus transport appears to be around 12–17 Hz (29). However, clinical trials have not shown greater efficacy of high-frequency oscillation with a more optimal oscillation frequency compared with standard physiotherapy in patients with chronic bronchitis (30) and CF patients in stable condition (31) or hospitalized (32).

Positive expiratory pressure mask breathing and flutter breathing

In the early 1980s, PEP mask breathing was introduced to further improve physiotherapy treatment modalities that aim to increase mucus transport. Expiration against a resistance may prevent airway collapse and improve collateral ventilation. Indeed, Falk et al. (33) showed that the addition of this technique to forced expiration or postural drainage increased mucus expectoration in CF. Other investigators were unable

to show additional short-term effects on mucus transport in CF (34) or chronic bronchitis (35). However, it has been demonstrated that PEP therapy was superior to standard treatment in preserving pulmonary function in the long term (36).

Flutter breathing is the addition of a variable, oscillating expiratory pressure and airflow at the mouth to facilitate clearance of mucus. Although in patients with CF, Konstan et al. (37) observed a fivefold increase in expectorated mucus compared with cough or postural drainage, others were unable to find differences in expectoration (38). Sputum rheology was significantly altered during flutter breathing, but this did not result in an increased sputum volume (38).

BREATHING RETRAINING AND BODY POSITIONING

'Breathing retraining' is an all-embracing term for a range of techniques such as active expiration, pursed lips breathing, relaxation therapy, specific body positions, inspiratory muscle training (IMT) and diaphragmatic breathing. The aims of these exercises vary considerably and include the improvement of (regional) ventilation and gas exchange, amelioration of debilitating effects on the ventilatory pump, improvement of respiratory muscle function, decreasing dyspnoea and improvement of exercise tolerance and quality of life. In patients with COPD and asthma, breathing retraining is aimed at: (i) reducing dynamic hyperinflation of the rib cage; (ii) increasing strength and endurance of the respiratory muscles; and (iii) optimizing the pattern of thoraco-abdominal motion.

Breathing retraining to reduce dynamic hyperinflation of the rib cage

The idea of decreasing dynamic hyperinflation of the rib cage is based on the assumption that this intervention will result in the inspiratory muscles working over a more advantageous part of their length–tension relationship. Moreover, it is expected to decrease the elastic work of breathing, because the chest wall moves over a more favourable part of its pressure–volume curve. In this way, the workload on the inspiratory muscles should diminish, along with the sensation of dyspnoea. Several treatment strategies aim to reduce the hyperinflated chest wall.

RELAXATION EXERCISES

The rationale for relaxation exercises arises from the observation that hyperinflation in (partial) reversible airway obstruction is, at least in part, caused by an increased activity of the inspiratory muscles during expiration (39). This increased activity may continue even after recovery from an acute episode of airway obstruction, and hence contributes to the dynamic hyperinflation. However, hyperinflation in COPD is mainly due to altered lung mechanics (loss of elastic recoil pressure and air trapping) and is not associated with increased activity of inspiratory muscles during expiration. Renfoe (40) showed in COPD patients that progressive relaxation resulted in immediate decrease of heart rate, respiratory rate, anxiety and dyspnoea scores compared with a control group, but only respiratory rate dropped significantly over time. Gift *et al.* (41) observed similar improvements in a randomized controlled trial with relaxation with audiotapes in comparison to a control group. Significantly larger reductions in breathing rate, anxiety and dyspnoea compared with the control group were found. Kolaczkowski *et al.* (42) observed that the combination of relaxation exercises and manual compression of the thorax improved excursion of the thorax and oxygen saturation significantly. A positive trend towards a reduction of symptoms is apparent in applying relaxation exercises.

PURSED LIPS BREATHING

Pursed lips breathing aims to improve expiration both by its active and prolonged expiration through half-opened lips and by preventing airway collapse. Compared to spontaneous breathing, pursed lip breathing reduces respiratory rate, dyspnoea and P_aCO_2, and improves tidal volume and oxygen saturation in resting conditions (43, 44). However, its application during (treadmill) exercise did not improve blood gases (45).

Some COPD patients use the technique instinctively, while other patients do not. The changes in minute ventilation and gas exchange were not significantly related to the patients who reported subjective improvement of the sensation of dyspnoea. The 'symptom benefit patients' had a more marked increase of tidal volume and decrease of breathing frequency (45), while others reported a reduced elastic recoil pressure in symptom benefit patients (44). Breslin (43) observed, during pursed lip breathing, an increase in rib cage and accessory muscle recruitment during the entire breathing cycle, while the tension–time index of the diaphragmatic contraction decreased. These changes might have contributed to the decrease in dyspnoea sensation.

In conclusion, pursed lips breathing is found to be effective in improving gas exchange and reducing dyspnoea. COPD patients not adopting pursed lips breathing spontaneously show variable responses. Those patients with loss of elastic recoil pressure seem to benefit more from practising this technique during exertion and episodes of dyspnoea.

RIB CAGE MOBILIZATION TECHNIQUES

Mobilization of rib cage joints appears a specific aim for physiotherapy as the rib cage seems rigid in obstructive lung disease. However, after lung transplantation, without any mobilization of the rib cage, a significant reduction of hyperinflation is observed (46). The persistent hyperinflation after heart–lung transplantation in CF patients (47) and non-CF patients (46) might be a target for rib cage mobilization. In patients with COPD, however, the basis for such treatment seems weak as altered chest wall mechanics are related primarily to irreversible loss of elastic recoil and airway obstruction. Rib cage mobilization will not be effective in patients with COPD with altered pulmonary mechanics and is therefore not recommended.

Breathing retraining to improve respiratory muscle function

Reduced endurance and strength of the inspiratory muscles are frequently observed in chronic lung disease and neuromuscular disorders and contribute to dyspnoea, exercise limitation and probably respiratory failure. Improvement of respiratory muscle function is aimed at reducing the relative load on the muscles (the fraction of the actual pressure and the maximal pressure; $P_I/P_{I,max}$) and hence may contribute to reduce dyspnoea and increase the maximal sustained ventilatory capacity. This might also imply an improvement of exercise capacity in patients with ventilatory limitation during exercise. Breathing retraining and body positions aim to improve the length–tension relationship or geometry of the respiratory muscles (in particular of the diaphragm) or increase strength and endurance of the inspiratory muscles. According to the length–tension relationship, the output of the muscle increases when operating at a greater length, for the same neural input. At the same time the efficacy of the contraction in moving the rib cage improves. Also the piston-like movement of the diaphragm increases and enhances lung volume changes.

CONTRACTION OF THE ABDOMINAL MUSCLES DURING EXPIRATION

Contraction of the abdominal muscles during expiration lengthens the diaphragm, allowing it to operate close to its optimal length. In addition, active expiration will increase elastic recoil pressure of the diaphragm and the rib cage. The release of this pressure after relaxation of the expiratory muscles will assist the next inspiration. In healthy subjects, this mechanism is brought into play only with increased ventilation. However, in patients with severe COPD, contraction of abdominal muscles becomes invariably linked to resting breathing (48). Active expiration increases transdiaphragmatic pressure (P_{di}) and $P_{I,max}$. The additional effects of active expiration to exercise training in patients with severe COPD were studied by Casciari *et al.* (49). They observed a significant increase in maximum oxygen uptake during a bicycle ergometer test after a period of additional breathing retraining during a training programme on a treadmill, as compared with the treadmill programme without breathing retraining.

Although active expiration seems to improve inspiratory muscle function and is commonly observed in resting breathing and during exercise in COPD patients, the significance of abdominal muscle activity remains poorly understood (48).

BODY POSITION

Relief of dyspnoea is often experienced by patients in different body positions. Forward leaning has been shown to be very effective in COPD (50) and is probably the most adopted body position by patients with lung disease. The effect of this position seems not to be related to severity of airway obstruction, changes in minute ventilation or improved oxygenation (50). Hyperinflation and paradoxical abdominal movement were indeed related to relief of dyspnoea in the forward leaning position (50). Alternatively, forward leaning is associated with a significant reduction in EMG activity of the scalenes and sternomastoid muscles, increase in transdiaphragmatic pressure and significant improvement in thoraco-abdominal movements (50). From these studies it was concluded that the subjective improvement of dyspnoea in patients with COPD was the result of the more favourable position of the diaphragm on its length–tension curve. In addition, forward leaning with arm support allows accessory muscles (pectoralis minor and major) to contribute significantly to rib cage elevation. Banzett *et al.* (51) showed that this position enhanced ventilatory capacity in healthy subjects. The same holds for the forward leaning position with head support, which allows the accessory neck muscles to assist inspiration.

ABDOMINAL BELT

The 'abdominal belt' was developed as an aid to support diaphragmatic function. Early studies in patients with emphysema reported an increase in the excursion of the diaphragm and a reduction of the activity of accessory muscles during application of the abdominal belt. However, its application in patients with severe COPD significantly shortened endurance time on a bicycle ergometer (52).

The abdominal belt is also used in patients with spinal cord injury, in whom it improves vital capacity (53). However, increases in expiratory flow and expiratory pressures during abdominal strapping were not consistently observed in these patients (54).

RESPIRATORY MUSCLE TRAINING

Recent studies in patients with COPD have shown natural adaptations of the diaphragm at cellular (increased proportion of type I fibres) and subcellular (shortening of the sarcomeres and increased concentration of mitochondria) levels, contributing to greater resistance to fatigue and to better functional muscle behaviour (55). Despite these cellular adaptations, both functional inspiratory muscle strength and inspiratory muscle endurance are compromised in COPD. IMT may further enhance these spontaneous adaptations.

Three types of training, i.e. 'inspiratory resistive training' (IRT), threshold loading (ITL) and 'normocapnic hyperpnoea' (NCH), are practised at the present time. During NCH the patient is asked to ventilate maximally for 15–20 min. In a randomized controlled trial, NCH with this new device was shown to enhance respiratory muscle endurance and exercise capacity as well as quality of life in COPD patients (56). During 'inspiratory resistive breathing' the patient inspires through a mouthpiece and adapter with an adjustable diameter or 'threshold loading'. Most studies observed that breathing against an inspiratory load (at least 30 per cent $P_{I,max}$) increased maximal inspiratory pressure and endurance capacity of the inspiratory muscles (see overview). A recent study in COPD patients showed significant increases in the proportion of type I fibres and size of type II fibres in the external intercostals after IMT (57). Also dyspnoea (58) and nocturnal

desaturation time (59) decreased, while exercise performance tended to improve. IMT in addition to exercise training has been shown to improve exercise capacity more than exercise training alone (60, 61). The additional effect of IMT on exercise performance seemed to be related to the presence of inspiratory muscle weakness. At present there are no data to support resistive or threshold loading as the training method of choice. Threshold loading enhances velocity of inspiratory muscle shortening (62). This might be an important additional effect as this shortens inspiratory time and increases time for exhalation and relaxation.

It is concluded that, in COPD, well-controlled IMT improves inspiratory muscle function, resulting in an additional decrease of dyspnoea and nocturnal desaturation time, and potentially in improvement of exercise capacity in patients with inspiratory muscle weakness. Training intensity should be at least 30 per cent of the maximal inspiratory pressure for 30 min/day.

In tetraplegic patients respiratory muscle training has also been shown to enhance inspiratory muscle function, dyspnoea and exercise performance (63, 64). In patients with neuromuscular disease, respiratory muscle dysfunction is more complex and dependent on the precise disease and its stage. It seems that such patients, with more than 25 per cent of the predicted value of pulmonary function left, are still trainable (65). Although inspiratory muscle function is commonly affected in these diseases, expiratory muscle function is often more impaired in tetraplegia and multiple sclerosis. Expiratory muscle training has also been shown to be beneficial in the latter condition. In the long term, the progressive nature of most neuromuscular diseases affecting the primary function of the muscle probably impedes the beneficial effects of training.

Breathing retraining to optimize thoraco-abdominal movements

Alterations of chest wall motion are common in patients with asthma and COPD. Several studies have described an increase in rib cage contribution to chest wall motion and/or asynchrony between rib cage and abdominal motion in these patients (66, 67). The mechanisms underlying these alterations are not fully elucidated, but appear to be related to the degree of airflow obstruction, hyperinflation of the rib cage, changes in diaphragmatic function and increased contribution of accessory inspiratory muscles to chest wall motion. Indeed, increased firing frequency of single motor units of scalene and parasternal muscles (68), as well as the diaphragm (69, 70), were observed in COPD patients compared with age-matched control subjects. In contrast to what is often suggested, diaphragm displacement and shortening during tidal breathing were not different in COPD patients compared with healthy subjects (71). This indicates that the diaphragm displacement (actively and passively) still contributes to tidal breathing.

Activity of accessory muscles is positively associated with the sensation of dyspnoea, whereas diaphragm activity is negatively related to dyspnoea sensation (72). Consequently, diaphragmatic breathing, or slow and deep breathing, is commonly applied in physiotherapy practice attempting to correct abnormal chest wall motion, decrease work of breathing, accessory muscle activity and dyspnoea, increase efficiency of breathing and improve distribution of ventilation.

DIAPHRAGMATIC BREATHING

During diaphragmatic breathing the patient is told to move the abdominal wall predominantly during inspiration and to reduce upper rib cage motion. This aims to improve chest wall motion and the distribution of ventilation, to decrease the energy cost of breathing, the contribution of rib cage muscles and dyspnoea and to improve exercise performance.

All studies show that during diaphragmatic breathing, COPD patients are able voluntarily to change the breathing pattern to more abdominal movement and less thoracic excursion (73, 74). However, diaphragmatic breathing can be accompanied by increased asynchronous and paradoxical breathing movements, while no permanent changes of the breathing pattern are observed (73, 74). Although abdominal and thoracic movement clearly changed, no changes in ventilation distribution were observed (74). In several studies, an increased work of breathing, enhanced oxygen cost of breathing and reduced mechanical efficiency of breathing have been found (75). In addition, dyspnoea worsened during diaphragmatic breathing in patients with severe COPD (75), whereas pulmonary function and exercise capacity remained unaltered.

In conclusion, there is no evidence from controlled studies to support the use of diaphragmatic breathing in COPD patients.

SLOW AND DEEP BREATHING

Since, for a given minute ventilation, alveolar ventilation improves when breathing at a slower rate and higher tidal volume, this type of breathing is encouraged for patients with impaired alveolar ventilation. Several authors have reported a significant drop of respiratory frequency, and a significant rise of tidal volume and P_aO_2 during imposed low-frequency breathing at rest in patients with COPD (see section on 'Pursed lips breathing', p. 189). Slow and deep breathing retraining as part of pulmonary rehabilitation during exercise training may add to more efficient breathing during exercise and hence reduce the ventilatory demand and dyspnoea (76).

Unfortunately, these effects are counterbalanced by an increased work of breathing. Indeed, Bellemare and Grassino (77) demonstrated that for a given minute ventilation, fatigue of the diaphragm developed earlier during slow and deep breathing. This breathing pattern resulted in a significant increase in the relative force of contraction of the diaphragm ($P_{di}/P_{di,max}$), forcing it into the critical zone of muscle fatigue.

In summary, slow and deep breathing improves breathing efficiency and oxygen saturation at rest. A similar tendency has been observed during exercise, but needs further research. However, this type of breathing is associated with a breathing pattern that is prone to induce respiratory muscle fatigue.

EXERCISE TRAINING AND PERIPHERAL MUSCLE TRAINING

Impaired exercise tolerance is a common finding in patients with respiratory disease. Reduced exercise capacity shows only a weak relation to impairment of lung function. Other factors, such as peripheral and respiratory muscle weakness and deconditioning, are now recognized as important contributors to reduced exercise tolerance. Recent randomized controlled studies on the efficacy of pulmonary rehabilitation reported significant improvements in maximal exercise capacity, walking distance and endurance capacity after pulmonary rehabilitation. In addition, improved quality of life and reduced symptoms were observed (78).

Although these programmes are comprehensive, most authors consider exercise training a mandatory part of the programme. Endurance training involves a larger muscle mass working at moderate intensity for a longer period of time. This is discussed elsewhere in more detail. Strength training, on the other hand, involves a smaller muscle mass working at high intensity for a shorter period. Resistance training is performed as three series of eight repetitions each at 70 per cent of the one repetition maximum three times a week. Randomized controlled trials in COPD patients found that weight-lifting resulted in significant increases in peripheral muscle performance, endurance exercise capacity and quality of life (79). It remains unclear whether either endurance muscle training or strength training, or a combination of the two, is to be preferred. In COPD patients with peripheral muscle weakness, strength training was shown to be equally as effective as endurance training on exercise capacity and quality of life (80). The combination of strength and endurance training improved peripheral muscle strength, exercise performance and quality of life in COPD patients with muscle weakness compared with either endurance training or strength training alone (81).

Recently, neuromuscular stimulation of lower limb muscles in patients with severe COPD has been shown to improve muscle strength, exercise performance and quality of life (82).

Exercise in the ICU

A primary role of the physiotherapist in the ICU is to maintain or restore the patient's ability to be 'upright and moving' (see Dean and Ross [83]). Mobilization enhances oxygen transport, muscle function and coordination of movement and is prescribed according to type, intensity, duration and frequency. Compared with the medically stable patient, mobilization for the less stable patient requires particularly close monitoring to assess readiness for changes in the prescription. For example, in the critically ill, the intensity of the stimulus from orthostatic stress from body positioning and exercise stress needs to be minimal at first. In addition, the duration of a mobilization session is reduced, and the frequency increased. The course of treatment often changes quickly during the course of recovery from critical illness.

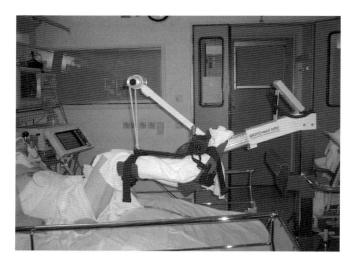

Figure 19.1 *Device for active and passive cycling in bedridden patients (Motomed Letto Enraf Nonius The Netherlands).*

Physiotherapy has an essential role in interventions to prevent and treat joint contractures and muscle atrophy (84, 85). Treatment modalities to prevent joint contractures are active or passive motion and splinting. It is not known for how long, over what range of motion or how frequently passive mobilizations should be performed. In clinical practice, one session a day of five to 10 repetitions of full range of motion (active or otherwise passive) is applied in uninjured joints. Twice daily might be necessary in injured extremities. Splinting is often used in patients with burn injury, trauma conditions and neurological conditions. From animal studies it is known that 30 min of stretch per day is sufficient to prevent loss of range of motion during immobilization (86).

Prevention of muscle atrophy is best obtained with active muscle contractions (87). Because some ICU patients are unable to perform voluntary contractions, passive stretching and electrical stimulation are suggested as alternative strategies. Passive stretching for at least 30 min/day has been shown to prevent loss of muscle weight and sarcomeres in series in an animal model (86). Dynamic intermittent stretching (continuous passive motion, Fig. 19.1) for 3 h/day prevented fibre atrophy and protein loss compared with twice-a-day passive stretching of less than 5 min per session (88). Indeed, electrical stimulation of the quadriceps, in addition to active limb mobilization, enhances muscle strength and decreases the number of days needed to transfer from bed to chair (89).

Key points

- Respiratory physiotherapy enhances airway clearance in respiratory disease associated with hypersecretion.
- Forced expiratory techniques are the most important treatment modalities to improve short-term airway clearance.

- Respiratory muscle training enhances strength, endurance and symptoms in various conditions associated with respiratory muscle weakness.
- Exercise training and peripheral muscle training are effective components of rehabilitation of patients with pulmonary disease.

REFERENCES

1. Vestbo J, Prescott E, Lange P, Copenhagen City Heart Study Group. Association of chronic mucus hypersecretion with FEV_1 decline and chronic obstructive pulmonary disease morbidity. *Am J Respir Crit Care Med* 1996; **153**: 1530–5.
2. Lieberman SL, Shefner JM, Young RR. Neurological disorders affecting respiration. In: Roussos C, ed. *The Thorax. Part C. Disease.* New York: Marcel Dekker 1995; 2135–75.
◆3. Thomas J, Cook DJ, Brooks D. Chest physical therapy management of patients with cystic fibrosis. A meta-analysis. *Am J Respir Crit Care Med* 1995; **151**: 846–50.
◆4. Jones AP, Rowe BH. Bronchopulmonary hygiene physical therapy for chronic obstructive pulmonary disease and bronchiectasis. *The Cochrane Library* 2000; **3**: 1–12.
5. Clarke SW, Jones JG, Oliver DR. Resistance to two-phase gas-liquid flow in airways. *J Appl Physiol* 1970; **29**: 464–71.
●6. Hasani A, Pavia D, Agnew JE, Clarke SW. Regional lung clearance during cough and forced expiration technique (FET): effects of flow and viscoelasticity. *Thorax* 1994; **49**: 557–61.
7. Hasani A, Pavia D, Agnew JE, Clarke SW. Regional mucus transport following unproductive cough and forced expiration technique in patients with airways obstruction. *Chest* 1994; **105**: 1420–5.
8. Bennett WD, Zeman KL. Effect of enhanced supramaximal flows on cough clearance. *J Appl Physiol* 1994; **77**: 1577–83.
9. Sivasothy P, Brown L, Smith IE, Shneerson JM. Effect of manually assisted cough and mechanical insufflation on cough flow of normal subjects, patients with chronic obstructive pulmonary disease (COPD), and patients with respiratory muscle weakness. *Thorax* 2001; **56**: 438–44.
10. Bach JR. Mechanical insufflation-exsufflation. Comparison with peak expiratory flows with manually assisted and unassisted coughing techniques. *Chest* 1993; **104**: 1553–62.
11. Warren VC. Glossopharyngeal and neck accessory muscle breathing in a young adult with C2 complete tetraplegia resulting in ventilator dependency. *Phys Ther* 2002; **82**: 590–600.
12. Singer M, Vermaat J, Hall G et al. Hemodynamic effects of manual hyperinflation in critically ill mechanically ventilated patients. *Chest* 1994; **106**: 1182–7.
●13. Ntoumenopoulos G, Presneill JJ, McElholum M, Cade JF. Chest physiotherapy for the prevention of ventilator-associated pneumonia. *Intensive Care Med* 2002; **28**: 850–6.
14. Fagevik Olsen M, Hahn I, Nordgren S et al. Randomized controlled trial of prophylactic chest physiotherapy in major abdominal surgery. *Br J Surg* 1997; **84**: 1535–8.
15. Algar FJ, Alvarez A, Salvatierra A et al. Predicting pulmonary complications after pneumonectomy for lung cancer. *Eur J Cardiothorac Surg* 2003; **23**: 201–8.
◆16. Thomas JA, McIntosh JM. Are incentive spirometry, intermittent positive pressure breathing and deep breathing excises effective in the prevention of postoperative pulmonary complications after abdominal surgery? A systematic overview and meta-analysis. *Phys Ther* 1994; **74**: 3–10.

17. Crowe JM, Bradley CA. The effectiveness of incentive spirometry with physical therapy for high-risk patients after coronary artery bypass surgery. *Phys Ther* 1997; **77**: 260–8.

18. Hall JC, Tarala R, Harris J *et al.* Incentive spirometry versus routine chest physiotherapy for prevention of pulmonary complications after abdominal surgery [see comments]. *Lancet* 1991; **337**: 953–6.

19. Gosselink R, Schrever K, De Leyn P *et al.* Recovery after thoracic surgery is not accelerated with incentive spirometry. *Crit Care Med* 2000; **28**: 679–83.

20. Wolff RK, Dolovich MB, Obminski G, Newhouse MT. Effects of exercise and eucapnic hyperventilation on bronchial clearance in man. *J Appl Physiol* 1977; **43**: 46–50.

●21. Oldenburg FA, Dolovich MB, Montgomery JM, Newhouse MT. Effects of postural drainage, exercise and cough on mucus clearance in chronic bronchitis. *Am Rev Respir Dis* 1979; **120**: 739–45.

22. Salh W, Bilton D, Dodd M, Webb AK. Effect of exercise and physiotherapy in aiding sputum expectoration in adults with cystic fibrosis. *Thorax* 1989; **44**: 1006–8.

23. Baldwin DR, Hill AL, Peckham DG, Knox AJ. Effect of addition of exercise to chest physiotherapy on sputum expectoration and lung function in adults with cystic fibrosis. *Respir Med* 1994; **88**: 49–53.

24. Rossman CM, Waldes R, Sampson D, Newhouse MT. Effect of chest physiotherapy on the removal of mucus in patients with cystic fibrosis. *Am Rev Respir Dis* 1982; **126**: 131–5.

●25. Sutton PP, Parker RA, Webber BA *et al.* Assessment of the forced expiration technique, postural drainage and directed coughing in chest physiotherapy. *Eur J Respir Dis* 1983; **64**: 62–8.

26. Gillespie DJ, Rehder K. Body position and ventilation-perfusion relationships in unilateral pulmonary disease. *Chest* 1987; **91**: 75–9.

27. Lamm WJE, Graham MM, Albert RK. Mechanism by which the prone position improves oxygenation in acute lung injury. *Am J Respir Crit Care Med* 1994; **150**: 184–93.

●28. van der Schans CP, Piers DA, Postma DS. Effect of manual percussion on tracheobronchial clearance in patients with chronic airflow obstruction and excessive tracheobronchial secretion. *Thorax* 1986; **41**: 448–52.

29. King M, Philips DM, Gross D *et al.* Enhanced tracheal mucus clearance with high frequency chest wall compression. *Am Rev Respir Dis* 1983; **128**: 511–15.

30. van Hengstum M, Festen J, Beurskens C *et al.* No effect of oral high frequency oscillation combined with forced expiration manoeuvres on tracheobronchial clearance in chronic bronchitis. *Eur Respir J* 1990; **3**: 14–18.

31. Natale JE, Pfeifle J, Homnick DN. Comparison of intrapulmonary percussive ventilation and chest physiotherapy. A pilot study in patients with cystic fibrosis. *Chest* 1994; **105**: 1789–93.

32. Arens R, Gozal D, Omlin KJ *et al.* Comparison of high frequency chest compression and conventional chest physiotherapy in hospitalized patients with cystic fibrosis. *Am J Respir Crit Care Med* 1994; **150**: 1154–7.

●33. Falk M, Kelstrup M, Andersen JB *et al.* Improving the ketchup bottle method with positive expiratory pressure (PEP), in cystic fibrosis. *Eur J Respir Dis* 1984; **65**: 423–32.

34. Lannefors L, Wollmer P. Mucus clearance with three chest physiotherapy regimes in cystic fibrosis: a comparison between postural drainage, PEP and physical exercise. *Eur Respir J* 1992; **5**: 748–53.

35. van Hengstum M, Festen J, Beurskens C *et al.* Effect of positive expiratory pressure mask physiotherapy (PEP) versus forced expiration technique (FET/PD) on regional lung clearance in chronic bronchitics. *Eur Respir J* 1991; **4**: 651–4.

36. McIlwaine PM, Wong LT, Peacock D, Davidson AGF. Long-term comparative trial of convential postural drainage and percussion versus positive expiratory pressure therapy in the treatment of cystic fibrosis. *J Pediatr* 1997; **131**: 570–4.

37. Konstan MW, Stern RC, Doershuk CF. Efficacy of the flutter device for airway mucus clearance in patients with cystic fibrosis. *J Pediatr* 1994; **124**: 689–93.

38. App EM, Kieselmann R, Reinhardt D *et al.* Sputum rheology changes in cystic fibrosis lung disease following two different types of physiotherapy: flutter vs autogenic drainage. *Chest* 1998; **114**: 171–7.

●39. Martin J, Powell E, Shore S, Emrich J, Engel LA. The role of the respiratory muscles in the hyperinflation of bronchial asthma. *Am Rev Respir Dis* 1980; **121**: 441–7.

40. Renfroe KL. Effect of progressive relaxation on dyspnea and state of anxiety in patients with chronic obstructive pulmonary disease. *Heart Lung* 1988; **17**: 408–13.

41. Gift AG, Moore T, Soeken K. Relaxation to reduce dyspnea and anxiety in COPD patients. *Nursing Res* 1992; **41**: 242–6.

●42. Kolaczkowski W, Taylor R, Hoffstein V. Improvement in oxygen saturation after chest physiotherapy in patients with emphysema. *Physiother Can* 1989; **41**: 18–23.

43. Breslin EH. The pattern of respiratory muscle recruitment during pursed-lips breathing in COPD. *Chest* 1992; **101**: 75–8.

44. Ingram RH, Schilder DP. Effect of pursed lips breathing on the pulmonary pressure-flow relationship in obstructive lung disease. *Am Rev Respir Dis* 1967; **96**: 381–8.

45. Mueller RE, Petty TL, Filley GF. Ventilation and arterial blood gas changes induced by pursed lips breathing. *J Appl Physiol* 1970; **28**: 784–9.

46. Pinet C, Estenne M. Effect of preoperative hyperinflation on static lung volumes after lung transplantation. *Eur Respir J* 2000; **16**: 482–5.

●47. Guignon I, Cassart M, Gevenois PA *et al.* Persistent hyperinflation after heart-lung transplantation for cystic fibrosis. *Am J Respir Crit Care Med* 1995; **151**(2 Part 1): 534–40.

●48. Ninane V, Rypens F, Yernault JC, De Troyer A. Abdominal muscle use during breathing in patients with chronic airflow obstruction. *Am Rev Respir Dis* 1992; **146**: 16–21.

49. Casciari RJ, Fairshter RD, Harrison A *et al.* Effects of breathing retraining in patients with chronic obstructive pulmonary disease. *Chest* 1981; **79**: 393–8.

50. Sharp JT, Druz WS, Moisan T *et al.* Postural relief of dyspnea in severe chronic obstructive pulmonary disease. *Am Rev Respir Dis* 1980; **122**: 201–11.

51. Banzett R, Topulos G, Leith DE, Natios C. Bracing arms increases the capacity for sustained hyperpnea. *Am Rev Respir Dis* 1983; **133**: 106–9.

52. Dodd DS, Brancatisano TP, Engel LA. Effect of abdominal strapping on chest wall mechanics during exercise in patients with severe chronic obstructive pulmonary disease. *Am Rev Respir Dis* 1985; **131**: 816–21.

53. Goldman JM, Rose LS, Williams SJ *et al.* Effect of abdominal binders on breathing in tetraplegic patients. *Thorax* 1986; **41**: 940–5.

54. Estenne M, Van Muylem A, Gorini M *et al.* Effects of abdominal strapping on forced expiration in tetraplegic patients. *Am J Respir Crit Care Med* 1998; **157**: 95–8.

◆55. Levine S, Kaiser L, Leferovich J, Tikunov B. Cellular adaptations in the diaphragm in chronic obstructive pulmonary disease. *N Engl J Med* 1997; **337**: 1799–806.

56. Scherer TA, Spengler C, Owassapian D et al. Respiratory muscle endurance training in chronic obstructive pulmonary disease. Impact on exercise capacity, dyspnea, and quality of life. Am J Respir Crit Care Med 2000; 162: 1709–14.

57. Ramirez-Sarmiento A, Orozco-Levi M, Guell R et al. Inspiratory muscle training in patients with chronic obstructive pulmonary disease: structural adaptation and physiologic outcomes. Am J Respir Crit Care Med 2002; 166: 1491–7.

58. Lisboa C, Villafranca C, Leiva A et al. Inspiratory muscle training in chronic airflow limitation: effect on exercise performance. Eur Respir J 1997; 10: 537–42.

59. Heijdra YF, Dekhuijzen PNR, van Herwaarden CLA et al. Nocturnal saturation improves by target-flow inspiratory muscle training in patients with COPD. Am J Respir Crit Care Med 1996; 153: 260–5.

●60. Dekhuijzen PNR, Folgering H, van Herwaarden CLA. Target-flow inspiratory muscle training during pulmonary rehabilitation in patients with COPD. Chest 1991; 99: 128–33.

61. Wanke T, Formanek D, Lahrmann H et al. The effects of combined inspiratory muscle and cycle ergometer training on exercise performance in patients with COPD. Eur Respir J 1994; 7: 2205–11.

62. Villafranca C, Borzone G, Leiva A, Lisboa C. Effect of inspiratory muscle training with intermediate load on inspiratory power output in COPD. Eur Respir J 1998; 11: 28–33.

63. Uijl SG, Houtman S, Folgering HT, Hopman MT. Training of the respiratory muscles in individuals with tetraplegia. Paraplegia 1999; 37: 575–9.

64. Liauw MY, Lin MC, Cheng PT et al. Resistive inspiratory muscle training: its effectiveness in patients with acute complete cervical cord injury. Arch Phys Med Rehabil 2000; 81: 752–6.

65. Wanke T, Toifl K, Merkle M et al. Inspiratory muscle training in patients with Duchenne muscular dystrophy. Chest 1994; 105: 475–82.

●66. Sharp JT, Danon J, Druz WS et al. Respiratory muscle function in patients with chronic obstructive pulmonary disease: its relationship to disability and to respiratory therapy. Am Rev Respir Dis 1974; 110: 154–68.

67. Sharp JT, Goldberg NM, Druz WS et al. Thoracoabdominal motion in COPD. Am Rev Respir Dis 1977; 115: 47–56.

68. Gandevia SC, Leeper JB, McKenzie DK, De Troyer A. Discharge frequencies of parasternal intercostal and scalene motor units during breathing in normal and COPD subjects. Am J Respir Crit Care Med 1996; 153: 622–8.

69. De Troyer A, Leeper JB, McKenzie DK, Gandevia SC. Neural drive to the diaphragm in patients with severe COPD. Am J Respir Crit Care Med 1997; 155: 1335–40.

70. Sinderby C, Beck J, Spahija JA et al. Voluntary activation of the diaphragm in health and disease. J Appl Physiol 1998; 85: 2146–58.

71. Gorman RB, McKenzie DK, Pride NB et al. Diaphragm length during tidal breathing in patients with chronic obstructive pulmonary disease. Am J Respir Crit Care Med 2002; 166: 1461–9.

72. Breslin GH, Garoutte BC, Celli BR. Correlations between dyspnea, diaphragm, and sternomastoid recruitment during inspiratory resistance breathing. Chest 1990; 98: 298–302.

73. Sackner MA, Gonzalez HF, Jenouri G, Rodriguez M. Effects of abdominal and thoracic breathing on breathing pattern components in normal subjects and in patients with COPD. Am Rev Respir Dis 1984; 130: 584–7.

74. Grimby G, Oxhoj H, Bake B. Effects of abdominal breathing on distribution of ventilation in obstructive lung disease. Clin Sci Mol Med 1975; 48: 193–9.

●75. Gosselink RAAM, Wagenaar RC, Sargeant AJ et al. Diaphragmatic breathing reduces efficiency of breathing in chronic obstructive pulmonary disease. Am J Respir Crit Care Med 1995; 151: 1136–42.

76. Casaburi R, Porszasz J, Burns MR et al. Physiologic benefits of exercise training in rehabilitation of patients with severe chronic obstructive pulmonary disease. Am J Respir Crit Care Med 1997; 155: 1541–51.

77. Bellemare F, Grassino A. Force reserve of the diaphragm in patients with chronic obstructive pulmonary disease. J Appl Physiol 1983; 55: 8–15.

◆78. Lacasse Y, Brosseau L, Milne S et al. Pulmonary rehabilitation for chronic obstructive pulmonary disease. Cochrane Database Syst Rev 2002; 3: CD003793.

79. Simpson K, Killian KJ, McCartney N et al. Randomised controlled trial of weightlifting exercise in patients with chronic airflow limitation. Thorax 1992; 47: 70–5.

●80. Spruit M, Gosselink R, Troosters T et al. Resistance vs endurance training in patients with COPD and peripheral muscle weakness. Eur Respir J 2002; 19: 1072–8.

81. Ortega F, Toral J, Cejudo P et al. Comparison of effects of strength and endurance training in patients with chronic obstructive pulmonary disease. Am J Respir Crit Care Med 2002; 166: 669–74.

●82. Neder JA, Sword D, Ward SA et al. Home-based neuromuscular electrical stimulation as a new rehabilitative strategy for severely disabled patients with chronic obstructive pulmonary disease (COPD). Thorax 2002; 57: 333–7.

◆83. Dean E, Ross J. Discordance between cardiopulmonary physiology and physical therapy. Toward a rational basis for practice. Chest 1992; 101: 1694–8.

84. Bamman MM, Caruso CF. Resistance exercise countermeasures for space flight: implications for training specificity. J Strength Cond Res 2000; 14: 45–9.

85. Shenkman B, Belozerova I, Nemirovskaya T et al. Time-course of human muscle fibre size reduction during head-down tilt bedrest. J Gravit Physiol 1998; 5: P71–2.

86. Williams PE. Use of intermittent stretch in the prevention of serial sarcomere loss in immobilised muscle. Ann Rheum Dis 1990; 49: 316–17.

87. Akima H, Ushiyama J-I, Kubo J et al. Resistance training during unweighting maintains muscle size and function in human calf. Med Sci Sports Exerc 2003; 35: 655–62.

●88. Griffiths RD, Palmer A, Helliwell T et al. Effect of passive stretching on the wasting of muscle in the critically ill. Nutrition 1995; 11: 428–32.

89. Zanotti E, Felicetti G, Maini M, Fracchia C. Peripheral muscle strength training in bed-bound patients with COPD receiving mechanical ventilation. Effect of electrical stimulation. Chest 2003; 124: 292–6.

20

Exercise in stable chronic obstructive pulmonary disease

ANTONIO PATESSIO, RICHARD CASABURI

INTRODUCTION

Before the pioneering work of Alvan Barach in the 1950s (1), patients with chronic obstructive pulmonary disease (COPD) were advised to avoid physical activity. For these patients, exercise elicits dyspnoea, a sensation of uncomfortable short- ness of breath. However, unlike some other unpleasant sensa- tions (e.g. cardiac angina), dyspnoea does not signal that tissue damage is taking place. Since then, a body of literature has been amassed (2–5), indicating that exercise tolerance improves as a result of exercise training programmes. Patients feel better and improve their exercise performance after these programmes, while their spirometric indices of airflow obstruc- tion do not change (6, 7); a substantial number of randomized, controlled trials demonstrate clearly that exercise programmes improve the ability to perform exercise (8). Psychological as well as physiological changes are the basis for these improvements.

PSYCHOLOGICAL BENEFITS OF EXERCISE PROGRAMMES

The psychological approach posits that patients can be desen- sitized to exertional dyspnoea (9, 10). Patients become desen- sitized to the sensation of dyspnoea, because they exercise in safe and protected environments and learn not to fear dys- pnoea brought about by exercise (10):

- Patients successfully participating in an exercise programme gain positive feedback from mastering something perceived as being difficult.

- Progressive exercise in a supervised programme with others having similar debilities calms unrealistic fears. This explanation would predict that generally inferior results would be obtained from home exercise programmes (11).
- Dyspnoeic stimuli are perceived as less intense when the patient's attention is focused on non-dyspnoeic stimuli. Thus, listening to music or exercising with a group of people distracts patients from respiratory sensations.

Psychological benefits from an exercise programme can be substantial, although there are few established guidelines to define the most efficient exercise programme parameters to achieve this goal. Intuitively, the setting, the exercise partners and the experience and dedication of the rehabilitation staff are of importance.

PHYSIOLOGICAL BENEFITS OF EXERCISE PROGRAMMES

Several studies have confirmed that patients with COPD can, indeed, achieve a physiological training effect from a well- designed programme of exercise training. Comprehensive reviews have reported the results of exercise programmes for COPD patients (12, 13). It is clear that patients completing an exercise programme feel that their exercise tolerance has increased. On effort-dependent measures of exercise endurance, performance is generally better. However, until recently, few studies have featured a control group, the design of the exercise programmes has varied widely and the adequacy of the pro- gramme has been difficult to evaluate (12). In particular,

Derby Hospitals NHS Foundation
Trust
Library and Knowledge Service

measures that are influenced by motivational factors, such as tests that measure the amount of work done in a given period of time (e.g. 6-min walk distance) or the length of the time for which a given work rate can be tolerated, are highly dependent on motivation. Modes of exercise in which performance can be improved by practice or strategy [e.g. pacing strategy on a motor-driven treadmill (14)] may also produce equivocal measures of physiological improvements in exercise capacity. As a result, most of the published literature cannot be used to determine the parameters of an exercise programme that are effective in improving the physiological ability to exercise.

More recently, however, several studies have appeared that confirm that patients with COPD can, indeed, achieve a physiological training effect from a well-designed programme of exercise training. Casaburi et al. (2) demonstrated that patients with predominantly moderate COPD respond to a programme of high-intensity training with reduced levels of blood lactate and pulmonary ventilation at a given heavy work rate. The same group demonstrated that substantial improvements in exercise tolerance can be obtained as a result of a rigorous programme of exercise training even in those patients with severe obstruction who are unable to elevate blood lactate levels. The improvements of exercise tolerance have been found to be accompanied by measurable physiological changes: (i) improved muscle function (including more rapid O_2 uptake kinetics following exercise onset) (15); and (ii) altered pattern of breathing: higher tidal volume and lower breathing frequency that lead to a reduced V_D/V_T and thus to a lower ventilatory requirement for exercise (15–16).

Maltais et al. have demonstrated that intensive training increases the levels of aerobic enzymes and the capillary density of leg muscle of patients with severe COPD (17, 18), by means of morphological and biochemical analysis of muscle biopsy specimens of thigh muscle.

EXERCISE PRESCRIPTION IN COPD

The design of an exercise training programme should take into consideration intensity, frequency and duration of exercise, factors that influence the degree of the training effect. However, well controlled trials have not been carried out to ascertain the optimal characteristics of these factors in patients with lung disease. Nevertheless, certain extrapolations from the responses of healthy subjects seem warranted: in middle aged non-athletes training sessions of 30 min, three times a week for 15 weeks significantly improve maximal oxygen uptake (19). Then, it seems reasonable to advise that exercise programmes for patients with lung disease should feature sessions three to five times per week with at least 30 min per session. Programmes should last at least 5 weeks and preferably longer.

The issue of exercise intensity is much more controversial. Intensity prescriptions suitable for healthy elderly subjects cannot be utilized for patients with chronic lung disease. Criteria based on predicted heart rate or oxygen uptake are especially problematic. Since these patients are usually ventilatory limited, peak effort is associated with a heart rate and oxygen uptake ($\dot{V}O_2$) considerably lower than predicted levels. Standard criteria that dictate an exercise intensity (e.g. 60 per cent of predicted maximum heart rate) may well be above the patient's peak exercise tolerance. On the other hand, basing the prescription on a similar percentage of the observed peak heart rate or $\dot{V}O_2$ sometimes leads to unreasonably low exercise intensity targets (e.g. below unloaded pedalling requirements). Calculating heart rate reserve is problematic since resting heart rate is often high and varies considerably day to day.

Moreover, some authors have suggested that most COPD patients with very severe airway obstruction are unable to exercise above a 'critical training intensity' (20–22). Belman and Kendregan (23) observed significant improvement in endurance time only in nine out of 15 patients exercised at a relatively low training level (30 per cent of maximal), after 6 weeks of four training sessions per week (23). However, other authors have reported the feasibility of training patients with pulmonary disease at near-maximal intensity (24–26) and, indeed, increased exercise endurance has been obtained in patients undergoing such programmes (6, 26). These results are based on the fact that patients with COPD have been found to be able to tolerate high fractions of their peak exercise tolerance for prolonged periods of time, probably because levels of pulmonary ventilation mildly below the limiting ventilation are well tolerated. Casaburi et al. (2) showed that the high-intensity training programme (80 per cent of peak work rate in an incremental test) was more effective than the low-intensity one (50 per cent of peak work rate) (2). Another study demonstrated that high-intensity training (more than 60 per cent of peak work rate) resulted in significant improvements of many physiological variables (27).

Therefore, a reasonable strategy for patients with COPD might be to keep the same duration and frequency characteristics of the training programme as for normal subjects and to utilize the maximal intensity tolerated without cardiovascular side-effects.

Selection criteria

Reduced exercise tolerance should be the main selection criterion for exercise training. Resting spirometric measures do not correlate well with $\dot{V}O_{2,max}$, but they can be broadly predictive of the range of work rates that a patient can perform. For example, patients with relatively good spirometry ($FEV_1 >50$ per cent of predicted) are generally not limited to any appreciable extent in performing basic daily activities; however, they may well benefit from exercise training in reference both to occupational demands and to undertaking more physically demanding hobbies or social activities. Even patients with more severe airway obstruction can regain greater autonomy in everyday life activities, e.g. caring for personal needs. Exclusion criteria should be a history of recent myocardial infarction, unstable or frequent angina, serious arrhythmias, orthopaedic problems or uncompensated metabolic disorders.

Assessment

Patients with chronic lung disease are often elderly and may have high coexisting impairment of other organ systems. This is especially true of patients with COPD. Such patients require a systematic assessment before an exercise programme can be safely undertaken. An evaluation by a physician, including a medical history, physical examination, basic blood tests (haematology and chemistry), chest X-ray and resting electrocardiogram (ECG), should be on record. A recent pulmonary function test and arterial blood gas analysis serve as objective evidence of disease severity. Patients should be in a stable phase of their disease and pharmacological therapy should be optimized. Since cigarette smoking is self-destructive behaviour and may subvert the therapeutic environment of the group, most programmes do not accept participants who have yet to stop smoking (though it is plausible that an exercise programme may be a useful adjunct to smoking cessation efforts). A cardiopulmonary exercise test (28) is quite useful for patients about to undertake an exercise programme. It provides the greatest information on factors limiting exercise performance, possible risks and whether lactic acidosis is present. Serial 12-lead ECGs allow detection of cardiac arrhythmias or ischaemia that might contraindicate vigorous exercise. The size of increment of the work rate should be chosen in such a way that the test lasts approximately 8–12 min. Whether or not a substantial amount of lactic acidosis is present can be estimated by non-invasive methods (29) or ascertained by means of an arterialized-venous sample taken within the second minute of recovery.

Breathlessness during exercise should be measured using category or continuous scales, since they are considered to be reproducible (though with great intersubject variability) (30, 31). Pulse oximetry can be used to detect exercise-induced hypoxemia. If arterial O_2 saturation drops below approximately 90 per cent, or arterial P_{O_2} falls below 55 torr, prescription of supplemental oxygen (via nasal cannula) should be mandatory during the exercise programme. Prescription of supplemental O_2 to patients with lesser degrees of hypoxemia during rehabilitative exercise may make the training programme will be more effective (see below). Cardiopulmonary exercise testing can also be used to establish an exercise intensity prescription. If testing is repeated after the exercise programme, an objective measure of benefit can be obtained.

In settings where cardiopulmonary exercise testing is not available, lower-technology testing modalities may be of use. A 'walking test' may provide an appropriate baseline assessment in these cases (32, 33), and standards for performance of these tests have been published recently (34). However, it must be stressed that these tests do not generally provide the safety assessment generated with cardiopulmonary exercise testing (e.g. ischaemia, arrhythmia, desaturation during exercise) nor can information regarding the mechanism of exercise limitation be derived.

Training session

The patient should start each session with a warm-up period of 3–5 min, performed at 0 watts on a cycle ergometer or at 0 per cent inclination on a treadmill at a speed chosen by the patient. It is advisable to use the first few exercise sessions as low-intensity 'warm-up' to ensure that disused muscles will not be inordinately sore. A reasonable approach to initiate a high-intensity exercise training programme is to target a work rate equal to 80 per cent of the peak work rate achieved in the pre-programme cardiopulmonary exercise test. If the exercise programme is not to be performed on a calibrated cycle ergometer (as it often is not), then a heart rate target equal to the heart rate observed at 80 per cent of the peak work rate achieved in the pre-programme cardiopulmonary exercise test can be selected. Based on the rehabilitation therapist's assessment, this initial intensity target may have to be adjusted up or down. Further, it may be appropriate to allow the patient to break the exercise session into two or more portions for the first few sessions. As the exercise programme proceeds and the patient's fitness improves, exercise intensity targets should be adjusted upward to maximize the training stimulus.

During these sessions the rehabilitation therapist should check the heart rate, rhythm, blood pressure and oxygen saturation of patients while they are exercising and teach them to monitor heart rate in order to provide a useful guide to quantify the physical activities they perform outside the hospital.

Since the physiological benefits of exercise training disappear over a 1- to 2-month period if regular exercise is not continued (35), a maintenance programme of exercise must be recommended.

Strength training

Strength (resistance) exercise training has started to receive attention as a means to combat skeletal muscle dysfunction, because of demonstrations that peripheral muscle weakness is common in COPD. Hamilton et al. (36) reported that strength scores of COPD patients averaged 81 per cent of those in a control population. Bernard et al. (37) found that lower extremity voluntary strength measures (one repetition maximum, 1 RM) for COPD patients averaged 73 per cent of those in a matched control group while thigh muscle cross-sectional size averaged 76 per cent of that of the control group (37). The rationale for including a resistance training component is not only to provide a countermeasure against this loss of muscle strength and size, but also to avoid a decrease in ability to perform daily functional activities, such as stair climbing and carrying objects. Loss of muscle force-generating potential has been shown to be significantly related to utilization of health care resources in COPD (38). Decreased strength has also been linked to falls in the healthy elderly (39), which frequently lead to broken bones and substantial morbidity.

Resistance training has been shown to improve muscle function and performance of functional activities in patients with COPD, although this finding is based on only a few published studies (40–44). These concepts have recently been reviewed by Storer (44). Simpson *et al.* (40) utilized an 8-week programme of resistance training for three muscle groups and reported improvements of 16–40 per cent in maximum voluntary strength versus no significant change in the control group. Bernard *et al.* (41) compared the results of aerobic exercise training with those of aerobic + resistance training. In this 12-week intervention, thigh muscle cross-sectional area increased 8 per cent, quadriceps muscle strength increased 20 per cent and pectoralis major strength increased 15 per cent in the aerobic + resistance training group. These increases were all significantly greater than those seen in the aerobic training only group.

As with endurance training, there have been no studies to establish an optimal resistance training programme for COPD patients. Extrapolations from programmes used to develop strength, power and endurance in healthy individuals (45), and the successful outcomes in COPD patients reported in the literature to date (40, 41), offer a template for programme design. A synthesis of this information would suggest a training frequency of 2–3 days/week, with two to three sets of eight to 10 repetitions utilizing loads progressing from 50 to 85 per cent of a current 1 RM assessment. Studies utilizing some combination of these guidelines have demonstrated substantial improvements in muscle strength (40, 41) and size (41). As with endurance training, a gradual introduction to resistance exercise training, perhaps with one set of eight to 10 repetitions using 50–60 per cent of 1 RM for major muscle groups, will avoid excessively sore muscles and allow the participant to establish a training base from which the rehabilitation specialist may progress.

Other considerations in the formulation of a resistance training programme for people with COPD include type of resistance used, the rest interval between sets or exercises, choice of exercises and safety considerations. Many types of resistance are available, including elastic resistance, machine weights, free weights and body weight. Choice of equipment is often dictated by what is available. However, almost any form of resistance will suffice, so long as it can be graded in its application, is safe to use and has some motivational appeal to the participant. Choice of exercises may be dictated by patient goals (e.g. improving ability to climb stairs in the patient's domicile) or by contraindications such as arthritic joints or osteoporosis (a particular problem in patients undergoing long-term corticosteroid therapy). Safety concerns in addition to those identified above for endurance exercise training include the need to use a biomechanically safe lifting technique. Further, periodic blood pressure measurements are needed in order to monitor the pressor response to the resistance exercise, and it may be necessary to periodically monitor oxygen saturation and level of dyspnoea. Further research will be needed to establish firm resistance training guidelines for COPD patients.

Arm exercise

The performance of many everyday tasks requires the concerted action of muscle groups that contribute to upper torso and arm positioning. Some of these muscles also support respiration.

In patients with severe chronic airflow obstruction, the diaphragm becomes less efficient in the generation of inspiratory pressure, and its function is supported by the muscles of the rib cage (46). When patients perform unsupported arm exercise, some of these muscles must decrease their support to respiration, affecting the pattern of ventilation (47). Celli *et al.* (48) have demonstrated in patients with severe chronic lung disease that unsupported arm exercise resulted in dyssynchronous thoraco-abdominal excursion that was not solely due to diaphragmatic fatigue. They concluded that unsupported arm exercise could shift work to the diaphragm and in some way lead to dyssynchrony. This hypothesis has been confirmed in other studies (49, 50), through the measurement of oesophageal and gastric pressures. Besides the mechanical consequences, unsupported arm exercise also involves additional metabolic cost. In fact, simple arm elevations result in a significant increase in $\dot{V}O_2$ and carbon dioxide production ($\dot{V}CO_2$) (51) as well as in heart rate and minute ventilation ($\dot{V}_E$). In healthy subjects, arm cranking is more demanding than leg cycling, as shown by higher $\dot{V}O_2$, $\dot{V}_E$, heart rate, blood pressure and lactate production (52–54) for the same work rate, and lower $\dot{V}O_2$, $\dot{V}_E$, cardiac output and lactate levels at maximal effort (51–57). These observations suggest that training the arms should enable the patients to perform more upper extremity work. In addition, the decreased ventilatory requirement for the same work improves the patient's capacity to perform arm activities. Several studies have shown that arm training results in improved performance and that the improved performance is, for the most part, task-specific (23, 58, 59).

NEW STRATEGIES TO IMPROVE EXERCISE TOLERANCE IN COPD

Given the demonstrated value of exercise training, recent research has focused on defining methods to enhance the effectiveness of exercise training programmes and, in addition, to define new approaches to improving muscle function. The rationale for such approaches has gained credence based on a recent demonstration that a substantial fraction of patients with moderate to severe COPD are limited in their exercise tolerance by leg muscle fatigue rather than by ventilatory limitation (60, 61). The quality of the evidence supporting the use of these strategies in the clinical management of COPD patients differs substantially among these techniques. It deserves to be mentioned that clinical trials designed to establish that a given intervention yields superior results compared with standard interventions are generally difficult to perform because of the rather wide variability of responses to exercise interventions among COPD patients.

Pressure support ventilation

Given the demonstration that higher exercise intensity during a training programme yields superior physiological manifestations of training programme benefits, if the work of breathing can be reduced, then patients who are limited in their exercise tolerance by respiratory muscle fatigue may be able to sustain higher exercise intensities during a training programme. Pressure support ventilation facilitates inspiratory muscle unloading and, although the apparatus may be somewhat unwieldy, may be used during exercise tasks utilizing stationary ergometers (e.g. treadmills, exercycles).

Keilty et al. (62) demonstrated that inspiratory pressure support allowed a treadmill task to be performed for a longer period of time before a given level of dyspnoea was experienced. Three randomized controlled trials have appeared recently, attempting to test the hypothesis that either proportional assist ventilation or nasal positive pressure ventilation improves the effectiveness of a rehabilitative exercise programme in COPD (63–65). These trials have had mixed results, perhaps in part because of the modest size of the study groups (intervention group sizes 10, 11 and 18 subjects). In one trial, significantly greater improvements in some measures of exercise tolerance and in manifestations of a physiological training effect were seen in the group receiving proportional assist ventilation (62). In the other two trials no significant benefit was discerned; in one it was noted that pressure support ventilation was not tolerated by some patients (64).

One-legged exercise

To the extent that exercise tolerance is limited by the metabolic demands of the exercise and the consequent ventilatory response, exercise of a smaller muscle mass may allow a high exercise intensity in that muscle group without engendering a limiting ventilatory requirement. Although the metabolic responses to single leg exercise have been explored (66, 67), whether training one leg at a time yields superior training effects has yet to be studied.

Interval training

Interval training involves repeated bouts of high-intensity exercise interspersed with recovery periods (light exercise or rest) (68). In healthy subjects, interval training with rest during the recovery period has been widely studied and, in some studies, has shown better results than continuous training (e.g. 68–73). Gorostiaga et al. (69) showed a greater increase in peak $\dot{V}O_2$ and peak work rate after an interval training programme than after continuous training. Gaesser et al. (70) showed that peak $\dot{V}O_2$ increased significantly only with interval training, and Poole et al. (71) showed that the lactate threshold exhibited greater improvements in interval training than in continuous training. Ahmaidi et al. (72) found that, in elderly people, interval training was more easily accepted and tolerated than continuous training.

Theoretical explanations for superior responses to interval training have been proposed. One or 2 min at high-intensity work rate induce high blood lactate levels due to the depletion of phosphocreatine and the use of oxygen myoglobin-bound reserves, but interspersed periods of sub-lactate threshold

work rates may facilitate lactate removal (68). When compared with the same total amount of work performed continuously, interval training has been shown to engender less lactate accumulation (73) and to prevent glycogen depletion by favouring the metabolism of lipids (68).

In patients with COPD, interval training has been shown to be capable of inducing physiological training effects (74–81). The most common interval training protocol studied in these patients is square-wave bilevel training, i.e. moderate- to high-intensity exercise alternated with low-intensity exercise (67, 74, 76–78, 80). Rehabilitation programmes that included bilevel interval training yielded a delay in lactate threshold, an increase in peak work rate and peak $\dot{V}O_2$ and improvements in quality of life (76, 78). Recently, Sala et al. (67) showed an increase in peak oxygen extraction ratio, reduced phosphocreatine recovery time and improved cellular bioenergetics after a bilevel cycling training programme. Coppoolse et al. (77) compared high-intensity bilevel interval training with moderate-intensity continuous training in a group of 21 COPD patients. The superiority of the interval training approach was not clearly demonstrated.

Anabolic drugs

Since muscle dysfunction has been identified in COPD (81) and implicated as a source of exercise intolerance in at least a portion of patients (60), pharmacological agents that improve muscle function can be seen as rational therapy. No practical pharmacological approach has been validated to date that improves the aerobic function of skeletal muscles. However, two classes of drugs are known to improve muscle strength: growth hormone (GH) and the anabolic steroids. Because of its high cost and its failure to consistently improve muscle function, practicality of GH administration has been questioned (82). These drugs may be considered drugs of abuse when used to enhance athletic performance, but may be appropriately used in patients with chronic disease, if efficacy and safety can be demonstrated.

Several studies published in recent years have demonstrated the effectiveness of anabolic steroids in healthy young men. Healthy eugonadal men responded to supraphysiological doses of testosterone enanthate (600 mg/week) with increased muscle mass and strength, and decreased fat mass (83). A recent study showed that the dose–response relationship for increase in muscle mass and strength and decrease in fat mass in healthy young men is linear (84), and defined the morphological and biochemical changes that occur in the muscle biopsy specimens of these subjects (85). There is accumulating evidence that older men whose testosterone levels are mildly low respond to testosterone replacement with increased lean body mass and strength and decreased fat mass (86–88). Testosterone supplementation in men with HIV wasting syndrome yields increased strength and lean body mass and decreased fat mass (89).

A few studies of anabolic steroid supplementation in COPD have been reported. Schols et al. (90) administered a relatively low dose of nandrolone every 2 weeks for 8 weeks; small increases in lean body mass and respiratory muscle strength were observed. Six months of stanozolol administration to 10 men with COPD resulted in increased body weight, lean body mass, but no endurance exercise changes (91). Forty-nine subjects completed a 4-month observational study of oxandrolone; body weight increased, but 6-min walk distance did not (92). Similarly, in a recent randomized placebo-controlled multi-centre trial of oxandrolone involving 142 underweight COPD subjects, an increase in lean mass and a decrease in fat mass were discerned; 6-min walk distance was unchanged (93). Finally, a recent study showed that 10 weeks of testosterone enanthate supplementation within the physiological range in COPD men with low testosterone levels significantly increased muscle mass and strength and decreased fat mass; these benefits were additive to those of strength training (94). It is considered that anabolic hormone supplementation may be a useful therapy in women with COPD and may be effective at doses lower than those used in men (95).

Oxygen supplementation

Three physiological effects of supplemental oxygen have the potential to increase exercise tolerance of the hypoxaemic COPD patient:

- hypoxic stimulation of the carotid bodies is reduced
- the pulmonary circulation vasodilates
- arterial oxygen content increases.

The latter two mechanisms have the potential to indirectly reduce carotid body stimulation at heavy levels of exercise by increasing oxygen delivery to the exercising muscles and reducing carotid body stimulation by lactic acidaemia. The predominant mechanism for oxygen's effect on exercise tolerance has recently been clarified (96).

Ambulatory oxygen therapy has widely been shown to increase exercise performance and to relieve exertional dyspnoea in COPD patients (e.g. 97–101). Recent studies indicate that reduction in hyperinflation plays an important role in the oxygen-linked relief of dyspnoea (97, 101). Interestingly, supplemental oxygen generally increases exercise tolerance in patients with only mild to moderate hypoxaemia (i.e. levels of hypoxaemia not severe enough to meet guidelines for long-term oxygen therapy) (97, 102, 103).

It seems plausible that breathing oxygen during rehabilitative exercise would allow higher exercise intensities and, therefore, superior training efficacy. However, for this strategy to work, it would be necessary that the oxygen supplementation actually increased arterial oxygen saturation and that rehabilitation participants were encouraged toward their highest tolerated exercise intensity. It can be speculated that a series of studies (104–107) failed to demonstrate benefits of supplemental oxygen because they did not adhere to these design features. A recently published study (108) differed in features of experimental design from some of these previous studies in that: (i) a double-blinded design was employed; (ii) sufficient supplemental oxygen was given during training to raise arterial oxygen saturation; (iii) subjects were urged to maximize their training work rates so that any increase in exercise tolerance produced by oxygen breathing would result in higher training intensity; and (iv) both effort-dependent and effort-independent measures of exercise tolerance were utilized to detect the magnitude of the training effect. This study involved 29 non-hypoxaemic patients with severe COPD (FEV_1 = 36 per cent of predicted). All exercised in a 7-week outpatient programme; during exercise they received by nasal cannula either O_2 (3 L/min) (n = 14) or compressed air (3 L/min) (n = 15). Exercise was on cycle ergometers for 45 min, three times per week; as the programme proceeded, work rate was progressively increased. Both groups had higher exercise tolerance (while breathing air) after training. However, the O_2-trained group increased training work rate more rapidly over the 7 weeks than the air-trained group. After training, exercise endurance increased significantly more in the O_2-trained group (213 per cent) than in the air-trained group (170 per cent). In a training programme of this design, supplemental O_2 provided during high-intensity rehabilitative training facilitates higher training intensity and yields superior gains in exercise tolerance.

Electrical muscle stimulation

Studies of transcutaneous electrical neuromuscular stimulation (TENS) in the COPD population have recently been reported. Rhythmic stimulation of the large muscles of the leg increases muscle metabolism and, at least in theory, has the potential to induce a training response if delivered in long enough sessions, if the sessions continue over a number of weeks and if the intensity of the induced 'exercise' is sufficient. Three small controlled studies of this technique in severe COPD patients have been reported, one a home-based intervention (109), one centre-based (110) and one in bed-bound patients (111) receiving mechanical ventilation. In all three, effort-dependent measures of leg strength improved; in two (109, 110), measures of exercise endurance improved as well. These early encouraging results need to be expanded to evaluate the magnitude of the metabolic response (and, thus, exercise intensity) engendered by the electrical stimulation and to seek evidence of muscle adaptations (e.g. via muscle biopsy).

CONCLUSION

It is well established that training increases exercise tolerance in patients with chronic lung disease. Physiological changes contribute to this improvement: reduction of lactic acidosis, minute ventilation and heart rate for a given work rate, and enhanced activity of mitochondrial enzymes and capillary density in the trained muscles. To obtain these results, training intensity should be the highest tolerated by the patient without cardiovascular side-effects. Among the new strategies that can be used to improve exercise tolerance, oxygen supplementation, even in patients who do not desaturate during exercise, seems the most promising. Exercise therapy should then play a central role in rehabilitation programmes (112) for patients with COPD.

Key points

- Exercise tolerance improves as a result of exercise training programmes.
- Physiological changes contribute to these improvements: reduction of lactic acidosis, minute ventilation and heart rate for a given work rate, and enhanced activity of mitochondrial enzymes and capillary density in the trained muscles.
- Exercise programmes should feature sessions three to five times per week with at least 30 min per session at maximal intensity tolerated without cardiovascular side-effects. Programmes should last at least 5 weeks and preferably longer.
- Reduced exercise tolerance should be the main selection criterion for exercise training. Exclusion criteria should be: a history of recent myocardial infarction, unstable or frequent angina, serious arrhythmias, orthopaedic problems and uncompensated metabolic disorders.
- Resistance training has been shown to improve muscle function and performance of functional activities in patients with COPD.
- Arm training enables patients to perform more upper extremity work.
- Among the new strategies to improve exercise tolerance, oxygen supplementation in patients who do not desaturate during exercise seems to be the most promising, since it allows higher exercise intensities and, therefore, superior training efficacy.
- Exercise therapy should play a central role in rehabilitation programmes for patients with COPD.

REFERENCES

●1. Barach AL, Bickerman HA, Beck G. Advances in the treatment of non-tuberculous pulmonary disease. *Bull NY Acad Med* 1952; **28**: 353–6.

●2. Casaburi R, Patessio A, Ioli F *et al.* Reduction in exercise lactic acidosis and ventilation as a result of exercise training in patients with obstructive lung disease. *Am Rev Respir Dis* 1991; **143**: 9–18.

●3. Cockcroft AE, Sanders MJ, Berry G. Randomized controlled trial of rehabilitation in chronic respiratory disability. *Thorax* 1981; **36**: 200–3.

●4. Sinclair DJM, Ingram CG. Controlled trial of supervised exercise training in chronic bronchitis. *Br Med J* 1980; **1**: 519–21.

●5. Holle RHO, Williams DV, Vandree JC *et al.* Increased muscle efficiency and sustained benefits in an outpatient community hospital-based pulmonary rehabilitation program. *Chest* 1988; **94**: 1161–8.

◆6. Ries AL. Position paper of the American Association of Cardiovascular and Pulmonary Rehabilitation. Scientific basis of pulmonary rehabilitation. *J Cardiopulm Rehabil* 1990; **10**: 418–41.

◆7. Casaburi R. Exercise training in chronic obstructive lung disease. In: Casaburi R, Petty TL, eds. *Principles and Practice of Pulmonary Rehabilitation.* Philadelphia: Saunders, 1993; 204– 24.

◆8. ACCP/AACVPR Pulmonary Rehabilitation Guidelines Panel. Pulmonary rehabilitation: joint ACCP/AACVPR evidence-based guidelines. American College of Chest Physicians. American Association of Cardiovascular and Pulmonary Rehabilitation. *Chest* 1997; **112**: 1363–96.

●9. O'Donnell DE, McGuire M, Samis L, Webb KA. The impact of exercise reconditioning on breathlessness in severe chronic airflow limitation. *Am J Respir Crit Care Med* 1995; **152**: 2005–13.

◆10. Haas F, Salazar-Schicchi J, Axen R. *Desensitization to Dyspnea in Chronic Obstructive Pulmonary Disease.* In: Casaburi R, Petty TL, eds. *Principles and Practice of Pulmonary Rehabilitation.* Philadelphia: Saunders, 1993; 241– 51.

●11. Puente-Maestu L, Sánz ML, Sánz P *et al.* Comparison of effects of supervised versus self-monitored training programmes in patients with chronic obstructive pulmonary disease. *Eur Respir J* 2000; **15**: 517–26.

●12. Kamischke A, Kemper DE, Castel MA *et al.* Testosterone levels in men with chronic obstructive lung disease with or without glucocorticoid therapy. *Eur Respir J* 1998; **11**: 41–5.

●13. Decramer M, Lacquet LM, Fagard R, Rogiers P. Corticosteroids contribute to muscle weakness in chronic airflow obstruction. *Am J Respir Crit Care Med* 1994; **150**: 11–16.

◆14. Chester EH, Belman MJ, Bahler RC *et al.* Multidisciplinary treatment of chronic pulmonary insufficiency. 3. The effect of physical training on cardiorespiratory performance in patients with chronic pulmonary disease. Chest 1977; 72(Suppl. 6): 695–702.

●15. Casaburi R, Porszasz J, Burns MR *et al.* Physiologic benefits of exercise training in rehabilitation of severe COPD patients. *Am J Respir Crit Care Med* 1997; **155**: 1541–51.

◆16. Casaburi R. Mechanisms of the reduced ventilatory requirement as a result of exercise training. Eur Respir Rev 1995; 5: 42–6.

●17. Maltais F, Leblanc P, Simard C *et al.* Skeletal muscle adaptation to endurance training in patients with chronic obstructive pulmonary disease. *Am J Respir Crit Care Med* 1996; **154**: 442–7.

●18. Jobin J, Maltais F, Doyon JF *et al.* Chronic obstructive pulmonary disease: capillarity and fiber-type characteristics of skeletal muscle. *J Cardiopulm Rehabil* 1998; **18**: 432–7.

●19. Siegel W, Blonquist G, Mitchell JH. Effects of a quantitated physical training program on middle-aged sedentary man. *Circulation* 1970; **41**: 19–29.

◆20. Casaburi R. Deconditioning. In: Fishman AP, ed. *Pulmonary Rehabilitation. Lung Biology in Health and Disease Series.* New York: Marcel Dekker; 1996; 213–30.

◆21. Weg JG. Therapeutic exercise in patients with chronic obstructive pulmonary disease. In: Wenger NK, ed. *Cardiovascular Clinics. Exercise and the Heart,* 2nd edn. Philadelphia: Davis FA, 1985; 261–75.

◆22. Hughes RL, Davison R. Limitations of exercise reconditioning in COLD. Chest 1983; 83: 241–9.

●23. Belman MJ, Kendregan BA. Exercise training fails to increase skeletal muscle enzymes in patients with chronic obstructive pulmonary disease. *Am Rev Respir Dis* 1981; **123**: 256–61.

●24. Ries AL, Kaplan RM, Limberg TM, Prewitt LM. Effects of pulmonary rehabilitation on physiological and psychosocial outcomes in patients with chronic obstructive pulmonary disease. *Ann Intern Med* 1995; **122**: 823–32.

●25. Ries AL, Archibald CJ. Endurance exercise training at maximal targets in patients with chronic obstructive pulmonary disease. *J Cardiopulm Rehab* 1987; **7**: 594–601.

●26. Punzal AP, Ries AL, Kaplan RM, Prewitt LM. Maximum intensity exercise training in patients with chronic obstructive pulmonary disease. *Chest* 1991; **100**: 618–23.

●27. Maltais F, Leblanc P, Jobin J *et al.* Intensity of training and physiologic adaption in patients with chronic obstructive pulmonary disease. *Am J Respir Crit Care Med* 1997; **155**: 555–61.

◆28. Brower R, Permutt S. Exercise and the pulmonary circulation. In: Whipp BJ, Wasseman K, eds. *Exercise: Pulmonary Physiology and Pathophysiology.* New York: Marcel Dekker, 1991; 201–20.

●29. Patessio A, Casaburi R, Carone M *et al.* Comparison of gas exchange, lactate, and lactic acidosis threshold in patients with chronic obstructive pulmonary disease. *Am Rev Respir Dis* 1993; **148**: 622–6.

●30. Adams L, Chronos N, Lane R, Guz A. The measurement of breathlessness induced in normal subjects. validity of 2 scaling techniques. *Clin Sci* 1985; **69**: 7–16.

●31. Mahler DA, Rosiello RA, Harver A *et al.* Comparison of clinical dyspnea ratings and psychophysical measurements of respiratory sensation in obstructive airway disease. *Am Rev Respir Dis* 1987; **135**: 1229–33.

●32. McGavin CR, Gupta SP, McHardy GJR. Twelve-minute walking test for assessing disability in chronic bronchitis. *Br Med J* 1976; **1**: 822–3.

●33. Butland JA, Pang J, Gross BR *et al.* Two-, six-, and 12-minute walking tests in respiratory disease. *Br Med J* 1982; **284**: 1607–8.

◆34. ATS Committee on Proficiency Standards for Clinical Pulmonary Function Laboratories. ATS statement: guidelines for the six-minute walk test. *Am J Respir Crit Care Med* 2002; **166**: 111–17.

●35. Coyle EF, Martin WH, Sinacore DR *et al.* Time course of loss adaptation after stopping prolonged intense endurance training. *J Appl Physiol* 1984; **57**: 1857–64.

●36. Hamilton ALKJ, Killian E, Summers Jones NL. Muscle strength, symptom intensity, and exercise capacity in patients with cardiorespiratory disorders. *Am J Respir Crit Care Med* 1995; **152**: 2021–31.

●37. Bernard S, Leblanc PF, Whittom F *et al.* Peripheral muscle weakness in patients with chronic obstructive pulmonary disease. *Am J Respir Crit Care Med* 1998; **158**: 629–34.

●38. Decramer M, Gosselink R, Troosters T, Verschueren Evers G. Muscle weakness is related to utilization of health care resources in COPD patients. *Eur Respir J* 1997; **10**: 417–23.

●39. Fiatarone MA, O'Neill EF, Doyle N *et al.* The Boston FICSIT study: the effects of resistance training and nutritional supplementation on physical frailty in the oldest old. *J Am Geriatr Soc* 1993; **41**: 333–7.

●40. Simpson K, Killian K, McCartney N *et al.* Randomised controlled trial of weight lifting exercise in patients with chronic airflow limitation. *Thorax* 1992; **47**: 70–5.

●41. Bernard S, Whittom F, Leblanc P *et al.* Aerobic and strength training in patients with chronic obstructive pulmonary disease. *Am J Respir Crit Car Med* 1999; **159**: 896–901.

●42. Spruit MA, Gosselink R, Troosters T *et al.* Resistance versus endurance training in patients with COPD and skeletal muscle weakness. *Eur Respir J* 2002; **19**: 1072–8.

●43. Ortega F, Toral J, Cejudo P *et al.* Comparison of effects of strength and endurance training in patients with chronic obstructive pulmonary disease. *Am J Respir Crit Care Med* 2002; **166**: 669–74.

◆44. Storer TW. Exercise in chronic pulmonary disease: resistance exercise prescription. *Med Sci Sports Exerc* 2001; 33(7 Suppl.): S680–S692.

◆45. Fleck SJ, Kraemer W. *Designing Resistance Training Programs*, 2nd edn. Champaign, IL: Human Kinetics, 1997.

●46. Martinez FJ, Couser J, Celli BR. Factors that determine ventilatory muscle recruitment in patients with chronic airflow obstruction. *Am Rev Respir Dis* 1990; **142**: 276–82.

●47. Tangri S, Woolf CR. The breathing pattern in chronic obstructive lung disease, during the performance of some common daily activities. *Chest* 1973; **63**: 126–7.

●48. Celli BR, Rassulo J, Make B. Dyssynchronous breathing associated with arm but not leg exercise in patients with COPD. *N Engl J Med* 1968; **314**: 1485–90.

●49. Criner GJ, Celli BR. Effect of unsupported arm exercise on ventilatory muscle recruitment in patients with severe chronic airflow obstruction. *Am Rev Respir Dis* 1988; **138**: 856–67.

●50. Celli BR, Criner GJ, Rassulo. Ventilatory muscle recruitment during unsupported arm exercise in normal subjects. *J Appl Physiol* 1988; **64**: 1936–41.

●51. Martinez FJ, Couser J, Celli BR. Factors influencing ventilatory muscle recruitment in patients with chronic airflow obstruction. *Am Rev Respir Dis* 1990; **142**: 276–82.

●52. Bobbert AC. Physiological comparison of three types of ergometry. *J Appl Physiol* 1960; **15**: 1007–14.

●53. Davis JA, Vodak P, Wilmore JH *et al.* Anaerobic threshold and maximal power for three modes of exercise. *J Appl Physiol* 1976; **41**: 549–50.

●54. Steinberg J, Astrand PO, Ekblom B *et al.* Hemodynamic response to work with different muscle groups, sitting and supine. *J Appl Physiol* 1967; **22**: 61–70.

●55. Reybrouck T, Heigenhouser GF, Faulkner JA. Limitations to maximum oxygen uptake in arm, leg and combined arm-leg ergometry. *J Appl Physiol* 1975; **38**: 774–9.

●56. Martin TW, Zeballos RJ, Weisman IM. Gas exchange during maximal upper extremity exercise. *Chest* 1991; **99**: 420–5.

●57. Epstein SK, Celli BR, Martinez FJ *et al.* Arm training reduces the VO$_2$ and VE cost of unsupported arm exercise and elevation in chronic obstructive pulmonary disease. *J Cardiopulm Rehabil* 1997; **17**: 171–7.

●58. Lake FR, Hendersen K, Briffa T *et al.* Upper limb and lower limb exercise training in patients with chronic airflow obstruction. *Chest* 1990; **97**: 1077–82.

●59. Ries AL, Ellis B, Hawkins RW. Upper extremity exercise training in chronic obstructive pulmonary disease. *Chest* 1988; **93**: 688–92.

◆60. Casaburi R. Limitation to exercise tolerance in chronic obstructive pulmonary disease look to the muscles of ambulation. *Am J Respir Crit Care Med* 2003; **15**: 409–10.

●61. Saey D, Debigare R, Leblanc P *et al.* Contractile leg fatigue after cycle exercise: a factor limiting exercise in patients with chronic obstructive pulmonary disease. *Am J Respir Crit Care Med* 2003; **15**: 425–30.

●62. Keilty SE, Ponte J, Fleming TA, Moxham J. Effect of inspiratory pressure support on exercise tolerance and breathlessness in patients with severe stable chronic obstructive pulmonary disease. *Thorax* 1994; **49**: 990–4.

●63. Hawkins P, Johnson LC, Nikoletou D *et al.* Proportional assist ventilation as an aid to exercise training in severe chronic obstructive pulmonary disease. *Thorax* 2002; **57**: 853–9.

●64. Bianchi L, Foglio K, Porta R *et al.* Lack of additional effect of adjunct of assisted ventilation to pulmonary rehabilitation in mild COPD patients. *Respir Med* 2002; **96**: 359–67.

●65. Johnson JE, Gavin DJ, Adams-Dramiga S. Effect of training with Heliox and noninvasive positive pressure ventilation on exercise ability in patients with severe COPD. *Chest* 2002; **122**: 464–72.

●66. Richardson RS, Sheldon J, Poole DC *et al.* Evidence of skeletal muscle metabolic reserve during whole body exercise in patients with chronic obstructive pulmonary disease. *Am J Respir Crit Care Med* 1999; **159**: 881–5.

●67. Sala E, Roca J, Marrades RM *et al.* Effects of endurance training on skeletal muscle bioenergetics in chronic obstructive pulmonary disease. *Am J Respir Crit Care Med* 1999; **159**: 1726–34.

●68. Billat VL. Interval training for performance: a scientific and empirical practice. Special recommendation for middle and long distance running. Part I: aerobic interval training. *Sports Med* 2001; **31**: 13–31.

●69. Gorostiaga EM, Walter CB, Foster C, Hickson RC. Uniqueness of interval and continuous training at the same maintained exercise intensity. *Eur J Appl Physiol* 1991; **63**: 101–7.

●70. Gaesser GA, Wilson LA. Effects of continuous and interval training on the parameters of power-endurance time relationship for high-intensity exercise. *Int J Sports Med* 1988; **9**: 417–21.

●71. Poole DC, Gaesser GA. Response of ventilatory and lactate thresholds to continuous and interval training. *J Appl Physiol* 1985; **58**: 1115–21.

●72. Ahmaidi S, Masse-Biron J, Adam B *et al.* Effects of interval training at the ventilatory threshold on clinical and cardio-respiratory responses in elderly humans. *Eur J Appl Physiol* 1998; **78**: 170–6.

●73. Fox EL, Robinson S, Wiegman DL. Metabolic energy sources during continuous and interval running. *J Appl Physiol* 1969; **27**: 174–8.

●74. Gimenez M, Servera E, Vergara P *et al.* Endurance training in patients with chronic obstructive pulmonary disease: a comparison of high versus moderate intensity. *Arch Phys Med Rehabil* 2000; **81**: 102–9.

●75. Larson JL, Covey MK, Wirtz SE *et al.* Cycle ergometer and inspiratory muscle training in chronic obstructive pulmonary disease. *Am J Respir Crit Care Med* 1999; **160**: 500–7.

●76. Vallet G, Ahmaidi S, Serres I *et al.* Comparison of two training programmes in chronic airflow limitation patients: standardized versus individualized protocols. *Eur Respir J* 1997; **10**: 114–22.

●77. Coppoolse R, Schols AMWJ, Baarends EM *et al.* Interval versus continuous training in patients with severe COPD. A randomized clinical trial. *Eur Respir J* 1999; **14**: 258–63.

●78. Fuchs-Climent D, Legallais D, Varray A *et al.* Quality of life and exercise tolerance in chronic obstructive pulmonary disease. Effect of a short and intensive inpatient rehabilitation program. *Am J Phys Med Rehabil* 1999; **78**: 330–5.

●79. Gosselink R, Troosters T, Decramer M. Exercise training in COPD patients: interval versus endurance training. *Eur Respir J* 1998; **12**: 2s.

◆80. Goldstein RS, Gort EH, Stubbing D *et al.* Randomised controlled trial of respiratory rehabilitation. *Lancet* 1994; **344**: 1394–7.

◆81. Casaburi R, Gosselink R, Decramer M *et al.* Skeletal muscle dysfunction in obstructive pulmonary disease. A Statement of the American Thoracic Society and European Respiratory Society. *Am J Respir Crit Care Med* 1999; **159**(4, Part 2): S1–40.

◆82. Casaburi R. Anabolic therapies in chronic obstructive pulmonary disease. *Monaldi Arch Chest Dis* 1998; **53**: 454–9.

●83. Bhasin S, Storer TW, Berman N *et al.* The effects of supraphysiological doses of testosterone on muscle size and strength in normal men. *N Engl J Med* 1996; **335**: 1–7.

●84. Bhasin S, Woodhouse L, Casaburi R *et al.* Testosterone dose–response relationships in healthy young men. *Am J Physiol Endocrinol Metab* 2001; **281**: E1172–81.

●85. Sinha-Hikim I, Artaza J, Gonzalez-Cadivid N *et al.* Testosterone-induced increase in muscle size in healthy, young men is associated with muscle fiber hypertrophy. *Am J Physiol Endocrinol Metab* 2002; **283**: E154–64.

●86. Tenover JS. Effects of testosterone supplementation in the aging male. *J Clin Endocrinol Metab* 1992; **75**: 1092–8.

●87. Urban RJ, Bodenburg YH, Gilkison C *et al.* Testosterone administration to elderly men increases skeletal muscle strength and protein synthesis. *Am J Physiol* 1995; **269** (*Endrocrinol Metabol* 1995; **32**): E820–6.

●88. Bakhshi V, Elliott M, Gentili A *et al.* Testosterone improves rehabilitation outcomes in ill older men. *J Am Geriatric Soc* 2000; **48**: 550–3.

●89. Bhasin S, Storer TW, Javanbakht M *et al.* Testosterone replacement and resistance exercise in HIV-infected men with weight loss and low testosterone levels. *J Am Med Assoc* 2000; **283**: 763–70.

●90. Schols AMW, Soeters PB, Mostert R *et al.* Physiologic effects of nutritional support and anabolic steroids in patients with chronic obstructive pulmonary disease. *Am J Respir Crit Care Med* 1995; **152**: 1268–74.

●91. Ferreira IM, Verreschi IT, Nery LE *et al.* The influence of 6 months of oral anabolic steroids on body mass and respiratory muscles in undernourished COPD patients. *Chest* 1998; **114**: 19–28.

●92. Yeh S-S, Deguzman B, Kramer T. Reversal of COPD-associated weight loss using the anabolic agent oxandrolone. *Chest* 2002; **122**: 421–8.

●93. Make B, Piquette C, Kramer T *et al.* Oxandrolone increases weight and muscle mass in underweight COPD patients (abstract). *Chest* 2002; **122**(Suppl.): 73S.

●94. Casaburi R, Consentino G, Bhasin S *et al.* A randomized trial of strength training and testosterone supplementation in men with chronic obstructive pulmonary disease. *Eur Respir J* 2001; **18**(Suppl. 33): 173S.

◆95. Casaburi R. Skeletal muscle dysfunction in chronic obstructive pulmonary disease. *Med Sci Sports Exercise* 2001; **33**(7): S662–70.

●96. Somfay A, Porszasz J, Lee SM, Casaburi R. Effect of hyperoxia on gas exchange and lactate kinetics following exercise onset in non-hypoxemic COPD patients. *Chest* 2002; **121**: 393–400.

●97. Somfay A, Porszasz J, Lee SM, Casaburi R. Effect of oxygen on hyperinflation and exercise endurance in non-hypoxemic COPD patients. *Eur Respir J* 2001; **18**: 77–84.

●98. Stein DA, Bradley BL, Miller W. Mechanisms of oxygen effects on exercise in chronic obstructive pulmonary disease. *Chest* 1982; **81**: 6–10.

●99. Bradley BL, Garner AE, Billiu K *et al.* Oxygen-assisted exercise in chronic obstructive lung disease: the effect on exercise capacity and arterial blood gas tensions. *Am Rev Respir Dis* 1978; **118**: 239–43.

●100. Dean NC, Brown JK, Himelman RB *et al.* Oxygen may improve dyspnea and endurance in patients with chronic obstructive pulmonary disease and only mild hypoxemia. *Am Rev Respir Dis* 1992; **148**: 941–5.

●101. O'Donnell DE, Bain DJ, Webb KA. Factors contributing to relief of exertional breathlessness during hyperoxia in chronic airflow limitation. *Am J Respir Crit Care Med* 1997; **155**: 530–5.

●102. Woodcock AA, Gross ER, Geddes DM. Oxygen relieves breathlessness in 'pink puffers'. *Lancet* 1981; **1**: 907–9.

●103. O'Donnell DE, D'Arsigny C, Webb KA. Effects of hyperoxia on ventilatory limitation during exercise in advanced chronic obstructive pulmonary disease. *Am J Respir Crit Care Med* 2001; **163**: 892–8.

●104. McDonald CF, Blyth CM, Lazarus MD *et al*. Exertional oxygen of limited benefit in patients with chronic obstructive pulmonary disease and mild hypoxemia. *Am J Respir Crit Care Med* 1995; **152**: 1616–19.

●105. Garrod R, Paul EA, Wedzicha JA. Supplemental oxygen during pulmonary rehabilitation in patients with COPD with exercise hypoxaemia. *Thorax* 2000; **55**: 539–43.

●106. Rooyackers JM, Dekhuijzen PN, Van Herwaarden CL, Folgering HT. Training with supplemental oxygen in patients with COPD and hypoxaemia at peak exercise. *Eur Respir J* 1997; **10**: 1278–84.

●107. Wadell K, Henriksson-Larsen K, Lundgren R. Physical training with and without oxygen in patients with chronic obstructive pulmonary disease and exercise-induced hypoxaemia. *J Rehabil Med* 2001; **33**: 200–5.

●108. Emtner M, Porszasz J, Burns M *et al*. Benefits of supplemental oxygen in exercise training in non-hypoxemic COPD patients. *Am J Respir Crit Care Med* 2003; **68**: 1034–42.

●109. Neder JA, Sword D, Ward SA *et al*. Home-based neuromuscular electrical stimulation as a new rehabilitative strategy for severely disabled patients with chronic obstructive pulmonary disease (COPD). *Thorax* 2002; **57**: 333–7.

●110. Bourjeily-Habr G, Rochester CL, Palermo F *et al*. Randomised controlled trial of transcutaneous electrical muscle stimulation of the lower extremities in patients with chronic obstructive pulmonary disease. *Thorax* 2002; **57**: 1045–9.

●111. Zanotti E, Felicetti G, Maini M, Fracchia C. Peripheral muscle strength training in bed-bound patients with COPD receiving mechanical ventilation: effect of electrical stimulation. *Chest* 2003; **124**: 292–6.

◆112. Lacasse Y, Wong E, Guyatt GH *et al*. Meta-analysis of respiratory rehabilitation in chronic obstructive pulmonary disease. *Lancet* 1996; **348**: 1115–19.

21

The role of collaborative self-management education in pulmonary rehabilitation

RICK HODDER

INTRODUCTION

Optimum therapy for chronic lung disease is similar to that for any chronic illness that has no cure and includes not only attempts to improve lung function (usually with limited success), but also, perhaps more importantly, management strategies to help patients best cope with the unavoidable consequences of this devastating disease. In the case of chronic obstructive pulmonary disease (COPD), the systemic effects of the disease, secondary physical deconditioning, the presence of co-morbid illness and disease-induced psychosocial stressors quickly emerge as major priorities for optimum management. Not surprisingly, therefore, patient education directed at promoting disease self-management has become an integral component in the therapy of many chronic diseases (1, 2), including COPD. For example, patient self-management education has been shown to reduce the frequency of asthma attacks and improve patient disability from this disease (3). The positive impact of patient and family education for chronic lung disease has been implicitly recognized by health care professionals through its almost obligatory inclusion in formalized pulmonary rehabilitation programmes (4–7). Despite this tacit endorsement of the value of patient education, a recent systematic review of pulmonary rehabilitation in COPD, concluded that the only essential component of pulmonary rehabilitation was exercise training, and that strong evidence supporting the value of other programme components including education, was lacking (8). In another

systematic review of patient education in COPD, but which did not include pulmonary rehabilitation programmes, the authors also concluded that there was insufficient evidence to support a stand alone role for patient education in COPD management, and that additional clinical trials were needed (9). However, the primary goal of pulmonary rehabilitation is not simply improved exercise tolerance, but rather to help the patient achieve the highest possible level of independent function, despite the challenges of living with chronic lung disease (6, 10, 11). This includes important elements of emotional and psychosocial functioning, and successful programmes help patients and their families to become better educated about the disease and its management and, most importantly, to become more self-sufficient and involved in their own care. This often involves effecting psychosocial changes and behaviour modification for these patients, such as improved adaptation to stress and improved coping strategies. In order to accomplish this holistic or whole-patient goal, pulmonary rehabilitation programmes must adopt a multidisciplinary approach consisting of several components which, in addition to exercise training and chest physiotherapy techniques, include education for the patients and their family/care-givers, as well as psychosocial support designed to address the often difficult psychological, emotional and social challenges faced by these individuals (12, 13).

This chapter will review the growing evidence supporting the role of patient and family education in pulmonary rehabilitation, as well as the educational aspects of psychosocial support for patients with chronic lung disease. Data from large hospital-based multidisciplinary pulmonary rehabilitation programmes, as well as from smaller, less resource-intensive programmes and from outpatient, ambulatory self-management programmes, will be reviewed. Emphasis will be placed on the concept of collaborative self-management education as an example of a more comprehensive approach to patient education and disease management (11, 14, 15). The challenge of disease self-management is also discussed in Chapter 36. Because almost all of the controlled clinical trial research into the value of patient education in chronic lung disease has dealt with COPD, this disease will be the main focus of the chapter. With few exceptions, pulmonary rehabilitation and education for patients with chronic pulmonary fibrosis would be expected to follow similar guidelines and be associated with similar outcomes compared to those for COPD (16, 17). The special problems associated with other non-COPD chronic lung conditions requiring pulmonary rehabilitation, and, in particular, the special interests of patients with neuromuscular disease, are dealt with elsewhere in this textbook (Chs 27–29).

INTERNATIONAL PERSPECTIVE ON PATIENT EDUCATION IN PULMONARY REHABILITATION

The Global Initiative for Obstructive Lung Disease (GOLD) (18) states that:

> the overall approach to managing stable COPD should be characterized by a stepwise increase in treatment, depending on the severity of the disease. For patients with COPD, health education can play a role in improving skills, ability to cope with illness, and health status … (and) it is effective.

This statement defines a basic principle of optimum COPD management, namely that education, not only for patients, but also for families, health care professionals and even the general public, should form the foundation upon which all other aspects of COPD management are based (Fig. 21.1).

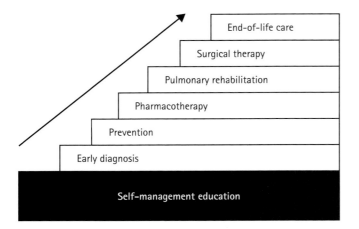

Figure 21.1   *The fundamental role for education in the stepwise management of COPD, emphasizing the pivotal role of self-management education.*

The experience of pulmonary rehabilitation in several countries has been recently summarized (13) and although the central role and value of patient education in COPD management is recognized by practitioners of pulmonary rehabilitation, there is currently considerable international variation in the availability, content and organizational aspects of patient education and rehabilitation for chronic pulmonary disease. The Canadian Lung Association (CLA; www.lung.ca) and the Canadian Thoracic Society (CTS), for example, have endorsed the central role of patient self-management education in the recent Canadian guidelines for COPD management (19). The CLA has also developed a national COPD patient education programme ('BreathWorks'), which includes patient educational materials, links to local resources and support groups and a telephone helpline. The CLA has also partnered with the Canadian COPD Alliance (CCA; www.lung.ca), a national forum designed to facilitate collaboration among groups working in the area of COPD (e.g. professional societies for nurses, respiratory therapists, physiotherapists, etc.), to create a national certification programme for a COPD educator. COPD educators are health care professionals (usually respiratory therapists or nurses) who are trained in the techniques of self-management education for patients with COPD, and who are also often certified asthma educators, employed in a variety of settings ranging from local clinics to formalized, multidisciplinary pulmonary rehabilitation programmes. In the United States, the American Lung Association has an extensive inventory of patient education resources (www.lungusa.org), and the National Lung Health Education Program (NLHEP) (20) is another educational initiative created to help facilitate earlier diagnosis of COPD, as well as to facilitate a coordinated effort to improve the overall level of public, patient and health care professional education about this disease. An extensive, practical overview of the components of a multidisciplinary pulmonary rehabilitation programme, including how to set up the educational components of such a programme and a description of clinical competency guidelines for pulmonary rehabilitation professionals, is available from the American Association of Cardiovascular and Pulmonary Rehabilitation (6). The British Thoracic Society (BTS) has recently updated its COPD guidelines and, in recognizing the value of patient education and self-management in COPD, has recommended that specific educational packages and self-management advice be developed for patients with this disease (21). The BTS has also developed useful educational material for patients (www.brit-thoracic.org.uk) and has partnered with industry to create the BTS COPD Consortium (www.brit-thoracic.org.uk/copd) which provides extensive educational material about COPD for patients and health care professionals. The European prospective on patient education in pulmonary rehabilitation is somewhat more difficult to assess, as the coordination of health care services of the different western European countries is still in progress. From the lay perspective, COPD educational initiatives are being coordinated by the European Network of COPD Patients' Associations (ENCPA), a subgroup of the European Foundation of Allergy and Airways Diseases Patients' Associations (EFA;

www.efanet.org). Recently, a European Respiratory Society (ERS) task force paper emphasized the multidisciplinary aspect of pulmonary rehabilitation and the scientific basis for management and evaluation of patients with chronic respiratory disease, and included a specific reference to education of the patient and family as an essential component of pulmonary rehabilitation (22). In 1998, a Japanese study comparing the organization and content of pulmonary rehabilitation programmes of North America, Europe and Japan observed that patient education was a significant component of pulmonary rehabilitation in 98 per cent of North American programmes and in 86 per cent of European programmes, whereas the figure was only 20 per cent for the Tokyo-based pulmonary rehabilitation programmes, which tended to be concerned primarily with long-term oxygen therapy (23). Information about pulmonary rehabilitation and patient education for chronic lung disease from other countries is scarce (13).

THE NEED FOR COLLABORATIVE SELF-MANAGEMENT EDUCATION IN PULMONARY REHABILITATION

Chronic obstructive pulmonary disease is a disease of loss: loss of youth, loss of physical vitality, loss of social interaction, loss of self-worth and, all too often, loss of hope. Daily activities affected by COPD include sleep and rest, mobility, self-care, home and family management, ability to enjoy hobbies, recreational activities, family/friends, and emotional, sexual, social and behavioural functioning. Thus, although primarily a respiratory disease, COPD has important systemic manifestations, including reduced exercise tolerance, fatigue, nutritional, emotional and psychosocial factors, which when added to the ageing process and co-morbid illness often present, strain the patient's ability to maintain a sense of self-worth and to maintain an active role within the family and community (24). Patients become fearful of not being able to maintain their independence, with resultant anxiety and even depression over becoming a burden to their families and upon society. Thus, like many chronic illnesses, COPD progressively imposes both physiological and psychological burdens that combine to result in an overall deterioration in the patient's quality of life (25).

The quality of life for family members and other caregivers of individuals with COPD is also influenced heavily by the disease and, as it evolves, this impact on the patient's family becomes part of the disease process itself, as care-givers of patients with chronic lung disease become overwhelmed by the chronicity of their burden (26). Frustrations of family members may arise from social losses, enforced job changes and shifting household responsibilities, which often disrupt family dynamics. These family tensions can lead to sentiments of over-dependency, resentment and even ambivalence, all of which may have negative impacts on the patient's quality of life and ability to cope with the burdens of chronic lung disease (27). Thus, in helping to optimally manage COPD,

the health care professional and pulmonary rehabilitation team must consider not only the pathophysiology and multiple exacerbations of this disease, but its psychosocial impact on patients and families as well.

A recent international survey entitled *Confronting COPD* clearly identified the need for patient and health care professional education about COPD (28). Conducted between November 2000 and January 2001, this survey included 3265 individuals with COPD in Canada, the USA, France, Italy, Germany, the Netherlands, Spain and the UK. The study observed that there is a high rate of undiagnosed COPD worldwide and, even for patients diagnosed with COPD, fewer than half felt that they were well informed about their condition and its treatment. The majority of patients were symptomatic: 68 per cent reported breathlessness with stairs; 51 per cent had daily breathlessness; and 24 per cent had breathlessness with talking. Despite this considerable symptomatic burden, 75 per cent of patients self-reported their disease as being only 'mild'. This suggests that COPD patients tend to under-appreciate the severity of their disease and to overestimate their degree of disease control, which can act as a barrier to successful management of this condition. This apparent disconnection between disease burden and perception of disease severity has been noted by others for both COPD (29) and asthma (30), and may reflect some resignation on the part of patients (and physicians), both of whom may have unnecessarily nihilistic expectations for what can be achieved with a modern, comprehensive approach to disease management, including the use of pulmonary rehabilitation and education about self-management strategies. This therapeutic nihilism may also contribute to the common observation that patient adherence to disease management plans, in particular those advocating regular exercise and behavioural modification, is poor, as is evident from the fact that more than 50 per cent of patients who begin programmes to promote lifestyle changes do not complete them (31).

These observations suggest several ways in which COPD management can be improved. First, there is a clear need for both health care professionals and patients to be educated that COPD is fundamentally different from asthma and that asthma management programmes will not work for COPD (21). To this end, educational efforts to raise public awareness of COPD itself, its risk factors and the benefits of early detection should be continued and expanded where deficient. Such efforts include smoking cessation and prevention strategies; increased use of influenza vaccinations and dissemination of state-of-the-art information on symptom-relief methods, including pharmacological and non-pharmacological strategies. Comprehensive COPD management mandates a multidisciplinary approach that requires resources and personnel beyond those usually available in an office or clinic-based environment. Thus educational efforts to promote greater awareness of local community patient/family support and rehabilitation resources are essential. If such resources do not exist, efforts to facilitate their development become important, as does education to promote the paradigm of a collaborative self-management approach to COPD therapy. Patients, the public and especially health care professionals need to be educated that modern, comprehensive management of COPD means that having this disease is no longer a hopeless case. In this regard, information about the significant patient gains, including health-related quality of life (HRQL), symptom control, exercise tolerance, reduction in exacerbations, improved

self-confidence, reduced anxiety, depression and improved social functioning, that can be achieved with a multidisciplinary, collaborative self-management approach to therapy needs to be widely disseminated. The many potential advantages that might accrue from a successful collaborative self-management education approach to COPD management, not only for patients and health care professionals, but also for the health care system itself, are listed in Box 21.1. Evidence from controlled clinical trials supporting these benefits from collaborative self-management education in COPD will be presented below.

Box 21.1   Potential advantages of a collaborative care and self-management education approach for COPD

Patient advantages

- Increased self-confidence from being better informed
- Reduced uncertainty, anxiety, depression
- Improved symptom control
- Improved health-related quality of life
- Improved adherence to a COPD management plan, including a regular exercise programme
- Enhanced self-efficacy and sense of being in control

Health care professional advantages

- Fewer unscheduled clinic visits
- Fewer emergency department visits
- Improved patient satisfaction

Health care system advantages

- Fewer emergency department visits
- Fewer hospital admissions
- Less time off work
- Reduced costs of care

DEFINING PATIENT EDUCATION AND COLLABORATIVE SELF–MANAGEMENT EDUCATION

Ideally, patient education involves not only teaching, but also promoting learning and behaviour modification. The goal is to help the patient and the patient's family, improve knowledge, increase self-confidence and learn to take charge of the disease by actions that facilitate prevention and control of symptoms through the adoption of healthy lifestyles. The differences between traditional patient education and collaborative self-management education approaches are listed in Table 21.1. The term 'collaborative self-management education' suggests a more comprehensive approach to patient education and disease management (14, 15). Whereas traditional patient education imparts disease-specific information and technical skills (e.g. inhaler technique), self-management education is different in that it teaches problem-solving skills and how to effect positive change. Collaboration refers to

Table 21.1   *Traditional patient education versus collaborative self-management education in COPD*

	Traditional patient education	Collaborative self–management education
Content	COPD information and technical skills (e.g. inhaler technique)	Problem-solving skills. How to identify and manage specific problems (e.g. a COPD exacerbation, progressive breathlessness, a panic attack)
Problem formulation	Exclusively disease-related (e.g. persisting breathlessness; cough and mucus)	Patient, family and health care professional identify problems specific to the individual and environment that may or may not be disease-related (e.g. lack of family/social/community support; worry over being a burden to spouse; family conflicts; poor self-image; depression; fear of death)
Education goals	Imparts COPD-specific knowledge that may lead to improved clinical outcomes (e.g. smoking cessation, rational use of bronchodilators)	Provides problem-solving skills relevant to COPD that empower the patient to have greater self-confidence and autonomy in the ability to make changes that will result in improved life quality (e.g. how to find local support groups; printed material; web-based COPD information)
	Emphasis on the importance of adherence to prescribed treatments (e.g. taking medications as prescribed, a regular exercise programme)	Provides specific assistance that facilitates increased self-management and self-efficacy to improve clinical, social and emotional outcomes (e.g. family support; links to pulmonary rehabilitation professionals and programmes; behaviour modification for enhanced adherence to regular exercise programme)
Who is the educator?	A health care professional (e.g. a physician, or clinic nurse)	A health care professional (e.g. pulmonary rehabilitation professional/COPD educator); a peer leader, or even other patients (often in a group setting)

regular interaction of the patient with family, care-givers, health care professionals, community resources and social support groups.

An important concept in self-management is self-efficacy, or the confidence that one can carry out a behaviour necessary to reach a desired goal (32). Self-efficacy is frequently poor for patients with chronic lung disease, in part because they lose the sense of autonomy over their lives as the disease and their dependence on others advance. The expectations that patients have for their own self-efficacy are important, because these expectations can affect their success in self-management or in a pulmonary rehabilitation programme (33). It has been demonstrated, for example, that empowering patients to believe that they can positively modify their behaviour will successfully increase their self-efficacy expectations, and improve exercise performance and adherence to treatment plans following pulmonary rehabilitation (33, 34). A positive impact of social support on psychological health and even survival in COPD has also been demonstrated (35, 36).

REQUIREMENTS FOR SUCCESSFUL COLLABORATIVE SELF-MANAGEMENT EDUCATION IN PULMONARY REHABILITATION

Building an effective self-management education partnership, whether clinic-based or as part of a formal pulmonary rehabilitation programme, depends upon particular attributes of both patients and health care professionals and upon certain key programme elements (Box 21.2).

Box 21.2   Essential requirements for a successful patient/family/health care professional partnership that promotes self-management in COPD

Patient/family/health care professional attributes

- A patient-focused management strategy (i.e. focus on relief of symptoms and psychosocial issues) rather than just a disease-focused approach (i.e. focus on drug therapy, inhaler technique, etc.)
- Good communication among patient, family and health care professionals
- Awareness of cultural, ethnicity issues
- Desire on the part of patients to take control of their own condition and to practise self-management
- Willingness of health care professional to empower patients to self-management
- Willingness of patients to effect behavioural change (e.g. quit smoking, exercise regularly)
- Ability of health care professional to elicit patient's true concerns (e.g. being a burden on family, loss of self-worth, fear of death)
- Ability of patient/family/health care professionals to identify potential barriers to successful self-management

Pulmonary rehabilitation programme elements[a]

Patient and family learning assessment

- Patient and family interview to assess:
  - prior educational and literacy level
  - educational needs (e.g. disease state knowledge)
  - learning styles
- Provision of educational materials on chronic lung disease
- Distribution of patient workbook

Core knowledge (COPD)

- Normal anatomy and physiology of respiratory system
- Pathophysiology of lung disease and basis for symptoms such as breathlessness
- Nature of COPD and differences from asthma
- Relevance of co-morbid illness to pulmonary rehabilitation, exercise training
- Description and rationale for medical tests, including blood tests, spirometry, exercise tests, chest radiography, blood gases and oxyhaemoglobin saturation measurement

Principles of pharmacological and non-pharmacological management of COPD

- Medication side-effects, indications, dosing, drug interactions and inhaler technique
- Importance of adherence to treatment plans
- Techniques for self-monitoring
- Breathing training and dyspnoea control techniques
- Relaxation techniques
- Activities of daily living and energy conservation techniques
- Principles of good nutrition
- Chest physical therapy and bronchial hygiene techniques
- Rationale, importance and principles for regular exercise
- Exercise prescription
- Ability to identify impending COPD exacerbation
- Development of an action plan for COPD exacerbations

Psychosocial elements

- Identification of family stressors, conflicts, fears
- Development of effective coping techniques
- Identification of anxiety and depression and referral for therapy when appropriate
- Assistance with behavioural modification and lifestyle changes
- Sexuality issues
- Cultural and ethnicity issues
- End-of-life issues
- Identification of social support needs and resources
- Identification of available local resources
  - COPD educator
  - patient support groups
- Printed, video, web-based educational resources

---

[a]Programme may be hospital, clinic or home-based.

Patient/family and health care professional attributes

Successful collaborative self-management of COPD requires a paradigm shift (particularly for physicians), from a predominantly drug-oriented approach to disease management to an appreciation of the essential role of non-pharmacological therapy for COPD. Important non-pharmacological therapies include regular exercise, good nutritional practices, chest physiotherapy techniques, behaviour modification and relaxation techniques, and psychosocial support techniques, which, however, are often poorly understood and poorly appreciated by physicians.

It is also essential that physicians come to realize that a patient-centred approach to disease management is more likely to be successful in improving patient quality of life than the traditional, but outdated, physician-centred and disease-centred approaches to therapy. For example, rather than focusing on the chest radiograph or FEV_1, a better approach is to concentrate on issues more in line with what patients consider to be most important to their quality of life, such as breathlessness, reduced exercise tolerance, fear, depression, self-image, stress on family, etc. In so doing, health care professionals will be following the sound advice of Sir William Osler, who, in paraphrasing Hippocrates, said: 'It is more important to know what sort of person this disease has, than to know what sort of disease this person has.' If health care professionals and patients can be better educated on how to get to know each other's perspectives on disease management, it will be much easier for them to establish a more meaningful and successful partnership. Patients also need to acquire certain skills that will enhance their ability to participate in a collaborative care strategy that values self-management. For example, they need to be educated that their agendas are as important as the physician's and on how they can make their needs heard. This is one of the main principles in support of the multidisciplinary team approach to patient education that typifies most pulmonary rehabilitation and successful collaborative self-management programmes.

Good communication between all parties is therefore essential to ensure successful collaborative self-management of chronic lung disease. Health care professionals should discipline themselves to take the time to listen to their patients' replies and questions, rather than forcing an artificial time-based agenda upon them. In this regard, physicians and other health care professionals must develop good patient assessment skills designed to elicit not only the patient's disease-related needs, but also psychosocial and learning needs. An understanding of particular cultural or ethnicity issues is also important. Health care professionals should learn to use interview strategies that will elicit and answer the patient's most important questions. For example, asking open-ended questions such as 'What worries you the most?' or 'What do you feel the future holds for you?', and specific, focused questions such as 'Who are your most important support persons?', 'Do you feel that you are a burden to your family?' or 'What is it that makes you the most breathless?' are likely to be more useful than simply asking about medication tolerance and benefits, or using unfocused questions such as 'How are things today?'. The advantage of having access to a COPD educator, or a pulmonary rehabilitation programme with dedicated patient-centred time is self-evident in this regard.

Health care professionals will be more comfortable and confident in empowering patients to acquire self-management skills if they are aware of local community resources (e.g. pulmonary rehabilitation programme, COPD educator), social support groups and other educational materials (print, video, web-based, etc.) that will assist with successful disease self-management for their patients. Patients and families also need to be made sufficiently self-confident that they willingly become more involved in disease self-management, always secure in the knowledge that help from health care professionals will be readily available. For example, patients must be hopeful that their symptoms will improve, so that they become motivated to change established counterproductive behaviours for healthier, more positive behaviours such as quitting smoking and adopting a regular exercise programme.

Collaborative self-management in chronic lung disease is more likely to be successful if the patient lives within a supportive family environment. As discussed earlier, the family or care-givers of patients with chronic lung disease experience significant stress themselves which may affect the success of attempts at self-management education in pulmonary rehabilitation. Either family members may be too supportive and not allow the patient to do much activity, or the chronic burden of living with the COPD patient can provoke resentment and apathy in the family and so hinder a supportive environment (26, 37). It is therefore important to realize that the family plays an important role in the rehabilitation process and should be included in the educational programme whenever possible (38), so that family members can be taught how to help patients to take more control of their disease management.

Programme elements

Regardless of the size and complexity of the programme and the setting in which self-management education occurs, the essential components of such programmes are well-defined (6) and are listed in Box 21.2. The initial steps of collaborative self-management education constitute an educational and psychosocial assessment of patients and family members or care-givers. This interview has several goals, including assessment of the prior education levels of patients and their family, and their learning needs and abilities. The styles of learning (e.g. hands-on, visual, verbal, written, small group or individual learning) most likely to be effective for the individuals are also assessed. Patients' prior knowledge of the disease process and the strategies to treat and to cope with the illness are also assessed, noting what has worked in the past and what has not. The use of a simple written or verbal pre-test may be helpful to objectify this process (6). Other aspects to be assessed at this initial stage include patients' hearing, vision and language proficiency, as well as any cultural issues that may be relevant to the learning process. The psychosocial assessment should include motivation level, coping strategies (e.g. alcohol use), presence of anxiety or depression, family stressors and conflict, the need for behavioural and lifestyle change and sexual dysfunction. This initial meeting also helps to acquaint patients and family members with the pulmonary rehabilitation team and, in so doing, to establish rapport, a sense of mutual respect and confidence and to reduce the anxiety and fear that are often present at this stage.

Various components of patient self-management education may be done by different health care professionals and members of the pulmonary rehabilitation team (e.g. physician, nurse, respiratory therapist, physiotherapist, occupational therapist, psychologist, nutritionist, social worker), depending on the topic being discussed and on the size and complexity of the rehabilitation team (see Ch. 18). In some small programmes, only one or two individuals in addition to a physician may responsible and provide an effective service (39, 40). Depending on the size of the programme, education may be done individually or in small groups. When teaching in a group setting, arranging the patients in a circular fashion without a table may help to create an atmosphere of shared problem-solving and facilitate discussion (Fig. 21.2). In general, information retention is more likely to be successful when a variety of teaching methods requiring the use of several senses are employed, including lectures, discussions, assigned reading, audiovisual material and hands-on demonstrations with practice. In the case of COPD, several patient-oriented educational materials are available, as described earlier in this chapter. Self-help books and manuals for COPD also exist as part of the GOLD (www.goldcopd.com), BTS COPD Consortium (www.brit-thoracic.org.uk/copd) and CLA BreathWorks (www.lung.ca) initiatives and in various formats (41, 42). The success of the education programme will depend on many factors, including the teaching and communication skills of the educator; the opportunity for patients and family members to contribute to the programme planning (i.e. a needs assessment); the clarity of the programme's teaching goals and objectives;

the adequacy of programme resources; and identification of potential barriers to learning (see below). The educational process may seem daunting for patients and their family at first, and the provision of a clearly written and illustrated rehabilitation patient workbook or handbook may be reassuring and can help as a source of reinforcement of the programme goals (43, 44).

The other components of a comprehensive self-management education programme listed in Box 21.2 are self-evident and follow logically. Self-management of chronic lung disease will be more effective when patient and family have a basic knowledge of both normal respiratory anatomy and physiology, as well as of how disease affects the body and causes symptoms. The influence of co-morbid illness (e.g. heart disease or arthritis) on the rehabilitation and training process is explained, as are the rudiments of medical tests and their interpretation. The principles of pharmacological and non-pharmacological treatments for chronic lung disease are reviewed, with an emphasis on the importance of non-drug treatments such as exercise training, energy conservation and symptom control strategies. Finally, various psychosocial issues that may affect learning or require special attention are explored. Such issues include patients' fears, anxieties and coping skills, family stressors and conflicts, sexuality issues and, if appropriate, any cultural or ethnicity issues that may influence learning. Upon completion of the education and rehabilitation programme, referral of the patient to a local support group (e.g. 'SOB – Shortness of Breath', 'Better Breathers', 'Huff and Puff' club, etc.) for ongoing educational and social support, and even exercise maintenance can be very helpful if these resources exist (43).

Once the initial assessment of the patient and family/caregiver has been completed, the rehabilitation team can begin to develop the necessary educational sessions (6, 45). This involves setting realistic learning goals which should include efforts to facilitate necessary behavioural and lifestyle changes that will lead to improved quality of life (for both patients and families), and which will help empower patients to take charge and become more active participants in their own health care by practising effective self-management strategies. Goal-setting should be done in simple terms that are easily understood and perceived as being relevant by the patient. Behaviour modification is thus an important ingredient in disease self-management (46, 47), and raising expectations for self-efficacy is key to achieving positive behavioural change in COPD patients. Patients can enhance their self-efficacy if they can be taught to do things that help themselves and so build their self-confidence and autonomy with self-management. As discussed earlier, acquisition of autonomy is directly related to improvements in HRQL (see also Ch. 15) and is probably more important than the actual behaviours that are taught (48). A meta-analysis of studies comparing behavioural modification methods with simple didactic teaching observed relatively small, non-significant effects with didactic methods, whereas behavioural modification techniques often resulted in large and clinically significant effects on health behaviour (47). Techniques used to enhance self-efficacy and facilitate

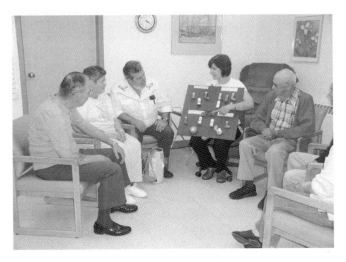

Figure 21.2 *Effective small group setting for patient education in chronic obstructive pulmonary disease (COPD).*

Box 21.3   Techniques for enhancing self-efficacy and successful behavioural change in COPD

- Explain the rationale for behaviour change
- Set realistic goals for behaviour change
- Help patients reduce the fear of changing behaviour (e.g. reassurance that exercise is safe)
- Facilitate family and social support for behaviour change
- Demonstrate how others have successfully changed behaviour
- Teach patients how to self-monitor for successful behavioural change
- Help patients practise the desired behaviour
- Practise positive reinforcement of behaviour change (i.e. provide rewards)

Box 21.4   Potential barriers to successful collaborative self-management education

Patient/family factors

- Low reading comprehension level
- Poor concentration or forgetfulness
- Anxiety and stress
- Excessive breathlessness and fatigue
- Unwilling or unable to take control
- Lack of adequate family or social support
- Cultural or ethnicity issues

Physician factors

- Lack of understanding, or fear of patient self-management
- Sense of too much time and cost
- Lack of motivation
- Insufficient support personnel (e.g. COPD educator)
- Lack of educational materials
- Lack of awareness of local resources (e.g. personnel, rehabilitation programme, educational materials)

Health care system factors

- Lack of awareness of system benefits and cost-effectiveness of this approach
- Inadequate community resource personnel
- Lack of educational material
- Local resources poorly publicized
- Inadequate financial resources
- Lack of a champion to lobby for change

---

positive behaviour modification are common components of many pulmonary rehabilitation programmes and are listed in Box 21.3. Such techniques include self-monitoring of specified goals, stimulus control, self-reinforcement, self-rewards, and reversal of negative behaviours.

Barriers to successful self-management education

Potential barriers to successful self-management education and possible solutions must also be appreciated by the health care professionals. Barriers to successful patient and family education may be related to the patient, the health care professional or the health care system itself (Box 21.4). As noted above, such patient factors include the level of education and reading skills, so that printed materials are often designed for a fairly basic literacy level, with abundant illustrations and video instruction if possible. Individualization of material through active demonstration of new skills (e.g. relaxation techniques) is essential. Teaching in a quiet environment with few distractions is helpful for patients who may be forgetful, or who have difficulty concentrating. Approaches that utilize humour, or that encourage open or group discussion of stressful feelings, may facilitate learning for patients burdened with anxiety and stress. For patients with excessive breathlessness and fatigue due to advanced disease, education sessions should be kept short and given after patients have had the opportunity to rest from other activities. The most important physician-related barriers to successful patient self-management education have been discussed above. Not infrequently, additional financial and resource-intensive barriers must be overcome. Local and national health care systems and their administrators may not appreciate the potential cost-effectiveness of a collaborative self-management approach to disease management, so that appropriate resources, including financial, facilities and personnel may not be readily available. In this regard, effective strategies for lobbying for positive change in support of educational programmes promoting self-management may be required, depending on local circumstances.

Setting for self-management education

Pulmonary rehabilitation and self-management education can occur in a variety of settings, depending on circumstances and the availability of local resources (39, 40). Patient education can begin in the acute hospital setting during COPD exacerbations; it can be part of a hospital-based multidisciplinary pulmonary rehabilitation programme, on either an outpatient or in-patient basis. Smaller, less resource-intensive programmes can be set up in outpatient clinics. Even the home environment can be suitable when patients cannot easily travel to a hospital or outpatient setting (49). Smaller pulmonary rehabilitation programmes will become increasingly important, because the majority of patients with chronic lung disease do not have adequate access to large-scale multidisciplinary programmes. For example, in Canada, where pulmonary rehabilitation is an established treatment modality, a 1998 national survey indicated that the existing rehabilitation programmes could serve less than 1 per cent of the rehabilitation needs of the Canadian COPD population (50).

WHAT IS THE EVIDENCE THAT PATIENT EDUCATION AND SELF-MANAGEMENT WORK IN COPD?

As discussed earlier, recent systematic reviews and meta-analyses of controlled trials suggest that the role of patient education in COPD management is uncertain (8, 9, 19, 21). However, there is a dichotomy between this view and those of practitioners of pulmonary rehabilitation, who recognize clear benefits attributable to patient and family education as an integral component of such programmes. This difference of opinion probably reflects the fact that data from controlled trials on patient education are sometimes found wanting due to the inherent difficulties in performing such trials. Quantifiable assessment of the value of education in COPD is difficult, because of the relatively long time required to achieve improvements in objective measurements of exercise capacity, and, perhaps even more importantly, because other end-points, such as HRQL and health care resource utilization, have only relatively recently been recognized as important outcome measures (25, 51). In addition, studies of patient education and self-management have not been double-blinded with respect to the interventions tested, because this is essentially impossible to accomplish in behavioural control clinical trials. Other problems with study analysis include varying periods of patient follow-up; often widely varying modes of education and self-management schemes; group vs. individual education; and the types of educational materials used (e.g. verbal instruction, written material, videos, etc.). As mentioned earlier, the patient's psychosocial status can also influence the success of self-management education and the success of pulmonary rehabilitation, and this has been infrequently considered in clinical trials. For example, in one study comparing an education-only programme to one that also included exercise training, patients who were the most depressed at baseline and who became less depressed during the programme experienced the greatest gains in exercise tolerance (52).

In order to review the evidence for the value of patient education and self-management education in COPD for the recent Canadian Thoracic Society COPD guidelines, a systematic literature review was conducted (19). The objectives of the review were to assess the effectiveness of self-management education interventions designed to develop self-care skills in adults with COPD and to identify the key components of an effective COPD self-management education intervention. Studies included in the review were restricted to: (i) randomized, controlled trials; (ii) quasi-experimental studies; (iii) prospective cohort or case–control trials. Primary outcomes sought in this review included HRQL scores, symptoms (e.g. dyspnoea), frequency and management of exacerbations, and health care resource utilization (e.g. emergency department visits, hospital admissions and unscheduled physician or clinic visits). Secondary outcomes included adherence, self-efficacy, skill development, patient knowledge and satisfaction, lung function and exercise capacity. The recent systematic review of self-management education in COPD from the

> **Box 21.5**   Levels of evidence
>
> Level 1: Evidence from one or more randomized trials
> Level 2: Evidence from one or more well-designed cohort or case–control studies
> Level 3: Consensus from expert groups based on clinical experience
>
> Evidence is further subdivided into the following categories:
>
> A. Good evidence to support a recommendation for use
> B. Moderate evidence to support a recommendation
> C. Poor evidence to support a recommendation for or against use
> D. Moderate evidence to support a recommendation against use
> E. Good evidence to support a recommendation against use

Cochrane Library (9), which also included non-randomized trials, was also included. The levels of evidence used in the current review are outlined in Box 21.5. All of the controlled trials reviewed used two basic trial designs: groups of patients with COPD of various degrees of severity (though not often well-described), randomized to an education-alone strategy, or to a strategy that included patient education plus exercise training; or a comparison of some form of formal patient education vs. 'usual care'. For this reason, specific trial details are not reported here.

Principle of collaborative self-management education

Collaborative self-management education is a valid and effective educational strategy in chronic disease management (level 1A)

The general principle of collaborative self-management in chronic illness has been evaluated by Lorig and co-workers (53, 54), who studied patients 40 years of age or older, with a physician-confirmed diagnosis of heart disease, lung disease, stroke or arthritis. Collaborative self-management consisted of the Chronic Disease Self-management Program, a community-based patient self-management education course. The content of the course has been published as *Living a Healthy Life with Chronic Conditions* (2) and was used as a text by participants. Topics covered included exercise; use of cognitive symptom management techniques; nutrition; fatigue and sleep management; use of community resources; use of medications; dealing with emotions of fear, anger, depression; communication with others, including health care professionals; problem-solving and decision-making. Each course was taught by a pair of trained lay leaders and the programme was given in seven weekly, 2.5-h sessions, similar to what occurs in many formal pulmonary rehabilitation programmes. Treatment subjects, when compared with controls, demonstrated improvement at

6 months in weekly minutes of exercise, frequency of cognitive symptom management, communication with physicians, self-reported health, fatigue, disability and social/role activities/limitations. They also had fewer hospitalizations and days in hospital. Most of these benefits were sustained at 1 year follow-up. Collaborative self-management for COPD patients has also recently been validated as an effective educational strategy by Bourbeau et al. (55) and is discussed in greater detail below.

Health–related quality of life (HRQL)

Self-management education in COPD can improve HRQL and health status (level 1A)

Chronic obstructive pulmonary disease-specific HRQL assessed using the St George's Respiratory Questionnaire (SGRQ) (56) has been measured in several studies (55, 57–59). Gallefoss and co-workers (58, 60) conducted a randomized trial of patient education vs. usual care in 62 outpatients patients with COPD, including a self-management plan for exacerbations for each patient. At 12 months after the intervention, HRQL as measured by the SGRQ was improved in the educated COPD group, but not in controls; however, this did not reach statistical or clinical significance. Using a similar trial design, Watson et al. (59) demonstrated that at 6 months the SGRQ activity and symptom domain scores were improved in the self-management education group compared with controls. When results from these two studies are combined, the SGRQ physical activity domain showed a significant and clinically relevant improved score (weighted mean difference, 10; 95 per cent confidence interval, -18.5 to -2.0) in favour of the patient education group (9). Preliminary results from EDU-CARE, a large, randomized, controlled trial from the Italian Association of Hospital Pulmonologists (61), have recently been reported (57). Results from this trial, which compares an educational intervention that includes telephone reinforcements vs. general advice and usual care in over 750 COPD patients, demonstrate that, at 6 months, patients in the educational group had a statistically significant improvement in the total SGRQ ($P < 0.0001$), and the magnitude of improvement was double the accepted threshold for clinical significance. The difference in the improvement between the educational and control groups was also statistically and clinically significant ($P = 0.0004$). Bourbeau et al. (55) conducted a multi-centre, randomized trial in patients with advanced COPD who had at least one COPD hospitalization in the previous year. Patients were randomized to a self-management education programme or to usual care. The intervention consisted of a comprehensive patient education programme, *Living Well with COPD* (42), administered through weekly visits by trained COPD educators over a 2-month period with monthly telephone follow-up. There were statistically significant and clinically meaningful improvements in the SGRQ total (-4.2; 95 per cent CI: -7.7 to -0.7) and impact (-6.2; -10.7 to -1.8) scores in the intervention group at 4 months. At 12 months follow-up, although SGRQ scores were still improved over baseline, only in the impact domain was this statistically and clinically significant (-4.7; -9.5–0.01).

Other trials of patient education in COPD using non-COPD-specific HRQL tools have in general failed to demonstrate significant impacts from patient education alone (62–64). Emery et al. (63) examined the effect of exercise and education on exercise endurance and psychological well-being in 79 elderly patients with COPD, randomly assigned to 10 weeks of exercise, education and stress management vs. education and stress management alone. Exercise endurance and indices of depression, anxiety and improved cognitive performance improved in the exercise plus education group, but not in the education-only group. Similar results have been reported by Ries et al. (65), emphasizing the crucial role for exercise training in pulmonary rehabilitation (8).

The importance of behavioural modification in the education of patients with COPD and its impact on HRQL have been demonstrated by Kunik et al. (66), who compared an educational intervention alone vs. a single 2-h session of cognitive behavioural therapy (CBT) in 56 elderly COPD patients. In this single blind, randomized trial, one group was given a single 2-h session of group CBT, designed to reduce symptoms of anxiety, with relaxation training, cognitive interventions and graduated practice, followed by homework and weekly calls for 6 weeks. The control group received 2 h of COPD education, followed by weekly calls. Compared with controls, the CBT group showed decreased depression and anxiety, but there was no difference in physical functioning between groups. Because 20–40 per cent of patients with COPD have high levels of anxiety and depression, these results suggest that CBT should probably be an important component of education programmes in COPD (27, 67).

Symptoms

Evidence supporting a role for self-management education in reducing symptoms in COPD is inconclusive (level 1C)

The effects of self-management education on COPD symptoms (e.g. dyspnoea) have been examined in two studies using different methodologies, but results were inconclusive (68, 69). Sassi-Dambron et al. (70) also assessed whether strategies for dyspnoea management alone might influence dyspnoea, exercise capacity and HRQL. In this trial, 89 patients with COPD were randomized to either a 6-week programme of dyspnoea management or to lectures on general health education. No exercise training was offered to either group. After 6 weeks, there were no significant differences between the study and control groups in any of the outcome measures, suggesting that dyspnoea management alone, without structured exercise training, is unlikely to improve this aspect of HRQL.

Health care resource utilization

Self-management education interventions can reduce health care resource utilization (level 1A)

A few studies have reported on the effects of self-management education on COPD-related utilization of health care resources and this topic is discussed further in Chapter 36. Dhein and co-workers have recently reported a favourable effect on hospitalization over 6 months for COPD in a randomized controlled trial comparing four 2-h outpatient education programmes with usual care (71, 72). In the COPD intervention group, self-monitoring of disease was significantly increased compared with the control group, and a significant reduction in the number of hospital days per patient per 6 months, from 7.1 to 4.3 ($P < 0.05$), was also seen in the intervention group. In the comprehensive self-management education trial by Bourbeau et al. (55) described earlier, hospital admissions for COPD exacerbations were significantly reduced, by 39.8 per cent, in the intervention group compared with the control group ($P = 0.01$). In addition, hospitalizations for other health problems were reduced by 57.1 per cent ($P = 0.01$) and emergency department visits were reduced by 41.0 per cent ($P = 0.02$) in the self-management education group.

Unscheduled physician and clinic visits have also been shown to be reduced in response to self-management education (55, 73). In the Bourbeau et al. (55) trial, unscheduled physician visits were reduced by 58.9 per cent ($P = 0.003$). In a study by Gallefoss and Bakke (73), during a 12 month follow-up, two times as many uneducated (control) COPD patients visited their primary care physicians compared with patients who received self-management education ($P = 0.001$), and the mean reduction in physician visits was 85 per cent in the educated COPD group compared with controls ($P < 0.0001$). This reduced health care resource utilization translated into reduced health care costs (74). This study was conducted in Norway, and, although not strictly comparable, translated into euros as follows: for every euro spent on patient education, a savings of 7.5 euros in overall health care costs was realized. In this trial, the number needed to educate to make one patient independent of the general practitioner was calculated to be 1.7 patients.

Frequency and management of COPD exacerbations

Self-management education may be associated with a reduction in the frequency of COPD exacerbations (level 1C), but does improve patient management of exacerbations (level 1B)

The frequency of exacerbations is a difficult outcome measure to study with confidence, mainly because it is highly dependent upon how a COPD exacerbation is defined. For example, the frequency of exacerbations that are infectious in origin are unlikely to be altered by any self-management intervention. However, self-management education can improve patient response to acute exacerbations of COPD, and because simple symptomatic exacerbations may often go unreported (75), it is possible that effective self-management education could provide patients with management strategies that would effectively preempt or control such flare-ups. In the study by Dhein and co-workers (71, 72), a self-management education intervention was associated with a significant reduction in the number of COPD exacerbations in the 6 months following patient education. In the EDU-CARE trial reported by Carone

et al. (57), at 6 months follow-up, the educational group had fewer exacerbations than the usual care group ($P = 0.01$). In the trial by Watson et al. (59), patients were randomized to receive a detailed self-management plan that provided advice on the management of COPD exacerbations in the form of an action plan plus a supply of prednisone and antibiotics. After 6 months, there were significant differences in self-management behaviour in the intervention group compared with controls. In response to worsening symptoms, 34 per cent in the intervention group vs. 7 per cent in the control group ($P = 0.014$) initiated prednisone therapy and 44 per cent (intervention) vs. 7 per cent ($P = 0.002$) initiated antibiotics.

Lung function and exercise capacity

Self-management education does not improve lung function, but can improve adherence to a regular exercise programme for patients with COPD (level 1C)

Although education alone might be expected to motivate some COPD patients to exercise more regularly and so improve exercise capacity, this has been difficult to demonstrate. Toshima et al. (76) reported a trial of comprehensive rehabilitation vs. education alone in patients with COPD. Patients were randomized to either an 8-week comprehensive rehabilitation programme, or to a four-session didactic education programme. The group receiving comprehensive rehabilitation showed improvements in exercise capacity, self-efficacy for walking and dyspnoea scores, whereas the education-only group showed no change in exercise capacity or symptom scores. Other studies have also suggested that patient education alone does not improve exercise performance (76–82).

Because exercise training is considered a cornerstone of pulmonary rehabilitation, behavioural modification to address problems with psychological functioning may influence the patient's ability to engage in, and benefit from, exercise training. Atkins et al. (83) evaluated the influence of behavioural modification added to exercise training on the patient's ability to follow an unsupervised walking programme. COPD patients were randomized to one of three behavioural modification groups, or to control groups who received only the walking prescription. In the behavioural modification groups, which met for seven sessions over 3 months, patients were trained to become aware of their own negative thoughts, feelings and behaviours, and to replace them with more positive cognition, and were also asked to give themselves 'rewards' contingent upon daily walking. At 3 months follow-up, the behavioural modification groups all showed significantly improved adherence to the walking prescription and improved exercise capacity compared with the control groups ($P < 0.02$).

The reported duration of positive behavioural modification changes is variable (84). Mall et al. (85) reported persisting benefits in exercise endurance and disease comprehension at 5 years follow-up in 32 per cent of COPD patients who completed an outpatient rehabilitation programme, while 32 per cent of patients had died and 36 per cent were worse. In the trial by Ries et al. (65), benefits of an educational + exercise programme for COPD that were clear at 6 months post-programme had diminished after only 12 months, suggesting that strategies to foster continuing behavioural change (e.g. an exercise maintenance programme), such as regular follow-up and referral to patient support clubs, are often necessary.

Patient satisfaction

Self-management education is associated with improved patient satisfaction with health care professionals (level 1B)

Patient satisfaction with their primary care physicians is important in disease management and, if significant, would be expected to enhance the success of self-management education initiatives, perhaps as a result of improved communication between patients, families and health care professionals. In the study of Gallefoss *et al.* (60) mentioned earlier, patient satisfaction with the handling of their disease by the primary care physicians was assessed before the self-management education intervention and again at 12 months. Prior to educational intervention, 85 per cent of COPD patients were satisfied with the care from their physicians. At 12 months, 100 per cent of COPD patients in the self-management education group were satisfied with the care received from their physicians, compared with 78 per cent of control patients ($P = 0.023$). This trial suggests that patient satisfaction may explain many of the positive effects of patient education, a hypothesis that requires further research.

Key points

- COPD is a systemic illness with important physiological, psychological and social manifestations that require a holistic, rather than merely a disease-oriented, management strategy for optimum patient benefit.
- Patient and family education and, in particular, collaborative self-management education have proved beneficial for patients with chronic lung disease and should be considered an essential component of pulmonary rehabilitation programmes, regardless of their size or complexity.
- The benefits of collaborative self-management education include:
  - improved health-related quality of life for patients with COPD (level 1A evidence)
  - reduced health care resource utilization for COPD (level 1A evidence)
  - improved patient satisfaction with health care professionals (level 1B evidence)
  - improved patient management of exacerbations (level 1B evidence)
  - improved adherence to regular exercise for patients with COPD (level 1C evidence)

- reduction in the frequency of COPD exacerbations (level 1C evidence)
- evidence supporting a role for self-management education in reducing symptoms such as dyspnoea in COPD is inconclusive (level 1C evidence)
- The structural components of collaborative self-management education have been well-defined and include:
  - assessment of learning needs/styles
  - assessment of psychosocial issues (e.g. coping strategies)
  - goal-setting and evaluation including self-monitoring
  - core disease knowledge
  - principles of pharmacological therapy
  - principles and rationale of non-pharmacological therapy (e.g. exercise training, behavioural modification)
- Recognition of the value of collaborative self-management education for chronic lung disease is growing globally.

REFERENCES

◆1. Partridge M. Patient education and the delivery of care. *Eur Respir Monograph* 2003; **8**: 449–58.

2. Lorig KR, Holman H, Sobel D *et al. Living a Healthy Life with Chronic Conditions.* Palo Alto, CA; Bull Publishing, 1993.

3. Gibson PG, Ram FS, Powell H. Asthma education. *Respir Med* 2003; **97**: 1036–44.

4. American Thoracic Society. Pulmonary rehabilitation. Official statement of the American Thoracic Society Board of Directors. *Am J Respir Crit Care Med* 1999; **159**: 1666–82.

5. Lacasse Y, Wong E, Guyatt G *et al.* A meta-analysis of respiratory rehabilitation in chronic obstructive pulmonary disease. *Lancet* 1996; **348**: 1115–19.

◆6. American Association of Cardiovascular and Pulmonary Rehabilitation. *Guidelines for Pulmonary Rehabilitation Programs,* 2nd edn. Champaign, IL: Human Kinetics, 1998.

7. ACCP/AACVPR Pulmonary Rehabilitation Guidelines Panel. American College of Chest Physicians. American Association of Cardiovascular and Pulmonary Rehabilitation. Pulmonary rehabilitation: joint ACCP/AACVPR evidence-based guidelines. *Chest* 1997; **112**: 1363–96.

●8. Lacasse Y, Guyatt GH, Goldstein RS. The components of a respiratory rehabilitation program: a systematic overview. *Chest* 1997; **111**: 1077–88.

●9. Monninkhof E, van der Valk P, van der Palen J *et al.* Self-management education for patients with chronic obstructive pulmonary disease: a systematic review. *Thorax* 2003; **58**: 394–8.

10. Kaplan R, Eakin E, Ries A. Psychosocial issues in the rehabilitation of patients with chronic obstructive pulmonary disease. In: Casaburi R, Petty T, eds. *Principles and Practice of Pulmonary Rehabilitation.* Philadelphia: WB Saunders, 1993; 351–65.

◆11. Bourbeau J, Nault D, Borycki E. *Comprehensive Management of Chronic Obstructive Pulmonary Disease.* Hamilton, London: BC Decker, 2002.

12. Cherniack N, Altose M, Homma I. *Rehabilitation of the Patient with Respiratory Disease.* New York: McGraw-Hill, 1999.

◆13. Hodgkin J, Celli B, Connors G, Pulmonary Rehabilitation. *Guidelines to Success.* Philadelphia: Lippincott, Williams & Wilkins, 2000; 635–91.

◆14. Bodenheimer T, Lorig K, Holman H *et al.* Patient self-management of chronic disease in primary care. *J Am Med Assoc* 2002; **288**: 2469–75.

◆15. Tiep B. Disease management of COPD with pulmonary rehabilitation. *Chest* 1997; **112**: 1630–56.

16. Bach J. Physical medicine interventions and rehabilitation of patients with neuromuscular weakness. In: Hodgkin J, Celli B, Connors G, eds. *Pulmonary Rehabilitation: Guidelines to Success.* Philadelphia: Lippincott, Williams & Wilkins, 2000; 591–608.

17. Novitch R. Rehabilitation in non-COPD lung disease. In: Hodgkin J, Celli B, Connors G, eds. *Pulmonary Rehabilitation: Guidelines to Success.* Philadelphia: Lippincott, Williams & Wilkins 2000, 609–20.

18. Pauwels R. GOLD: global strategy for the diagnosis, management and prevention of chronic obstructive pulmonary disease. *Am J Respir Crit Care Med* 2001; **163**: 1256–76.

19. O'Donnell D, Aaron S, Bourbeau J. Canadian Thoracic Society recommendations for management of chronic obstructive pulmonary disease. *Can Respir J* 2003; **10**(Suppl. A).

20. Petty TL. Strategies in preserving lung health and preventing COPD and associated diseases. The National Lung Health Education Program (NLHEP). *Chest* 1998; **113**: 123S–163S.

21. British Thoracic Society. Chronic obstructive pulmonary disease: national clinical guideline on management of chronic obstructive pulmonary disease in adults in primary and secondary care. *Thorax* 2004; **59**(Suppl. I): 1–232.

22. ERS Task Force. Position paper: selection criteria and programs for pulmonary rehabilitation in COPD patients. *Eur Respir J* 1997; **10**: 744–57.

23. Kida K, Jinno S, Nomura K *et al.* Pulmonary rehabilitation program survey in North America, Europe and Tokyo. *J Cardiopulm Rehabil* 1998; **18**: 301–8.

24. Agusti A, Noguera A, Sauleda J *et al.* Systemic effects of chronic obstructive pulmonary disease. *Eur Respir J* 2003; **21**: 347–60.

25. Carone M, Donner C, Jones P. Health status measurement: an increasingly important outcome evaluation in COPD patients. *Monaldi Arch Chest Dis* 2001; **56**: 297–8.

26. Stuifbergen A. The impact of chronic illness on families. *Fam Community Health* 1987; **4**: 43–51.

27. Sandhu HS. Psychosocial issues in chronic obstructive pulmonary disease. *Clin Chest Med* 1986; **7**: 629–42.

●28. Rennard S, Decramer M, Calverley PM *et al.* Impact of COPD in North America and Europe in 2000: subjects' perspective of Confronting COPD International Survey. *Eur Respir J* 2002; **4**: 799–805.

29. Vermeire PA. The burden of chronic obstructive pulmonary disease. *Respir Med* 2002; **96**(Suppl. C): S3–10.

30. Price D, Wolfe S. Delivery of asthma care: patients use and views on healthcare services, as determined from a nationwide interview survey. *J Asthma* 2000; **5**: 141–4.

31. Kaplan R, Toshima M, Atkins C *et al.* Adherence to prescribed regimens for patients with chronic obstructive pulmonary disease. In: O'Keene JK, Shumaker SA, eds. *Handbook of Health Behavior Change.* New York: Springer, 1990; 126–43.

32. Bandura A. *Self-Efficacy. The Exercise of Control.* New York, NY: WH Freeman, 1997.

33. Kaplan R, Ries A, Prewitt L *et al.* Self-efficacy expectations predict survival for patients with chronic obstructive pulmonary disease. *Health Psychol* 1994; **13**: 366–8.

34. Kaplan R, Simon H. Compliance in medical care. Reconsideration of self-prediction. *Ann Behav Med* 1990; **12**: 66–71.

35. Kaplan RM, Ries AL, Prewitt LM *et al.* Self-efficacy expectations predict survival for patients with chronic obstructive pulmonary disease. *Health Psychol* 1994; **13**: 366–8.

36. Grodner S, Prewitt L, Jaworski B *et al.* The impact of social support in pulmonary rehabilitation of patients with chronic obstructive pulmonary disease. *Ann Behav Med* 1996; **18**: 139–45.

37. Cossette S, Levesque L. Caregiving tasks as predictors of mental health of wife caregivers of men with chronic obstructive pulmonary disease. *Res Nurs Health* 1993; **46**: 251–63.

◆38. Gilmartin M. Patient and family education. *Clin Chest Med* 1986; **7**: 619–28.

39. Tietsort J. A storefront program for pulmonary rehabilitation. In: Casaburi R, Petty T, eds. *Principles and Practice of Pulmonary Rehabilitation.* Philadelphia: WB Saunders, 1993; 474–7.

40. Kravetz H. How the office-based pulmonary rehabilitation program works. In: Casaburi R, Petty T, eds. *Principles and Practice of Pulmonary Rehabilitation.* Philadelphia: WB Saunders, 1993; 483–6.

◆41. Hodder R, Lightstone S. *Every Breath I Take: A Guide to Living with COPD.* Toronto: Key Porter Books Limited 2003.

◆42. Levasseur C, Beaucage D, Borycki E *et al. Living Well with COPD.* Toronto: The Piper Group (from Boehringer-Ingelheim Canada), 1998.

43. Petty T, Tiep B, Burns M. *Essentials of Pulmonary Rehabilitation: A 'Do It Yourself' Program.* Lomita, CA: Pulmonary Education and Research Foundation, 1991.

44. Tiep B, Chow M. *Pulmonary Activation Program: Rehabilitation Guidebook.* Pomona, CA 1991.

45. Tiep B. Pulmonary rehabilitation program organization. In: Casaburi R, Petty T, eds. *Principles and Practice of Pulmonary Rehabilitation.* Philadelphia: WB Saunders, 1993; 302–16.

46. Todd W, Ladon E. Disease management: maximising treatment adherence and self-management. *Dis Manage Health Outcomes* 1998; **3**: 1–10.

47. Mazzuca S. Does patient education in chronic disease have therapeutic value? *J Chronic Dis* 1982; **35**: 521–9.

48. Smeets F. Patient education and quality of life. *Eur Respir J* 1997; **7**: 85–7.

49. Wijkstra P, van der Mark T, Kraan J *et al.* Long-term effects of home rehabilitation on physical performance in chronic obstructive pulmonary disease. *Am J Respir Crit Care Med* 1996; **153**: 1234–41.

50. Brooks D, Lacasse Y, Goldstein R. Pulmonary rehabilitation programs in Canada: a national survey. *Am J Respir Crit Care Med* 1998; **157**: A787.

51. Lacasse Y, Wong E, Guyatt GH *et al.* Health status measurement instruments in chronic obstructive pulmonary disease. *Can Respir J* 1997; **4**: 152–64.

52. Toshima M, Blumberg E, Ries A *et al.* Does rehabilitation reduce depression in patients with chronic obstructive pulmonary disease? *J Cardiopulmonary Rehabil* 1992; **12**: 261–9.

●53. Lorig KR. Evidence suggesting that a chronic disease self-management program can improve health status while reducing hospitalization. *Med Care* 1999, 37, 5–14.

54. Lorig KR, Sobel D, Ritter P *et al.* Effect of a self-management program on patients with chronic disease. *Eff Clin Pract* 2001; **4**: 256–62.

●55. Bourbeau J, Julien M, Maltais F *et al.* Reduction of hospital utilization in patients with chronic obstructive pulmonary disease: a disease-specific self-management intervention. *Arch Intern Med* 2003; **163**: 585–91.

56. Jones P. Health status measurement in chronic obstructive pulmonary disease. *Thorax* 2001; **56**: 880-7.

57. Carone M, Donner C. EduCare, an educational program for COPD, reduces exacerbations and improves quality of life. *Am J Respir Crit Care Med* 2003; **167**: A967.

●58. Gallefoss F, Bakke PS, Rsgaard PK. Quality of life assessment after patient education in a randomized controlled study on asthma and chronic obstructive pulmonary disease. *Am J Respir Crit Care Med* 1999; **159**: 812-17.

59. Watson PB, Town GI, Holbrook N *et al.* Evaluation of a self-management plan for chronic obstructive pulmonary disease. *Eur Respir J* 1997; **10**: 1267-71.

60. Gallefoss F, Bakke PS. Patient satisfaction with healthcare in asthmatics and patients with COPD before and after patient education. *Respir Med* 2000; **94**: 1057-64.

61. Carone M, Bertolotti G, Ceveri I *et al.* EDU-CARE, a randomised, multicentre, parallel group study on education and quality of life in COPD. *Monaldi Arch Chest Dis* 2002; **57**: 25-9.

●62. Blake RL Jr, Vandiver TA, Braun S *et al.* A randomized controlled evaluation of a psychosocial intervention in adults with chronic lung disease. *Fam Med* 1990; **22**: 365-70.

63. Emery CF, Schein RL, Hauck ER *et al.* Psychological and cognitive outcomes of a randomized trial of exercise among patients with chronic obstructive pulmonary disease. *Health Psychol* 1998; **17**: 232-40.

64. Littlejohns P, Baveystock CM, Parnell H *et al.* Randomised controlled trial of the effectiveness of a respiratory health worker in reducing impairment, disability, and handicap due to chronic airflow limitation. *Thorax* 1991; **46**: 559-64.

●65. Ries A, Kaplan R, Limberg T *et al.* Effects of pulmonary rehabilitation on physiologic and psychosocial outcomes in patients with chronic obstructive pulmonary disease. *Ann Intern Med* 1995; **122**: 823-32.

66. Kunik ME, Braun U, Stanley MA *et al.* One session cognitive behavioural therapy for elderly patients with chronic obstructive pulmonary disease. *Psychol Med* 2001; **31**: 717-23.

67. van Ede Y, Yzermans C, Brouwer H. Prevalence of depression in patients with chronic obstructive pulmonary disease: a systematic review. *Thorax* 1999; **54**: 688-92.

68. Solomon DK, Portner TS, Bass GE *et al.* Clinical and economic outcomes in the hypertension and COPD arms of a multicenter outcomes study. *J Am Pharmaceut Assoc* 1998; **38**: 574-85.

69. Gourley G, Portner T, Gourley D *et al.* Humanistic outcomes in the hypertension and COPD arms of a multicenter outcomes study. *J Am Pharm Assoc* 1998; **38**: 586-97.

70. Sassi-Dambron DE, Eakin EG, Ries AL *et al.* Treatment of dyspnea in COPD. A controlled clinical trial of dyspnea management strategies. *Chest* 1995; **107**: 724-9.

71. Worth H, Dhein Y, Schacher C *et al.* A comparison of the outcome of patient education in asthma and COPD. *Am J Respiratory Crit Care Med* 2003; **167**: A965.

72. Dhein Y, Munks-Lederer C, Worth H. Evaluation of a structured education programme for patients with COPD under outpatient conditions: a pilot study. *Pneumologie* 2003; **57**: 591-7.

73. Gallefoss F, Bakke PS. Impact of patient education and self-management on morbidity in asthmatics and patients with chronic obstructive pulmonary disease. *Respir Med* 2000; **94**: 279-87.

●74. Gallefoss F, Bakke PS. Cost-benefit and cost-effectiveness analysis of self-management in patients with COPD - a 1-year follow-up randomized, controlled trial. *Respir Med* 2002; **96**: 424-31.

75. Seemungal T, Donaldson G, Bhowmik A *et al.* Time course and recovery of exacerbations in patients with chronic obstructive pulmonary disease. *Am J Respir Crit Care Med* 2000; **161**: 1608-13.

●76. Toshima MT, Kaplan RM, Ries AL. Experimental evaluation of rehabilitation in chronic obstructive pulmonary disease: short-term effects on exercise endurance and health status. *Health Psychol* 1990; **9**: 237-52.

77. Ashikaga T, Vacek PM, Lewis SO. Evaluation of a community-based education program for individuals with chronic obstructive pulmonary disease. *J Rehabil* 1980; **46**: 23-7.

78. Janelli LM, Scherer Y, Schmieder L. Can a pulmonary health teaching program alter patients' ability to cope with COPD? *Rehabil Nurs* 1991; **16**: 199-202.

79. Howland J, Nelson E, Barlow P *et al.* Chronic obstructive airway disease; impact of health education. *Chest* 1986; **90**: 233-8.

80. Scherer YK, Schmieder LE, Shimmel S. The effects of education alone and in combination with pulmonary rehabilitation on self-efficacy in patients with COPD. *Rehabil Nurs* 1998; **23**: 71-7.

81. Emery CF, Schein RL, Hauck ER *et al.* Psychological and cognitive outcomes of a randomized trial of exercise among patients with chronic obstructive pulmonary disease. *Health Psychol* 1998; **17**: 232-40.

82. Howard J, Davies J, Roghmann K. Respiratory teaching of patients: how effective is it? *J Adv Nur* 1987; **12**: 207-14.

●83. Atkins C, Kaplan R, Timms R *et al.* Behavioral exercise programs in the management of chronic obstructive pulmonary disease. *J Consult Clin Psychol* 1984; **52**: 591-603.

84. Foglio K, Bianchi L, Ambrosino N. Is it really useful to repeat outpatient pulmonary rehabilitation programs in patients with chronic airway obstruction? *Chest* 2001; **119**: 1696-704.

85. Mall T, Medeiros M. Objective evaluation of results of a pulmonary rehabilitation program in a community hospital. *Chest* 1988; **94**: 1156-60.

22

Treatment of tobacco dependence

KARL FAGERSTRÖM, STEPHEN I. RENNARD

INTRODUCTION

According to World Health Organization (WHO) estimates, there are currently 1.1 billion tobacco smokers worldwide, representing about one-third of the entire population aged 15 years and over. Assuming that current trends in tobacco use continue, by 2030 the number of smokers worldwide will have grown to 1.64 billion, with a corresponding increase in tobacco-related diseases and deaths.

As tobacco consumption rises, there is generally a lag of approximately 30–40 years before a resulting increase in smoking-related mortality. Currently, tobacco use causes an estimated three million annual deaths worldwide, of which 1.9 million occur in the developed world (1). Although the rate of increase in smoking-related mortality in the developed world shows sign of slowing among men, it continues to accelerate among women. Moreover, with the massive expansion over recent decades in tobacco consumption in the developing world, smoking-related mortality is set to rise substantially. Without concerted action, it is estimated that the number of deaths worldwide will grow to 10 million annually by 2030, with 70 per cent of these occurring in developing countries. Tobacco is predicted to become the leading single cause of death by the 2020s, causing more than one in every eight deaths, and COPD's share of this death toll is steadily increasing. Half of all lifetime smokers will die prematurely as a result of tobacco use (2). Many others will experience tobacco-related morbidity.

SOME PATHOPHYSIOLOGY OF TOBACCO DEPENDENCE

There is now little doubt that a majority of the people who smoke tobacco do so to experience the psychopharmacological properties of the nicotine present in tobacco and that a significant proportion of habitual tobacco users become addicted to the drug nicotine.

The fundamental pharmacological effect of nicotine is through its action on the nicotinic acetylcholinergic receptors (nAChRs). These receptors are either homo- or hetero-pentamers that form an ion channel. As more than 15 gene products can form monomeric components of nicotinic receptors, there are a large number of theoretically possible combinations, many of which are present physiologically (3). Several specific receptor subtypes have been suggested to play an important role in nicotine addiction (4). The nicotinic receptors are distinct from the muscarinic receptors, which bind acetylcholine but not nicotine and are members of the G-protein coupled receptor family. Nicotinic receptors are believed to function primarily as modulators regulating the release of other neurotransmitters. The action of nicotinic receptors in modulating dopamine and norepinephrine (noradrenaline) release has been suggested to be of particular importance in nicotine addiction and in the perceived psychoactive actions of nicotine. In contrast, peripheral nicotinic receptors, which can modulate autonomic nervous system function, are not thought to contribute directly to the subjective pleasurable effects or the dependence characterizing smoking. By activation of central nAChRs, beneficial effects of nicotine such as cognitive enhancement, and increased control over arousal and negative emotions may occur (5). A schematic and highly hypothetical illustration of nAChR status as a function of state of addiction or neuroadaptation is shown in Fig. 22.1(a)–(d).

Under normal conditions a certain number of nAChRs are available for the cholinergic transmission (Fig. 22.1a). When initially exposed to tobacco smoke, some of these receptors are blocked after initial stimulation, leaving the nAChR system partially blocked (Fig. 22.1b). With continued smoking this blockade serves as a stimulus for upregulation to

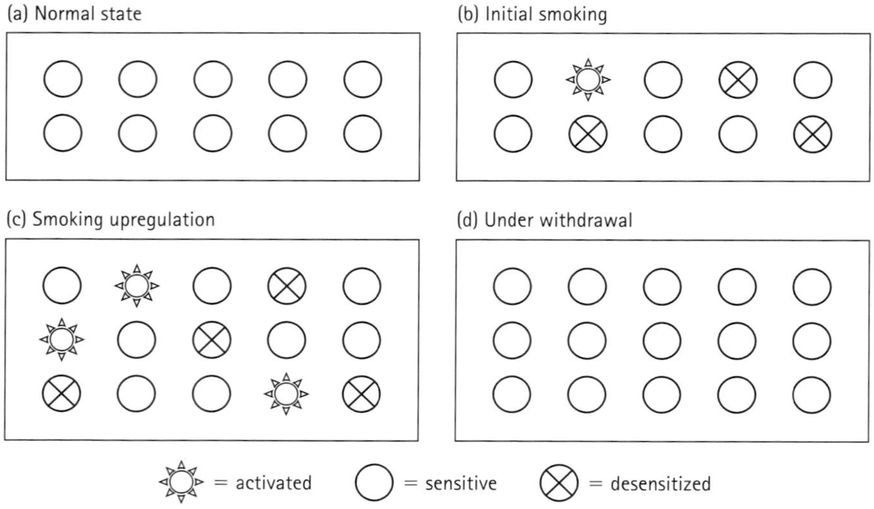

(a) Normal state

(b) Initial smoking

(c) Smoking upregulation

(d) Under withdrawal

☀ = activated   ◯ = sensitive   ⊗ = desensitized

Figure 22.1 *The status of the neuronal nicotinic acetylcholinergic receptors as a function of degree of tobacco dependence and neuroadaptation.*

compensate for the antagonistic effect of nicotine (Fig. 22.1c). The upregulation is dependent on the mode of administration. Chronic infusion of nicotine has been associated with more upregulation than injections (6). It is thought that those who smoke more often and with short intervals are administering nicotine in a way that is more conducive to receptor upregulation compared with those smoking just a few cigarettes per day with long intervals between. Finally, if nicotine administration is stopped, the system will have too many nAChRs, which may result in a hypercholinergic activity and withdrawal symptoms (Fig. 22.1d). The task for the cholinergic nervous system when nicotine administration is stopped is to re-adapt to a nicotine-free state. Unfortunately for the smoker, some of the changes following nicotine administration may be very long-lasting (7, 8).

The neuropharmacological correlates for tolerance may, at least partially, have to do with the process of neuroadaptation. The number of receptors or degree of upregulation is probably related to the long-term tolerance, while the more acute tolerance may be linked to the actual state of the receptor, whether it is in a sensitized or desensitized state.

MANAGEMENT OF TOBACCO DEPENDENCE

In a chest unit, about half of the patients are smokers, but among COPD patients 80–90 per cent are current or former smokers. For many of the respiratory disorders, smoking is part of the aetiology and should thus also be part of the management and treatment of the disease. This is particularly true for COPD where therapies other than treating the tobacco smoking have little effect on the long-term direction of the disease (9).

Smoking is a condition with features that are somewhat foreign and uncommon for physicians to deal with. Most conditions that physicians work with are biologically determined and often involve tissue damage. Smoking is often seen as a psychosocial phenomenon. Today, however, tobacco smoking

is regarded as a disorder by most authorities (10). Tobacco smoking can be regarded as a chronic relapsing disorder like peptic ulcers but, as with peptic ulcers, there are also effective treatments available.

There are many variables, e.g. environmental and genetic factors, that determine who will develop disease from smoking, e.g. COPD and lung cancer. One of the commonly overlooked factors is the propensity to become a smoker and the degree of dependence that develops. A series of twin studies have consistently demonstrated a genetic predisposition to become a smoker and to remain a smoker (11). Several candidate genes have been suggested (12). In a representative population study on degree of nicotine dependence in healthy and COPD smokers, it was found that COPD smokers were significantly more dependent (13). It has also been observed that the dependence is stronger in smokers with lung cancer than in healthy smokers (14). The smokers seen in the chest unit might be more dependent and therefore have more difficulties giving up than other smokers. This calls for more aggressive and innovative solutions to their smoking problem. Simple brief advice is seldom enough to break these heavily addicted patients' tobacco dependence.

Most physicians have just too short a time to spend with their patients, often not more than a few minutes per patient. In order to be efficient with the little time available, doctors often feel a need to use that time to convey important information to the patient, often in an authoritative one-way manner. This style is also generally the most effective way to transfer information, but is less effective in changing attitudes. In this case, true discussion is more likely to increase willingness and motivation to change smoking habits. Attitudes, in particular to smoking, a drug use that most smokers like and identify with, are more difficult to change than, for example, increasing the knowledge of asthma with consequential behavioural change. Thus a different strategy is needed, particularly since COPD patients are not usually approaching physicians asking for help to stop smoking. Unfortunately a common background is that the patient has been advised several times already by physicians and has

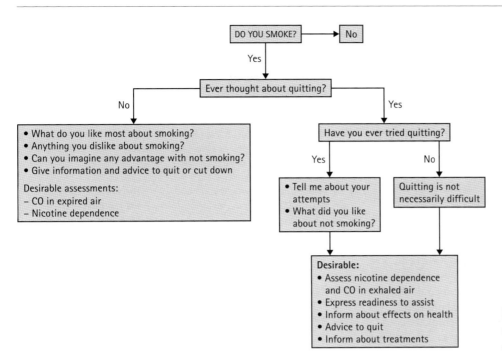

Figure 22.2 *Algorithm for a semi-structured interview with a smoker. Adapted from Rollnick et al. (15).*

failed repeatedly. These repeated failures may have damaged the patient's self-esteem and self-confidence so much that in order to have a better balance between attitude and behaviour they may say they are no longer willing to stop. This can be seen as an accommodation to reality: 'There's no point in trying again when I will fail anyway.'

In order to best help such smokers, physicians need to establish a good rapport with the smoker for whom smoking is a very sensitive topic. Often patients expect that doctors will tell them to stop smoking in a direct and clear way that will make them embarrassed and defensive. Therefore, an approach is called for in which smoking is discussed in an unthreatening, respectful and empathetic way.

Adequate information is currently available to suggest the benefit of a structured approach to the smoking patient. This approach includes a semi-structured interview together with an assessment of nicotine dependency and a biological measure of smoking: exhaled carbon monoxide.

Semi-structured interview

One aim of the conversation with the patient is to gather information on the current situation. In order for that to happen, listening becomes an important skill for the physician. The physician could begin by giving the patient a chance to talk about something unthreatening, e.g. what he or she likes or dislikes about smoking. Try to have the patient think about what could be good about stopping or reducing smoking by asking, for example, 'Would there be any benefits to your health if you did not smoke at all?' Patients are generally better persuaded by reasons which they feel they have discovered themselves than by those put into their minds by others, including their doctor.

Motivation for quitting and self-confidence in quitting are two constructs that can provide important information about the patient's readiness to quit. The physician could ask, 'How important is it for you to stop smoking?'; or, assuming the patient had already made up his or her mind to give up smoking: 'How confident are you that you will succeed?' Both questions should be answered on a 10-point scale, with 10 equal to 'very important' and 'entirely certain', respectively. This would give a picture how the smoker views an attempt to stop and what needs to be strengthened. Sometimes the patient is low in both motivation and self-confidence, in which case encouraging the patient to attempt to quit may not be a good idea. Probably more often with COPD patients the motivation is reasonably strong but the self-confidence in the ability to quit may be low. In order to obtain more information on the lack of self-confidence and how it can be strengthened, the physician could ask, 'You gave me a low 3 on self-confidence; what would need to happen for you to get from your current 3 to a 7?' The same sort of question can, of course, be asked in relation to motivation. If the readiness to give up is good, patients should rate themselves high on both variables (15).

Figure 22.2 shows an algorithm indicating how a conversation with a patient might proceed. The first step in any intervention is to establish whether the patient smokes or not. While this may be the most important modifiable health-related activity, it is asked far too seldom. In the US, guidelines suggest that this question be asked at every visit and be recorded, much as a vital sign.

It can be assessed by simply asking: 'Are you smoking?' This is better than asking, 'Are you a smoker?', since those smoking just a few cigarettes per day may not see themselves as smokers. If the answer is 'yes', the next question could be something like: 'Have you ever thought about quitting?' If patients have not thought about quitting, it is likely that they have a positive attitude towards smoking. Soft questions to follow up with are: 'What do you like most about smoking?' and 'Can you imagine any advantage in not smoking?'

If the smoker has thought about quitting, a further question could be: 'Why have you thought about quitting?' It is important that the patient is stimulated to give reasons why quitting is desirable rather than the physician putting the arguments into the smoker's mouth. After reinforcing the reasons for quitting, the next question could be: 'Have you ever tried?' If the smoker has tried, the natural continuation is: 'Tell me about your attempts.' The information gleaned from this could be important when dealing with future attempts to quit. Another question to ask is: 'What did you like about not smoking?' Here, try to stimulate the smoker to remember, or, if the attempt was too short, to imagine what could have been positive. If smokers have not tried to quit, it may be because they think it is too difficult to give up. In that case it could be valuable to find out what might increase their self-confidence (15).

In summary, the challenge in talking to smokers is to let them, rather than the clinician, do most of the talking. Clinicians should merely give them small prompts to keep them on relevant subjects and try to be respectful, understanding and empathetic.

Assessing the strength of the dependence and carbon monoxide concentrations in exhaled air

The strength of dependency can vary significantly. The degree of dependence has, for example, been found to predict success in cessation, withdrawal symptoms and need for pharmacological treatment (16). To get a diagnosis of dependence is therefore essential to guide the clinician.

Historically, the number of cigarettes smoked has served as the only measure of dependence. Today research has shown that number of cigarettes by itself is not the best measure of nicotine dependence. Biochemical measures, such as nicotine and its major metabolite cotinine, have more recently been used as indicators of dependence. However, nicotine has a short half-life of approximately 2 h and nicotine concentrations are therefore very dependent on time of day and when the last cigarette was smoked. Cotinine, a metabolite of nicotine with a half-life of 15–20 h, therefore has its advantages. Both can be analysed from blood plasma, saliva and urine. For cotinine, concentrations in plasma of <40 ng/mL are considered non-smoking levels. An 'average' smoker's level is around 200 ng/mL but can go all the way up to 1000 ng/mL (17). To date, sophisticated laboratory equipment has been necessary to determine these levels, but simpler devices for salivary and urinary determinations are being developed with a reasonable accuracy and quantitative grading. NicoMeter (a stick) is marketed in the USA (Serex Inc., Maywood, NY, USA) but not yet in Europe; while Smokescreen (Mermaid Diagnostics Ltd, Birmingham, UK), a syringe system, is available in Europe.

An indication of degree of dependence can also be obtained by questionnaires. The Fagerström Test for Nicotine

Table 22.1 *Fagerström test for nicotine dependence*

Questions	Answers	Points
1. How soon after you wake up do you smoke your first cigarette?	Within 5 min	3
	6–30 min	2
	31–60 min	1
	After 60 min	0
2. Do you find it difficult to refrain from smoking in places where it is forbidden, e.g. in church, at the library, in the cinema?	Yes	1
	No	0
3. Which cigarette would you hate most to give up?	The first one in the morning	1
	All others	0
4. How many cigarettes/day do you smoke?	10 or less	0
	11–20	1
	21–30	2
	31 or more	3
5. Do you smoke more frequently during the first hours after waking than during the rest of the day?	Yes	1
	No	0
6. Do you smoke if you are so ill that you are in bed most of the day?	Yes	1
	No	0

Dependence (FTND) is a widely used and researched short (six items) questionnaire (12). The information can be obtained in an interview or smokers can fill in the questionnaire themselves (Table 22.1). The scores range from 0 to 10 and the average in representative samples of smokers is usually between 3–4 points. The two most important questions relate to time to first cigarette in the morning and number of cigarettes smoked per day. These two questions alone give almost as much information as the whole questionnaire (18). Another strong, but relatively infrequent, indicator of dependence is nocturnal smoking. These smokers usually score very high on the FTND (19).

In the WHO's International Classification of Diseases and Injuries, diagnostic criteria are given for tobacco dependence. Here tobacco dependence can only be determined qualitatively (10).

Assessing the carbon monoxide (CO) in exhaled air can also be an indicator of dependence. The assessment of CO can be seen as an indicator of total smoke intake. If the CO intake is high, one can, with good reasons, assume that intake of nicotine and other toxins is also high. The CO concentration in the body can easily be obtained by having the smoker breathe into a CO analyser (Bedfont Scientific Ltd, Rochester, Kent; and MicroMedical Ltd, Kent, UK). The measurement of CO is in parts per million, which can easily be converted to COHb. In the absence of a CO analyser, COHb can of course be obtained from analysis of a blood sample. To demonstrate the 'CO effect' in smokers is of great motivational value. The recommended procedure is that therapists first obtain a reading for themselves, showing the normal CO concentration of 1–3 ppm. Smokers then blow into the machine, when they will invariably see a much higher reading of, on average, 10–20 ppm

Derby Hospitals NHS Foundation Trust

Library and Knowledge Service

(2–5 per cent COHb). CO has a half-life of approximately 4 h. Readings in the morning are therefore much lower than in the afternoon (20). One or certainly 2 days after the last cigarette, the CO is normal. This rapid normalization is very rewarding for the subject to see. After normalization, CO assessment can be used for control purposes. The elevated smoking CO value can be used to inform the smoker of the benefits of quitting. This is a little tricky. Reductions in CO may improve exercise performance as they improve O_2 delivery (21, 22).

However, while acute high levels of CO are toxic, chronic low levels may not be very toxic (23, 24). In fact, CO may have an anti-inflammatory action and serve to mitigate development of disease (25–27). This raises the interesting possibility that reduced CO devices (in a harm reduction strategy) may, in some respects, be worse!

TREATMENT

Behavioural

Treatment for tobacco smoking can be either behavioural or pharmacological. Among the behavioural methods, cognitive behaviour therapy is probably the most effective procedure but it is also expensive and seldom available. Fortunately, simpler counselling methods that can easily be applied by physicians and nurses without special training are also effective. Content and procedures with good efficacy are (28):

- the general problem-solving approach
- rapid smoking (inhaling from a cigarette approximately every seventh second until nausea or vomiting occurs)
- availability of social support.

Today there are also programmes on the internet that are believed to be effective, particularly those which are interactive.

It is encouraging to learn that there is a good association between stopping smoking and the number of minutes the doctor spends with the patient, as well as the number of sessions, the number of personnel involved and the duration of the treatment (29, 30). In order for a treatment to be maximally effective, it should also have a pharmacological component, particularly for the more nicotine-dependent subjects.

Pharmacological

NICOTINE REPLACEMENT

Nicotine is absorbed rapidly from cigarette smoke, which delivers a nicotine aerosol into the alveoli of the lung, from where it enters the arterial circulation and is rapidly distributed to body tissues. It takes only about 10 s for nicotine to reach the brain. Nicotine levels then fall, owing to uptake by peripheral tissues and, later, to elimination of nicotine from the body. Arteriovenous differences during cigarette smoking are substantial (31). The pharmacological relevance of this observation is that rapid delivery of nicotine results in a more intense pharmacological response, because of the higher arterial levels entering the brain rapidly. Nicotine levels in the brain decline between cigarettes, providing an opportunity for re-sensitization of receptors so that positive reinforcement can occur with successive cigarettes without too much development of tolerance. None of the available nicotine replacement (NR) products can mimic the pharmacological effects of a cigarette.

The rationale for NR is that when the smoker stops smoking cigarettes, the administration of nicotine from a different modality, such as a gum, will decrease the withdrawal symptoms during the initial phase of smoking abstinence. The pharmacological dependence on cigarettes is more or less transferred to the nicotine replacement product, enabling subjects to focus their resources for the cessation attempt on the behavioural aspects of coping with the urges from a strongly ingrained habit. Usually, the pharmacological dependence is not fully maintained because of a lower nicotine dose than during smoking. After a variable period of 2–6 months the nicotine supplementation can be tapered off gradually. In essence, the nicotine dependence is transferred, tapered and eliminated.

Transdermal systems.   There are three main nicotine patches on the market. The main difference between the patches is their drug-release kinetics: 24-h patches (Niquitin and Nicotinell) produce a more even, sustained blood level of nicotine throughout the entire day and night, whereas the 16-h patch (Nicorette) provides nicotine replacement during waking hours only. The two patches designed for 24-h application contain and deliver higher total amounts of nicotine than the 16-h patches. Peak plasma nicotine concentrations, which are normally reached within 4–9 h after patch application, vary between 13 and 23 ng/mL. Trough levels normally range between 2 and 11 ng/mL (32).

Recently a comparative pharmacokinetic study of these three patches has been carried out. This study showed a higher steady state and maximum nicotine concentration for the 24-h patches relative to the 16-h patches. Among the 24-h patches, Niquitin showed a higher relative dose of nicotine (AUC) and maximum concentration compared with Nicotinell (33). If more than one patch is used, a proportional dose linearity can be expected. Steady state is normally reached on the second day.

Acute systems (nicotine gum).   After a single dose, the increment is approximately 4–5 ng/mL for the 2 mg strength, and 6–7 ng for the 4 mg strength. After a single dose, the time to maximum concentration is achieved after approximately 30 min. When one piece was chewed hourly for 12 h, the trough levels were 4.3 and 7.9 ng/mL for 2 and 4 mg strengths, respectively (34), but in unpublished data, higher figures have been reported. In clinical trials with highly encouraged gum use, the nicotine concentrations achieved were about one-third of the baseline nicotine levels when smoking with 2 mg strength, and two-thirds with 4 mg strength. In routine practice, gum use is usually within five to 10 pieces/day, and the nicotine concentration therefore rarely exceeds 10 ng/mL for the 2 mg strength and 15 ng/mL for the 4 mg strength.

Nicotine nasal spray. One dose consists of 1 mg, 0.5 mg to each nostril. The spray is the fastest-acting of the NR products. It takes less than 10 min to reach maximum concentration and the increment of a dose is about 3–5 ng/mL. If used regularly, one, two or three times per hour, the nicotine concentrations after 12 h are 6, 13 and 18 ng/mL, respectively. Although the spray is faster than the gum, it is slower than nicotine uptake from a cigarette (35).

Oral inhaler. The oral inhaler, a mouthpiece 90 mm long and 10 mm wide, contains a porous plug that is saturated with 10 mg nicotine plus 10 per cent menthol to mask the nicotine taste and reduce irritation. It is a flexible ad lib dosing form, but offers more habit replacement than any of the other NR products.

When room temperature air is sucked through the porous plug, the nicotine concentration is 2 μmol/L. A puff of 50 mL (similar to an ordinary puff on a cigarette) releases about 0.1 μmol/L, while a cigarette would give about 1 umol/l. With higher ambient temperature, the concentration of nicotine increases, but will not reach the yield of a cigarette. The oral inhaler is therefore a relatively weak nicotine dosing system that requires the subject to work hard to reinforce the levels of nicotine. In a study where nicotine was radioactively labelled, it was found that only very minute amounts are inhaled into the lungs. Most of the nicotine was deposited buccally or in the upper respiratory tract (36). With ordinary use the inhaler gives about the same nicotine concentrations as 2 mg gum.

Sublingual tablet. The sublingual tablet contains 2 mg nicotine. The tablet should be kept under the tongue and be allowed to dissolve over approximately 20 min. The sublingual tablet is roughly bioequivalent to 2 mg nicotine gum. Highly dependent smokers are recommended to use two tablets (37).

Lozenges. Like nicotine gum, nicotine from the lozenge is absorbed slowly through the buccal mucosa and delivered into systemic circulation. The amount of nicotine absorbed per lozenge appears to be somewhat higher than that delivered by gum. Single-dose studies demonstrated 8–10 per cent higher C_{max} values and 25–27 per cent higher $AUC_{0-\infty}$ values from 2 and 4 mg lozenges (Niquitin) compared with gums at both 2 and 4 mg dose levels, which is probably due to the residual nicotine retained in the gum (38). There is also a 1 mg lozenge (Nicotinell) for lighter smokers available in some countries. The indication for the lozenge allocates smokers to the 2 or 4 mg dose based on whether the first cigarette of the day is smoked within 30 min after waking or not.

Efficacy

There is ample evidence that NRT is effective in helping smokers to quit. It is by far the most extensively and rigorously tested smoking cessation treatment. The most recent update by the Cochrane review summarizes 49 trials of nicotine gum, 24 of the transdermal nicotine patch, four of nicotine spray and four of nicotine inhalators. The overall odds ratio for abstinence with NR compared with placebo was 1.73 (95 per cent confidence interval [CI], 1.60–1.86). All administration

forms appear be equally effective. These odds were maintained regardless of the intensity of additional support or the setting in which the NR was offered (30).

It is important to realize that in these studies continuous abstinence (the strictest criterion was 'not a single puff allowed') over the long term has been required to count as success. Randomization to treatment groups and objective verification of smoking status are other requirements. Generally, the active/placebo difference has been larger in clinic-like settings than in general practice settings with minimal interventions. Success rates have also been found to be associated with degree of dependence.

Underdosing is a common feature with gum as with the other acute administration forms. Another reason for the better success rates in clinical trials is probably related to the better information the subjects receive on how to use replacement. This is particularly relevant for the gum, which is a surprisingly complex pharmaceutical to use. The nicotine bound to the polacrilex resin is released only with chewing. It must be absorbed across the buccal mucosa, however, so swallowing must be suppressed. Swallowed nicotine can lead to local gastrointestinal side-effects, but has limited systemic effect due to high first-pass metabolism in the liver. In a trial where the effect of a run-in week of gum use before quitting smoking was tested, significantly more use of product and fewer side-effects were reported. There was also a trend towards better success rates (39).

From the data available, it seems that the more replacement products used, preferably on a fixed schedule, the better the results, and that the 4 mg strength produces better results among highly dependent smokers than 2 mg gum.

With patches the users have no control over the nicotine dose, but because of simple instructions and ease of use, compliance with patches is usually better than with other NR products. The efficacy of nicotine patches has been found to be very robust across settings, countries and type of patient. Eight weeks of patch use has been shown to be as effective as longer courses of treatment, and there is no evidence that tapered use is better than abrupt withdrawal (40). Since there is no dose adjustment possible with patches but smokers vary in their dependence, it has been logical to try higher doses. In the largest well controlled smoking cessation study (26), a higher dose, 25 mg, was compared with the normal 15 mg dose of the 16-h patch. A small but significant effect of the higher dose was found. Similarly, in a recent review of studies involving higher patch doses, only a small effect in favour of higher dose was found (41). However, when nicotine patch dose has been tailored to the smokers' pre-treatment nicotine concentration, very encouraging results have been obtained (42).

For the 2 and 4 mg lozenges (Niquitin) there is only one trial reported. In this trial the 4 mg strength was given to highly dependent smokers smoking their first cigarette within 30 min after waking up. After 1 year the success rate in the highly dependent groups was 6 per cent on placebo and 15 per cent on 4 mg lozenge. For the less dependent smokers using placebo and a 2 mg lozenge, the percentages were 10 and 18, respectively (38).

Combining NR products

The rationale for concurrent combination of nicotine medications is that the provision of nicotine using different forms and modes of delivery can give improved symptom relief and possibly enhanced cessation outcomes than either product used alone by more adequately providing both higher daily levels of nicotine and the on-demand doses so readily provided by cigarettes. The nicotine patch, which delivers nicotine in a passive form, produces relatively steady levels of drug. A patch provides a general reduction of withdrawal symptoms and craving after application. However, this steady-state nicotine dosing does not allow users to respond to 'breakthrough' cravings with acute nicotine doses. These cravings, while usually brief, can be quite intense and are likely to be significant contributors to relapse (43). Most studies testing the efficacy of combined NR have found it to be more effective than single product use (44).

Safety

The safety of NR medications when used alone has been well demonstrated in numerous clinical trials. However, as with many medications, the adverse events and other pharmacological effects of nicotine are related to dose and speed of delivery. In general, nicotine-delivering medications provide lower doses per unit or per hour than are typically obtained by cigarette smoking, and the rate of nicotine infusion to arterial blood is substantially slower for nicotine medications than that achieved from inhaled cigarette smoke. Despite the fact that nicotine can produce adverse effects, severe acute adverse effects rarely occur when people are smoking, or using NR products, because tobacco users quickly learn not to exceed nicotine concentrations that are at the threshold for producing effects such as nausea or light-headedness (45). In fact, when replacing cigarettes with NR, a common problem is failure to comply with administration regimens that would provide enough nicotine to adequately relieve withdrawal symptoms.

The most frequently reported side-effect when using nicotine patches is local skin reaction. These reactions are usually mild and can be easily tolerated, although hypersensitivity, disseminated and local contact sensitization have been reported with all 24-h patches. It has been found that sleep disturbance is somewhat more common with 24-h patches than the 16-h patch (32). When sleeping problems occur with 24-h patches, the patch can be taken off in the evening. With the acute systems the most common side-effects consist mostly of local symptoms in the mouth, throat and stomach. After adequate instructions, most smokers learn how to use the products properly. Local irritation in the mouth and throat, indigestion and hiccups are the most common side-effects. Also, constant chewing can produce side-effects such as oral or throat soreness, ache in chewing muscles, and hypertrophy of the masseter muscles, and can exacerbate dental problems and temporomandibular joint disease.

BUPROPION

Bupropion sustained release (SR) is a unique, non-nicotine treatment hypothesized to act upon neurological pathways involved in nicotine dependence. Bupropion SR is a norepinephrine (noradrenaline) and dopamine reuptake inhibitor with some antagonistic effect on the nicotinic receptor. Its precise mechanism of action in smoking cessation is not definitively known (46).

The clinical efficacy of bupropion SR has been established in several well controlled trials (47). The 300 mg daily dose was significantly more effective than a 100 mg daily dose at promoting short- and long-term abstinence. Bupropion SR has also been shown to be effective for smoking cessation in patients with cardiovascular disease and COPD (48). Furthermore, the efficacy of bupropion SR does not vary significantly with patients' age, sex, history of depression or alcoholism, or degree of dependence on smoking.

Besides being effective at improving smoking cessation rates when administered for short treatment periods (7–12 weeks), bupropion SR administered for 12 months was effective in delaying relapse in patients who stopped smoking within 7 weeks of bupropion SR initiation (49). In another study, bupropion SR enhanced long-term smoking cessation rates in patients who were failures from a previous trial (50).

Bupropion SR is generally well tolerated. The most common adverse events associated with bupropion SR treatment for smoking cessation are dry mouth and insomnia, which were reported approximately twice as frequently with bupropion SR than with placebo in controlled clinical trials. The most medically important serious adverse event reported with bupropion is seizure, which occurs infrequently and is associated with risk factors such as the presence of a seizure disorder (e.g. epilepsy) or an eating disorder (e.g. bulimia or anorexia nervosa). When bupropion is administered as outlined in the product information, the rate of seizure is approximately 0.1 per cent (51).

Administration of bupropion.   Steady-state plasma concentrations of bupropion and its active metabolites are achieved at approximately 8 days after initiation of therapy. To maximize the chances of therapeutic success, bupropion therapy should be initiated 1–2 weeks before the target quit date to allow steady-state drug and metabolite levels to be attained. For the first 3–7 days, 150 mg/day of bupropion is given and thereafter the dose should increase to 300 mg/day except where the 150 mg dose is preferable, e.g. in elderly and low-weight smokers. The treatment duration is normally 7–12 weeks.

COMPARABLE EFFICACY OF BUPROPION AND NRT

Nicotine replacement and bupropion seem to be equally effective with close to doubling long-term quit rates. Smoking cessation guidelines classify both as first-line treatments, and treats them as equally efficacious (28).

In a recent meta-analysis of 33 studies with nicotine patches and seven with bupropion the long-term efficacy was evaluated. The relative risks against placebo for being abstinent at 12 months follow up after quitting were 1.73 for nicotine patch and 1.76 for bupropion (52). Two medications currently available have potential for therapeutic support of smoking cessation (53). These medications are clonidine, an antihypertensive with central anti-norepinephrine actions, and the tricyclic antidepressant nortriptyline. Neither is approved specifically for smoking cessation. Both, however, have been evaluated in several clinical trials, and based on the weight of evidence, guidelines suggest the clinician experienced in their use consider them as second-line treatments. A number of other psychoactive compounds have been tested. Available evidence does not support their use.

WHAT CAN BE DONE WITH SMOKERS WHO CANNOT OR DO NOT WANT TO QUIT?

What advice can be given to smokers who have failed in their attempts to quit? Generally, if a certain approach or method has failed, it would be wise to offer something different or new as methods that have previously failed are often associated with low or negative expectations. The new method could involve more intensive intervention, e.g. professional help with medications or behavioural treatment.

Another approach could be to offer a less dramatic programme of reducing smoking for those not willing and able to stop smoking abruptly. There are two possible benefits with reducing smoking. First, and most important, it can be a way to gradually, rather than abruptly, quit smoking altogether. Quitting in this less traumatic way could take anything from weeks to months. The other possible benefit is to reduce the harm done to the patient from smoking. Tobacco smoking lends itself very well to a harm reduction approach, since for COPD and respiratory disorders in general there is a strong relationship between amount smoked and disease risk.

Nicotine replacement products and bupropion can also be used to aid reduction in smoking. With bupropion, one study found bupropion to be more effective than placebo in reducing smoking (54). For NR there are several studies (e.g. 55) that have shown positive effects in reducing smoking, but there is also a study with NR mailed to the participating subjects that showed no effect (56).

A concern with these studies is that smokers who reduce may become less motivated to quit. An unexpected 'bonus' in the studies to date, however, is that many smokers previously unwilling to quit became motivated to do so (54, 55).

What are the benefits of the harm reduction approach for COPD patients?

In a study by Rennard *et al.* (57), 15 heavy smokers (>40 cigarettes/day) who were not interested in quitting were evaluated. The study goal was to reduce the number of cigarettes smoked daily by 50 per cent, and smokers were instructed to use at least 10 pieces of 2 mg nicotine gum per day. Cigarette smoking declined rapidly within the first week, from a mean of 51 to 19 cigarettes/day. This reduction was maintained for the 9 weeks of the study with no evidence of a loss of treatment effect over time. Mean exhaled CO levels decreased from 49 ppm at baseline to 27 ppm at 4 weeks, and remained at this level until week 9. Bronchoscopy at week 9 showed a decline in airways inflammation using a visual index, a decline in alveolar macrophage and a decrease in neutrophil elastase.

Wennike *et al.* (58) found that reduced smoking aided by the oral inhaler produced an 11 per cent reduction in inhaled steroids, and a reduction in bronchial hyperreactivity was observed at the 4-month follow-up. In a case study (17 cases) all five patients who could maintain a substantial reduction in smoking for 18 months showed improved lung function (59).

In a single case with emphysema and COPD, an 8-month smoking reduction period resulted in complete cessation with considerable improvement in lung function (60). In a population study with a 30-year follow-up, smokers who reduced smoking had a reduced rate of $FEV_{0.75}$ decline compared with continuous smokers (61). However in another prospective population study looking at hospitalization for COPD, no effect was seen among reducers compared with non-reducers (62).

There are concerns that taking nicotine from NR products while smoking at the same time could increase nicotine concentrations and cause adverse effects. In order to investigate this, Fagerström and Hughes (63) reviewed all studies with concurrent use of cigarettes and use of acute NR products. The smokers titrated their nicotine levels quite well with acute forms of NR. No increase in nicotine blood concentration was found. The reduction in cigarettes was not paralleled by the same reduction in CO. Thus there seems to be some compensatory smoking, so that the smokers smoke their remaining cigarettes more intensively. It thus seems that an assessment of CO is a necessity in harm/smoking reduction studies for securing reduction in harm. A sizeable reduction in cigarettes smoked, e.g. 20 per cent, may produce little or no reduced harm if CO intake is a valid indicator. There is a growing agreement among clinicians and researchers that a 50 per cent reduction in number of cigarettes smoked may need to be obtained before true harm reduction can be reasonably ascertained. However, when reductions in CO can be achieved, oxygen delivery is likely to be improved, due to increased carrying capacity of haemoglobin. In patients with coronary artery disease, this effect can have an acute benefit on exercise performance (21). Regarding adverse effects, they were few and mild with concurrent smoking and use of NR, and an increase in cardiac toxicity was not observed (21, 64, 65).

Where harm reduction strategies will fit into clinical management remains to be determined. Adverse effect of such strategies could include providing a disincentive to quitting, providing a seemingly 'safer' way to start smoking and, possibly, eroding the social impetus fostering cessation. The topic of harm reduction has been reviewed by the Institute of Medicine in the United States and their report suggests that it should be part of all comprehensive tobacco control programmes (66). Clinicians should at least be aware of such approaches as, unfortunately, many patients with significant smoke-induced disease will be unable or unwilling to quit.

Key points

- Many smokers suffer from the tobacco dependence disorder that involves structural changes in the brain.
- Giving up smoking is the most important intervention for COPD patients.
- Many COPD smokers are highly dependent on tobacco and may have co-morbidity such as depression that makes stopping smoking particularly difficult.
- When obtaining the background information and doing counselling, physicians should adopt an unthreatening, respectful and empathetic style.
- There are effective pharmacological treatments that will increase benefit.
- Be prepared to find alternatives, such as quitting gradually, for those not interested or able to quit abruptly. A harm reduction approach, e.g. NR used concurrently with smoking, may be a good aid to reduce cigarette consumption, although clinical benefits remain to be clearly established.

REFERENCES

●1. World Health Organization *Tobacco or Health; A Global Status Report*. Geneva: World Health Organization 1997.
2. Peto R. Smoking and death. *Br Med J* 1994; **309**: 937–9.
3. Picciotto MR, Caldarone BJ, Brunzell DH *et al*. Neuronal nicotinic acetylcholine receptor subunit knockout mice: physiological and behavioral phenotypes and possible clinical implications. *Pharmacol Ther* 2001; **92**: 89–108.
4. Picciotto MR, Corrigall WA. Neuronal systems underlying behaviors related to nicotine addiction: neural circuits and molecular genetics. *J Neurosci* 2002; **22**: 3338–41.
5. Sherwood N. Effects of nicotine on human psychomotor performance. *Hum Psychopharmacol* 1993; **8**: 155–84.
6. Ulrich YM, Hargreaves KM, Flores CM. A comparison of multiple injections versus continuous infusion of nicotine for producing up-regulation of neuronal [^{3}H]–epibatidine binding sites. *Neuropharmacology* 1997; **36**: 1119–25.
7. Van de Kamp JL, Collins AC. Prenatal nicotine alters nicotinic receptor development in the mouse brain. *Pharmacol Biochem Behav* 1994; **47**: 889–900.
8. Balfour DJ. Neural mechanisms underlying nicotine dependence. *Addiction* 1994; **89**: 1419–23.
●9. Anthonisen NR, Connett JE, Kiley GP. Effects of smoking intervention and use of an inhaled anticholinergic bronchodilator on the rate of decline in FEV1. The lung health study. *J Am Med Assoc* 1994; **272**: 1497–505.
10. The World Health Organization. *The ICD-10 Classification of Mental, Behavioural Disorders*. Geneva: World Health Organization, 1992.
11. Li MD, Cheng R, Ma JZ, Swan GE. A meta-analysis of estimated genetic and environmental effects on smoking behavior in male and female adult twins. *Addiction* 2003; **98**: 23–31.
●12. Rossing MA. Genetic influences on smoking: candidate genes. *Environ Health Perspect* 1998; **106**: 231–8.

13. Jimenez-Ruiz CA. Smoking characteristics. differences in attitudes and dependence between healthy smokers and smokers with COPD. *Chest* 2001; **119**: 1365–70.
14. Kubik A, Zatloukal P, Boyle P *et al*. A case-control study of lung cancer among Czech women. *Lung Cancer* 2001; **31**: 111–21.
15. Rollnick S, Mason P, Butler C *et al*. *Health Behaviour Change; a Guide for Practitioners*. Churchill Livingstone, London 1999.
16. Fagerström K-O, Schneider N. Measuring nicotine dependence: a review of the Fagerström Tolerance Questionnaire. *J Behav Med* 1989; **12**: 182.
17. Etter JF, Duc TV, Perneger TV. Saliva cotinine levels in smokers and non-smokers. *Am J Epidem* 2000; **151**: 251–8.
●18. Heatherton TF, Kozlowski LT, Frecker RC *et al*. The Fagerström test for nicotine dependence: a revision of the Fagerström tolerance questionnaire. *Br J Addiction* 1991; **86**: 1119–27.
19. Kunze U, Schoberberger R, Schmeiser-Rieder A *et al*. Alternative nicotine delivery systems (ANDS) – public health aspects. *Wiener Klinische Wochenschrift* 1998; **110**: 811–16.
20. Jarvis MJ, Belcher W, Vessey C. Low cost carbon monoxide monitors in smoking assessment. *Thorax* 1986; **41**: 886–7.
21. Mahmarian JJ, Moye LA, Nasser GA. Nicotine patch therapy in smoking cessation reduces the extent of exercise-induced myocardial ischemia. *J Am Coll Cardiol* 1997; **30**: 125–30.
22. McDonough P, Moffatt RJ. Smoking-induced elevations in blood carboxyhaemoglobin levels. Effect on maximal oxygen uptake. *Sports Med* 1999; **27**: 275–83.
23. Committee of the Environmental and Occupational Health Assembly of the American Thoracic Society. Health effects of outdoor air pollution. *Am J Respir Crit Care Med* 1996; **153**: 3–50.
24. Committee of the Environmental and Occupational Health Assembly of the American Thoracic Society. Health effects of outdoor air pollution. Part 2. *Am J Respir Crit Care Med* 1996; **153**: 477–98.
25. Otterbein LE, Mantell LL, Choi AM. Carbon monoxide provides protection against hyperoxic lung injury. *Am J Physiol* 1999; **276**: L688–94.
26. Otterbein LE, Zuckerbraun BS, Haga M *et al*. Carbon monoxide suppresses arteriosclerotic lesions associated with chronic graft rejection and with balloon injury. *Nat Med* 2003; **9**: 183–90.
27. Song R, Kubo M, Morse D *et al*. Carbon monoxide induces cytoprotection in rat orthotopic lung transplantation via anti-inflammatory and anti-apoptotic effects. *Am J Pathol* 2003; **163**: 231–42.
●28. Fiore MC, Bailey WC, Cohen SJ. *Treating Tobacco Use and Dependence. Clinical Practice Guideline*. Rockville, MD: US Department of Health and Human Services, 2000.
●29. Fiore MC, Bailey WC, Cohen SJ. *Smoking Cessation. Guideline Technical Report no. 18*. Publication No. AHCPR 97-No. 4. Rockville, MD: US Department of Health and Human Services, Public Health Service, Agency for Health Care Policy and Research, 1997.
●30. Cochrane Tobacco Addiction Group. Online. www.dphpc.ox.ac.uk/cochrane_tobacco/index.html. Oxford: Department of Primary Health Care, University of Oxford.
31. Henningfield JE, Stapleton JM, Benowitz NL *et al*. Higher levels of nicotine in arterial than in venous blood after cigarette smoking. *Drug Alcohol Depend* 1993; **33**: 23–9.
32. Fagerström K-O, Sachs DPL. Medical management of tobacco dependence: a critical review of nicotine skin patches. *Current Pulmonol* 1995; **16**: 223–38.
33. Fant RV, Henningfield JE, Shiffman S *et al*. A pharmacokinetic crossover study to compare the absorption characteristics of three transdermal nicotine patches. *Pharmacol Biochem Behav* 2000; **67**: 479–82.

34. Benowitz NL, Jacob P III, Savanapridi C. Determinants of nicotine intake while chewing nicotine polacrilex gum. *Clin Pharmacol Ther* 1987; **41**: 467–73.

35. Benowitz NL, Zevin S, Jacob P III. Sources of variability in nicotine and cotinine levels with use of nicotine nasal spray. *Br J Clin Pharmacol* 1997; **43**: 259–67.

36. Bergström M, Nordberg A, Lunell E. Regional deposition of inhaled 11C-nicotine vapour in the human airway as visualized by positron emission tomography. *Clin Pharmacol Ther* 1995; **57**: 309–17.

37. Molander L, Lunell E. Pharmacokinetic investigation of a nicotine sublingual tablet. *Eur J Clin Pharmacol* 2001; **56**: 813–19.

38. Shiffman S, Dresler CM, Hajek P *et al*. Efficacy of a nicotine lozenge for smoking cessation. *Arch Intern Med* 2002; **162**: 1267–76.

39. Herrera N, Franco R, Herrera L *et al*. Nicotine gum, 2 and 4 mg, for nicotine dependence: a double-blind placebo-controlled trial within a behaviour modification support program. *Chest* 1995; **106**: 447–51.

40. Tonnesen P, Paoletti P, Gustavsson G *et al*. Higher dosage nicotine patches increase one-year smoking cessation rates: results from the European CEASE trial. Collaborative European Anti-Smoking Evaluation. *Eur Resp J* 1999; **13**: 238–46.

41. Hughes JR, Lesmes GR, Hatsukami DK *et al*. Are higher doses of nicotine replacement more effective for smoking cessation. *Nicotine Tobacco Res* 1999; **1**: 169–74.

42. Sachs DPL, Benowitz NL, Bostrom AG, Hansen MD. *Percent Serum Replacement & Success of Nicotine Patch Therapy*. Presented at ATS International Conference, Seattle, WA, USA.

43. Killen JD, Fortmann SP. Craving is associated with smoking relapse: findings from three prospective studies. *Exp Clin Psychopharmacol* 1997 1995; **5**: 137–42.

44. Sweeney C, Fant R, Fagerström KO *et al*. Combination nicotine replacement therapy for smoking cessation. *CNS Drugs* 2001; **15**: 453–67.

45. Zevin S, Jacop P, Benowitz N. Dose-related cardiovascular and endocrine effects of transdermal nicotine. *Clin Pharmacol Therapeutics* 1998; **64**: 87–95.

46. Johnston AJ, Ascher J, Landbetter R *et al*. Pharmacokinetic optimisation of sustained-release bupropion for smoking cessation. *Drugs* 2002; **62**(Suppl. 2): 11–24.

47. Hurt RD, Sachs DP, Glover ED *et al*. A comparison of sustained release bupropion and placebo for smoking cessation. *N Engl J Med* 1997; **337**: 1195–202.

48. Tashkin DP, Kanner R, Bailey W. Smoking cessation in patients with chronic obstructive pulmonary disease. *Lancet* 2001; **357**: 1571–5.

49. Hays JT, Hurt RD, Rigotti N *et al*. Sustained-release bupropion for pharmacologic relapse prevention after smoking cessation. *Ann Intern Med* 2001; **135**: 423–33.

50. Gonzales DH, Nides MA, Ferry LH *et al*. Bupropion SR as an aid to smoking cessation in smokers treated previously with bupropion. *Clin Pharmacol Ther* 2001; **9**: 438–44.

51. Aubin HJ. Tolerability and safety of sustained-release bupropion in the management of smoking cessation. *Drugs* 2002; **62**: 45–52.

52. Fagerström K-O. Clinical treatment of tobacco dependence: the endurance of pharmacologic efficacy. (Monograph.) *J Clin Psychiatry* 2003; **18**: 35–40.

53. Fiore MC. US public health service clinical practice guideline: treating tobacco use and dependence. *Respir Care* 2000; **45**: 1200–62.

54. Hatsukami D, Rennard S, Malcolm R *et al*. A multicenter study examining the effects of Zyban vs placebo as an aid to smoking reduction leading to cessation among smokers unwilling to quit. *Poster at the Annual European Meeting of the Society for Research on Nicotine and Tobacco, September 19–22, Paris*. 2001.

55. Bolliger C, Zellweger P, Danielsson T *et al*. Smoking reduction with oral nicotine inhalers: Double blind, randomised clinical trial of efficacy and safety. *Br Med J* 2000; **321**: 329–33.

56. Etter J-F, Laszlo E, Zellweger JP *et al*. Nicotine replacement to reduce cigarette consumption in smokers who are unwilling to quit: a randomized study. *J Clin Psychpharmacol* 2002; **22**: 1–9.

57. Rennard S, Daughton D, Fujita J. Short-term smoking reduction is associated with reduction in measures of lower respiratory tract inflammation in heavy smokers. *Eur Respir J* 1990; **3**: 752–9.

58. Wennike PJ, Bremann L, Tonnesen P. Does smoking cessation/reduction improve asthma regulation. *Poster at the Annual Meeting of the ERS, Berlin, September 20–25*. 2001.

59. Jimenez-Ruiz C, Solano S, Viteri S *et al*. Harm reduction – a treatment approach for resistant smokers with tobacco-related symptoms. *Respiration* 2002; **69**: 452–5.

60. Fagerström K-O. From reduced smoking to quitting: improvements in COPD symptoms and lung function. A case report. *Nicotine Tobacco Res* 2001; **3**: 93–4.

61. Pelkonen M, Notkola IL, Tulkiainen H *et al*. Smoking cessation, decline in pulmonary function and total mortality: a 30 year follow up study among Finnish cohorts of the Seven Countries Study. *Thorax* 2001; **56**: 703–9.

62. Godtfredsen NS, Vestbo J, Osler M *et al*. Risk of hospital admission for COPD following smoking cessation and reduction: a Danish population study. *Thorax* 2002; **57**: 967–72.

63. Fagerström K-O, Hughes J. Nicotine concentrations with concurrent use of cigarettes and nicotine replacement: A review. *Nicotine Tobacco Res* 2002; (Suppl.): 73–79.

64. Joseph AM, Norma SM, Ferry LH. The safety of transdermal nicotine as an aid to smoking cessation in patients with cardiac disease. *N Engl J Med* 1996; **335**: 1792–8.

65. Working Group for the Study of Transdermal Nicotine in Patients with Coronary Artery Disease. Nicotine replacement therapy for patients with coronary artery disease. *Arch Intern Med* 1994; **154**: 989–95.

●66. Stratton K, Shetty P, Wallace R, Bondurant S (eds). *Clearing the Smoke: Assessing the Science Base for Tobacco Harm Reduction*. Washington, DC: National Academy Press, 2001.

23

Nutrition and metabolic therapy

ANNEMIE M. W. J. SCHOLS, EMIEL F. M. WOUTERS

INTRODUCTION

Nutritional screening and therapy are considered essential components of pulmonary rehabilitation nowadays. In particular, systemic manifestations of chronic obstructive pulmonary disease (COPD), such as weight loss, muscle wasting and altered muscle metabolism, are potential targets for intervention. This chapter demonstrates the rationale and efficacy of nutritional support strategies to reverse weight loss and discusses the effects of nutritional supplementation and pharmacological anabolic stimuli as part of a pulmonary rehabilitation programme to treat muscle wasting. Furthermore, we address the perspective for metabolic modulation to enhance the response to exercise training.

TREATMENT OF WEIGHT LOSS

The association between underweight and increased mortality risk has been well established in numerous retrospective studies ranging from selected COPD patients to population-based samples (1–3). Two prospective studies even showed, in COPD patients with a body mass index (BMI) below 25 kg/m^2, that weight gain was associated with decreased mortality risk (2, 4). Based on these studies it can be concluded that not only underweight COPD patients should be considered for caloric supplementation but also patients with a BMI $<25 \text{ kg/m}^2$ and involuntary weight loss. It is not fully understood why COPD patients become underweight but weight loss, specifically loss of fat mass, is generally the result of a negative energy balance. Weight loss may occur independently of the severity of the airflow obstruction, but is more prevalent in the emphysematous subtype (5). In contrast to many other chronic diseases and conditions, elevated daily energy expenditure has been measured in free-living ambulatory COPD patients and patients participating in a rehabilitation programme (6, 7). This disease-specific increase in energy metabolism has been attributed to increased oxygen cost of respiratory muscle activity and decreased muscle efficiency during leg exercise. It is as yet unclear whether this increased energy metabolism is predominantly due to mechanical factors or also to abnormalities in muscle energy and substrate metabolism.

An obvious choice to improve energy balance might be to decrease energy expenditure. However, according to the GOLD (Global Initiative for Chronic Obstructive Lung Disease) guidelines, exercise training is a key intervention of evidence-based pulmonary rehabilitation to improve limited functional abilities and maintain an active lifestyle (8). Since COPD patients may have an elevated energy metabolism and should at the same time be advised to increase exercise, restricting energy output will be hard to realize and is not desirable. This implies that COPD patients who suffer from weight loss, and even weight-stable patients at risk, should be encouraged to increase their apparently normal energy intake during pulmonary rehabilitation. This could avoid weight loss, specific loss of muscle mass, and a related decrease in functional ability, or could help them regain weight. Besides optimizing the treatment of patients who are already underweight, it is therefore important to detect and reverse involuntary weight loss in order to avoid functional decline.

Efficacy of nutritional supplementation

Treatment of weight loss may be achieved by increasing dietary intake per se or by altering dietary habits to include different (energy-dense) foods and optimum timing of meals/snacks in relation to symptoms and activity patterns. In a controlled clinical setting, we showed that nutritional supplementation is feasible and effectively induces weight gain and functional improvement when integrated as part of a pulmonary rehabilitation programme (9). However, in the home setting, it is more difficult for patients to balance their energy expenditure. Goris *et al.* (10) measured energy balance over a period of 3 months in underweight COPD patients by careful measurement of dietary intake and daily activity using accelerometers. Remarkably an inverse relationship was found between physical activity (measured with accelerometers) and body weight gain. This observation fits with a recent study in normal and underweight patients showing that 7 weeks of outpatient pulmonary rehabilitation, consisting mainly of endurance walking exercise, without nutritional supplementation, resulted in a negative energy balance and a significant weight loss of 0.5 kg (11).

These observations stress the importance of carefully assessing dietary habits and activity pattern prior to implementing a dietary supplementation regimen and regular supervision of compliance and dietary intake by a nurse or a dietician to ensure that patients actually meet the prescribed dietary intake. When oral nutritional supplements are considered, it is important to realize that there are limitations to the caloric amount of supplements that can be given daily and that patients may start to compensate their normal dietary intake. Also the portion size and distribution of supplements during the day are important things to consider. Distribution of supplementation appears more effective at the end of the afternoon or evening than in the morning (10). While, overall, patients tolerate a caloric load up to 500 kcal, it was shown in a subgroup of severely underweight patients that, in contrast to placebo or a liquid supplement of 250 kcal, exercise capacity measured with a submaximal exercise test was decreased 1 h after ingestion of a 500 kcal supplement (12).

Substrate oxidation and ventilation are intrinsically related, and theoretically meal-related dyspnoea and impaired ventilatory reserves might restrict the carbohydrate content of nutritional support in respiratory disease. Earlier studies indeed showed adverse effects of a carbohydrate-rich energy overload (970 kcal) on CO_2 production and exercise capacity (13), but these results were not confirmed when using a normal energy load (500 kcal) (14). Recent studies show that carbohydrate-rich supplements may even have positive effects. In one study, a fat-rich supplement caused an acute increase in dyspnoea, while no effect on this symptom was seen after an equicaloric carbohydrate-rich supplement (12). A clinical trial investigating the effects of nutritional supplementation during pulmonary rehabilitation, using the same carbohydrate-rich supplement as in Vermeeren *et al.* (12), showed a positive relationship between total carbohydrate intake and exercise performance measured with an incremental shuttle-walk test (11).

Caloric supplementation vs. dietary change

Nutritional interventions for COPD patients have focused mainly on therapeutic caloric support. Furthermore, studies investigating the effect of dietary supplementation were often conducted among severe COPD cases, in whom, besides a negative energy balance, a specific negative protein balance is also often observed that may complicate the efficacy of nutritional support. Sometimes increasing energy intake among severe COPD cases is difficult to accomplish, and if energy intake is not increased, weight and functionality will certainly not improve. Interventions should also be extended to prevention and early treatment of weight loss, i.e. before patients are extremely wasted. This means expanding the target group to include primary care patients before they have become underweight, and putting more emphasis on dietary change than on medically prescribed supplementation.

TREATMENT OF MUSCLE WASTING

Protein

The normal metabolic response to semi-starvation is a decreased resting metabolic rate and altered substrate oxidation (i.e. increased fatty acid oxidation and decreased protein turnover) to favour loss of fat mass and limit loss of protein to preserve fat-free mass. In contrast, increased resting energy requirements, elevated whole-body protein turnover rates and a decreased lipolytic response after beta-adrenergic stimulation have been observed in some of the COPD patients (15–17). These metabolic adaptations are reflected in body compositional studies showing that weight loss is accompanied by significant loss of fat-free mass and that muscle wasting may also occur in normal weight-stable subjects (18). It is specifically the loss of fat-free mass (consisting predominantly of muscle mass) that is related to impaired skeletal muscle strength and exercise capacity (19, 20). It has even been shown that muscle mass is a better predictor of survival in COPD than body weight (21).

From a nutritional point of view, wasting of muscle mass is due to an impaired balance between protein synthesis (anabolism) and protein breakdown (catabolism). Besides decreased dietary intake and abnormalities in substrate metabolism, however, other non-nutritive factors, including physical inactivity, alterations in the neuroendocrine response and presence of a systemic inflammatory response, may contribute to a negative protein balance in COPD. From a therapeutic perspective it is important to know the relative contribution of these factors to muscle wasting of the individual patients to judge the efficacy of nutritional support. While increasing energy intake can compensate elevated energy requirements and vice-versa, uncontrolled protein breakdown cannot be overcome by only increasing protein synthesis and vice-versa. Muscle protein synthesis rate was decreased in a group of underweight clinically stable patients with emphysema while protein breakdown rate was normal (22). Several studies have therefore investigated in underweight COPD patients the effects of pharmacological anabolic stimuli to promote protein synthesis, including anabolic steroids and growth hormone. These studies were indeed able to document a significant gain in muscle mass after intervention (23–25), illustrating that there is room for specific stimulation of protein synthesis in these patients. No studies have yet specifically investigated the ability to induce or enhance muscle weight gain by nutritional modulation of protein synthesis rates. This may be achieved by increasing protein intake and optimization of essential amino acid intake. It has been clearly shown in other wasting conditions that adequate intake of protein is also a prerequisite for optimal efficacy of anabolic drugs (26) as well as resistance exercise training (27).

Amino acids

Amino acids are the building blocks of protein and several studies to date have reported an abnormal plasma amino acid pattern in COPD. Of interest are the consistently reduced plasma levels of branched-chain amino acids (BCAAs) in underweight COPD patients and in those with low muscle mass (28, 29). There are some indications that low plasma BCAAs in COPD patients are due to specific alterations in leucine metabolism, possibly mediated by altered insulin regulation (29). Leucine is an interesting nutritional substrate since it not only serves as precursor, but also activates signalling pathways that enhance activity and synthesis of proteins involved in messenger RNA translocation to upregulate protein synthesis in skeletal muscle (30).

Polyunsaturated fatty acids

Despite anabolic nutritional and/or pharmacological stimulation, (muscle) weight gain is limited in some COPD patients. As in other chronic inflammatory disorders, poor therapeutic response was related to presence of systemic inflammation (31). Disproportionate muscle wasting linked to systemic inflammation and unresponsive to nutritional supplementation is commonly referred to as the cachexia syndrome. Current insight into the molecular mechanisms of cachexia indicates a complex interaction between inflammatory mediators, oxidative stress and growth factors, not only involved in an imbalance between muscle protein synthesis and breakdown, but also in processes that govern muscle plasticity, such as skeletal muscle fibre degeneration, apoptosis and regeneration (32). New insights into the molecular regulation of muscle wasting may, in the near future, provide novel nutritional or pharmacological therapies by specifically targeting crucial mediators of the intracellular signalling pathways involved.

At present, from a nutritional and metabolic perspective, specific interest has recently been focused on fatty acid modulation since fatty acid composition of inflammatory and immune cells is sensitive to change according to the fatty acid composition of the diet. The n-3 polyunsaturated fatty acids (PUFAs) eicopentanaenoic acid (EPA) and docosahexaenoic acid (DHA) are found in high proportions in oily fish and fish oils. The n-3 PUFAs are structurally and functionally distinct from the n-6 PUFAs. Typically human inflammatory cells contain high proportions of the n-6 PUFAs, arachidonic acid

and low proportions of n-3 PUFAs. The significance of this difference is that arachidonic acid is the precursor of 2-series prostaglandins and 4-series leukotrienes, which are highly active mediators of inflammation. Feeding fish oil results in partial replacement of arachidonic acid in inflammatory cell membranes by EPA. This change leads to a decreased production of arachidonic acid-derived mediators. This response alone is a potentially beneficial anti-inflammatory effect of PUFA. Supplementation of the diet of healthy volunteers with fish oil-derived n-3 PUFAs resulted in decreased monocyte and neutrophil chemotaxis and decreased production of proinflammatory cytokines (33). Clinical studies have reported that fish oil supplementation has beneficial effects on the systemic inflammatory response and disease activity in conditions such as rheumatoid arthritis and inflammatory bowel disease (33).

Besides encouraging effects of PUFA supplementation with respect to decreased systemic inflammatory response, uncontrolled clinical trials observed body weight gain in patients suffering from cancer cachexia (34). The latter may be related to other effects of n-3 PUFAs which occur downstream of altered eicosanoid production, or may be independent of this activity. Nuclear factor kappa B (NF-κB) is a critical mediator of the intracellular signalling events triggered by TNF-α and other inflammatory cytokines, including skeletal muscle-specific gene expression (33). Recent studies have shown that n-3 PUFAs can downregulate the activity of NF-κB. A recent multicentre trial compared a protein- and energy-dense nutritional supplement enriched with n-3 fatty acids and antioxidants with an equicaloric and isonitrogenous control supplement on weight, fat-free mass and quality of life in advanced pancreatic cancer patients suffering from involuntary weight loss (35). No difference was seen in treatment response between the two groups. The authors ascribed this disappointing result to obvious non-compliance, since a post hoc correlation analysis in the enriched group, but not in the control group, showed a positive association between supplement intake and weight gain.

Clearly more clinical trials are required to investigate the potential role of n-3 fatty acid-enriched supplements in cachexia in cancer or other chronic wasting conditions like COPD.

NUTRITIONAL MODULATION TO ENHANCE THE RESPONSE TO EXERCISE

Amino acids

In addition to fostering a general higher rate of postprandial protein synthesis, increased availability of amino acids also enhances the stimulation of protein synthesis that occurs in response to exercise (36). The magnitude of stimulation, however, appears to depend on the timing of administration of amino acids relative to the period of exercise (36). Positive effects of protein synthesis have been shown when protein-rich supplements are given either immediately before or directly after exercise training.

Besides stimulation of protein synthesis, BCAAs are also important precursors for glutamate (GLU), which is one of the most important non-essential amino acids in muscle. BCAAs derived from net protein breakdown and by uptake into the muscle pool undergo transamination to yield branched-chain ketoacid and GLU. Intracellular GLU is involved in numerous metabolic processes, including substrate phosphorylation and replenishment of tricarboxylic acid (TCA) intermediates to preserve high-energy phosphates at rest and during exercise. Moreover, intracellular GLU is known as an important precursor for antioxidant glutathione (GSH) and glutamine (GLN) synthesis in muscle (37). Recently, a consistently reduced muscle GLU status of severe COPD patients was reported (37, 38), which further decreased during a submaximal exercise bout (39). While muscle redox potential (GSSG [oxidized glutathione]/GSH) increases after endurance exercise training in healthy subjects, patients with COPD showed a reduced ability to adapt in this way, as reflected by a lower capacity to synthesize GSH (40). These observations provide a perspective for amino acid supplementation to modulate exercise-induced protein synthesis as well as exercise-induced oxidative stress.

Creatine

Besides muscle wasting, intrinsic abnormalities in peripheral skeletal muscle morphology and metabolism have been described in COPD patients, pointing towards a decreased oxidative capacity. These abnormalities include muscle fibre-type shifts from the oxidative type I fibres to the glycolytic type IIx fibres (41), accompanied by a decrease in oxidative enzymes involved in carbohydrate and fatty acid oxidation (42). Detailed information on substrate metabolism at the whole-body and skeletal muscle levels in COPD is lacking. Nevertheless, the metabolic adaptations have clinical consequences, as illustrated, for example, by a decreased mechanical efficiency (43) and an enhanced lactic acid production during exercise (44) relative to healthy control subjects. In addition, nuclear magnetic resonance studies using single limb exercise models showed a rapid decline and impaired recovery of phosphocreatine stores (45). Phosphocreatine is an energy store that is used immediately after onset of exercise for rapid anaerobic muscle performance and it would be interesting to see if creatine supplementation as part of a rehabilitation programme is reflected in improved skeletal muscle performance in COPD.

Positive effects of endurance exercise training illustrate that decreased muscle oxidative capacity in COPD is at least partly reversible (45), although, again, detailed information on the effect of endurance training on substrate metabolism in COPD is lacking. While the overall effects of endurance-type exercise are positive, the available studies also clearly show that it is difficult to enhance this response by modulating exercise type and intensity only (46, 47). It is therefore tempting to explore the potential of nutritional modulation on muscle substrate metabolism to enhance improvement of exercise capacity in COPD.

The muscle fibre-type shift from type I to type IIx, together with the enhanced lactic acid production during exercise,

points towards a decreased oxidative capacity for fatty acids specifically. This suggestion is consistent with the finding that 3-hydroxyacyl-coenzyme A dehydrogenase (HADH; an enzyme involved in the β-oxidation of fatty acids) was shown to be decreased in COPD (42), whereas phosphofructokinase (a glycolytic enzyme) was found to be increased in some studies (42, 48). The decreased fat oxidative capacity in COPD can also be explained by the shift in muscle fibre type. Furthermore, reduced uncoupling protein 3 (UCP3) content has been found in the peripheral musculature of patients with COPD. This protein may play an important role in mitochondrial fatty acid maintenance (49). Future studies are clearly needed to further explore the presence and mechanisms of decreased fat oxidative capacity in COPD. Moreover, these studies may be a further trigger to explore the potential of nutritional modulation on muscle substrate metabolism to enhance improvement of exercise capacity.

PUFAs, particularly those of the n-3 family and the n-6 family, have been shown to specifically alter expression of genes involved in substrate metabolism. They may upregulate the expression of genes encoding proteins involved in fatty acid oxidation while simultaneously downregulating genes encoding proteins of lipid synthesis (50). Therefore, PUFAs can be of potential interest in improving oxidative capacity in COPD. PUFAs govern oxidative gene expression by activation of the nuclear hormone peroxisome proliferator-activated receptors (the so-called PPARs) (51). This is also the basis for the use of PPAR agonists in overcoming disturbances in substrate metabolism in insulin resistant disorders (i.e. the metabolic syndrome).

Anabolic steroids

Anabolic steroids could be an additional mode of intervention to improve the response to exercise training, in particular to enhance muscle weight gain, since anabolic steroids interact with the IGF-1 system (52) and may stimulate protein synthesis in the presence of enough protein intake (26). However, other mechanisms may also contribute to the physiological effects of anabolic steroids. Anabolic steroids counteract catabolic effects of glucocorticoids and may also increase erythropoietic function (26). Three controlled studies investigated the effect of oral (oxandrolone) and intramuscular (nandrolone decanoate) administration of anabolic steroids on body composition in underweight COPD patients and reported a gain in fat-free mass after 1–6 months of treatment (23–25). We also investigated the efficacy of anabolic steroids as part of a pulmonary rehabilitation programme relative to rehabilitation alone on skeletal muscle function and exercise capacity. Besides a significant improvement in fat-free mass, improvements in muscle function were associated with improvements in erythropoietic parameters (25). The use of low-dose oral glucocorticoids as maintenance medication significantly impaired the response to pulmonary rehabilitation with respect to respiratory muscle function and exercise, which could be restored by nandrolone decanoate treatment (25). This observation is in line with positive effects of nandrolone decanoate in other diseases requiring long-term systemic glucocorticoid treatment (53).

NUTRITIONAL SUPPORT AS INTEGRATED PART OF COPD MANAGEMENT

In this chapter we have tried to show that nutrition is an essential component of pulmonary rehabilitation, but that it is important to time both the type and duration of nutritional support appropriately. In overweight COPD patients ($25 < BMI < 30\,kg/m^2$) the emphasis of pulmonary rehabilitation should be on exercise to improve muscle oxidative capacity and a healthy diet to maintain a stable weight. There is no reason to put these patients on a weight-losing diet since, remarkably, all available COPD studies show that being overweight is associated with a better prognosis than being normal weight ($20 < BMI < 25\,kg/m^2$). This is less clear for obese patients, and certainly when patients experience obesity-related symptoms or complications, a weight-losing diet can be considered in this subgroup, but preferably in combination with exercise to improve oxidative capacity and limit the loss of fat-free mass. In normal-weight COPD patients, it is important to monitor body weight regularly, to be able to start nutritional intervention at an early stage, at the onset of involuntary weight loss. When this specific group (at risk for muscle wasting) starts with a pulmonary rehabilitation programme, it is important to take into consideration the fact that regular exercise elevates energy requirements that may need to be compensated. Therefore, it is preferable, specifically in patients who have already experienced involuntary weight loss, to adjust dietary intake and dietary habits first, before starting with the rehabilitation programme. Obviously in (weight-losing) underweight COPD patients ($BMI < 21\,kg/m^2$), nutritional intervention should initially precede, and later be combined with, an appropriate exercise programme.

Besides optimal timing of nutritional and metabolic therapy, successful intervention relies on a motivated patient, a supportive social environment and optimal communication between the various care-givers within the multidisciplinary rehabilitation team.

Key points

- Nutritional supplementation should be considered not only in underweight COPD patients ($BMI < 21\,kg/m^2$) but also in normal-weight patients suffering from involuntary weight loss ($21 < BMI < 25\,kg/m^2$).
- Successful nutritional intervention requires optimal incorporation of nutritional supplements in the daily dietary and activity pattern of the COPD patient, and therefore a multidisciplinary treatment approach.

- Protein- and carbohydrate-enriched supplements are preferable to fat-rich supplements to enhance efficacy of pulmonary rehabilitation.
- Anabolic steroids may enhance muscle weight gain in COPD, particularly in patients requiring long-term systemic glucocorticoid treatment.

REFERENCES

1. Wilson DO, Rogers RM, Wright EC, Anthonisen NR. Body weight in chronic obstructive pulmonary disease. The National Institutes of Health Intermittent Positive-Pressure Breathing Trial. *Am Rev Respir Dis* 1989; **139**: 1435–8.

●2. Schols AM, Slangen J, Volovics L, Wouters EF. Weight loss is a reversible factor in the prognosis of chronic obstructive pulmonary disease. *Am J Respir Crit Care Med* 1998; **157**: 1791–7.

●3. Landbo C, Prescott E, Lange P et al. Prognostic value of nutritional status in chronic obstructive pulmonary disease. *Am J Respir Crit Care Med* 1999; **160**: 1856–61.

4. Prescott E, Almdal T, Mikkelsen KL et al. Prognostic value of weight change in chronic obstructive pulmonary disease: results from the Copenhagen City Heart Study. *Eur Respir J* 2002; **20**: 539–44.

5. Engelen MP, Schols AM, Lamers RJ, Wouters EF. Different patterns of chronic tissue wasting among patients with chronic obstructive pulmonary disease. *Clin Nutr* 1999; **18**: 275–80.

6. Baarends EM, Schols AM, Pannemans DL et al. Total free living energy expenditure in patients with severe chronic obstructive pulmonary disease. *Am J Respir Crit Care Med* 1997; **155**: 549–54.

7. Slinde F, Ellegard L, Gronberg AM et al. Total energy expenditure in underweight patients with severe chronic obstructive pulmonary disease living at home. *Clin Nutr* 2003; **22**: 159–65.

8. Pauwels RA, Buist AS, Calverley PM et al. Global strategy for the diagnosis, management, and prevention of chronic obstructive pulmonary disease. NHLBI/WHO Global Initiative for Chronic Obstructive Lung Disease (GOLD) Workshop summary. *Am J Respir Crit Care Med* 2001; **163**: 1256–76.

●9. Creutzberg EC, Wouters EF, Mostert R et al. Efficacy of nutritional supplementation therapy in depleted patients with chronic obstructive pulmonary disease. *Nutrition* 2003; **19**: 120–7.

●10. Goris AH, Vermeeren MA, Wouters EF et al. Energy balance in depleted ambulatory patients with chronic obstructive pulmonary disease: the effect of physical activity and oral nutritional supplementation. *Br J Nutr* 2003; **89**: 725–9.

●11. Steiner MC, Barton RL, Singh SJ, Morgan MD. Nutritional enhancement of exercise performance in chronic obstructive pulmonary disease: a randomized controlled trial. *Thorax* 2003; **58**: 745–51.

12. Vermeeren MA, Wouters EF, Nelissen LH et al. Acute effects of different nutritional supplements on symptoms and functional capacity in patients with chronic obstructive pulmonary disease. *Am J Clin Nutr* 2001; **73**: 295–301.

13. Ferreira I, Brooks D, Lacasse Y, Goldstein R. Nutritional intervention in COPD: a systematic overview. *Chest* 2001; **119**: 353–63.

14. Akrabawi SS, Mobarhan S, Stoltz RR, Ferguson PW. Gastric emptying, pulmonary function, gas exchange, and respiratory quotient after feeding a moderate versus high fat enteral formula

meal in chronic obstructive pulmonary disease patients. *Nutrition* 1996; **12**: 260–5.

15. Schiffelers SL, Blaak EE, Baarends EM *et al.* Beta-adrenoceptor-mediated thermogenesis and lipolysis in patients with chronic obstructive pulmonary disease. *Am J Physiol Endocrinol Metab* 2001; **280**: E357–64.

16. Engelen MPKJ, Deutz NEP, Wouters EFM, Schols AMWJ. Enhanced levels of whole-body protein turnover in patients with chronic obstructive pulmonary disease. *Am J Respir Crit Care Med* 2000; **162**: 1488-92.

17. Creutzberg EC, Schols AM, Bothmer Quaedvlieg FC, Wouters EF. Prevalence of an elevated resting energy expenditure in patients with chronic obstructive pulmonary disease in relation to body composition and lung function. *Eur J Clin Nutr* 1998; **52**: 396-401.

18. Schols AM, Soeters PB, Dingemans AM *et al.* Prevalence and characteristics of nutritional depletion in patients with stable COPD eligible for pulmonary rehabilitation. *Am Rev Respir Dis* 1993; **147**: 1151-6.

19. Bernard S, LeBlanc P, Whittom F *et al.* Peripheral muscle weakness in patients with chronic obstructive pulmonary disease. *Am J Respir Crit Care Med* 1998; **158**: 629-34.

20. Baarends EM, Schols AM, Mostert R, Wouters EF. Peak exercise response in relation to tissue depletion in patients with chronic obstructive pulmonary disease. *Eur Respir J* 1997; **10**: 2807-13.

21. Marquis K, Debigare R, Lacasse Y *et al.* Midthigh muscle cross-sectional area is a better predictor of mortality than body mass index in patients with chronic obstructive pulmonary disease. *Am J Respir Crit Care Med* 2002; **166**: 809-13.

22. Morrison WL, Gibson JN, Scrimgeour C, Rennie MJ. Muscle wasting in emphysema. *Clin Sci (Lond)* 1988; **75**: 415-20.

23. Ferreira IM, Verreschi IT, Nery LE. The influence of oral anabolic steroids on body mass and respiratory muscles in undernourished COPD patients. *Chest* 1998; **114**: 19-28.

24. Yeh SS, Deguzman B, Kramer T. Reversal of COPD-associated weight loss using the anabolic agent oxandrolone. *Chest* 2002; **122**: 421-8.

●25. Creutzberg EC, Wouters EF, Mostert R *et al.* A role for anabolic steroids in the rehabilitation of patients with COPD?: a double-blind, placebo-controlled, randomized trial, *Chest* 2003; **124**: 1733-42.

26. Basaria S, Wahlstrom JT, Dobs AS. Clinical review 138: anabolic-androgenic steroid therapy in the treatment of chronic diseases. *J Clin Endocrinol Metab* 2001; **86**: 5108-17.

27. Borsheim E, Tipton KD, Wolf SE, Wolfe RR. Essential amino acids and muscle protein recovery from resistance exercise. *Am J Physiol Endocrinol Metab* 2002; **283**: E648-57.

28. Yoneda T, Yoshikawa M, Fu A *et al.* Plasma levels of amino acids and hypermetabolism in patients with chronic obstructive pulmonary disease. *Nutrition* 2001; **17**: 95-9.

29. Engelen MP, Wouters EF, Deutz NE *et al.* Factors contributing to alterations in skeletal muscle and plasma amino acid profiles in patients with chronic obstructive pulmonary disease. *Am J Clin Nutr* 2000; **72**: 1480-7.

30. Anthony JC, Anthony TG, Kimball SR, Jefferson LS. Signaling pathways involved in translational control of protein synthesis in skeletal muscle by leucine. *J Nutr* 2001; **131**: 856S-60S.

●31. Creutzberg EC, Schols AM, Weling-Scheepers CA *et al.* Characterization of nonresponse to high caloric oral nutritional therapy in depleted patients with chronic obstructive pulmonary disease. *Am J Respir Crit Care Med* 2000; **161**(3 Part 1): 745-52.

32. Debigare R, Cote CH, Maltais F. Peripheral muscle wasting in chronic obstructive pulmonary disease. Clinical relevance and mechanisms. *Am J Respir Crit Care Med* 2001; **164**: 1712-17.

33. Calder PC. Polyunsaturated fatty acids, inflammation, and immunity. *Lipids* 2001; **36**: 1007-24.

34. Barber MD, Ross JA, Voss AC *et al.* The effect of an oral nutritional supplement enriched with fish oil on weight-loss in patients with pancreatic cancer. *Br J Cancer* 1999; **81**: 80-6.

●35. Fearon KC, von Meyenfeldt MF, Moses AG *et al.* Effect of a protein and energy dense n-3 fatty acid enriched oral supplement on loss of weight and lean tissue in cancer cachexia: a randomised double blind trial. *Gut* 2003; **52**: 1479-86.

36. Levenhagen DK, Gresham JD, Carlson MG *et al.* Postexercise nutrient intake timing in humans is critical to recovery of leg glucose and protein homeostasis. *Am J Physiol Endocrinol Metab* 2001; **280**: E982-93.

37. Engelen MP, Schols AM, Does JD *et al.* Altered glutamate metabolism is associated with reduced muscle glutathione levels in patients with emphysema. *Am J Respir Crit Care Med* 2000; **161**: 98-103.

38. Pouw EM, Schols AM, Deutz NE, Wouters EF. Plasma and muscle amino acid levels in relation to resting energy expenditure and inflammation in stable chronic obstructive pulmonary disease. *Am J Respir Crit Care Med* 1998; **158**: 797-801.

39. Engelen MP, Wouters EF, Deutz NE *et al.* Effects of exercise on amino acid metabolism in patients with chronic obstructive pulmonary disease. *Am J Respir Crit Care Med* 2001; **163**: 859-64.

40. Rabinovich RAE, Ardite T, Troosters N *et al.* Reduced muscle redox capacity after endurance training in patients with chronic obstructive pulmonary disease. *Am J Respir Crit Care Med* 2001; **164**: 1114-18.

41. Gosker HR. van Mameren H, van Dijk PJ *et al.* Skeletal muscle fibre-type shifting and metabolic profile in patients with chronic obstructive pulmonary disease. *Eur Respir J* 2002; **19**: 617-25.

42. Maltais F, LeBlanc P, Whittom F *et al.* Oxidative enzyme activities of the vastus lateralis muscle and the functional status in patients with COPD. *Thorax* 2000; **55**: 848-53.

43. Baarends EM, Schols AM, Akkermans MA, Wouters EF. Decreased mechanical efficiency in clinically stable patients with COPD. *Thorax* 1997; **52**: 981-6.

44. Maltais FA, Simard A, Simard C *et al.* Oxidative capacity of the skeletal muscle and lactic acid kinetics during exercise in normal subjects and in patients with COPD. *Am J Respir Crit Care Med* 1996; **153**: 288-93.

45. Sala E, Roca J, Marrades RM *et al.* Effects of endurance training on skeletal muscle bioenergetics in chronic obstructive pulmonary disease. *Am J Respir Crit Care Med* 1999; **159**: 1726-34.

46. Coppoolse R, Schols AM, Baarends EM *et al.* Interval versus continuous training in patients with severe COPD: a randomized clinical trial. *Eur Respir J* 1999; **14**: 258-63.

47. Ortega F, Toral J, Cejudo P *et al.* Comparison of effects of strength and endurance training in patients with chronic obstructive pulmonary disease. *Am J Respir Crit Care Med* 2002; **166**: 669-74.

48. Jakobsson P, Jorfeldt L, Henriksson J. Metabolic enzyme activity in the quadriceps femoris muscle in patients with severe chronic obstructive pulmonary disease. *Am J Respir Crit Care Med* 1995; **151**(2 Part 1): 374-7.

49. Gosker HR, Schrauwen P, Hesselink MK *et al.* Uncoupling protein-3 content is decreased in peripheral skeletal muscle of patients with COPD. *Eur Respir J* 2003; **22**: 88-93.

50. Clarke SD. Polyunsaturated fatty acid regulation of gene transcription: a mechanism to improve energy balance and insulin resistance. *Br J Nutr* 2000; **83**(Suppl. 1): S59-S66.

51. Schoonjans K, Staels B, Auwerx J. The peroxisome proliferator activated receptors (PPARS) and their effects on lipid metabolism

and adipocyte differentiation. *Biochim Biophys Acta* 1996; **1302**: 93–109.

52. Lewis MI, Horvitz GD, Clemmons DR, Fournier M. Role if IGF-1 and IGF-binding proteins within diaphragm muscle in modulating the effects of nandrolone. *Am J Physiol Endocrinol Metab* 2001; **282**: E483–90.

●53. Crawford BA, Liu PY, Kean MT *et al*. Randomized placebo-controlled trial of androgen effects on muscle and bone in men requiring long-term systemic glucocorticoid treatment. *J Clin Endocrinol Metab* 2003; **88**: 3167–76.

24

Pharmacological management in chronic respiratory diseases

RACHEL A. BROWN, CLIVE P. PAGE

INTRODUCTION

Following the diagnosis of a chronic respiratory disease, the use of drugs is almost always paramount to the process of rehabilitation. Although drugs are rarely able to provide a cure, they can be successfully used to gain sufficient control of a disease in order to alleviate symptoms and increase quality of life, and, in the case of asthma, perhaps alter the outcome of the disease. Drugs therefore constitute a major part of disease management in asthma and chronic obstructive pulmonary disease (COPD).

Advances in the pharmacological therapy of asthma have resulted in a high level of control over this disease, with the majority of asthmatics now able to lead a normal life. Conversely, the therapy of COPD is far less successful, with current treatment providing some symptomatic relief and increased quality of life but unable to slow the disease progression. Although both diseases are characterized by airflow obstruction, the airflow obstruction in asthma is variable and responds well to bronchodilator drugs when required. By contrast, the airflow obstruction in COPD is generally fixed and bronchodilator drugs can only, at best, partially reverse the obstruction.

Differences in the pathogenesis and pathology of asthma and COPD are considered to be responsible for the variation in responses to pharmacological therapies that are administered with the aim of controlling airflow obstruction. In particular, it is the specific inflammatory features that distinguish asthma from COPD that are held accountable for this variation.

In asthma, several factors can contribute to airflow obstruction. Many asthmatics are atopic, and inhalation of allergen results in acute bronchoconstriction, which is directly caused by the products of IgE-mediated airway mast cell degranulation, such as histamine, leukotrienes and prostaglandins (early-phase response) (1, 2). Non-allergenic factors can also trigger acute bronchoconstriction (non-atopic asthma), such as exercise, cold air and pollutants. Following this early-phase response, various mast cell-derived mediators generate an inflammatory response in a matter of hours, resulting in a more prolonged airflow limitation (late-phase response) (2). Various types of cells infiltrate the airways, predominantly eosinophils, the inflammatory products of which are thought to contribute to this airways obstruction. Chronic inflammation in asthmatic airways is thought to contribute to airways hyperresponsiveness, where a wide variety of both endogenous and exogenous stimuli are able to induce bronchoconstriction in asthmatics that have little or no activity in healthy subjects (3). This is a hallmark of asthma that is less prominent in patients with COPD.

The causes of the airflow obstruction in COPD are considerably different from those in asthma. The causative factor in more than 80 per cent of cases of COPD is cigarette smoking. Cigarette smoke is a complex mixture of a vast range of chemical compounds, many of which can cause tissue damage (4). Thus, a long-term heavy smoking habit generally results in chronic inflammation involving the entire tracheobronchial tree, and at least 20 per cent of heavy smokers (>20 pack-years) develop chronic airflow obstruction due to a combination of chronic bronchitis, chronic bronchiolitis and emphysema (5). The inflammatory profile observed in the airways and lungs of COPD subjects is markedly different from that observed in asthmatics. Neutrophils tend to be the predominant inflammatory cell that infiltrates the airways and lungs (as opposed to eosinophils in asthma), and are currently thought to be significant source of inflammatory mediators implicated in the pathogenesis and pathology of COPD (6).

Thus, it is these differences in the pathogenesis and pathology of asthma and COPD that have governed the need for different pharmacological approaches in order to treat both conditions in the most effective manner possible. The introduction of inhaled corticosteroids has revolutionized the therapy of asthma, whilst it is now clear that drugs in this class are of little benefit in COPD. Corticosteroids are highly effective at controlling the inflammation in asthma, and thus the long-term pathological consequences of asthma. Corticosteroids inhibit many cellular processes associated with the excessive recruitment and inflammatory activity of eosinophils in asthmatic airways, which is considered to be their major mechanism of action (7). By contrast, numerous studies have failed to demonstrate any real therapeutic benefit of corticosteroids in COPD patients, and they are not recommended for use in the treatment of this disease (8). In particular, several large multicentre studies with corticosteroids conducted over years have shown no effect on the progressive decline in lung function, confirming these observations. However, corticosteroids are considered to be of benefit in acute exacerbations (8) and may also reduce the frequency (9). The reasons for the poor efficacy of corticosteroids in COPD remain to be established. It is recognized that the inflammation in COPD is largely attributed to the excessive and chronic accumulation of neutrophils, and corticosteroids are unable to effectively suppress the inflammatory activity of neutrophils. This may therefore contribute to the poor efficacy of corticosteroids in COPD. Furthermore, some reports even suggest that corticosteroids can augment the activity of neutrophils by delaying spontaneous apoptosis (as opposed to inducing apoptosis of eosinophils), an important mechanism by which inflammation can be resolved (10).

Thus, asthma is generally a highly controllable condition although a significant minority of asthmatics suffer severe persistent asthma. By contrast, there is an urgent need for novel pharmacological therapies in COPD that are able to target the underlying inflammation. Various novel therapies for the treatment of both asthma and COPD are currently under clinical investigation, and these will also be reviewed in addition to the current recommended pharmacological therapy of asthma and COPD in the next section.

ASTHMA

Aims of pharmacological therapy

In conjunction with numerous non-pharmacological therapies, such as limiting exposure to environmental allergens, current pharmacological asthma therapy has two main aims. The first is to control symptoms sufficiently so that patients can lead an entirely normal life, such that they are able to work and participate in everyday activities such as sport. Drugs administered with this aim are classed as 'relievers'. The second aim is to control the underlying inflammation such that decline in lung function, severe attacks and death are all prevented and drugs used for this purpose are classed as 'controllers'.

It is recommended that treatment follows a stepwise progression with the number of therapies increased until satisfactory control over the asthma has been achieved, which is then stepped down once control has been achieved for several months in order to ensure the lowest incidence of side effects (11).

Current pharmacological therapy

RELIEVERS

The initial aim of asthma therapy is to provide symptomatic relief, either as a 'rescue' therapy during an acute exacerbation when the airways constrict in response to a wide range of stimuli, or through affording a level of 'bronchoprotection' through prophylactic administration in order to prevent the bronchoconstriction occurring in the first place in response to such stimuli. Several classes of drugs can achieve this, but the drug of choice to perform these tasks in asthma is a β_2-adrenoceptor agonist.

β_2-Agonists are derivatives of epinephrine (adrenaline) and were developed to have a greater selectivity for β_2-adrenoceptors than epinephrine, in addition to being less susceptible to degradation by catechol-O-methyl transferase (COMT). β_2-Agonists activate β_2-adrenoceptors present on airway smooth muscle, which results in muscle relaxation. β_2-Adrenoceptors are G_s-protein coupled receptors and the major signalling pathway activated following agonists binding these receptors present upon airway smooth muscle results in the formation of the second messenger cyclic-$3',5'$-adenosine monophosphate (cAMP) from ATP. cAMP activates protein kinase A (PKA), which in turn activates multiple pathways through phosphorylating a variety of proteins including myosin light chain kinase (MLCK), the consequence of this being muscle relaxation (12, 13).

In asthmatic airways, airway smooth muscle contraction can result from a wide range of stimuli and consequently β_2-agonists are considered to be functional antagonists, given that their main action is not to induce bronchodilation per se, but to limit or prevent the occurrence of bronchoconstriction through the ongoing antagonism of various spasmogens.

Several short-acting β_2-agonists are available for use as bronchodilator agents and include salbutamol, terbutaline and fenoterol, which are routinely administered by inhalation through the use of inhaler devices. A variety of drug formulations and delivery systems are available, providing a number of options for a patient to maximize the efficacy of the drug being administered (14). Direct delivery of β_2-agonists to the lung by inhalation achieves a high concentration of the drug at the target site within seconds, whilst reducing the incidence of side-effects by minimizing systemic exposure.

The bronchodilatory effects of short-acting β_2-agonists occur within minutes and can last for up to 6 h (as measured by FEV_1), whilst the bronchoprotective effects have a shorter duration of action (up to 4 h), as demonstrated by a number of studies with asthmatic subjects exposed to various spasmogens (15–19). Presumably, under the latter conditions the concentration of drug is not high enough to oppose the effects of these stimuli, yet is high enough to elevate the FEV_1 under basal conditions. Thus, for patients with moderate or severe asthma or those with nocturnal asthma, long-acting β_2-agonists such as salmeterol and formoterol are more suitable, as the bronchodilatory activity of these drugs lasts for up to 12 h and they are bronchoprotective for a similar length of time (20, 21). Thus, twice-daily administration of long-acting β_2-agonists can provide continuous symptomatic relief.

Adverse effects that may occur following the use of inhaled β_2-agonists include muscle tremor and tachycardia. Under certain circumstances, β_2-agonists are administered orally or intravenously, e.g. in severe asthma and status asthmaticus. In these situations the incidence of adverse effects is greater in comparison to inhaled administration.

β_2-Adrenoceptors are not exclusive to airway smooth muscle cells and are present on other resident airway cells such as mast cells, in addition to inflammatory cells that infiltrate the airways. Consequently, it is thought that a number of other pharmacological effects of β_2-agonists occur in asthmatic airways in addition to bronchodilation. Various studies have investigated the effects of β_2-agonists on inflammatory cells *in vitro* and are summarized in Table 24.1.

Numerous studies investigating the direct effects of β_2-agonists on inflammatory cells in asthmatic subjects have produced conflicting results as to whether β_2-agonists do indeed possess anti-inflammatory properties. Elevation of cAMP in inflammatory cells usually suppresses their inflammatory functions (44). Thus, it is thought that β_2-agonists possess anti-inflammatory properties by virtue of their ability to elevate cAMP following β_2-adrenoceptor activation [in addition to putative non-β_2-adrenoceptor-mediated effects(45)]. It is generally accepted that the *in vitro* observations concerning

mast cells extend to the clinical setting (22). However, the anti-inflammatory effects of β_2-agonists on other inflammatory cells *in vivo*, such as eosinophils, are still unclear and remain to be established (45).

Although β_2-agonists are highly efficacious in achieving immediate symptomatic relief in acute exacerbations of asthma, some long-term problems have been associated with the chronic use of these drugs, in particular the 'prophylactic' therapeutic approach taken with long-acting β_2-agonists. These include decreases in the bronchodilator and bronchoprotective effects of β_2-agonists, in addition to an increase in airways hyperresponsiveness. However, the mechanisms underlying the unwanted effects of β_2-agonists after chronic administration remain unclear and therefore further research is required to clarify the long-term effects of chronic β_2-agonist administration.

Although β_2-agonists are the mainstay reliever therapy in asthma, a variety of other bronchodilator drugs besides β_2-agonists are available for use, such as anticholinergics. Inhaled anticholinergics can be used as an adjunct to β_2-agonists, but are not as effective as β_2-agonists at inducing bronchodilation in asthmatics. They also appear to be of more benefit as rescue medication in acute asthma attacks than in the management of chronic asthma, and so may be useful in the former setting (46). Anticholinergic drugs have a longer onset of action than β_2-agonists (1–2 h, as against minutes) and the physiological response to these drugs in asthmatics is highly variable. Anticholinergic drugs in clinical use for asthma include ipratropium bromide and oxitropium bromide. The mechanism of action involves inhibition of intrinsic vagal cholinergic tone of airway smooth muscle through antagonism at M_3 receptors, present on airway smooth muscle, in addition

Table 24.1 *In vitro effects of β_2-agonists on inflammatory cells*

Cell type	Effect of short-acting β_2-agonists	Effect of long-acting β_2-agonists
Mast cell	Inhibit degranulation and inflammatory mediator release (22)	Inhibit degranulation and inflammatory mediator release (22)
Monocyte	Attenuate cytokine release (23, 24) No effect on IL-1-β or LTB_4 release (26)	Attenuate cytokine release (23–25) Inhibit thromboxane B_2 release (25) No effect on IL-1β or LTB_4 release (26)
Macrophage	No effect on thromboxane B_2 release (25) No effect on IL-1β or LTB_4 release (26) Inhibit TNF-α and IL-6 secretion (27)	Inhibit thromboxane B_2 release (25) No effect on IL-1β or LTB_4 release (26) Inhibit proteinase and superoxide release (28)
Eosinophil	Inhibit eosinophil peroxidase and LTC_4 release (29, 30) Inhibit superoxide production (31–33)	No effect on eosinophil peroxidase and LTC_4 release (29) Inhibit superoxide production (31) Inhibit chemotaxis (34)
Neutrophil	Small inhibitory effect on respiratory burst (35–37) Inhibit chemotaxis (38)	Small inhibitory effect on respiratory burst (35–37)
T-lymphocyte	Inhibit cytokine release (IL-3, IL-4, IL-5, IFN-γ and GM-CSF) (40, 41) Inhibit proliferation (41)	Inhibit cytokine release (IL-2, -3, -4, -5, GM-CSF and IFN-γ (39–41)) Inhibit proliferation (39, 41)
Basophil	No reported effects	Inhibit IL-4 and IL-13 release (42) Inhibit IgE-induced histamine release (42, 43)

GM-CSF, granulocyte–macrophage colony-stimulating factor; IgE, immunoglobulin E; IL, interleukin; INF, interferon; LTB, leukotriene B; LTC, leukotriene C; TNF, tumour necrosis factor.

to reflex bronchoconstriction caused by inhaled irritants. However they also block M_1 (ganglionic) receptors and presynaptic M_2 autoreceptors, the latter being an undesirable effect as blockade of M_2 receptors facilitates acetylcholine release. Very recently, the longer-acting and more efficacious anticholinergic tiotropium bromide has become available for clinical use in COPD, although its efficacy in asthma remains to be established (47). Tiotropium bromide exhibits greater selectivity for M_1 and M_3 receptors than its predecessors and, as it dissociates very slowly from these receptors, is significantly longer-acting than ipratropium bromide and oxitropium bromide. Tiotropium bromide may therefore be of greater therapeutic benefit in asthma (48). Adverse effects that may occur with inhaled anticholinergic drugs include dryness of the mouth and a bitter taste.

CONTROLLERS

In addition to the administration of pharmacological agents to provide symptomatic relief, various drugs are used to control the underlying inflammation. The first-line agents used to achieve this are corticosteroids. Inhaled corticosteroids are highly efficacious at suppressing the inflammation that occurs in asthma and are used as a matter of course in all but the mildest asthma. They are therefore recommended for use in any patient needing to use a β_2-agonist more than three times a week. The use of corticosteroids in asthmatic patients improves lung function significantly. In consequence, symptoms and exacerbations are reduced, which in turn leads to a decreased requirement for bronchodilator therapy. Corticosteroids thus afford a high level of control over asthma and prevent many of the long-term detrimental effects of asthma on lung function.

Corticosteroids, or more specifically glucocorticoids, suppress numerous aspects of the inflammation present in asthmatic airways by targeting many different inflammatory and resident cell types both directly and indirectly. Some important direct cellular effects of glucocorticoids are summarized in Box 24.1.

Glucocorticoids used in asthma therapy are synthetic derivatives of endogenous glucocorticoids, which are lipid-soluble hormones that perform a range of physiological functions including suppression of inflammation. Synthetic glucocorticoids were developed to possess greater anti-inflammatory effects whilst minimizing unwanted mineralocorticoid effects. They act on the intracellular glucocorticoid receptor (GR). The GR is complexed with various proteins, including heat shock protein 90 (hsp90). When the glucocorticoid molecule binds its receptor, the GR dissociates from hsp90, enabling it to translocate to the nucleus where it binds to DNA via specific nucleotide palindromic sequences known as glucocorticoid response elements (GREs). GREs are located within the promoter region of target genes and the GR binds to these regions as a dimer. Thus, the end result of GR binding GREs is either activation or inhibition of gene transcription, otherwise known as transactivation or transrepression (49).

The former effect of glucocorticoids is only considered to play a minor role in the anti-inflammatory effects of these

Box 24.1 Experimental effects of glucocorticoids on inflammatory and resident airway cells associated with pathology of asthma

Eosinophil

Inhibit eosinophil survival by inhibiting effects of granulocyte–macrophage colony-stimulating factor (GM-CSF) and interleukin-5 (52, 53), probably a result of inducing apoptosis (54)
Enhance phagocytic clearance of apoptotic eosinophils by macrophages (55)

Macrophage

Inhibit cytokine and inflammatory mediator release from alveolar macrophages *in vitro* (56–59) and *in vivo* (60)

Dendritic cell

Inhibit the development of dendritic cells from peripheral blood precursors (61)
Reduce the number of tissue dendritic cells in an animal model of allergic airway inflammation (62)

T-lymphocyte

Inhibit secretion of cytokines (63–65)
Induce apoptosis (66)

Mast cell

Suppress mast cell activation through inhibiting mast cell secretion of IL-4 (67)

Epithelial cell

Inhibit transcription of adhesion molecules, chemokines, cytokines and other inflammatory proteins such as cyclooxygenase-2 (COX-2) (55)
Increase rate of phagocytosis of apoptotic eosinophils (68)

Endothelial cell

Inhibit airway microvascular leakage, possible through inducing expression of vasocortin (69)

Airway smooth muscle cell

Increase β_2-adrenoceptor expression (70)

Mucus-secreting cells

Decrease mucus secretion from submucosal gland cells (71)
Reduce goblet cell hyperplasia in a murine model of asthma (72)

drugs in asthma. The expression of anti-inflammatory proteins, such as lipocortin-1, interleukin-1ra (IL-1ra), IL-10 and IκB-α, is increased and thus contributes to the anti-inflammatory actions of glucocorticoids (49). Interestingly, glucocorticoids also upregulate expression of the β_2-adrenoceptor, thereby limiting potential downregulation of this receptor following chronic use of β_2-agonists (50).

Transrepression of genes encoding for proinflammatory proteins is thought to be the major mechanism by which glucocorticoids mediate anti-inflammatory effects, as the expression of numerous inflammatory mediators is decreased. These include IL-1–IL-6, IL-8, IL-11, IL-13, tumour necrosis factor-α (TNF-α), granulocyte–macrophage colony-stimulating factor (GM-CSF), RANTES, MIP-1-α, MCP-1, MCP-3, MCP-4 and eotaxin. The expression of various adhesion molecules is decreased, including intercellular adhesion molecule-1 (ICAM-1), vascular cell adhesion molecule-1 (VCAM-1) and E-selectin, in addition to various signalling enzymes, namely inducible nitric oxide synthase (iNOS), cyclooxygenase-2 (COX-2) and phospholipase A_2 (PLA_2) (51). Transrepression occurs through two mechanisms: GR binding DNA and also non-genomic mechanisms. The latter effects are currently thought to occur more frequently and generally involve the direct binding to, and inhibition of, transcription factors such as NF-κB and AP-1, as well as inhibition of certain cell signalling molecules, such as mitogen-activated protein (MAP) kinases (49) (Box 24.1).

The observed experimental effects of glucocorticoids are generally supported by clinical findings. Glucocorticoids have been extensively studied in asthmatic subjects and reduce the number and activity of inflammatory cells in the airways, as measured by studying biopsy, bronchoalveolar lavage and sputum samples. Cells observed to become reduced in number include eosinophils, mast cells, CD4+ T-lymphocytes and macrophages. The attenuation of inflammatory cell activity consequently allows for the repair and restitution of the airway epithelium, which is often damaged and disrupted in asthmatic airways, in addition to a reduction of goblet cell hyperplasia (73, 74).

Synthetic glucocorticoids used in the therapy of asthma include beclomethasone, budesonide and fluticasone and are administered by inhalation, although they are sometimes given orally in the short-term management of acute asthma exacerbations and also in severe asthma for better control. Side-effects that may arise from inhaled use are not common, but include dysphonia and oral candidiasis. The commonly used doses of inhaled glucocorticoids are generally not absorbed sufficiently to cause systemic side-effects, but oral administration can stunt growth in children and cause osteoporosis in adults.

In addition to glucocorticoids, several other types of drugs may be used as add-on therapies to provide further control over asthma. These include theophylline, leukotriene-receptor antagonists and synthesis inhibitors, sodium cromoglycate and nedocromil sodium.

Theophylline belongs to the methylxanthine class of drugs, other members of which include caffeine and theobromine. Theophylline is a weak non-selective inhibitor of phosphodiesterase (PDE) enzymes, which results in airway smooth muscle relaxation. However, theophylline and its derivative, aminophylline, require oral administration as they lack efficacy when administered by inhalation. Also, the bronchodilator action occurs within a very narrow therapeutic window (plasma level of 10–20 g/mL), which unfortunately coincides with a dose that will frequently produce adverse effects, namely nausea and vomiting, but sometimes serious cardiovascular and CNS

effects as well (75). As a result of these effects, theophylline has limited use as a bronchodilator drug. In addition, its use has also declined with the introduction of inhaled glucocorticoids. However, it has recently become apparent that lower doses of theophylline (plasma level <10 μg/mL) have anti-inflammatory and immunomodulatory actions, such as inhibition of eosinophil recruitment and activation in the airways (76–83). This has led to lower doses of theophylline being recommended that achieve a plasma concentration of 5–15 g/mL, which then enables patients to benefit from the anti-inflammatory effects of theophylline with the advantage of a lower incidence of adverse effects.

The mechanisms by which theophylline exerts anti-inflammatory effects are unclear. It is not thought that these effects are mediated via inhibition of PDE isoenzymes, as selective PDE-4 inhibitors do not share some of the effects of theophylline (84, 85). A number of alternative possibilities have been suggested and include adenosine receptor antagonism, although it is not clear which cell types and adenosine receptors are involved. Conflicting data have arisen with regard to whether this is antagonism at the A_1 (86), A_{2a} or A_{2b} (87) receptor, and to confuse things even further, theophylline may be acting as an A_3 agonist on eosinophils, which results in the inhibition of degranulation (88). Theophylline has also been shown to inhibit eosinophil survival and induce apoptosis (84, 89). Another mechanism that may be of importance is the immunomodulatory ability of theophylline to augment CD8+ T-cell function whilst concomitantly inhibiting CD4+ T-cell recruitment to the airways (83).

In summary, therefore, although it is not yet clear exactly how theophylline mediates its anti-inflammatory and immunomodulatory effects, it is likely that the use of theophylline in asthma will become more widespread, simply as a steroid-sparing drug, or possibly as a first-line therapy in its own right.

Leukotriene receptor antagonists and synthesis inhibitors are the latest addition to the range of second-line therapies available for use in the treatment of asthma. The role of cysteinyl leukotrienes (LTC_4, LTD_4 and LTE_4) in the pathology of asthma is well established (90). The effects of leukotrienes include bronchial smooth muscle contraction, eosinophil recruitment, increased vascular permeability, mucus secretion and decreased mucociliary clearance. Thus, as the persistent generation of leukotrienes is a feature of asthma, reducing their activity became a desirable therapeutic target. One approach was to develop an inhibitor of 5-lipoxygenase, the first enzyme required in the biosynthesis of leukotrienes from arachidonic acid. The only inhibitor of 5-lipoxygenase in clinical use is zileuton (91). The other approach taken was to develop antagonists of the cysteinyl leukotriene receptor, $CysLT_1$. This approach yielded several compounds that are now in clinical use and include montelukast, pranlukast and zafirlukast (92). Both classes of drugs are administered orally and produce few, if any, adverse effects, although there is an association with zileuton and liver toxicity, which requires monitoring if zileuton is prescribed.

Anti-leukotriene therapy, however, has not displayed the efficacy that was originally anticipated. The therapeutic effects of these drugs are still less than the effects that can be achieved with low doses of glucocorticoids (93, 94) and attempts to use anti-leukotriene drugs as a monotherapy results in loss of asthma control (95). Thus, anti-leukotriene drugs cannot be substituted for glucocorticoids, but used only as an add-on therapy in order to improve asthma control where needed.

The cromones are another class of drugs that can be used as an add-on therapy, or sometimes as first-line agents. Sodium cromoglycate and nedocromil sodium attenuate the early- and late-phase asthmatic response and reduce airways hyper-responsiveness (96, 97). Both drugs are administered orally and have minor side-effects. Although traditionally referred to as 'mast cell stabilizers', this is probably only one mechanism of action out of several, which remain to be established as the activity of other inflammatory cells is inhibited by these drugs. Similar to theophylline, there is some evidence that adenosine receptor antagonism may be involved (98).

Sodium cromoglycate appears to be a beneficial therapeutic agent in mild allergic asthma and is accepted as a first-line agent, particularly in children. Nedocromil sodium is used in a similar manner, although it appears to have a broader spectrum of activity than sodium cromoglycate and is effective against non-immunological stimuli such as exercise (99), and is also helpful in managing cough through an inhibitory effect on airway sensory nerves (100).

Future pharmacological therapy

Despite the therapeutic advances made following the introduction of inhaled glucocorticoids in the treatment of asthma, a small but significant proportion of asthmatic sufferers are unable to gain control over their asthma through the use of glucocorticoids, or any of the other drugs that are currently available (101). In addition to steroid-resistant asthmatics, the chronic use of glucocorticoids in children is also undesirable (102). Thus, given that the incidence of asthma itself is on the increase (103), considerable efforts are being made to find novel pharmacological therapies for the management of asthma, in addition to drugs that can prevent the development of asthma.

Current approaches to achieve these objectives include the development of drugs to inhibit the recruitment and activity of eosinophils, inhibitors of IgE, chemokines, various cytokines, including IL-4, IL-5 and IL-13, several adhesion molecules and cell-signalling molecules, and also direct inhibitors of inflammatory mediators implicated in asthma. Consequently, many products of these areas of research have reached clinical development, and the future of asthma treatment looks promising (104).

CHRONIC OBSTRUCTIVE PULMONARY DISEASE

Aims of pharmacological therapy

The ideal aims of COPD therapy are to relieve airflow obstruction and slow the progression of the disease by suppressing the underlying inflammation. However, as described earlier, current treatment of COPD at best only achieves partial symptomatic relief, and as glucocorticoids have little or no efficacy in COPD, there are no effective treatments available to reduce the underlying inflammation. Thus, the current aims of COPD therapy are simply to reduce symptoms throughout the inevitable progression of the disease.

Current therapy

In comparison to the wide range of effective therapies for asthma, the drugs available for the treatment of COPD are very limited both in number and efficacy. The therapy of COPD follows a stepwise progression related to the severity of the disease using the few drugs that are available. International guidelines for the treatment of COPD have recently been set out by the Global Initiative for Chronic Obstructive Lung Disease (GOLD) (105). In the case of smoking-induced COPD, the first strategy is, of course, smoking cessation. This is the only action that may slow the disease progression, although it is recognized that cigarette smoking is highly addictive and a notoriously difficult habit to refrain from, even with nicotine replacement therapy and the recent nicotine cessation therapy, bupropion (106). Nicotine can now be administered in numerous forms, from chewing gum to patches, and can provide both physical and psychological assistance for the determined smoker making a serious attempt to quit smoking. Bupropion is an atypical antidepressant that has been licensed for smoking cessation relatively recently. Although its mechanism of action is unclear, it is now considered to be the first-line pharmacological treatment for nicotine addiction. Thus, the use of these drugs is probably the only pharmacological treatment of smoking associated COPD that may affect the course of the disease, albeit in a minority of patients.

Following attempts at smoking cessation, various bronchodilators are used to improve airflow limitation. In contrast to the treatment of asthma, anticholinergics such as ipratropium bromide and the recently developed tiotropium bromide are generally the drugs of choice in the therapy of COPD. Administered by inhalation, these drugs are prescribed as a maintenance therapy, whilst short-acting β_2-agonists such as salbutamol, which are less effective in COPD than in asthma, are prescribed for occasional use for extra symptom control (107). Longer-acting β_2-agonists have recently been found to have an additive effect when administered with an anticholinergic and the combined therapy is used in patients with more severe COPD (108). Theophylline is frequently used as a third-line therapy (105).

Although COPD is an inflammatory disease, the use of corticosteroids to reduce the inflammation is controversial. Neither oral nor inhaled corticosteroids are able to slow the decline in FEV_1 (105). Some patients do respond, but it is thought that these patients have coexistent asthma (109). However, one benefit of inhaled corticosteroids is that they appear to reduce the number of exacerbations in patients with severe COPD, and so may be of benefit to some patients (110).

Other pharmacological treatments of COPD include influenza vaccines and antibiotics to reduce the number of exacerbations, and K_1-antitrypsin (K_1-AT) augmentation therapy for use in patients with K_1-AT deficiency-induced COPD. Mucolytic agents such as carbocysteine are of benefit in a minority of patients with viscous sputum. A variety of non-pharmacological treatments exist, with the aim of improving lung function and survival in COPD patients, and include oxygen therapy and pulmonary rehabilitation (exercise, education and physiotherapy), in addition to various surgical techniques such as lung volume reduction surgery (105). In summary, therefore, there is a severe lack of effective pharmacological therapies for the treatment of COPD, and consequently the overall outlook is very poor for patients following the diagnosis of this disease.

Future pharmacological therapy

In recent years, the urgent need for new pharmacological treatments of COPD has seen an upsurge in research activity. Hence, there are now many drugs currently under investigation for use in the therapy of COPD, and many of these are undergoing clinical trials and may be approved for use in the near future. With the introduction of tiotropium bromide, less emphasis has been placed on finding new bronchodilator drugs and has focused upon treating the underlying inflammation. There are three main areas of investigation with the aim of reducing inflammatory aspects of COPD: the first is developing inhibitors of proinflammatory mediators such as TNF-α and LTB_4; the second is directly targeting inflammatory mediators themselves, such as neutrophil elastase; and the third is the use of anti-inflammatory drugs with a more general action, such as PDE-4 inhibitors.

Firstly, various proinflammatory mediators have been implicated in the pathogenesis and pathology of COPD. One important inflammatory mediator implicated in COPD is LTB_4. Several receptor antagonists of the potent neutrophil chemoattractant LTB_4 are in clinical development. Two receptor subtypes for LTB_4 have been identified. BLT_1 is the receptor expressed on granulocytes and monocytes, and consequently selective antagonists against this receptor have been developed (107). Two studies have shown these antagonists can inhibit the neutrophil chemotactic activity of sputum from COPD patients (111, 112), and so may reduce neutrophil migration to the airways and lungs. Zileuton is also under investigation, although the side-effects of this drug are problematic.

Inhibitors of another major neutrophil chemoattractant, IL-8, are also in clinical development. The same study investigating LTB_4 (112) showed a blocking antibody to IL-8 inhibited the neutrophil chemotactic activity of sputum from COPD patients, and a separate study demonstrated inhibition of neutrophilia *in vivo* with a similar antibody that is now in clinical trials (113). The contribution of LTB_4 and IL-8 to the total chemotactic activity in patients with COPD has been shown to be approximately 47 and 31 per cent, respectively, and thus inhibitors of LTB_4 and IL-8 administered in combination

could significantly reduce neutrophil infiltration and associated inflammation (112). In addition to a blocking antibody, small-molecule inhibitors of the IL-8 receptor involved in chemotaxis, CXCR2, are also in clinical development (114). A CXCR2 antagonist may also inhibit monocyte haptotaxis and thus be of further benefit by reducing the pulmonary macrophage population.

TNF-K is another proinflammatory cytokine significantly implicated in the pathogenesis of COPD. It has many proinflammatory effects, elimination of which would be highly desirable. Infliximab is a humanized monoclonal antibody against TNF-K that is currently in clinical trials for COPD, and has already been shown to be effective in rheumatoid arthritis. Another drug originally developed for rheumatoid arthritis that is also in clinical development for COPD is etanercept, a soluble TNF receptor (107).

Drugs under investigation that directly target inflammatory mediators include antioxidants and proteinase inhibitors. Oxidative stress is a pathological feature of COPD and results from exposure to cigarette-derived oxidants and reactive oxygen species derived from inflammatory cells. Oxidants have many pathological effects such as inactivation of antiproteinases, injury to the epithelium and lung matrix and increased gene expression of proinflammatory mediators. They also increase sequestration of neutrophils from pulmonary microvasculature into the lungs. Thus antioxidants such as stable glutathione compounds, superoxide dismutase analogues and selenium-based drugs are now in pre-clinical development (115). Inhibitors of oxidative stress resulting from iNOS activity are also under investigation and some selective inhibitors of iNOS are now in development for clinical use (116).

Proteinases such as neutrophil elastase are heavily implicated in the pathogenesis of emphysema and the inflammation present in the upper and central airways. Thus, inhibition of the excessive proteolytic activity that occurs in COPD would be very desirable. It may seem that the obvious course of action is to produce recombinant endogenous inhibitors such as K_1-AT or secretory leukocyte protease inhibitor (SLPI) and administer these to COPD patients. However, the manufacture of large amounts of protein is required and at a very high cost, so this therapeutic approach has so far been limited to patients with K_1-AT deficiency. A more attractive alternative has been to develop small-molecule proteinase inhibitors. ONO5046 and FR901277, for example, are highly potent inhibitors of serine proteinases and are now in clinical trials (117).

Inhibitors of macrophage cysteine proteinases (cathepsins K, L, S) are also in development, in addition to inhibitors of matrix metalloproteinases (MMPs), namely MMP-9, which has elastolytic activity (107).

Finally, although not a direct inhibitor, retinoic acid has been shown to reverse elastase-induced emphysema in rats, and retinoic acid receptor agonists are being investigated in patients with emphysema (118). In addition to direct inhibitors of proinflammatory and inflammatory mediators, a less specific approach to resolve the inflammation in COPD has been to develop more general anti-inflammatory drugs with multiple effects. Much attention has centred upon PDE-4 inhibitors. As described above, PDE-4 inhibitors have a broad-spectrum anti-inflammatory effect upon leucocytes that express PDE-4, which in the context of COPD is inclusive of neutrophils, macrophages and CD8+ T-lymphocytes (119). Cilomilast was shown to improve FEV$_1$ in patients with COPD and has now reached phase III clinical trials (120). However, to date, it has proved difficult to separate the nausea and gastrointestinal side-effects of PDE-4 inhibitors from the therapeutic effects and this may limit their use, although PDE-4 inhibitors that do not induce nausea and vomiting have been described recently (121). Although originally intended to be administered orally, investigations into administering PDE-4 inhibitors by the inhaled route are also underway.

Other types of anti-inflammatory drugs under investigation include inhibitors of nuclear factor-kappa B (NF-8B), which inhibit secretion of various cytokines and MMPs such as IL-8 and TNF-K, and adhesion molecule blockers that reduce inflammatory cell recruitment. Inhibitors of p38 MAP kinase, which possess broad-spectrum anti-inflammatory activity, have also been developed, as well as phosphatidylinositol 3-kinase inhibitors, which have been shown to inhibit neutrophil migration and activation (107). The broad-spectrum anti-inflammatory cytokine IL-10 is also under investigation.

Thus, the huge interest in developing new treatments for COPD has yielded many promising new drugs, which may possess the ability to slow the progression of the disease by targeting the underlying inflammation and lead to much brighter prospects for patients following the diagnosis of COPD.

Key points

- A wide range of pharmacological therapies are currently available for the treatment of obstructive airway diseases such as asthma and COPD.
- An excellent level of control over asthma is now attainable through the administration of glucocorticoid drugs that are able to control the underlying inflammation, and hence the disease progression.
- In addition to glucocorticoids, both short-acting and long-acting β$_2$-agonists are successfully used to provide additional control over airways obstruction, either on an 'as needed' basis or prophylactically.
- Glucocorticoids exhibit little or no efficacy in the treatment of COPD.
- Bronchodilator drugs including anticholinergics and β$_2$-agonists are only partially able to reverse the airways obstruction.
- A variety of novel anti-inflammatory drugs are currently under investigation for the treatment of COPD and a number of these are now undergoing clinical testing.

REFERENCES

1. Bingham CO, Austen KF. Mast-cell responses in the development of asthma. *J Allergy Clin Immunol* 2000; **105**: S527–34.
2. Pearlman DS. Pathophysiology of the inflammatory response. *J Allergy Clin Immunol* 1999; **104**: S132–7.
3. O'Byrne PM, Inman MD. Airway hyperresponsiveness. *Chest* 2003; **123**: 411S–16S.
4. Rodgman A, Smith CJ, Perfetti TA. The composition of cigarette smoke: a retrospective, with emphasis on polycyclic components. *Hum Exp Toxicol* 2000; **19**: 573–95.
5. Barnes PJ. Molecular genetics of chronic obstructive pulmonary disease. *Thorax* 1999; **54**: 245–52.
6. Stockley RA. Neutrophils and the pathogenesis of COPD. *Chest* 2002; **121**: 151S–5S.
7. van der Velden VH. Glucocorticoids: mechanisms of action and anti-inflammatory potential in asthma. *Med Inflamm* 1998; **7**: 229–37.
8. Pauwels RA, Buist AS, Calverley PM *et al.* (the Gold Scientific Committee). Global strategy for the diagnosis, management, and prevention of chronic obstructive pulmonary disease. NHLBI/WHO Global Initiative for Chronic Obstructive Lung Disease (GOLD) Workshop summary. *Am J Respir Crit Care Med* 2001; **163**: 1256–76.
9. Jones PW, Willit LR, Burge PS, Calverley PM. Disease severity and the effect of fluticasone propionate on chronic obstructive pulmonary disease exacerbations. *Eur Respir J* 2003; **21**: 68–73.
10. Haslett C. Granulocyte apoptosis and its role in the resolution and control of lung inflammation. *Am J Respir Crit Care Med* 1999; **160**: S5–11.
11. National Heart, Lung, and Blood Institute/World Health Organization. *Global Initiative for Asthma: Global Strategy for Asthma Management and Prevention. Workshop Report.* Bethesda, MD: NHLBI/WHO, 1995.
12. Johnson M. The beta-adrenoceptor. *Am J Respir Crit Care Med* 1998; **158**(5 Part 3): S146–53.
13. Spina D, Page CP, O'Connor BJ. β$_2$-adrenoceptors. In: *Drugs for the Treatment of Respiratory Diseases.* Cambridge: Cambridge University Press, 2003; 56–104.
14. Cipolla D, Farr S, Gonda I, Otulana B. Delivery of biologics to the lung. In: Hansel TT, Barnes PJ, eds. *New Drugs for Asthma, Allergy and COPD.* (Progress in Respiratory Research, Vol. 31). Basel: Karger, 2001; 20–3.
15. Larj MJ, Bleecker ER. Effects of beta2-agonists on airway tone and bronchial responsiveness. *J Allergy Clin Immunol* 2002; **110**(6 Suppl.): S304–12.
16. Ahrens RC, Harris JB, Milavetz G *et al.* Use of bronchial provocation with histamine to compare the pharmacodynamics of inhaled albuterol and metaproterenol in patients with asthma. *J Allergy Clin Immunol* 1987; **79**: 876–82.
17. Gongora HC, Wisniewski AF, Tattersfield AE. A single-dose comparison of inhaled albuterol and two formulations of salmeterol on airway reactivity in asthmatic subjects. *Am Rev Respir Dis* 1991; **144**(3 Part 1): 626–9.
18. Anderson SD, Rodwell LT, Du Toit J, Young IH. Duration of protection by inhaled salmeterol in exercise-induced asthma. *Chest* 1991; **100**: 1254–60.
19. Malo JL, Ghezzo H, Trudeau C *et al.* Duration of action of inhaled terbutaline at two different doses and of albuterol in protecting against bronchoconstriction induced by hyperventilation of dry cold air in asthmatic subjects. *Am Rev Respir Dis* 1989; **140**: 817–21.

20. Pearlman DS, Chervinsky P, Laforce C et al. A comparison of salmeterol with albuterol in the treatment of mild-to-moderate asthma. N Engl J Med 1992; **327**: 1420–5.

21. Lötvall J. The long and short of β₂-agonists. Pulm Pharmacol Ther 2002; **15**: 497–501.

22. Weston MC, Peachell PT. Regulation of human mast cell and basophil function by cAMP. Gen Pharmacol 1998; **31**: 715–19.

23. Pennings HJ, Dentener MA, Buurman WA, Wouters EFM. Salbutamol and salmeterol modulate cytokine production by peripheral blood monocytes. Eur Resp J 1995; 8(Suppl. 19): 1871.

24. Pantelidis P, Hayes KL, Vardey C, Du Bois RM. Modulation of monocyte cytokine secretion by β₂-agonists: a comparison of salbutamol and salmeterol. Eur Resp J 1995; 8(Suppl. 19): 2692.

25. Baker AJ, Palmer J, Johnson M, Fuller RW. Inhibitory actions of salmeterol on human airway macrophages and blood monocytes. Eur J Pharmacol 1994; **264**: 301–6.

26. Zetterlund A, Linden M, Larsson K. Effects of beta2-agonists and budesonide on interleukin-1beta and leukotriene B4 secretion: studies of human monocytes and alveolar macrophages. J Asthma 1998; **35**: 565–73.

27. Izeboud CA, Monshouwer M, van Miert AS, Witkamp RF. The beta-adrenoceptor agonist clenbuterol is a potent inhibitor of the LPS-induced production of TNF-alpha and IL-6 in vitro and in vivo. Inflamm Res 1999; **48**: 497–502.

28. Joseph M, Tonnel AB, Capron A, Dessaint JP. The interaction of IgE antibody with human alveolar macrophages and its participation in the inflammatory processes of lung allergy. Agents Actions 1981; **11**: 619–22.

29. Munoz NM, Rabe KF, Vita AJ et al. Paradoxical blockade of beta adrenergically mediated inhibition of stimulated eosinophil secretion by salmeterol. J Pharmacol Exp Ther 1995; **273**: 850–4.

30. Leff AR, Herrnreiter A, Naclerio RM et al. Effect of enantiomeric forms of albuterol on stimulated secretion of granular protein from human eosinophils. Pulm Pharmacol Ther 1997; **10**: 97–104.

31. Ezeamuzie CI, al-Hage M. Differential effects of salbutamol and salmeterol on human eosinophil responses. J Pharmacol Exp Ther 1998; **284**: 25–31.

32. Dent G, Giembycz MA, Evans PM et al. Suppression of human eosinophil respiratory burst and cyclic AMP hydrolysis by inhibitors of type IV phosphodiesterase: interaction with the beta adrenoceptor agonist albuterol. J Pharmacol Exp Ther 1994; **271**: 1167–74.

33. Hadjokas NE, Crowley JJ, Bayer CR, Nielson CP. Beta-adrenergic regulation of the eosinophil respiratory burst as detected by lucigenin-dependent luminescence. J Allergy Clin Immunol 1995; **95**: 735–41.

34. Tool AT, Mul FP, Knol EF et al. The effect of salmeterol and nimesulide on chemotaxis and synthesis of PAF and LTC4 by human eosinophils. Eur Respir J Suppl 1996; **22**: 141–5s.

35. Anderson R, Feldman C, Theron AJ et al. Anti-inflammatory, membrane–stabilizing interactions of salmeterol with human neutrophils in vitro. Br J Pharmacol 1996; **117**: 1387–94.

36. Ottonello L, Morone P, Dapino P, Dallegri F. Inhibitory effect of salmeterol on the respiratory burst of adherent human neutrophils. Clin Exp Immunol 1996; **106**: 97–102.

37. Mirza ZN, Kato M, Kimura H et al. Fenoterol inhibits superoxide anion generation by human polymorphonuclear leukocytes via beta-adrenoceptor-dependent and -independent mechanisms. Ann Allergy Asthma Immunol 2002; **88**: 494–500.

38. Silvestri M, Oddera S, Lantero S, Rossi GA. Beta 2-agonist-induced inhibition of neutrophil chemotaxis is not associated with modification of LFA-1 and Mac-1 expression or with impairment

39. of polymorphonuclear leukocyte antibacterial activity. Respir Med 1999; **93**: 416–23.

39. Sekut L, Champion BR, Page K et al. Anti-inflammatory activity of salmeterol: down-regulation of cytokine production. Clin Exp Immunol 1995; **99**: 461–6.

40. Borger P, Hoekstra Y, Esselink MT et al. Beta-adrenoceptor-mediated inhibition of IFN-gamma, IL-3, and GM-CSF mRNA accumulation in activated human T lymphocytes is solely mediated by the beta2-adrenoceptor subtype. Am J Respir Cell Mol Biol 1998; **19**: 400–7.

41. Holen E, Elsayed S. Effects of beta2 adrenoceptor agonists on T-cell subpopulations. APMIS 1998; **106**: 849–57.

42. Gibbs BF, Vollrath IB, Albrecht C et al. Inhibition of interleukin-4 and interleukin-13 release from immunologically activated human basophils due to the actions of anti-allergic drugs. Naunyn Schmiedebergs Arch Pharmacol 1998; **357**: 573–8.

43. Kleine-Tebbe J, Frank G, Josties C, Kunkel G. Influence of salmeterol, a long-acting beta 2-adrenoceptor agonist, on IgE-mediated histamine release from human basophils. J Invest Allergol Clin Immunol 1994; **4**: 12–17.

44. Torphy TJ. Phosphodiesterase isozymes: molecular targets for novel antiasthma agents. Am J Respir Crit Care Med 1998; **157**: 351–70.

45. Johnson M. Effects of beta2-agonists on resident and infiltrating inflammatory cells. J Allergy Clin Immunol 2002; **110**(6 Suppl.): S282–90.

46. Jacoby DB, Fryer AD. Anticholinergic therapy for airway diseases. Life Sci 2001; **68**: 2565–72.

47. Hansel TT, Barnes PJ. Tiotropium bromide. a novel once-daily anticholinergic bronchodilator for the treatment of COPD. Drugs Today (Barc) 2002; **38**: 585–600.

48. O'Connor BJ, Towse LJ, Barnes PJ. Prolonged effect of tiotropium bromide on methacholine-induced bronchoconstriction in asthma. Am J Respir Crit Care Med 1996; **154**(4 Part 1): 876–80.

49. Pelaia G, Vatrella A, Cuda G et al. Molecular mechanisms of corticosteroid actions in chronic inflammatory airway diseases. Life Sci 2003; **72**: 1549–61.

50. Barnes PJ. Beta-adrenergic receptors and their regulation. Am J Respir Crit Care Med 1995; **152**: 838–60.

51. Umland SP, Schleimer RP, Johnston SL. Review of the molecular and cellular mechanisms of action of glucocorticoids for use in asthma. Pulm Pharmacol Ther 2002; **15**: 35–50.

52. Wallen N, Kita H, Weiller D, Gleich GJ. Glucocorticoids inhibit cytokine-mediated eosinophil survival. J Immunol 1991; **147**: 3490–5.

53. Lamas AM, Leon OG, Schleimer RP. Glucocorticoids inhibit eosinophil responses to granulocyte-macrophage colony-stimulating factor. J Immunol 1991; **147**: 254–9.

54. Druilhe A, Letuve S, Pretolani M. Glucocorticoid-induced apoptosis in human eosinophils: mechanisms of action. Apoptosis 2003; **8**: 481–95.

55. Walsh GM, Sexton DW, Blaylock MG. Corticosteroids, eosinophils and bronchial epithelial cells: new insights into the resolution of inflammation in asthma. J Endocrinol 2003; **178**: 37–43.

56. Linden M, Brattsand R. Effects of a corticosteroid, budesonide, on alveolar macrophage and blood monocyte secretion of cytokines: differential sensitivity of GM-CSF, IL-1 beta, and IL-6. Pulm Pharmacol 1994; **7**: 43–7.

57. Fuller RW, Kelsey CR, Cole PJ et al. Dexamethasone inhibits the production of thromboxane B2 and leukotriene B4 by human alveolar and peritoneal macrophages in culture. Clin Sci (Lond) 1984; **67**: 653–6.

58. Martinet N, Vaillant P, Charles T et al. Dexamethasone modulation of tumour necrosis factor-alpha (cachectin) release by activated normal human alveolar macrophages. Eur Respir J 1992; **5**: 67–72.

59. Standiford TJ, Kunkel SL, Rolfe MW et al. Regulation of human alveolar macrophage- and blood monocyte-derived interleukin-8 by prostaglandin E2 and dexamethasone. Am J Respir Cell Mol Biol 1992; **6**: 75–81.

60. Bergstrand H, Bjornson A, Blaschke E et al. Effects of an inhaled corticosteroid, budesonide, on alveolar macrophage function in smokers. Thorax 1990; **45**: 362–8.

61. van den Heuvel MM, van Beek NM, Broug-Holub E et al. Glucocorticoids modulate the development of dendritic cells from blood precursors. Clin Exp Immunol 1999; **115**: 5778–83.

62. Nelson DJ, Mcwilliam AS, Haining S, Holt PG. Modulation of airway intraepithelial dendritic cells following exposure to steroids. Am J Respir Crit Care Med 1995; **151**: 475–81.

63. Stam WB, Van Oosterhout AJ, Nijkamp FP. Pharmacologic modulation of Th1- and Th2-associated lymphokine production. Life Sci 1993; **53**: 1921–34.

64. Choy DK, Ko F, Li ST et al. Effects of theophylline, dexamethasone and salbutamol on cytokine gene expression in human peripheral blood CD4+ T-cells. Eur Respir J 1999; **14**: 1106–12.

65. Snijdewint FG, Kapsenberg ML, Wauben-Penris PJ, Bos JD. Corticosteroids class-dependently inhibit in vitro Th1- and Th2-type cytokine production. Immunopharmacology 1995; **29**: 93–101.

66. Melis M, Siena L, Pace E et al. Fluticasone induces apoptosis in peripheral T-lymphocytes: a comparison between asthmatic and normal subjects. Eur Respir J 2002; **19**: 257–66.

67. Yoshikawa H, Tasaka K. Suppression of mast cell activation by glucocorticoid. Arch Immunol Ther Exp (Warsz) 2000; **48**: 487–95.

68. Walsh GM, Sexton DW, Blaylock MG. Corticosteroids, eosinophils and bronchial epithelial cells: new insights into the resolution of inflammation in asthma. J Endocrinol 2003; **178**: 37–43.

69. Boschetto P, Rogers DF, Fabbri LM, Barnes PJ. Corticosteroid inhibition of airway microvascular leakage. Am Rev Respir Dis 1991; **143**: 605–9.

70. Mak JC, Nishikawa M, Barnes PJ. Glucocorticosteroids increase beta 2-adrenergic receptor transcription in human lung. Am J Physiol 1995; **268**(1 Part 1): L41–6.

71. Shimura S, Sasaki T, Ikeda K et al. Direct inhibitory action of glucocorticoid on glycoconjugate secretion from airway submucosal glands. Am Rev Respir Dis 1990; **141**(4 Part 1): 1044–9.

72. Blyth DI, Pedrick MS, Savage TJ et al. Induction, duration, and resolution of airway goblet cell hyperplasia in a murine model of atopic asthma: effect of concurrent infection with respiratory syncytial virus and response to dexamethasone. Am J Respir Cell Mol Biol 1998; **19**: 38–54.

73. Barnes PJ, Pedersen S, Busse WW. Efficacy and safety of inhaled corticosteroids. Am J Respir Crit Care Med 1998; **157**: S1–53.

74. Caramori G, Adcock I. Pharmacology of airway inflammation in asthma and COPD. Pulm Pharmacol Ther 2003; **16**: 247–77.

75. Weinberger M, Hendeles L. Theophylline in asthma. N Engl J Med 1996; **334**: 1380–8.

76. Ward AJ, Mckenniff M, Evans JM et al. Theophylline – an immunomodulatory role in asthma? Am Rev Respir Dis 1993; **147**: 518–23.

77. Sullivan P, Bekir S, Jaffar Z et al. Anti-inflammatory effects of low-dose oral theophylline in atopic asthma. Lancet 1994; **343**: 1006–8.

78. Kidney J, Dominguez M, Taylor PM et al. Immunomodulation by theophylline in asthma. Demonstration by withdrawal of therapy. Am J Respir Crit Care Med 1995; **151**: 1907–14.

79. Djukanovic R, Finnerty JP, Lee C et al. The effects of theophylline on mucosal inflammation in asthmatic airways: biopsy results. Eur Respir J 1995; **8**: 831–3.

80. Finnerty JP, Lee C, Wilson S et al. Effects of theophylline on inflammatory cells and cytokines in asthmatic subjects: a placebo-controlled parallel group study. Eur Respir J 1996; **9**: 1672–7.

81. Lim S, Tomita K, Carramori G et al. Low-dose theophylline reduces eosinophilic inflammation but not exhaled nitric oxide in mild asthma. Am J Respir Crit Care Med 2001; **164**: 273–6.

82. Yasui K, Komiyama A. New clinical applications of xanthine derivatives: modulatory actions on leukocyte survival and function. Int J Hematol 2001; **73**: 87–92.

83. Spina D. Theophylline and PDE4 inhibitors in asthma. Curr Opin Pulm Med 2003; **9**: 57–64.

84. Yasui K, Hu B, Nakazawa T et al. Theophylline accelerates human granulocyte apoptosis not via phosphodiesterase inhibition. J Clin Invest 1997; **100**: 1677–84.

85. Banner KH, Hoult JR, Taylor MN et al. Possible contribution of prostaglandin E2 to the antiproliferative effect of phosphodiesterase 4 inhibitors in human mononuclear cells. Biochem Pharmacol 1999; **58**: 1487–95.

86. Nyce JW, Metzger WJ. DNA antisense therapy for asthma in an animal model. Nature 1997; **385**: 721–5.

87. Fozard JR. The case for a role for adenosine in asthma: almost convincing? Curr Opin Pharmacol 2003; **3**: 264–9.

88. Ezeamuzie CI. Involvement of A(3) receptors in the potentiation by adenosine of the inhibitory effect of theophylline on human eosinophil degranulation: possible novel mechanism of the anti-inflammatory action of theophylline. Biochem Pharmacol 2001; **61**: 1551–9.

89. Ohta K, Yamashita N. Apoptosis of eosinophils and lymphocytes in allergic inflammation. J Allergy Clin Immunol 1999; **104**: 14–21.

90. Borish L. The role of leukotrienes in upper and lower airway inflammation and the implications for treatment. Ann Allergy Asthma Immunol 2002; **88**(4 Suppl. 1): 16–22.

91. Carter GW, Young PR, Albert DH et al. 5-lipoxygenase inhibitory activity of zileuton. J Pharmacol Exp Ther 1991; **256**: 929–37.

92. Peters SP. Leukotriene receptor antagonists in asthma therapy. J Allergy Clin Immunol 2003; **111**(1 Suppl.): S62–70.

93. Bleecker ER, Welch MJ, Weinstein SF et al. Low-dose inhaled fluticasone propionate versus oral zafirlukast in the treatment of persistent asthma. J Allergy Clin Immunol 2000; **105**(6 Part 1): 1123–9.

94. Laviolette M, Malmstrom K, Lu S et al. Montelukast added to inhaled beclomethasone in treatment of asthma. Montelukast/Beclomethasone Additivity Group. Am J Respir Crit Care Med 1999; **160**: 1862–8.

95. Ducharme FM. Inhaled glucocorticoids versus leukotriene receptor antagonists as single agent asthma treatment: systematic review of current evidence. BMJ 2003; **326**: 621.

96. Norris AA. Pharmacology of sodium cromoglycate. Clin Exp Allergy 1996; **26**(Suppl. 4): 5–7.

97. Szefler SJ, Nelson HS. Alternative agents for anti-inflammatory treatment of asthma. J Allergy Clin Immunol 1998; **102**(4 Part 2): S23–35.

98. Church MK, Holgate ST. Adenosine-induced bronchoconstriction and its inhibition by nedocromil sodium. J Allergy Clin Immunol 1993; **92**(1 Part 2): 190–4.

99. Spooner CH, Saunders LD, Rowe BH. Nedocromil sodium for preventing exercise-induced bronchoconstriction. Cochrane Database Syst Rev 2002; **1**: CD001183.

100. Barnes PJ. Effect of nedocromil sodium on airway sensory nerves. *J Allergy Clin Immunol* 1993; **92**(1 Part 2): 182–6.

101. Wenzel S. Severe asthma: epidemiology, pathophysiology and treatment. *Mt Sinai J Med* 2003; **70**: 185–90.

102. Robinson JD, Angelini BL, Krahnke JS, Skoner DP. Inhaled steroids and the risk of adrenal suppression in children. *Expert Opin Drug Saf* 2002; **1**: 237–44.

103. Beasley R. The burden of asthma with specific reference to the United States. *J Allergy Clin Immunol* 2002; **109**(5 Suppl.): S482–S489.

104. Hansel TT, Barnes PJ. Novel drugs for treating asthma. *Curr Allergy Asthma Report* 2001; **1**: 164–73.

105. Pauwels RA, Buist AS, Calverley PM *et al.* (the Gold Scientific Committee). Global strategy for the diagnosis, management, and prevention of chronic obstructive pulmonary disease. NHLBI/WHO Global Initiative for Chronic Obstructive Lung Disease (GOLD) Workshop summary. *Am J Respir Crit Care Med* 2001; **163**: 1256–76.

106. George TP, O'Malley SS. Current pharmacological treatments for nicotine dependence. *Trends Pharmacol Sci* 2004; **25**: 42–8.

107. Barnes PJ. New treatments for COPD. *Nat Rev Drug Discov* 2002; **1**: 437–46.

108. van Noord JA, de Munck DR, Bantje TA *et al.* Long-term treatment of chronic obstructive pulmonary disease with salmeterol and the additive effect of ipratropium. *Eur Respir J* 2000; **15**: 878–85.

109. Papi A, Romagnoli M, Baraldo S *et al.* Partial reversibility of airflow limitation and increased exhaled NO and sputum eosinophilia in chronic obstructive pulmonary disease. *Am J Respir Crit Care Med* 2000; **162**: 1773–7.

110. Alsaeedi A, Sin DD, Mcalister FA. The effects of inhaled corticosteroids in chronic obstructive pulmonary disease: a systematic review of randomized placebo-controlled trials. *Am J Med* 2002; **113**: 59–65.

111. Crooks SW, Bayley DL, Hill SL, Stockley RA. Bronchial inflammation in acute bacterial exacerbations of chronic bronchitis. The role of leukotriene B4. *Eur Respir J* 2000; **15**: 274–80.

112. Woolhouse IS, Bayley DL, Stockley RA. Sputum chemotactic activity in chronic obstructive pulmonary disease: effect of alpha (1)-antitrypsin deficiency and the role of leukotriene B (4) and interleukin 8. *Thorax* 2002; **57**: 709–14.

113. Yang XD, Corvalan JR, Wang P *et al.* Fully human anti-interleukin-8 monoclonal antibodies: potential therapeutics for the treatment of inflammatory disease states. *J Leukoc Biol* 1999; **66**: 401–10.

114. Hay DW, Sarau HM. Interleukin-8 receptor antagonists in pulmonary diseases. *Curr Opin Pharmacol* 2001; **1**: 242–7.

115. Macnee W. Oxidants/antioxidants and Copd. *Chest* 2000; **117**: 303–17S.

116. Hobbs AJ, Higgs A, Moncada S. Inhibition of nitric oxide synthase as a potential therapeutic target. *Annu Rev Pharmacol Toxicol* 1999; **39**: 191–220.

117. Ohbayashi H. Neutrophil elastase inhibitors as treatment for COPD. *Expert Opin Invest Drugs* 2002; **11**: 965–80.

118. Mao JT, Goldin JG, Dermand J *et al.* A pilot study of all-trans-retinoic acid for the treatment of human emphysema. *Am J Respir Crit Care Med* 2002; **165**: 718–23.

119. Souness JE, Aldous D, Sargent C. Immunosuppressive and anti-inflammatory effects of cyclic AMP phosphodiesterase (PDE) type 4 inhibitors. *Immunopharmacology* 2000; **47**: 127–62.

120. Compton CH, Gubb J, Nieman R *et al.* Cilomilast, a selective phosphodiesterase-4 inhibitor for treatment of patients with chronic obstructive pulmonary disease: a randomised, dose-ranging study. *Lancet* 2001; **358**: 265–70.

121. Gale DD, Landells LJ, Spina D *et al.* Pharmacokinetic and pharmacodynamic profile following oral administration of the phosphodiesterase (PDE) 4 inhibitor V11294A in healthy volunteers. *Br J Clin Pharmacol* 2002; **54**: 478–84.

PART 4

Delivering pulmonary rehabilitation: specific problems

Derby Hospitals NHS Foundation
Trust
Library and Knowledge Service

25

Rehabilitation in asthma

KAI-HÅKON CARLSEN

INTRODUCTION

Asthma is a very common chronic disorder. It is the most common chronic illness of childhood. The lifetime prevalence of asthma in children has increased markedly over the last 30–40 years, presently varying from 2–3 to over 30 per cent throughout the world (1); and also among young adults asthma prevalence has increased over recent years. Sunyer *et al.* (2) demonstrated, in a study from 15 industrialized countries, an increased relative risk of 2.4 of having asthma in adult age for those born in 1966 vs. 1946 (2). During childhood, acute asthma attacks are the most common cause of admission to hospital, although modern anti-inflammatory treatment seems to decrease the risk of readmission to hospital after starting treatment, especially in children above 4–5 years of age (3, 4).

It is thus obvious that asthma causes severe illness, and the burden for asthmatic children and their families was well described by Lenny *et al.* (5) some years ago. They described a composite burden on several levels and on several levels of medical care. Firstly there is an increased burden on the sick child and the family, consisting of symptoms during the day and night, admissions to hospital, days away from school, much time spent on medication, and increased financial costs for the family. However, asthma also represents an increased burden on the community, due to medication costs, costs of general care, costs due to admissions to hospital, and costs associated with patients and family members being away from school and work (5). Taylor and Newacheck (6) reported, from an American national study of more than 17 000 households, that there were 2.7 million children with asthma, 7.3 million days restricted to bed, 1.9 million days in hospital, 10.1 million days away from school, and 12.9 million contacts with a doctor. Furthermore, they reported that 30 per cent of

children with asthma suffered from reduced ability to undertake daily physical activity due to their asthma, compared with only 4 per cent of the remainder of children (6).

Rehabilitation has therefore become increasingly important in the care of the asthmatic patients and has become a natural part of the management of children, as well as the adult patients, with asthma.

Asthma and allergy have a strong hereditary influence. Much effort has therefore been put into assessing the possibilities of preventing these disorders. A hierarchy of different levels of prevention has been suggested. Primary prevention has been defined as the prevention of the allergy or asthma itself; secondary prevention as the prevention of further manifestations of atopic manifestations after the first; and tertiary prevention as the prevention of further progression of asthma, prevention of remodelling of the airways, and reduction of symptoms and consequences of the disease to a minimum (7). Rehabilitation is an important part of tertiary prevention.

Pulmonary rehabilitation has been defined by a Task Force of the European Respiratory Society as 'a process which systematically uses scientifically based diagnostic management and evaluation options, to achieve the optimal daily functioning and health related quality of life of individual patients suffering from impairment and disability due to chronic respiratory diseases as measured by clinically and/or physiologically relevant outcome measures' (8). Although this task force was looking at the rehabilitation of chronic obstructive lung disease, the definition may also encompass asthma. Other definitions have underlined the need for a multidisciplinary approach to achieve these goals (9). The need for rehabilitation has been more focused upon in relation to chronic obstructive lung disease, but as asthma is a very complex condition with several different clinical presentations and causes, it clearly needs a

---

Box 25.1 Elements of rehabilitation of asthma

- The diagnostic process
  - lung function measurements
  - bronchial responsiveness
  - assessment of exercise-induced bronchoconstriction
  - work physiology; maximum oxygen uptake
  - assessment of compliance with treatment
  - psychological functioning
  - social functioning and need for social and economical support
  - assessment of educational needs
- Optimal treatment of asthma
- Education
  - asthma schools
  - individual education
  - written management plan
- Physical training
- Climate therapy
  - high-altitude training
  - change of climate

---

multidisciplinary approach and guidelines for the rehabilitation process. This chapter presents multidisciplinary approaches to the rehabilitation of children, adolescents and adults with asthma.

MEASURES OF REHABILITATION OF ASTHMA

Rehabilitation of asthma is truly a multidisciplinary task with several components of care. The different approaches are presented in Box 25.1 and combine optimal pharmacological treatment with educational measures on several aspects to help patients master their illness. A further important measure is physical training, and a procedure called 'climate therapy' has also been employed as part of the rehabilitation process. This includes prolonged stays in high-altitude environments, travel from cold to warm climates and speleotherapy as used in middle and eastern Europe. An effective rehabilitation programme would include several aspects of these measures at the same time. Mastering of illness is a key issue in this context, and the rehabilitation process can be envisaged as a multidisciplinary approach to dealing with asthma and its consequences.

DIAGNOSTIC MEASURES BEFORE AND DURING REHABILITATION

Before starting rehabilitation of an asthma patient, it is important to assess the severity of the patient's asthma and

functional ability. The diagnosis of asthma is still clinical and based upon a combination of case history and clinical examination. The diagnosis of asthma should be ensured before starting rehabilitation measures. Lung function assessment with maximum expiratory flow volume loops and the response to inhaled β_2-agonists should be performed routinely. Measurements of diurnal variability of peak expiratory flow rate are also useful in the monitoring of patients, particularly adult patients, as these can be unreliable in children (10). Exercise testing with standardized assessment of exercise-induced bronchoconstriction is preferable. In addition, determination of physical fitness with measurement of maximum oxygen uptake ($\dot{V}O_{2,max}$) may be useful. It is important to standardize exercise assessment with respect to the environmental conditions (temperature, humidity) (11), exercise load (12) and exercise duration (13).

During exercise testing with measurement of $\dot{V}O_{2,max}$, it is possible to measure tidal breathing flow volume loops. This is a useful way to determine what can be obtained by physical training in relationship to lung function. The tidal flow volume loops during exercise are compared with the maximal lung function measurements taken before exercise and possible flow limitation is assessed (14). Figure 25.1 demonstrates tidal flow volume loops during different stages of exercise compared with the maximum expiratory flow volume loop.

Non-specific bronchial responsiveness to metacholine or histamine (15) is a useful measure in the follow-up of asthma patients. Exercise testing is valuable before starting asthma rehabilitation, and also later to assess the effect of rehabilitation. Although increased non-specific bronchial responsiveness is not diagnosis-specific for asthma (11), it is useful in the monitoring of disease severity. Sont *et al.* (16) observed improved effects on airways inflammation and airways remodelling when employing measurements of non-specific bronchial responsiveness to metacholine as a tool in monitoring the treatment of asthma patients.

Compliance with treatment has been shown to vary in asthma patients, and has been shown to decrease markedly with time over longer periods of treatment (17). In order to understand the severity of asthma during ongoing treatment, and to be able to monitor the effect of rehabilitation measures, attempts to determine the compliance should be undertaken. This may be difficult without specific measures. Improvement of compliance with treatment is best obtained by good communication with the patient and by instituting educational measures that increase patients' understanding of the mechanisms and treatment of asthma.

It is important that the approaches to the patient and to the initiatives taken are multidisciplinary. This is also true for the initial assessment. The needs of asthmatic patients are manifold, and assessment should take into account patients' social relationships, psychological functioning, control of illness at school or at work, and need for physical training.

Diagnostic procedures should also include assessment of the need for educational measures to pass on knowledge to patients that is important for mastering of their illness, including tackling acute exacerbations and asthma attacks.

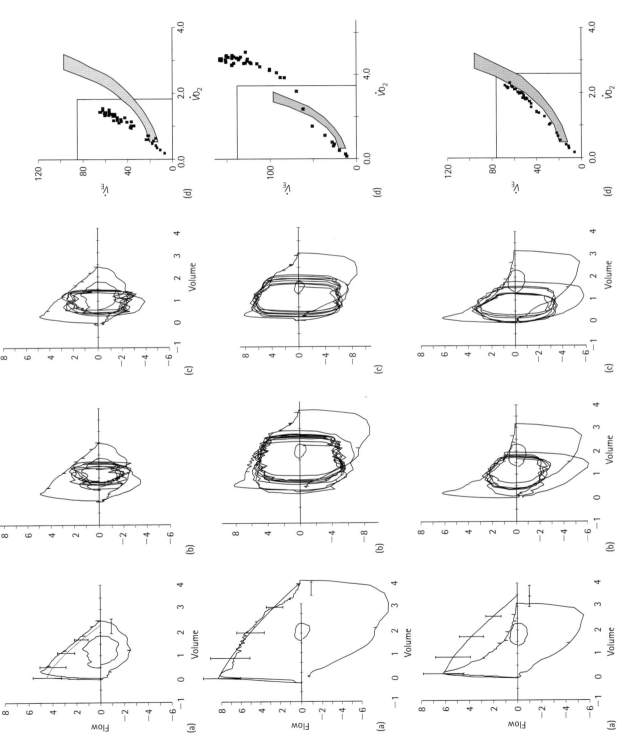

Figure 25.1 Tidal breathing flow volume loops obtained during exercise and compared to the maximum expiratory flow volume loops obtained before exercise (14). (a) Before start of exercise; (b) mid-exercise; (c) end of exercise; (d) minute ventilation ($\dot{V}_E$, y-axis) vs. oxygen uptake ($\dot{V}O_2$, x-axis). **Row 1** – an asthma patient with a low level of physical fitness. The patient does not take out his ventilatory reserve (b, c), and ventilation increases more than oxygen uptake (d). **Row 2** – an asthma patient of high physical fitness. The patient is a competitive junior athlete. The figure demonstrates the way the patient fully employs his maximum ventilatory reserve (c). Oxygen uptake increases normally with ventilation (d). **Row 3** – a patient with chronic obstructive lung disease and bronchiectasis. The patient is well trained and is training regularly. His tidal breathing during exercise demonstrates flow limitation even early during exercise (b). The patient uses his full inspiratory reserve (c). Oxygen uptake increases parallel with ventilation (d).

OPTIMAL TREATMENT OF ASTHMA

Rehabilitation measures should be multidisciplinary and take into account the circumstances of the patient's life. An important condition for successful rehabilitation is optimal pharmacological treatment of asthma. Furthermore, increased knowledge of the illness and improved understanding of pathogenetic mechanisms and treatment principles can play a substantial part in rehabilitation measures. Physical training is an essential part of rehabilitation. For some patients, psychological and social measures may also be important.

Pharmacological treatment of asthma is an important part of asthma care and of the rehabilitation process. In recent years, many guidelines for the treatment of asthma have been published, both on a global level (18) and on regional (19) and national levels (20). Some of these are evidence-based in their literature reviews and grade the level of their recommendations (20). These guidelines may provide a good basis for obtaining optimal asthma treatment in our patients. Anti-inflammatory treatment, in particular inhaled steroids, has been important for asthma treatment and for helping patients master their illness. This is reflected by the previously mentioned reduction in readmissions to hospital among asthmatic children in the Oslo and Gothenburg area (3, 4). Side-effects are few, and even if these may include slightly reduced growth in asthmatic children (21–23), the reduction in growth usually occurs early during treatment (24), and it has been reported that children with asthma, treated with inhaled budesonide, reached predicted adult height (25).

It is of particular importance for children and adolescents to take part in physical activity to ensure normal development (26). Pharmacological treatment should therefore aim to deal with exercise-induced bronchoconstriction (EIB). Anti-inflammatory treatment with inhaled steroids (even low-dose) (27) or leukotriene antagonists is important in this respect (28). Inhaled steroids show an effect on EIB after 1 week's treatment, as measured by reduction in FEV_1 after exercise (29), whereas an effect upon peripheral bronchial obstruction was obtained after 4 weeks of treatment (29). Usually, the optimal effect of inhaled steroids is obtained after 3–4 weeks (30). Leukotriene antagonists usually have a beneficial effect upon EIB after only 2–3 days (28, 31) and the effect can be sustained without developing tolerance for longer periods of time (28).

Steinshamn *et al.* (32) demonstrated that while the leukotriene antagonist, montelukast, had a beneficial effect upon EIB, the drug also improved running time to exhaustion and reduced the Borg score for exhaustion, but did not affect minute ventilation and oxygen pulse in adult asthmatics. Also, short-acting inhaled β_2-agonists taken 15 min before exercise improve EIB (33), whereas long-acting inhaled β_2-agonists have a controlling effect for up to 12 h (34–36). This is of therapeutic benefit in children, as physical activity is a normal part of their play and daily activities, and they usually do not plan their physical activity in advance.

Modern asthma treatment enables asthma patients to live a more normal daily life than was the case in the past. With optimal treatment the daily consequences of the illness become less severe and the quality of life improves. The medical management makes it easier for patients to access other measures of rehabilitation.

EDUCATIONAL MEASURES AND ASTHMA SCHOOLS

Asthma is a multifactorial disease with many causes and different clinical presentations. The clinical presentation of asthma varies with age, between different individuals, and also in a single asthmatic patient over time (37). The treatment of asthma is also composite, with several different drugs, different devices for inhalation, and different uses of the drugs according to disease activity or the occurrence of exacerbations. Patients need knowledge about the illness in order to be able to administer proper treatment, and health personnel active in asthma care have a responsibility for passing on this knowledge. Patients and their families need to be educated about the disease, its causative and provoking factors, and the medication and equipment used in its treatment. They also need a written plan for treatment. Education is an integral part of good asthma care and rehabilitation, and can improve patients' ability to cope with the illness, improving their quality of life and, at the same time, reducing the costs associated with asthma and the utilization of health care. This obvious need for education has led to the creation of asthma education programmes and asthma schools in many countries. Among the first organized asthma education programmes were the asthma summer camps, where teaching about asthma and its treatment was combined with physical activity and proper asthma care (38, 39), creating an optimal environment for teaching.

The various education plans for asthmatic children and adults differ in extent and content, ranging from systematic telephone contacts between asthma health care workers and parents of asthmatic children after acute admissions to hospital, to more systematic and extensive education programmes developed for adult asthmatic patients and patients with chronic obstructive lung disease (40). It was postulated that children admitted to emergency departments with acute asthma would benefit from educational measures. A Cochrane systematic review with meta-analysis was undertaken to assess this matter using published randomized clinical trials. In all, eight trials consisting of 1407 patients with education handled by researchers or nurses were included in the review. This systematic review could not establish any firm evidence that educational measures reduced subsequent emergency department visits, hospital admissions or unscheduled doctor visits in children admitted to hospital for acute asthma (41). Another systematic Cochrane review assessed the effect of written self-management plans for asthmatic children and adults (42). In this review only six randomized trials met the inclusion criteria, and the results were too inconsistent and the trials too small to draw any conclusions as to the effect of written management plans on asthma control (42). In another Cochrane review, written management plans based upon peak expiratory flow and symptoms were of similar value, but written plans combined with intensive education were superior to those combined with less intensive education (43).

On the other hand, several other studies of systematic education concerning asthmatic children and their parents, as well as adult patients, have demonstrated beneficial results. Gallefoss and co-workers undertook several randomized studies investigating the effect of systematic education on patients with asthma and chronic obstructive lung disease (40, 44–47). They established that non-smokers with a long history of asthma and a recent asthma attack were especially motivated to take part in an asthma school (47). Furthermore, a 1-year follow-up study in asthmatic patients who had participated in asthma school demonstrated improved lung function and symptoms and reduced costs in the group receiving education (44). Gallefoss *et al.* (46) further demonstrated in a randomized trial that two 2-h group sessions together with one to two individual sessions with a nurse or physiotherapist improved quality of life and lung function in asthma patients, but not in patients with chronic obstructive lung disease. Similar results were recently reported by Yilmaz and Akkaya (48), and a randomized controlled Russian study of 252 asthmatic children aged 4–14 years demonstrated clinical benefits from an asthma education programme (49).

Based on the vast number of studies investigating the effect of asthma education, further systematic Cochrane reviews have been performed on more thorough education programmes than the written management plans discussed above. In one review including 12 randomized studies, limited education (information only) in adults did not reduce hospital admissions or doctor visits, improve lung function, or reduce the need for asthma medication (50). Another systematic review assessed written self-management education combined with general health practitioners reviews. Self-management education was compared with usual care in 22 studies, and was found to reduce hospitalizations (odds ratio 0.57; 95 per cent confidence interval 0.38–0.88); emergency room visits (0.71, 0.57–0.90); unscheduled visits to the doctor (0.57, 0.40–0.82); days off work or school (0.55, 0.38–0.79); and nocturnal asthma (0.53, 0.39–0.72). Measures of lung function were little changed. Self-management programmes that involved a written action plan showed a greater reduction in hospitalization than those that did not (OR, 0.35; 95 per cent CI 0.18–0.68). People who managed their asthma by self-adjustment of their medications using an individualized written plan had better lung function than those whose medications were adjusted by a doctor (51).

One review was undertaken in asthmatic children aged 2–18 years. This systematic review included randomized controlled trials or controlled clinical trials of educational programmes for the self-management of asthma in children and adolescents that reported lung function, morbidity, self-perception of asthma control, or utilization of health care services. Thirty-two out of 45 identified trials were eligible, totalling 3706

patients aged 2–18 years. Education in asthma was associated with improved lung function (standardized mean difference 0.50, 95 per cent confidence interval 0.25–0.75) and self-efficacy (0.36, 0.15–0.57) and reduced absenteeism from school (−0.14, −0.23 to −0.04), number of days of restricted activity (−0.29, −0.33 to −0.09), and number of visits to an emergency department (−0.21, −0.33 to −0.09). The effect on morbidity was greatest with the programmes with strategies based on peak flow, interventions targeted at the individual, and participants with severe asthma. The reviewers concluded that educational programmes should be considered a part of the routine care of young people with asthma (52, 53).

Based upon the randomized trials, systematic reviews and meta-analyses of the effects of patient education as a rehabilitation tool in the care of asthmatic patients, one may conclude that educational measures matter in improving quality of life, lung function, symptoms and costs of asthma treatment. However, it seems that more thorough education programmes are superior to those with a minimum of educational measures.

PHYSICAL TRAINING

Development of asthma

Physical activity and training play an important part in the rehabilitation of asthmatic children and adults, but physical activity and fitness may have some influence in the development of asthma in schoolchildren and adolescents. In a recent Danish study it was found that low physical fitness during childhood was associated with the development of asthma in young adulthood (54). Furthermore, in a study from Oslo we found that bronchial responsiveness was inversely related to number of training hours per week (55). Recently it has been pointed out that there is a relationship between body mass index (BMI) or obesity and the prevalence of asthma (56). This has been found, in particular, among girls (57, 58), but it is also of interest that in a study among adults, β_2-receptor polymorphism and BMI were related to adult onset of asthma in sedentary women, but not in physically active women, suggesting a gene–environment interaction for asthma involving physical activity level (59). Thus several studies suggest a relationship between the development of asthma and low physical activity level in both children and adults, especially girls and women.

Physical fitness in children with mild to moderate asthma has been found to be comparable to that of healthy children (60–62). However, up to 30 per cent of children with asthma suffer from some limitation in physical activity in their daily life, and when on their regular asthma treatment, compared with 5 per cent of other children (6). Strunk *et al.* (26) reported that the level of physical fitness has an impact upon the self-assessment of asthmatic children, and that cardiovascular fitness correlates with psychological functioning in asthmatic children. It has been maintained that, because of its importance, the level of physical fitness and functioning in asthmatic children should be assessed in order to identify patients in whom appropriate measures should be taken (63).

The relationship between physical training and the possible development of asthma may be better understood by studying effects of strenuous exercise in athletes. Mediator release from eosinophils and neutrophils increased in both healthy and asthmatic athletes after heavy exercise. Serum eosinophil cationic protein (s-ECP) and serum myeloperoxidase (s-MPO) increased significantly 2–4 h after heavy exercise, but not after moderate exercise in Norwegian Olympic cross-country skiers (64). Heavy exercise may increase bronchial responsiveness. This increase in bronchial responsiveness has previously been demonstrated in Norwegian competitive swimmers after heavy swimming exercise (65). Inflammatory changes with lymphoid aggregates in bronchial biopsies were demonstrated more frequently in heavily trained young skiers without asthma, but with increased airways responsiveness to cold air, compared with control subjects (66).

It seems that heavy and repeated physical endurance training over prolonged time periods in combination with non-optimal environmental conditions may contribute to the development of asthma among top athletes. This was first described among cross-country skiers in Norway (67) and Sweden (68, 69), and later among endurance athletes in summer sports (70) and other types of sport (71, 72).

Environmental conditions

The lessons from athletes teach us that intense physical activity in combination with untoward environmental circumstances may cause deterioration of asthma instead of improving the general condition. Cold dry air provokes EIB and increases bronchial hyperresponsiveness. Drobnic et al. (73) reported that indoor swimming pools had high concentrations of chlorine and chlorine products, and recently Bernard et al. (74) reported epithelial injury in the airways due to repeated swimming in indoor pools and the relationship to chlorides by measuring serum surfactant associated proteins A and B (SP-A and SP-B) and 16 kDa Clara cell protein (CC16). They reported that regular attendance in indoor swimming pools increased lung epithelial permeability. EIB and total asthma prevalence were significantly related to regular swimming pool attendance (74). Thus environmental conditions in relationship to physical activity may have an impact upon respiratory health.

Physical training in the rehabilitation of asthma

Seemingly, there may be a conflict between recommending asthmatic children to exercise and to be physically active, and the possible role of high-intensity endurance training in the development of bronchial hyperresponsiveness and asthma in top athletes. Physical exercise has been considered by many as a natural part of the therapeutic approach to asthma. To benefit from physical training, the asthmatic patient must be able to control EIB. This may include treatment according to the principles outlined previously. The training should also be performed with thorough warm-up, with an intensity of approximately 50 per cent of maximum exercise load. One common recommendation has been to perform the training at a submaximal exercise level.

Most studies exploring the effect of physical training upon asthma have concerned asthmatic children and adolescents. Most studies are observational open studies, but several have included control groups in a randomized manner. Table 25.1 gives an overview of relevant studies and reports with assessment of level of evidence (75). Matsumoto et al. (76) found improved aerobic capacity in asthmatic children with swimming training over 6 weeks compared with a non-training control group, but no change in bronchial responsiveness to histamine. This was confirmed by Robinson et al. (77) and in adults (78–81). A recent systematic review and meta-analysis included 226 subjects from eight studies, of which six were in children aged 8 years or older who had participated in physical training for at least two 20-min sessions a week for at least 4 weeks (82). Subjects who exercised regularly, more than 20 min twice a week for at least 8 weeks, had increased $\dot{V}_{O_2,max}$, peak ventilation and maximum heart rate, whereas no changes were found in lung function or symptom score. Thus it was concluded that physical training improves physical fitness and endurance performance, but does not improve bronchial responsiveness, lung function and symptoms in asthmatic patients (82).

CLIMATE THERAPY

High-altitude therapy has traditionally been employed in the treatment of chronic lung diseases. This was the case before specific therapy was available for tuberculosis, and it has long been customary for children with chronic asthma to go for shorter or longer time periods into the mountains. Children from the Netherlands have gone to Switzerland, in particular Davos; in Italy children still go to Misurina; and in Norway there has been a hospital for asthmatic children at the mountainous ski resort of Geilo since the mid-1930s. Experience taught that such treatment was beneficial for the children, and now there is also scientific support for this presumption.

In Italy, Atillio Boner and his group have demonstrated in numerous publications that prolonged stays for up to half a year in the mountains have improved lung function, inflammation markers and bronchial hyperresponsiveness in asthmatic children, especially in children allergic to mites (83–85). He has also reported an additional effect of inhaled steroids (86). A Dutch study investigated the effect of 10 weeks' stay at high altitude, and found an improvement in bronchial responsiveness, lung function, symptoms and inflammation markers over and above the effect of inhaled steroids (87). Similar findings in a Norwegian study over 4–6 weeks were found for exercise-induced asthma and symptoms (88). In the Norwegian study a combination of rehabilitation measures were used: physical training, regular controlled medications, teaching

Table 25.1 Physical training as part of rehabilitation of asthma (level of evidence is given)

Type of study, level of evidence (in brackets)	Reference	Number of patients	Physical activity measure	End-point	Effect
Prospective open, No control group (3)	Emtner et al. (79)	26 adults	Swimming training 10 weeks	Lung function Exercise-induced asthma Metacholine responsiveness Exercise tolerance	V X Y V
Follow-up, open (3)	Emtner et al. (78)	58 adults	10 weeks' training Follow-up 3 years	Continuous physical training Lung function Exercise-induced asthma Metacholine responsiveness Symptoms	39/58 Y Y Y X
Randomized controlled, open (2−)	Cochrane and Clark (80)	36 adults	3 months' training	Histamine responsiveness Borg score for exertion $\dot{V}O_{2,max}$ Anaerobic threshold O_2 pulse	Y X V V V
Open, controlled two groups with and without training (2−)	Bundgaard et al. (81)	16/11	2 months	$\dot{V}O_{2,max}$ Exercise-induced asthma	V Y
Single blind, controlled, with and without training (2)	Matsumoto et al. (76)	8/8	6 weeks' swimming training	Histamine responsiveness Exercise-induced asthma Aerobic capacity	Y X V
Open, controlled, asthma and non-asthma (2−)	Robinson et al. (77)	8/7 asthma/non-asthma	12 weeks' indoor training	$\dot{V}O_{2,max}$ $\dot{V}_{E,peak}$ Symptom score	V X X
Meta-analysis, asthma and non-asthma (1+)	Ram et al. (82)	8 studies 226 (>8 years) asthma/non-asthma	>8 weeks >20 min twice per week	$\dot{V}O_{2,max}$, $\dot{V}_{E,peak}$, HR_{max} Lung function Symptom score	V Y Y

V, increased; X, reduced; Y, not changed; HR_{max}, maximum heart rate; $\dot{V}O_{2,max}$, maximum oxygen uptake; $\dot{V}_{E,peak}$, peak ventilation.
Levels of evidence [Harbour and Miller (75)]: 1++, high-quality meta-analyses, systematic reviews of RCTs, or RCTs with a very low risk of bias; 1+, well conducted meta-analyses, systematic reviews of RCTs, or RCTs with a low risk of bias; 1−, meta-analyses, systematic reviews or RCTs, or RCTs with a high risk of bias; 2++, high-quality systematic reviews of case–control or cohort studies, or high-quality case–control or cohort studies with a very low risk of confounding, bias, or chance and a high probability that the relationship is causal; 2+, well conducted case–control or cohort studies with a low risk of confounding, bias or chance and a moderate probability that the relationship is causal; 2−, case–control or cohort studies with a high risk of confounding, bias or chance and a significant risk that the relationship is not causal; 3, non-analytic studies, e.g. case reports, case series; 4, expert opinion.

about asthma and asthma treatment, and the effect of high altitude.

In middle and eastern Europe, another form for climate therapy has been used: speleotherapy. This consists of letting the patients stay for some hours down in salt mines on a daily basis. Although there have been numerous anecdotal reports on the effect of this type of treatment, a systematic Cochrane database review concluded that there was not enough evidence to make a judgment on this type of treatment (89).

CONCLUSIONS

Rehabilitation of asthma consists of a multitude of measures. Optimal medical treatment is the basis for successful rehabilitation. In order to understand the disease, and to know what are the correct measures to take at different disease stages, asthma education is important, but the success rate differs according to the extent of educational measures. It is crucial to get control of exercise-induced asthma. Physical training is important for improving general fitness and quality of life, but does not improve bronchial responsiveness or asthma activity per se. Thus rehabilitation of asthma consists of an integration of several different measures to be applied in a planned manner.

Key points

- Diagnostic measures before and during rehabilitation (monitoring) include a wide variety of assessments, such as clinical assessment, lung function measurements, bronchial responsiveness and assessment of exercise-induced bronchoconstriction, possible exercise limitation due to reduced lung function, and assessment of physical fitness, either by measuring $\dot{V}O_{2,max}$ or $\dot{V}_{E,peak}$, or by assessing fitness during exercise test for exercise-induced bronchoconstriction.
- Measures of rehabilitation are as follows:
  - *Pharmacological treatment of asthma*: this includes optimal treatment according to international (Global Initiative for Asthma) or national guidelines, preferably based upon evidence-based assessment; it should also aim at controlling exercise-induced asthma
  - *Education and asthma schools*: education about asthma illness, mechanisms and treatment; can be based upon individual teaching plans or systematized organized asthma education for patients and/or parents
  - *Environmental control*: includes environmental control in the home, kindergartens, schools and workplace; environmental control should include both exposure to relevant allergens for the single patient and general exposure to an inferior indoor environment

  - *Physical training in the rehabilitation of asthma*: participation in organized training groups enhances participation in physical training; this is important for improved quality of life, and getting control of asthma
  - *Climate therapy*: therapy involving a change of climate, e.g. high-altitude stays in the Italian and Swiss Alps, as well as in Norway, has been shown to improve allergen control and control of inflammation as well as bronchial responsiveness; it also includes travel from northern climates to the south during winter.

REFERENCES

1. Worldwide variations in the prevalence of asthma symptoms: the International Study of Asthma and Allergies in Childhood (ISAAC). *Eur Respir J* 1998; **12**: 315–35.
2. Sunyer J, Anto JM, Tobias A, Burney P. Generational increase of self-reported first attack of asthma in fifteen industrialized countries. European Community Respiratory Health Study (ECRHS). *Eur Respir J* 1999; **14**: 885–91.
3. Jonasson G, Lodrup Carlsen KC, Leegaard J *et al.* Trends in hospital admissions for childhood asthma in Oslo, Norway, 1980–95. *Allergy* 2000; **55**: 232–9.
4. Wennergren G, Strannegard IL. Asthma hospitalizations continue to decrease in schoolchildren but hospitalization rates for wheezing illnesses remain high in young children. *Acta Paediatr* 2002; **91**: 1239–45.
◆5. Lenney W, Well NEJ, O'Neill BA. The burden of paediatric asthma. *Eur Respir Rev* 1994; **4**: 49–62.
6. Taylor WR, Newacheck PW. Impact of childhood asthma upon health. *Pediatrics* 1992; **90**: 657–62.
◆7. Wahn U, Warner JA, de Weck A *et al.* (eds). *European Allergy White Paper Update.* Barcelona: UCB Institute of Allergy, 1999.
◆8. Donner CF, Muir JF. Selection criteria and programmes for pulmonary rehabilitation in COPD patients. Rehabilitation and Chronic Care Scientific Group of the European Respiratory Society. *Eur Respir J* 1997; **10**: 744–57.
◆9. Fishman AP. Pulmonary rehabilitation research. *Am J Respir Crit Care Med* 1994; **149**(3 Part 1): 825–33.
10. Brand PL, Duiverman EJ, Waalkens HJ *et al.* Peak flow variation in childhood asthma: correlation with symptoms, airways obstruction, and hyperresponsiveness during long-term treatment with inhaled corticosteroids. Dutch CNSLD Study Group. *Thorax* 1999; **54**: 103–7.
11. Carlsen KH, Engh G, Mørk M, Schrøder E. Cold air inhalation and exercise-induced bronchoconstriction in relationship to metacholine bronchial responsiveness. Different patterns in asthmatic children and children with other chronic lung diseases. *Respir Med* 1998; **92**: 308–15.
12. Carlsen KH, Engh G, Mørk M. Exercise-induced bronchoconstriction depends on exercise load. *Respir Med* 2000; **94**: 750–5.
13. Silverman M, Anderson SD. Standardization of exercise tests in asthmatic children. *Arch Dis Child* 1972; **47**: 882–9.
◆14. Johnson BD, Reddan WG, Pegelow DF *et al.* Flow limitation and regulation of functional residual capacity during exercise in a

physically active aging population. *Am Rev Respir Dis* 1991; **143**: 960–7.

15. Hargreave FE, Ryan G, Thomsom NC *et al.* Bronchial responsiveness to histamine or metacholine in asthma: measurement and clinical significance. *J Allergy Clin Immunol* 1981; **68**: 347–55.

16. Sont JK, Han J, van Krieken JM *et al.* Relationship between the inflammatory infiltrate in bronchial biopsy specimens and clinical severity of asthma in patients treated with inhaled steroids. *Thorax* 1996; **51**: 496–502.

●17. Jonasson G, Carlsen KH, Mowinckel P. Asthma drug adherence in a long term clinical trial. *Arch Dis Child* 2000; **83**: 330–3.

18. Global Initiative for Asthma/National Heart, Lung and Blood Institute. *Global Strategy for Asthma Management and Prevention*, 2nd edn. Bethesda, MD: National Institutes of Health, 2002.

19. Dahl R, Bjermer L. Nordic consensus report on asthma management. Nordic Asthma Consensus Group. *Respir Med* 2000; **94**: 299–327.

20. British Thoracic Society/Scottish Intercollegiate Guidelines Network. British guideline on the management of asthma. *Thorax* 2003; **58**(Suppl. 1): 1–94.

21. Doull IJM, Freezer NJ, Holgate ST, Doull IJ. Growth of prepubertal children with mild asthma treated with inhaled beclomethasone dipropionate. *Am J Respir Crit Care Med* 1995; **151**: 1715–19.

22. Tinkelman DG, Reed CE, Nelson HS, Offord KP. Aerosol beclomethasone dipropionate compared with theophylline as primary treatment of chronic, mild to moderately severe asthma in children. *Pediatrics* 1993; **92**: 64–77.

23. The Childhood Asthma Management Program Research Group. Long-term effects of budesonide or nedocromil in children with asthma. *N Engl J Med* 2000; **343**: 1054–63.

24. Doull IJ, Campbell MJ, Holgate ST. Duration of growth suppressive effects of regular inhaled corticosteroids. *Arch Dis Child* 1998; **78**: 172–3.

●25. Agertoft L, Pedersen S. Effect of long-term treatment with inhaled budesonide on adult height in children with asthma. *N Engl J Med* 2000; **343**: 1064–9.

●26. Strunk RC, Mrazek DA, Fukuhara JT *et al.* Cardiovascular fitness in children with asthma correlates with psychologic functioning of the child. *Pediatrics* 1989; **84**: 460–4.

27. Jonasson G, Carlsen KH, Hultquist C. Low-dose budesonide improves exercise-induced bronchospasm in schoolchildren. *Pediatr Allergy Immunol* 2000; **11**: 120–5.

28. Villaran C, O'Neill SJ, Helbling A *et al.* Montelukast versus salmeterol in patients with asthma and exercise-induced bronchoconstriction. *J Allergy Clin Immunol* 1999; **104**(3 Part 1): 547–53.

29. Henriksen JM, Dahl R. Effects of inhaled budesonide alone and in combination with low-dose terbutaline in children with exercise-induced asthma. *Am Rev Respir Dis* 1983; **128**: 993–7.

30. Waalkens HJ, van Essen-Zandvliet EE, Gerritsen J *et al.* The effect of an inhaled corticosteroid (budesonide) on exercise-induced asthma in children. Dutch CNSLD Study Group. *Eur Respir J* 1993; **6**: 652–6.

31. Leff JA, Busse WW, Pearlman D *et al.* Montelukast, a leukotriene-receptor antagonist, for the treatment of mild asthma and exercise-induced bronchoconstriction. *N Engl J Med* 1998; **339**: 147–52.

32. Steinshamn S, Sandsund M, Sue-Chu M, Bjermer L. Effects of montelukast on physical performance and exercise economy in adult asthmatics with exercise-induced bronchoconstriction. *Scand J Med Sci Sports* 2002; **12**: 211–17.

33. Anderson SD. Drugs and the control of exercise-induced asthma. *Eur Respir J* 1993; **6**: 1090–2.

34. Green CP, Price JF. Prevention of exercise induced asthma by inhaled salmeterol xinafoate. *Arch Dis Child* 1992; **67**: 1014–17.

35. Carlsen KH, Røksund O, Olsholt K *et al.* Overnight protection by inhaled salmeterol on exercise-induced asthma in children. *Eur Respir J* 1995; **8**: 1852–5.

36. Boner AL, Spezia E, Piovesan P *et al.* Inhaled formoterol in the prevention of exercise-induced bronchoconstriction in asthmatic children. *Am J Respir Crit Care Med* 1994; **149**: 935–9.

37. Aas K. Heterogeneity of childhood asthma. *Allergy* 1981; **36**: 3–14.

38. Lord A, St Leger LH, Ridge DT, Elisha D. The value of asthma camps for young people in Victoria, Australia. *Contemp Nurse* 2001; **11**: 133–41.

39. Sorrells VD, Chung W, Schlumpberger JM. The impact of a summer asthma camp experience on asthma education and morbidity in children. *J Fam Pract* 1995; **41**: 465–8.

●40. Gallefoss F, Bakke PS. Impact of patient education and self-management on morbidity in asthmatics and patients with chronic obstructive pulmonary disease. *Respir Med* 2000; **94**: 279–87.

41. Haby MM, Waters E, Robertson CF *et al.* Interventions for educating children who have attended the emergency room for asthma. *Cochrane Database Syst Rev* 2001; **1**: CD001290.

◆42. Toelle BG, Ram FS. Written individualised management plans for asthma in children and adults. *Cochrane Database Syst Rev* 2002; **3**: CD002171.

43. Powell H, Gibson PG. Options for self-management education for adults with asthma. *Cochrane Database Syst Rev* 2003; **1**: CD004107.

●44. Gallefoss F, Bakke PS. Cost-effectiveness of self-management in asthmatics: a 1-yr follow-up randomized, controlled trial. *Eur Respir J* 2001; **17**: 206–13.

45. Gallefoss F, Bakke PS. How does patient education and self-management among asthmatics and patients with chronic obstructive pulmonary disease affect medication? *Am J Respir Crit Care Med* 1999; **160**: 2000–5.

●46. Gallefoss F, Bakke PS, Rsgaard PK. Quality of life assessment after patient education in a randomized controlled study on asthma and chronic obstructive pulmonary disease. *Am J Respir Crit Care Med* 1999; **159**: 812–17.

47. Gallefoss F, Bakke PS, Wang IJ *et al.* Smoking status, disease duration, and educational level in females, are related to asthma school participation. *Eur Respir J* 2000; **15**: 1022–5.

48. Yilmaz A, Akkaya E. Evaluation of long-term efficacy of an asthma education programme in an out-patient clinic. *Respir Med* 2002; **96**: 519–24.

49. Maslennikova GY, Morosova ME, Salman NV *et al.* Asthma education programme in Russia: educating patients. *Patient Educ Couns* 1998; **33**: 113–27.

◆50. Gibson PG, Powell H, Coughlan J *et al.* Limited (information only) patient education programs for adults with asthma. *Cochrane Database Syst Rev* 2002; **2**: CD001005.

51. Gibson PG, Coughlan J, Wilson AJ *et al.* Self-management education and regular practitioner review for adults with asthma. *Cochrane Database Syst Rev* 2000; **2**: CD001117.

◆52. Guevara JP, Wolf FM, Grum CM, Clark NM. Effects of educational interventions for self management of asthma in children and adolescents. Systematic review and meta-analysis. *Br Med J* 2003; **326**: 1308–9.

◆53. Wolf FM, Guevara JP, Grum CM et al. Educational interventions for asthma in children. Cochrane Database Syst Rev 2003; 1: CD000326.

●54. Rasmussen F, Lambrechtsen J, Siersted HC et al. Low physical fitness in childhood is associated with the development of asthma in young adulthood: the Odense schoolchild study. Eur Respir J 2000; 16: 866–70.

55. Nystad W, Stigum H, Carlsen KH. Increased level of bronchial responsiveness in inactive children with asthma. Respir Med 2001; 95: 806–10.

56. Figueroa-Munoz JI, Chinn S, Rona RJ. Association between obesity and asthma in 4–11 year old children in the UK. Thorax 2001; 56: 133–7.

57. Castro-Rodriguez JA, Holberg CJ, Morgan WJ et al. Increased incidence of asthma-like symptoms in girls who become overweight or obese during the school years. Am J Respir Crit Care Med 2001; 163: 1344–9.

58. von Kries R, Hermann M, Grunert VP, von Mutius E. Is obesity a risk factor for childhood asthma? Allergy 2001; 56: 318–22.

●59. Barr RG, Cooper DM, Speizer FE et al. Beta(2)-adrenoceptor polymorphism and body mass index are associated with adult-onset asthma in sedentary but not active women. Chest 2001; 120: 1474–9.

60. Bevegard S, Eriksson BO, Graff-Lonnevig V et al. Respiratory function, cardiovascular dimensions and work capacity in boys with bronchial asthma. Acta Paediatr Scand 1976; 65: 289–96.

61. Hedlin G, Graff-Lonnevig V, Freyschuss U. Working capacity and pulmonary gas exchange in children with exercise-induced asthma. Acta Paediatr Scand 1986; 75: 947–54.

62. Santuz P, Baraldi E, Filippone M, Zacchello F. Exercise performance in children with asthma: is it different from that of healthy controls? Eur Respir J 1997; 10: 1254–60.

63. Strunk RC, Rubin D, Kelly L et al. Determination of fitness in children with asthma. Use of standardized tests for functional endurance, body fat composition, flexibility, and abdominal strength. Am J Dis Child 1988; 142: 940–4.

64. Rønsen O, Hem E, Edvardsen E et al. Changes in airways inflammatory markers during high intensity training in elite cross-country skiers. Eur Respir J 1995; 8: 473s.

●65. Carlsen KH, Oseid S, Odden H, Mellbye E. The response to heavy swimming exercise in children with and without bronchial asthma. In: Oseid S, Carlsen KH, eds. Children and Exercise XIII. Champaign, Illinois: Human Kinetics, 1989; 351–60.

66. Sue-Chu M, Larsson L, Moen T et al. Bronchoscopy and bronchoalveolar lavage findings in cross-country skiers with and without 'ski asthma'. Eur Respir J 1999; 13: 626–32.

67. Heir T, Oseid S. Self-reported asthma and exercise-induced asthma symptoms in high-level competetive cross-country skiers. Scand J Med Sci Sports 1994; 4: 128–33.

68. Larsson K, Ohlsson P, Larsson L et al. High prevalence of asthma in cross-country skiers [see comments]. Br Med J 1993; 307: 1326–9.

69. Sue-Chu M, Larsson L, Bjermer L. Prevalence of asthma in young cross-country skiers in central Scandinavia. Differences between Norway and Sweden. Respir Med 1996; 90: 99–105.

●70. Helenius IJ, Tikkanen HO, Haahtela T. Occurrence of exercise-induced bronchospasm in elite runners. Dependence on atopy and exposure to cold air and pollen. Br J Sports Med 1998; 32: 125–9.

71. Weiler JM, Metzger J, Donnelly AL et al. Prevalence of bronchial responsiveness in highly trained athletes. Chest 1986; 90: 23–8.

72. Weiler JM, Layton T, Hunt M. Asthma in United States Olympic athletes who participated in the 1996 Summer Games. J Allergy Clin Immunol 1998; 102: 722–6.

73. Drobnic F, Freixa A, Casan P et al. Assessment of chlorine exposure in swimmers during training. Med Sci Sports Exerc 1996; 28: 271–4.

●74. Bernard A, Carbonnelle S, Michel O et al. Lung hyperpermeability and asthma prevalence in schoolchildren: unexpected associations with the attendance at indoor chlorinated swimming pools. Occup Environ Med 2003; 60: 385–94.

◆75. Harbour R, Miller J. A new system for grading recommendations in evidence-based guidelines. Br Med J 2001; 323: 334–6.

●76. Matsumoto I, Araki H, Tsuda K et al. Effects of swimming training on aerobic capacity and exercise induced bronchoconstriction in children with bronchial asthma. Thorax 1999; 54: 196–201.

77. Robinson DM, Egglestone DM, Hill PM et al. Effects of a physical conditioning programme on asthmatic patients. NZ Med J 1992; 105: 253–6.

78. Emtner M, Finne M, Stalenheim G. A 3-year follow-up of asthmatic patients participating in a 10-week rehabilitation program with emphasis on physical training. Arch Phys Med Rehabil 1998; 79: 539–44.

79. Emtner M, Herala M, Stalenheim G. High-intensity physical training in adults with asthma. A 10-week rehabilitation program. Chest 1996; 109: 323–30.

80. Cochrane LM, Clark CJ. Benefits and problems of a physical training programme for asthmatic patients. Thorax 1990; 45: 345–51.

81. Bundgaard A, Ingemann-Hansen T, Schmidt A et al. Effect of physical training on peak oxygen consumption rate and exercise-induced asthma in adult asthmatics. Scand J Clin Laboratory Invest 1982; 42: 9–13.

◆82. Ram FS, Robinson SM, Black PN. Effects of physical training in asthma: a systematic review. Br J Sports Med 2000; 34: 162–7.

83. Boner AL, Peroni DG, Piacentini GL, Venge P. Influence of allergen avoidance at high altitude on serum markers of eosinophil activation in children with allergic asthma. Clin Exp Allergy 1993; 23: 1021–6.

●84. Boner AL, Niero E, Antolini I et al. Pulmonary function and bronchial hyperreactivity in asthmatic children with house dust mite allergy during prolonged stay in the Italian Alps (Misurina, 1756 m). Ann Allergy 1985; 54: 42–5.

85. Peroni DG, Boner AL, Vallone G et al. Effective allergen avoidance at high altitude reduces allergen-induced bronchial hyperresponsiveness. Am J Respir Crit Care Med 1994; 149: 1442–6.

86. Boner AL, Comis A, Schiassi M et al. Bronchial reactivity in asthmatic children at high and low altitude. Effect of budesonide. Am J Respir Crit Care Med 1995; 151: 1194–200.

●87. Grootendorst DC, Dahlen SE, van den Bos JW et al. Benefits of high altitude allergen avoidance in atopic adolescents with moderate to severe asthma, over and above treatment with high dose inhaled steroids. Clin Exp Allergy 2001; 31: 400–8.

88. Carlsen KH, Oseid S, Sandnes T et al. Asthma and mountain air (Astma og fjellluft). Tidsskr Nor Laegeforen 1991; 111: 935–7.

89. Beamon S, Falkenbach A, Fainburg G, Linde K. Speleotherapy for asthma. Cochrane Database Syst Rev 2000; 2: CD001741.

26

Guidelines for rehabilitation in the management of chronic obstructive pulmonary disease

ANDREW L. RIES

INTRODUCTION AND RATIONALE FOR PULMONARY REHABILITATION

Standard medical therapy is important in alleviating symptoms of chronic obstructive pulmonary disease (COPD), particularly the frightening symptom of breathlessness. However, patients are still left to cope with the consequences of a chronic, largely irreversible condition. Such individuals – who are frequently dyspnoeic, depressed, dysfunctional, disabled, desperate and difficult to deal with – often attend physician's offices, emergency rooms or hospitals, in part because of their inability to cope with their distressing symptoms. Pulmonary rehabilitation enhances standard medical therapy with multidisciplinary programmes that typically include education, physiotherapy techniques, psychosocial support and exercise training (1–10).

Pulmonary rehabilitation incorporates the broad philosophy of rehabilitation medicine, namely improving disability and restoring the individual to the highest possible level of independent function. Specific objectives focus on improving physical and psychological health as well as social functioning.

The expanding knowledge base and complexity of medical practice for chronic diseases in an ageing population emphasizes the importance of a close working relationship between pulmonary physicians and allied health professionals. Rehabilitation is a well-established treatment option for many acute and chronic medical conditions in which complex interactions of physical, psychological, social and environmental factors contribute to disability. Such conditions are best treated with input from multiple specialities directed towards the needs of the individual patient (7–17).

Patients are encouraged to become more knowledgeable about their disease, more actively involved in self-management and more independent in daily activities. As pulmonary rehabilitation attempts to reverse the patient's disability, key outcomes include psychological status and health-related quality of life.

DEFINITION

In 1974, the American College of Chest Physicians' Committee on Pulmonary Rehabilitation adopted the following definition (18):

> Pulmonary rehabilitation may be defined as an art of medical practice wherein an individually tailored, multidisciplinary programme is formulated which through accurate diagnosis, therapy, emotional support, and education, stabilizes or reverses both the physio- and psychopathology of pulmonary diseases and attempts to return the patient to the highest possible functional capacity allowed by his pulmonary handicap and overall life situation.

This definition highlights three important features of successful rehabilitation programmes:

- *individual* – patients with disabling COPD require individual assessment of their needs, individual attention, and a programme designed to meet their individual goals
- *multidisciplinary* – pulmonary rehabilitation programmes provide access to information from a variety of health care disciplines which is integrated into a comprehensive programme
- *attention to physio- and psychopathology* – programmes must pay attention to the patient's psychological and emotional issues as well as helping to address physiological impairments.

A more recent definition from an NIH workshop on pulmonary rehabilitation research is as follows (19):

> Pulmonary rehabilitation is a multidimensional continuum of services directed to persons with pulmonary disease and their families, usually by an interdisciplinary team of specialists, with the goal of achieving and maintaining the individual's maximum level of independence and functioning in the community.

Both of these definitions highlight the multidimensional aspects of pulmonary rehabilitation which requires skills associated with a variety of health professionals with a focus on a comprehensive care plan based on the individual patient.

REHABILITATION TEAM

Rehabilitation programmes take advantage of the wealth of expertise available in allied health professions that can complement the expertise of physicians (20). Team members:

- evaluate patients
- set specific goals
- organize and deliver treatments
- assess progress
- develop an individualized home maintenance programme
- provide liaison with the referring physician as well as other health providers.

The key to success is the dedicated team, able to relate to disabled pulmonary patients, rather than one specific programme model or group of professionals. Smaller programmes often have a key health professional, who, with the support of a medical director, coordinates other individuals with complementary expertise. This key individual might have a background in nursing, respiratory therapy, physical therapy or exercise science. Larger programmes may have a team of several health professionals who work closely together to deliver care.

The principle is that skills from several disciplines, under the direction of a physician medical director, are brought together to develop an integrated treatment plan. The terms multidisciplinary, interdisciplinary and transdisciplinary are often used interchangeably (16, 17). Nevertheless, it is useful to understand the conceptual differences among these terms.

Multidisciplinary team

The multidisciplinary team includes professionals from varying specialities, who work in parallel with the same patients, usually in the same health care setting. Each member assesses and treats, communicating their plans to the other team members at regular conferences. This model generally includes a team leader, who coordinates the team, and a case manager who in smaller teams is the same person. Decisions are typically made by one or two team members, with significant input from the other disciplines.

An advantage of a multidisciplinary team is the ability to integrate input from several different specialities into a plan for the management of a particular patient. A disadvantage of this approach is that team members work independently with each patient so that the end result is the aggregate of individual contributions rather than the product of an integrated team effort. This may lead to some fragmentation, which diminishes the overall effectiveness of the team, unless clear documentation is supplied and clear communication occurs.

Interdisciplinary team

The interdisciplinary team emphasizes a total team approach to decision-making and goal-setting at a patient's case conference. Although professionals in each speciality conduct separate assessments, they all converge to set goals, plan treatment and evaluate the patient's progress (17). In addition, the patient and family or partner are often included in the process. This structure is more time-consuming, but may provide greater efficiency in the utilization of staff. It may result in greater patient and staff satisfaction, fewer errors in conceptualizing the therapeutic programme and an overall decrease in health care costs.

Transdisciplinary team

The transdisciplinary model is the least frequently used form of team organization, in which team members work across the boundaries of their professional disciplines, with each one sharing responsibility for all areas of patient care. It is based on practical issues and individual expertise rather than on speciality training or formal discipline. In this model health care professionals fulfil their responsibilities interchangeably in assessment, treatment and evaluation. Each team member becomes a 'pulmonary rehabilitation specialist' rather than being a nurse, therapist or other specialist based on their formal training, licence or official certification.

In a truly transdisciplinary model, one team member may be able to develop and implement a rehabilitation treatment plan that includes elements from another discipline. For instance, a physical therapist may develop expertise in respiratory therapy techniques, such as breathing retraining or oxygen therapy, or a respiratory therapist may supervise exercise training.

Regardless of the model used, it is important to each team member to appreciate the aspects of rehabilitation that may be outside their initial training and expertise. With experience, the team adapts transdisciplinary characteristics regardless of the formal organizational model. When that same team incorporates new, less experienced professionals, it may revert to a more traditional multidisciplinary approach while the new staff members gain experience in pulmonary rehabilitation.

PATIENT SELECTION AND EVALUATION

The success of pulmonary rehabilitation is determined, at least in part, by appropriate patient selection (Box 26.1). The principles of rehabilitation, although determined mainly among patients with COPD, may be applied equally to patients

---

Box 26.1   Patient selection for pulmonary rehabilitation

- Chronic lung disease, obstructive or restrictive
- Disability from lung disease
- Motivation to be actively engaged in rehabilitation
- Stable on standard medical therapy
- Realistic treatment goals
- Absence of co-morbid conditions that would interfere with rehabilitation

---

Box 26.2   Components of a comprehensive pulmonary rehabilitation programme

- Initial evaluation
  - pulmonary function tests to diagnose and measure pulmonary impairment
  - exercise evaluation:
    assess exercise tolerance
    evaluate oxygen requirements
    determine training prescription
  - psychosocial assessment and health-related quality of life
- Education and training in self-management
- Respiratory therapy and chest physiotherapy
  - bronchial hygiene
  - breathing retraining techniques:
    pursed lip breathing
    diaphragmatic breathing
  - use of equipment
  - oxygen therapy
- Psychosocial support
- Exercise training
  - endurance
  - strength
  - upper extremity

---

with other types of chronic lung diseases, such as pulmonary fibrosis, cystic fibrosis, bronchiectasis, thoracic restriction and neuromuscular weakness (21). Eligibility relates more closely to disability and motivation than lung function.

The ideal patient is clinically stable, has realistic goals and is motivated to make the necessary behavioural changes (22). Patients with mild disease may not require a comprehensive care programme and some with severe disease may be too limited to benefit from an ambulatory programme. Resting hypercapnia is not a contraindication to successful rehabilitation (23).

Rehabilitation programmes support the patient but do not assume responsibility for primary medical care. They are part of the comprehensive management of patients with chronic pulmonary disease. Patients should be stable before beginning a programme so that treatment can extend the patient's level of function. Co-morbidities such as heart disease, psychiatric illness or joint disease must be addressed to avoid their interfering with the rehabilitation programme.

The initial evaluation includes taking the medical history and assessing psychosocial needs (Box 26.2). Communication with the primary care physician is also important. A careful initial evaluation will result in appropriate individual goals that are compatible with the expectations of the patient and the physician as well as the programme's objectives. Key family members or partners should be included in setting treatment goals.

Psychosocial assessment and health–related quality of life

Psychological, emotional and social issues are common among patients with chronic lung disease as they struggle to deal with symptoms which are often poorly understood (24–27). Secondary impairments, such as depression, fear, anxiety and dependency, often affect the pulmonary symptoms reported by patients (28).

Dyspnoea is a frightening symptom that leads to a cycle of reduced exertion, resulting in more dyspnoea, worsening fear and anxiety, which further aggravate the dyspnoea until the patient avoids any physical activity associated with these unpleasant symptoms. In the extreme, patients become house bound. Jensen (29) reported that high stress and low social support were better predictors of subsequent hospitalization than severity of airflow among patients with COPD. Therefore, the initial evaluation should include an assessment of the patient's psychological state, cognition, family and social

support, activities of daily living and employment history. Key support individuals may provide valuable insights. Many programmes also measure baseline dyspnoea and health-related quality of life, at the time of enrolment and subsequently at the time of follow-up. There are now a variety of general and disease-specific scales that are valid, reproducible and interpretable. A detailed account of approaches to the measurement of dyspnoea and health-related quality of life is found in Chapters 14 and 15, respectively.

Pulmonary function and exercise evaluation

Pulmonary function testing helps to characterize and quantify respiratory impairment. Spirometry and lung volume measurements are the most common measures. They can be supplemented with other tests as needed. Exercise testing is useful to assess exercise tolerance, evaluate the cause of exercise limitation and identify exercise-induced hypoxaemia. The exercise test can also be used to establish a safe and appropriate prescription for subsequent training (30, 31).

Measures of pulmonary function correlate weakly with exercise capacity. It is therefore important to exercise patients directly rather than predicting exercise tolerance from pulmonary mechanics. Exercise testing is easiest as a pre-programme baseline, when testing with the type of exercise used for training, such as treadmill testing for a walking programme. Workload, heart rate, electrocardiogram and arterial oxygenation should be monitored during the test. Other measurements, such as minute ventilation and expired gas analysis, depend on the interest and expertise of the staff, but are not essential for all programmes. Exercise testing protocols must take into account the variations in stable patients and the improvements that follow repeat testing (33).

Many pulmonary rehabilitation programmes utilize simpler tests of exercise capacity, such as timed distance (6 min) or shuttle-walk test (32–36). Such measures have standardized procedures (37). It is important to distinguish between maximal exercise tolerance and submaximal endurance. Although the 6-min walk test was developed from a field test of maximal exercise tolerance, an important goal in rehabilitation is paced walking. Therefore some programmes emphasize a paced, submaximal strategy for walking tests. Walking tests use limited monitoring equipment other than for oxygen saturation and heart rate. Recommended methods typically exclude monitoring equipment during the test. In order to establish a valid baseline, walking tests should be repeated two to three times.

Because the changes in arterial oxygenation during exercise are unpredictable (38), it is important to assess oxygen saturation during exercise before beginning a training programme. Measurement of arterial blood gases at rest and during exercise is most accurate but requires invasive arterial blood sampling. Therefore pulse oximetry is often used for continuous monitoring. Although extremely convenient, the precision of pulse oximetry for the assessment of arterial oxygenation is (95 per cent confidence interval) $\pm 4\%$ S_aO_2 (39).

Although a training prescription is often determined from an exercise test, patients sometimes demonstrate better than predicted exercise tolerance during training. Reasons for this include the absence of a mouthpiece as well as familiarity with the exercise equipment. Therefore it is important to re-evaluate exercise tolerance during the rehabilitation programme.

PROGRAMME COMPONENTS

Programmes typically include education and training, respiratory and chest physiotherapy, psychosocial support and exercise conditioning (Box 26.2). Many clinicians consider exercise conditioning to be the central feature of pulmonary rehabilitation. However, during exercise training, patients may also receive coaching on breathing retraining as well as psychosocial support. In a systematic review of the literature, Lacasse et al. (40) concluded that there was sufficient evidence to support the inclusion of exercise training and psychosocial support in pulmonary rehabilitation programmes, but that additional research was needed to further evaluate the types and intensity of exercise training as well as the role of education.

Education and training

Successful pulmonary rehabilitation depends upon the understanding and active involvement of both patients and their partners. Education is an integral component (36) at all levels of disease severity (41). A detailed review of education in pulmonary rehabilitation is found in Chapter 21. Education

alone may not improve health status or exercise capacity; however, education in self-management may reduce visits to the emergency room as well as admissions to hospital with COPD exacerbations (see Chapter 36). It is difficult to change attitudes and behaviour among individuals with severe, disabling chronic lung disease. Patients require specific, individualized strategies and instruction should match the patient's learning ability, respiratory condition and treatment. For instance, education is likely to differ among non-COPD conditions such as interstitial lung disease, lung volume reduction surgery, lung transplantation and lung cancer (42–44).

Respiratory therapy and chest physiotherapy instruction

As part of a comprehensive rehabilitation programme, each patient's needs for respiratory care techniques and patients should be taught their proper use. These may include chest physiotherapy for mucociliary clearance and secretion control, breathing techniques such as pursed lip and diaphragmatic breathing for the relief of dyspnoea, and the correct use of respiratory care equipment, such as nebulizers, metered dose inhalers and oxygen (45, 46).

BRONCHIAL HYGIENE

Patients with increased secretions or reduced secretion clearance may be more susceptible to retained secretions. Coughing and chest physiotherapy techniques are routinely required for secretion control. These techniques are especially important during respiratory exacerbations, which are usually characterized by an increase in secretions.

BREATHING RETRAINING TECHNIQUES

Diaphragmatic and pursed lip breathing help to control breathlessness and improve the ventilatory pattern by slowing the respiratory rate and increasing the tidal volume. Such techniques prevent dynamic airway compression, improve respiratory synchrony between abdominal and thoracic muscles and thereby improve gas exchange (47–49). The improvement in dyspnoea is a more consistent finding than changes in airflow (49). As pointed out by Miller (48), it is difficult to distinguish the separate contributions of each of the various methods as they are usually integrated with other programme components.

However, the most consistent physiological change observed after breathing training in patients with COPD is an increase in tidal volume and a decrease in respiratory rate. These techniques help patients to control their dyspnoea.

OXYGEN

Supplemental oxygen therapy is beneficial for patients with significant resting arterial hypoxaemia from either acute or chronic causes of lung disease. Long-term, continuous oxygen therapy has been clearly shown to improve survival and reduce morbidity in hypoxaemic patients with COPD (50–52). Possible benefits of supplemental oxygen for non-hypoxaemic patients or for patients with hypoxaemia only under certain conditions, such as exercise and sleep, are less clearly defined. Maintaining patients on oxygen presents a number of problems (53). Physically disabled and older patients may need assistance in handling, using and caring safely for such equipment. Therefore, it is important to assess each patient's oxygen requirements and to provide instruction in the most appropriate techniques.

Psychosocial support

Psychosocial support is essential to combat feelings of depression, hopelessness and inability to cope (54). Patients may show symptoms of anxiety, particularly fear of dyspnoea, denial, anger and isolation to the point of becoming sedentary. They also become dependent upon family members, friends and medical services to provide for their needs. They may be overly concerned with physical problems and psychosomatic symptoms. Sexual dysfunction and fear of sexual activities are common but often unspoken (55–57). Patients may also demonstrate cognitive or neuropsychological dysfunction, possibly related to the effects of hypoxaemia on the brain.

Psychosocial support is best provided by warm and enthusiastic staff, able to communicate effectively with patients and devote the necessary effort to motivate them. Family and friends can be included in programme activities to better cope with the patient's disease. Both individual and group therapy are used, as well as psychotropic drugs if psychological dysfunction is severe.

As dyspnoea is closely associated with anxiety, relaxation training is incorporated into pulmonary rehabilitation programmes. With progressive muscle relaxation techniques, patients are instructed to sequentially tense and then relax 16 different muscle groups. In a randomized controlled trial of this approach, Renfroe (58) noted greater reduction in dyspnoea and anxiety in the study group, compared with control subjects. Changes in dyspnoea correlated significantly with changes in anxiety.

Exercise

Exercise is an essential component of pulmonary rehabilitation (1, 59, 60). Accepted benefits include increased endurance, maximum oxygen consumption and task performance. The optimal methods of training are the subject of ongoing research. Of the various components in a comprehensive pulmonary rehabilitation programme, exercise is the most demanding in terms of personnel, equipment and expertise. One should be careful in applying principles derived from healthy individuals or cardiac patients to patients with chronic lung disease, as the factors that limit exercise may be quite different.

Exercise techniques should be simple and inexpensive. Benefits from exercise training are largely muscle- and task-specific so that training should be directed towards the activity most likely to benefit (59–61). Patients increase their exercise capacity in the absence of changes in lung function. Exercise training also provides an opportunity for patients to extend their capacity for physical work and to practise

methods that minimize dyspnoea, such as breathing and relaxation techniques.

Training should utilize methods easily adapted to the home setting. Walking programmes have the added benefit of encouraging patients to expand their social horizons. In inclement weather, patients can walk indoors, in shopping malls. Cycling and swimming are also effective exercise modalities. Patients should be encouraged to incorporate regular exercise into activities such as golf and gardening, that they enjoy, with an emphasis on increasing endurance to allow patients to become more functional within their physical limits. As patients gain experience and confidence, their exercise level can be increased. Strength training is often used to address the skeletal muscle dysfunction that is frequently observed in patients with chronic lung disease (46, 62). A detailed review of exercise training in lung disease can be found in Chapter 20.

EXERCISE-INDUCED HYPOXAEMIA

Patients who may or may not be hypoxaemic at rest may desaturate on exercise (38). Since exercise desaturation cannot be predicted from resting saturation or pulmonary mechanics, it is important to measure saturation during exercise in order to decide whether oxygen is necessary for safe training. With the availability of portable systems for ambulatory oxygen delivery, hypoxaemia is not a contraindication to exercise training.

UPPER EXTREMITY TRAINING

Many patients with chronic lung disease report disabling dyspnoea for daily activities involving the upper extremities, such as lifting or self-grooming, at work levels much lower than those used for the lower extremities. Compared with lower extremity exercise, upper extremity exercise is accompanied by a higher ventilatory demand for a given level of work (63, 64). This added ventilatory load associated with upper extremity work may lead to dyssynchronous abdominal/thoracic breathing (65). Since exercise training is specific to the muscles and tasks involved in training, upper extremity exercises may be important in helping pulmonary patients with common daily activities (66).

SETTING

Pulmonary rehabilitation has been successful in in-patient, outpatient, community-based or home settings. In-patient programmes are used for more disabled or unstable patients unable to travel to an outpatient setting (e.g. for patients recovering from an acute exacerbation or intensive care unit stay). They have also been used for more intensive treatment schedules in centres that attract patients who live far away. Outpatient and community-based programmes are directed towards stable, ambulatory patients who may be treated individually or in small groups. In home-based programmes, staff travel to the patient's home to supervise care.

Regardless of the setting or schedule of treatment sessions, the primary goal of pulmonary rehabilitation is to assist the patient in establishing a treatment regimen for daily use at home. The description of programme 'sessions' refers only to the supervised sessions provided by the health professionals to help establish the daily care programme. The long-term success of pulmonary rehabilitation depends upon patients' willingness and ability to effect a lifestyle change on their own. Therefore, it is essential that the recommended approaches be consistent with their daily life and home environment rather than depending on equipment that may not be available for regular use.

Key points

- Pulmonary rehabilitation is an effective, well-established treatment option that enhances standard medical therapy and helps patients with chronic lung disease to gain control of their condition, alleviate symptoms, optimize function and reduce the medical, psychological, social and economic burdens of their disease.
- The primary goal is to restore the patient to the highest possible level of independent function.
- Three important features are: (i) individual assessment with attention to developing realistic individual goals; (ii) use of a multidisciplinary team that incorporates and integrates input from a variety of health care disciplines; and (iii) attention to psychosocial as well as physical problems.
- The ideal patient is one with chronic lung disease who has been appropriately evaluated, is stable on standard medical treatment, and is motivated to be actively involved in his or her own care to improve health status.
- Patients with any type of chronic lung disease may be appropriate candidates for pulmonary rehabilitation.
- Selection should be based on the degree of disability rather than on any arbitrary lung function criteria.
- Key programme components include education and training for patients and their partners, instruction in respiratory and chest physiotherapy techniques, exercise and psychosocial support.

REFERENCES

◆1. ACCP-AACVPR Pulmonary Rehabilitation Guidelines Panel. Pulmonary rehabilitation: joint ACCP/AACVPR evidence-based guidelines. *Chest* 1997; **112**: 1363–96.

◆2. ACCP-AACVPR Pulmonary Rehabilitation Guidelines Panel. Pulmonary rehabilitation: joint ACCP/AACVPR evidence-based guidelines. *J Cardiopulm Rehabil* 1997; **17**: 371–405.

◆3. American Thoracic Society. Pulmonary rehabilitation – 1999. *Am J Respir Crit Care Med* 1999; **159**: 1666–82.

4. American Thoracic Society. Standards for the diagnosis and care of patients with chronic obstructive pulmonary disease (COPD) and asthma. *Am Rev Respir Dis* 1995; **152**: S78–121.

5. British Thoracic Society Standards of Care Subcommittee on Pulmonary Rehabilitation. Pulmonary rehabilitation. *Thorax* 2001; **56**: 827–34.

●6. Lacasse Y, Wong E, Guyatt GH et al. Meta-analysis of respiratory rehabilitation in chronic obstructive pulmonary disease. *Lancet* 1996; **348**: 1115–19.

◆7. Casaburi R, Petty TL. *Principles and Practice of Pulmonary Rehabilitation.* Philadelphia: WB Saunders, 1993.

◆8. Hodgkin JE, Celli BR, Connors GL. *Pulmonary Rehabilitation – Guidelines to Success.* Philadelphia: Lippincott Williams & Wilkins, 2000.

◆9. Ries AL. Position paper of the American Association of Cardiovascular and Pulmonary Rehabilitation: scientific basis of pulmonary rehabilitation. *J Cardiopulm Rehabil* 1990; **10**: 418–41.

◆10. American Association of Cardiovascular and Pulmonary Rehabilitation. *Guidelines for Pulmonary Rehabilitation Programs.* Champaign: Human Kinetics, 1998.

11. Ries AL. Rehabilitation in chronic obstructive pulmonary disease and other respiratory disorders. In: Fishman A, ed. *Pulmonary Diseases and Disorders.* New York: McGraw-Hill, 1997; 709–19.

12. Pashkow FJ, Dafoe W. *Clinical Cardiac Rehabilitation: A Cardiologist's Guide.* Baltimore: Williams & Wilkins, 1990.

13. Pollock M. *Heart Disease and Rehabilitation.* New York: John Wiley, 1986.

14. Kemp B, Brummel-Smith K, Ramsdell JW. *Geriatric Rehabilitation.* Boston: Little, Brown, 1990.

15. Fordyce WE. *Behavioral Methods for Chronic Pain and Illness.* St. Louis: Mosby, 1976.

16. Cole KD, Ramsdell JW. Issues in interdesciplinary team care. In: Kemp B, Brummel-Smith K, Ramsdell JW, eds. *Geriatric Rehabilitation.* Boston: Little, Brown, 1990; 371–85.

17. Lyth JR. Models of the team approach. In: Fletcher GF, Banja JD, Jann BB, Wolf SL, eds. *Rehabilitation Medicine: Contemporary Clinical Perspectives.* Philadelphia: Lea & Febinger, 1992; 225–42.

18. American Thoracic Society. Pulmonary rehabilitation. *Am Rev Respir Dis* 1981; **124**: 663–6.

◆19. Fishman AP. Pulmonary rehabilitation research: NIH workshop summary. *Am J Respir Crit Care Med* 1994; **149**: 825–33.

20. Ries AL, Squier HC. The team concept in pulmonary rehabilitation. In: Fishman A, ed. *Pulmonary Rehabilitation.* New York: Marcel Dekker, 1996: 55–65.

21. Foster S, Thomas HM. Pulmonary rehabilitation in lung disease other than chronic obstructive pulmonary disease. *Am Rev Respir Dis* 1990; **141**: 601–4.

22. Connors GA, Hodgkin JE, Asmus RM. A careful assessment is crucial to successful pulmonary rehabilitation. *J Cardiopulmon Rehabil* 1988; **11**: 435–8.

23. Foster S, Lopez D, Thomas HM. Pulmonary rehabilitation in COPD patients with elevated PCO2. *Am Rev Respir Dis* 1988; **138**: 1519–23.

◆24. Dudley DL, Glaser EM, Jorgenson BN, Logan DL. Psychosocial concomitants to rehabilitation in chronic obstructive pulmonary disease: Part 1. Psychosocial and psychological considerations. *Chest* 1980; **77**: 413–20.

◆25. Dudley DL, Glaser EM, Jorgenson BN, Logan DL. Psychosocial concomitants to rehabilitation in chronic obstructive pulmonary disease: Part 2. Psychosocial treatment. *Chest* 1980; **77**: 544–51.

◆26. Dudley DL, Glaser EM, Jorgenson BN, Logan DL. Psychosocial concomitants to rehabilitation in chronic obstructive pulmonary disease: Part 3: dealing with psychiatric disease (as distinguished from psychosocial or psychophysiologic problems). *Chest* 1980; **77**: 677–84.

27. Sandhu HS. Psychosocial issues in chronic obstructive pulmonary disease. *Clin Chest Med* 1986; **7**: 629–42.

28. Dales RE, Spitzer WO, Schechter MT, Suissa S. The influence of psychological status on respiratory symptom reporting. *Am Rev Respir Dis* 1989; **139**: 1459–63.

29. Jensen PS. Risk, protective factors, and supportive interventions in chronic airway obstruction. *Arch Gen Psychiatry* 1983; **40**: 1203–7.

◆30. Ries AL. The role of exercise testing in pulmonary diagnosis. *Clin Chest Med* 1987; **8**: 81–9.

◆31. American Thoracic Society-American College of Chest Physicians. ATS/ACCP statement on cardiopulmonary exercise testing. *Am J Respir Crit Care Med* 2003; **167**: 211–77.

◆32. American Thoracic Society. ATS Statement: guidelines for the six-minute walk test. *Am J Respir Crit Care Med* 2002; **166**: 111–17.

33. Sciurba FC, Slivka WA. Six-minute walk testing. *Sem Respir Crit Care Med* 1998; **19**: 383–92.

34. Steele B. Timed walking tests of exercise capacity in chronic cardiopulmonary illness. *J Cardiopulmonary Rehabil* 1996; **16**: 25–33.

35. Singh SJ, Morgan MDL, Scott S *et al*. Development of a shuttle walking test of disability in patients with chronic airways obstruction. *Thorax* 1992; **47**: 1019–24.

36. Revill SM, Morgan MDL, Singh SJ, Hardman AE. The endurance shuttle walk: a new field test for the assessment of endurance capacity in chronic obstructive pulmonary disease. *Thorax* 1999; **54**: 213–22.

37. Elpern EH, Stevens D, Kesten S. Variability in performance of timed walk tests in pulmonary rehabilitation programs. *Chest* 2000; **118**: 98–105.

●38. Ries AL, Farrow JT, Clausen JL. Pulmonary function tests cannot predict exercise-induced hypoxemia in chronic obstructive pulmonary disease. *Chest* 1988; **93**: 454–9.

39. Ries AL, JT F, JL C. Accuracy of two ear oximeters at rest and during exercise in pulmonary patients. *Am Rev Respir Dis* 1985; **132**: 685–9.

40. Lacasse Y, Guyatt GH, Goldstein RS. The components of a respiratory rehabilitation program. *Chest* 1997; **111**: 1077–88.

41. Neish CM, Hopp JW. The role of education in pulmonary rehabilitation. *J Cardiopulmonary Rehabil* 1988; **11**: 439–41.

42. Crouch R, MacIntyre NR. Pulmonary rehabilitation of the patient with nonobstructive lung disease. *Respir Care Clin N Am* 1998; **4**: 59–67.

43. Palmer SM, Tapson VF. Pulmonary rehabilitation in the surgical patient: lung transplantation and lung volume reduction surgery. *Respir Care Clin N Am* 1998; **4**: 71–83.

44. Ries AL. Pulmonary rehabilitation in patients with thoracic neoplasm. In: Aisner J, Arriagada R, Green MR *et al*. eds. *Comprehensive Textbook of Thoracic Oncology*. Baltimore: Williams & Wilkins, 1996; 1019–29.

45. Rochester DF, Goldberg SK. Techniques of respiratory physical therapy. *Am Rev Respir Dis* 1980; **122**(Suppl.):133–46.

46. Gigliotti F, Romagnoli I, Scano G. Breathing retraining and exercise conditioning in patients with chronic obstructive pulmonary disease (COPD): a physiological approach. *Respir Med* 2003; **97**: 197–204.

◆47. Ries AL, Bullock PJ, Larsen CA *et al*. *Shortness of Breath, A Guide to Better Living and Breathing*. St Louis: Mosby, 2001.

48. Miller WF. Physical therapeutic measures in the treatment of chronic bronchopulmonary disorders: methods for breathing training. *Am J Med* 1958; **24**: 929–40.

49. Faling LJ. Pulmonary rehabilitation – physical modalities. *Clin Chest Med* 1986; **7**: 599–618.

50. Anthonisen NR. Long-term oxygen therapy. *Ann Intern Med* 1983; **99**: 519–27.

●51. Medical Research Council Working Party. Long-term domiciliary oxygen therapy in chronic hypoxic cor pulmonale complicating chronic bronchitis and emphysema. *Lancet* 1981; **1**: 681–6.

●52. Nocturnal Oxygen Therapy Trial Group. Continuous or nocturnal oxygen therapy in hypoxemic chronic obstructive lung disease: a clinical trial. *Ann Intern Med* 1980; **93**: 391–8.

53. Tiep BL. Oxygen therapy for the mobile patient. *J Cardiopulmon Rehabil* 1988; **11**: 442–8.

54. Light RW, Merrill EJ, Despars JA *et al*. Prevalence of depression and anxiety in patients with COPD: relationship to functional capacity. *Chest* 1985; **87**: 35–8.

55. Fletcher EC, Martin RJ. Sexual dysfunction and erectile impotence in chronic obstructive pulmonary disease. *Chest* 1982; **81**: 413–21.

56. Timms RM. Sexual dysfunction and chronic obstructive pulmonary disease. *Chest* 1982; **81**: 398–400.

57. Curgian LM, Gronkiewicz CA. Enhancing sexual performance in COPD. *Nurse Pract* 1988; **13**: 34–8.

58. Renfroe KL. Effect of progressive relaxation on dyspnea and state anxiety in patients with chronic obstructive pulmonary disease. *Heart Lung* 1988; **17**: 408–13.

59. Ries AL. The importance of exercise in pulmonary rehabilitation. *Clin Chest Med* 1994; **15**: 327–37.

60. Gosselink, Troosters, Decramer M. Exercise training in COPD patients: the basic questions. *Eur Respir J* 1997; **10**: 2884–91.

◆61. Casaburi R. Exercise training in chronic obstructive lung disease. In: Casaburi R, Petty TL, eds. *Principles and Practice of Pulmonary Rehabilitation*. Philadelphia: WB Saunders, 1993; 204–24.

62. Spruit MA, Gosselink R, Troosters T *et al*. Resistance versus endurance training in patients with COPD and peripheral muscle weakness. *Eur Respir J* 2002; **19**: 1072–8.

63. Reybrouck T, Heigenhauser GF, Faulkner JA. Limitations to maximum oxygen uptake in arm, leg, and comgined arm-leg ergometry. *J Appl Physiol* 1975; **38**: 774–9.

64. Vokac Z, Bell H, Bautz-Holter E, Rodahl K. Oxygen uptake/heart rate relationship in leg and arm exercise, sitting and standing. *J Appl Physiol* 1975; **39**: 54–9.

●65. Celli BR, Rassulo J, Make BJ. Dyssynchronous breathing during arm but not leg exercise in patients with chronic airflow obstruction. *N Engl J Med* 1986; **314**: 1485–90.

66. Ries AL, Ellis B, Hawkins RW. Upper extremity exercise training in chronic obstructive pulmonary disease. *Chest* 1988; **93**: 688–92.

27

Rehabilitation in thoracic wall deformities

J. M. SHNEERSON

INTRODUCTION

Pulmonary rehabilitation techniques have been widely used in thoracic wall deformities, but for many of these there are few data about their effectiveness or their precise indications. Rehabilitation should be tailored to the individual's needs rather than be provided as a fixed combination of treatments, which may be of little relevance to the person's situation. The definition of rehabilitation as the process of disabled people acquiring knowledge and skills so that they can improve their physical and psychosocial function emphasizes the importance of patient involvement in the rehabilitation process, whereas the view of rehabilitation as the application of measures to reduce the impact of an impairment or disability regards it as a process which carers perform on behalf of patients. Both approaches may be useful in varying degrees in different people, as long as the aims of the rehabilitation programme are clearly defined and individually assessed.

Patients who have skeletal disorders affecting their thoracic cage often have other disabilities as well. The skeletal abnormality may, for instance, be secondary to muscle weakness caused by previous poliomyelitis or a muscular dystrophy, in which limb muscle weakness may cause difficulty in walking. This may be a more prominent disability than the respiratory problems. The person's quality of life is nevertheless only partially determined by these physical limitations, but also varies with the pattern of the patient's activities, the relative values that the individual places on each of these and the psychological adjustments and reactions to the physical limitations. These all need to be taken into account when planning a rehabilitation programme for those with thoracic wall deformities.

SYMPTOMS

The most prominent respiratory symptoms in thoracic wall deformities are breathlessness, sleep disturbance and fatigue.

Breathlessness

It is common in these disorders for mild shortness of breath on exertion to be present, but if this worsens it suggests a change in the deformity or the development of a complication of this. The severity of breathlessness is related to the percentage of the maximal pressure that can be generated by the inspiratory muscles during breathing (1). Any worsening of lung or chest wall compliance or increase in airflow obstruction, for instance, because of intercurrent chest infections or the development of asthma, may worsen breathlessness and even precipitate respiratory failure.

Diaphragmatic weakness is suggested by the development of orthopnoea since in the supine position the abdominal contents are drawn into the thorax by the negative intrathoracic pressure, which is transmitted across the passive diaphragm (2). While sitting and standing, the abdominal contents fall during inspiration, due to gravity, and they are raised by abdominal muscle contraction in expiration.

Breathlessness appearing at night may also be due to arousals at the end of central sleep apnoeas or hypopnoeas, or occasionally as part of Cheyne–Stokes respiration (3, 4).

Sleep disturbance

Arousal at the end of central sleep apnoeas is due to hypoxia and hypercapnia, and while the arousals tend to protect the arterial blood gas levels they lead to fragmentation of sleep and thereby to excessive daytime sleepiness (5), deteriorating concentration and short-term memory. Irritability and mood lability usually occur later.

Early morning headaches are due to carbon dioxide retention during sleep, particularly rapid eye movement (REM) sleep which predominates towards the end of the night. Hypercapnia causes cerebral vasodilatation and an increase in the intracranial pressure. The headaches usually wear off within 20–30 min of waking, as the P_{CO_2} falls with the increase in ventilation after sleep (6).

Sleep may also be disrupted by discomfort due to the thoracic wall deformity. A scoliosis or thoracic kyphosis often causes aching or pain, particularly if the sleeping position remains unchanged.

Fatigue

Physical tiredness during the day should be distinguished from excessive daytime sleepiness due to sleep fragmentation. It may be the result of limitation in the oxygen supply to the tissues because of either arterial hypoxia or a reduction in cardiac output due to, for instance, to pulmonary hypertension.

IMPACT OF PHYSICAL LIMITATIONS

The impact of these symptoms, such as breathlessness, on the quality of life depends on the degree to which it interferes with the interests or activities that are of value to the individual. These priorities may develop before the deformity becomes apparent. The ability to modify one's interests in the light of the physical limitations caused by the deformity are central to this. Physicians and other health care workers are prone to over-emphasize the impact of physical disabilities on the quality of life of those with thoracic wall and neuromuscular disorders (7, 8); in fact, people with physical disabilities often adapt their ambitions according to their physical limitations and have quite different perceptions of the impact of their deformity.

The main areas where physical limitations may influence patient lifestyle and where rehabilitation programmes may be of benefit are as follows:

- activities of daily living – breathlessness due to the thoracic wall deformity may, for instance, prevent the person from shopping, cooking or carrying out housework

- education – the non-respiratory physical disability may preclude attendance at mainstream schools (9)
- employment – modern regulations about the rights of physically disabled people have reduced the impact of thoracic wall deformities on employment, but nevertheless physically active jobs may be unsuitable for these people, and fatigue as well as breathlessness may limit the types of jobs that are suitable
- mobility – difficulty in walking and climbing stairs may pose problems, but physical aids can be invaluable. A wheelchair which carries a portable ventilator may enable a patient with respiratory failure to remain mobile and to travel widely.

PATHOPHYSIOLOGY OF RESPIRATORY IMPAIRMENT

The degree to which deformities of the thoracic wall affect respiratory function depends on the nature of the deformity (Box 27.1). Ventilatory failure is common following a thoracoplasty for previous tuberculosis (10) and with a thoracic scoliosis (11) or kyphosis of early onset (12). It is uncommon in ankylosing spondylitis and does not occur in pectus carinatum, pectus excavatum or in the straight back syndrome. Nevertheless most of the thoracic wall deformities have similar pathophysiological features (Fig. 27.1).

Lung development
The formation of the normal number of alveoli is impaired if a thoracic wall deformity develops before the age of around 4 years, by which time the normal number of alveoli have been formed. Congenital and infantile idiopathic scoliosis, early-onset kyphosis and asphyxiating thoracic dystrophy may all be associated with this complication.

Lung volumes
Thoracic wall deformities almost invariably cause a restrictive defect with reduction in total lung capacity (TLC), functional residual capacity (FRC), residual volume and vital capacity. The exception is ankylosing spondylitis in which FRC and TLC are not reduced (13).

Box 27.1   Thoracic wall deformities associated with ventilatory failure

- Scoliosis
  - congenital
  - idiopathic (if early onset)
  - neurofibromatosis
  Secondary to:
    - poliomyelitis
    - spinal muscular atrophy
    - Duchenne's muscular dystrophy
- Kyphosis (if early onset)
- Thoracoplasty (usually post-tuberculosis)

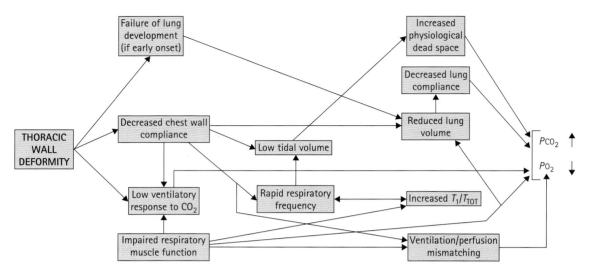

Figure 27.1   *Flow chart showing the effects of thoracic wall deformities on ventilation.*

Chest wall and lung compliance

The abnormal configuration of the thoracic cage reduces the compliance of the chest wall. Lung compliance falls, mainly because of the small lung volume. These compliance changes lead to a pattern of rapid shallow breathing which minimizes the work of breathing, but increases the dead space ventilation and thereby reduces the alveolar ventilation.

Respiratory muscle function

The contractility of the respiratory muscles is normal in thoracic wall deformities unless there is an underlying neuromuscular disorder. The force of contraction of the muscles is reduced when they operate other than at their optimal length. Distortion of the rib cage also puts the inspiratory muscles at a mechanical disadvantage, particularly in scoliosis and after a thoracoplasty.

Ventilatory drive

The central ventilatory drive is normal in thoracic wall deformities, but this cannot be translated into a normal degree of alveolar ventilation because of the abnormal respiratory mechanics and impaired respiratory muscle function (14). Once chronic hypercapnia develops, the increase in cerebrospinal fluid bicarbonate concentration reduces the sensitivity to hypercapnia and this is further impaired by sleep deprivation.

Blood gases

Mild hypoxia is common in thoracic wall deformities due to ventilation/perfusion mismatching, but hypoventilation may occur later, initially during sleep. It may develop insidiously or suddenly during an intercurrent illness such as a chest infection.

Exercise

During exercise, the tidal volume increases initially and this is followed by a rapid increase in respiratory rate (15). This increases the dead space to tidal volume ratio with a risk of alveolar hypoventilation. The arterial P_{O_2} may be maintained during exercise, but the pulmonary artery pressure rises

rapidly and in proportion to the reduction in pulmonary vascular bed. This is, in turn, related to the degree of the restrictive defect caused by the thoracic wall deformity (16).

Right heart failure and polycythaemia

Right heart failure develops as a result of pulmonary hypertension due to hypoxic pulmonary vasoconstriction and the reduced pulmonary vascular bed, which increases pulmonary vascular resistance. Hypoxia increases the sympathetic activity, which leads to renal vasoconstriction, activation of the renin–angiotensin–aldosterone system and thereby to sodium and water retention. The acidosis associated with hypercapnia increases the excretion of hydrogen ions by the renal tubules through absorption of sodium and bicarbonate. The additional erythropoietin secretion in response to renal hypoxia increases red cell formation, blood viscosity and, consequently, the pulmonary and systemic vascular resistance.

Sleep

During sleep the respiratory drive falls and the upper airway resistance increases (17). In REM sleep all the chest wall muscles, except the diaphragm, are inhibited and this predisposes to hypoventilation, particularly if diaphragm function is impaired due to abnormal configuration of the rib cage, as in scoliosis, and following a thoracoplasty. Repeated arousals due to hypoxia and hypercapnia lead to sleep fragmentation, which reduces the respiratory drive and predisposes to hypoventilation in non-REM sleep and subsequently in wakefulness as well.

PSYCHOLOGICAL TECHNIQUES

The physical limitations imposed by thoracic wall deformities commonly generate complex psychological responses. At one extreme, some patients wish to attain control of their limitations and their environment and they regard difficulties as opportunities to make a better future. This type of coping reaction requires adjustments and adaptations to their lifestyle to take into account the more restricted range of physical activities, and an acceptance of this and an enjoyment of what can still be carried out. Maintenance of contact with other people, both socially and in order to find out more about their disorder and what can be done to help, is a feature of this type of response. In contrast, those who feel that they are victims of their condition feel largely helpless to alter it or their environment. They have difficulty in adjusting their lifestyle and ambitions, and often become socially isolated.

Most people with thoracic wall deformities fall somewhere in between these polar responses. Their reaction depends on their personality before the deformity became apparent. The ability to cope with other problems earlier in life correlates with coping more successfully with the respiratory difficulties associated with a thoracic wall deformity. Emotional development may, however, be arrested if the deformity develops in childhood and leads to low self-esteem and restriction of social contacts. This is particularly prominent if the deformity arises suddenly, e.g. following trauma or surgery.

Mood disturbances mainly due to anxiety or depression are less frequent in thoracic wall deformities than might be expected. In a study of 116 subjects who had had poliomyelitis, only 15.8 per cent were depressed (18). This was related to social isolation and difficulties in accepting the effects of the underlying disorder.

The ability to improve the type of coping behaviour is an important part of rehabilitation. Education of the family and other carers so that they understand the situation and the feelings of the patient, and encouragement of social contacts are both important. The patient should be given as much realistic hope as possible (19) and the setting of achievable goals, which are not too taxing physically, is useful.

The ability of patients to return to the home with their family or other carers who understand their problems is an important part of rehabilitation and needs to be combined with, and not subservient to, the provision of optimal medical care. The emphasis on safety and dependence on health care professionals and equipment, which is common in hospitals and other institutions, is counterproductive. An atmosphere geared to increase the independence of patients is much more motivating and improves self-esteem. Ventilatory support, for instance, should be seen as a means of returning home and maintaining independence so that the patient's important activities can be carried out, as well as a mechanism of safeguarding respiration during sleep. The ability to travel with the ventilator outside the home and abroad, if desired, may be as important in improving the quality of life as technical advances in the ventilator itself.

If, despite these measures, anxiety and depression persist, careful selection of medication may be helpful. Most of the tricyclic antidepressants have a respiratory sedative effect and this may precipitate ventilatory failure in patients with severe respiratory impairment due to their thoracic wall deformity. Selective serotonin reuptake inhibitors (SSRIs) are, in general, preferable to tricyclic antidepressants, but the latter may be safe if they are taken at night and if patients reliably use ventilatory support throughout the night. Psychological techniques such as cognitive behavioural therapy can improve coping strategies and, in general, have been shown to have more prolonged benefits than drug treatment. In practice, the shortage of trained psychologists limits the availability of this type of treatment in many countries.

PHYSIOTHERAPY

The physiotherapist should recognize inefficient patterns of movement and attempt to teach patients how to correct them. If coordination and efficiency of movement can be improved, oxygen consumption falls and a greater range of activities can be performed without any increase in muscle strength or improvement in ventilatory function. Breathlessness is particularly common in exercise involving the arms, as the shoulder muscles in particular are used both as accessory respiratory muscles and during the arm exercise itself. Incoordination between these two competing priorities can easily disrupt respiration. Similarly, synchronization of leg and respiratory movements, particularly during walking and climbing stairs, may often reduce breathlessness.

Patients often walk too fast and become breathless because the increase in oxygen consumption raises their ventilatory requirements. Advice about reducing the speed of movement, particularly walking, is important.

The adoption of certain positions improves the efficiency of respiration and reduces breathlessness. Standing, leaning forwards and resting the arms on a surface may all be helpful. Energy can also be conserved with physical aids, such as a walking stick or handrail. Ventilatory support is a type of physical aid which reduces the work of breathing.

The physiotherapist has an important role in improving patients' confidence and coping strategies and in encouraging relaxation. This reduces the oxygen consumption and, if the respiratory muscles relax, the compliance of the chest wall increases. Patients should also be advised to assist their activities by planning rest periods between times when exercise is unavoidable. In those in whom the thoracic wall deformity is secondary to poliomyelitis, the progression of the post-poliomyelitis syndrome can be slowed or arrested by avoiding overuse of the affected muscles (20).

COUGH ASSISTANCE

A normal cough requires a deep inspiration, closure of the glottis and then a rapid forceful expiration as the glottis opens. In people with thoracic wall deformities, the depth of inspiration is limited, and if there is an underlying neuromuscular disorder, glottic function and expiration may also be abnormal (21). Conventional physiotherapy techniques to assist expectoration such as huffing may be required. A deep inspiration may be achieved by frog breathing (see below), breath stacking while using a ventilator, particularly if this is volume preset, or by specially designed cough assistance machines (e.g. insufflator-exsufflator; J Emerson Co, Cambridge, MA USA). These devices provide an approximately square wave of positive pressure to inflate the lungs and, by either a manual or an automatic switch, are then changed to generate a sudden negative pressure. This assists exhalation of air together with sputum or any other material in the airways. Manual thoracic or abdominal compression can be provided to assist expiration.

These techniques are of value particularly in those with neuromuscular disorders (22, 23), but in thoracic wall deformities without any underlying neuromuscular condition there is little benefit (24). In scoliosis, the abnormal chest shape makes manually assisted coughing and mechanical insufflation difficult to carry out effectively.

BREATHING TECHNIQUES

Improvement in the respiratory pattern both during rest and on exertion has been attempted through development of specific breathing exercises. Pursed lip breathing has been shown to be useful in emphysema, but not in thoracic wall deformities. 'Diaphragmatic' breathing and deep breathing exercises have been recommended in these conditions, but it is virtually impossible to selectively activate the diaphragm voluntarily. Nevertheless this type of exercise does encourage abdominal expansion during inspiration, and deep breathing exercises open distal airways and prevent subsegmental lung collapse and thereby increase lung compliance. The greater range of chest wall movements may also increase chest wall compliance and reduce the work of breathing (25). Deep breathing exercises and diaphragmatic breathing also reduce the respiratory frequency, which may reduce the work of breathing and increase alveolar ventilation.

Frog breathing is a technique which is of value mainly in those with neuromuscular disorders. The upper airway muscles are used to gulp air into the trachea and trap it below the glottis. This increases the vital capacity and maximum insufflation capacity without any activity of the muscles of the thorax and abdomen (26). It improves the cough, loudness of speech, and may prevent basal lung collapse in neuromuscular disorders, including tetraplegia (27, 28), poliomyelitis (29) and Duchenne's muscular dystrophy (30). It has not been shown to be of benefit in thoracic wall deformities without any underlying neuromuscular disorder.

EXERCISE TRAINING

Whole-body training

There is little evidence regarding the effectiveness of whole-body exercise training of the type that has been used extensively in COPD. The principle of whole-body exercise is that cardiovascular fitness improves with better oxygen delivery to the tissues. This is largely independent of any improvement in respiratory mechanics or respiratory muscle function. It may

be limited by cardiac abnormalities, e.g. cardiomyopathies associated with the thoracic wall deformity, and by difficulties in undertaking exercise because of disabilities affecting the limbs.

In one study, an exercise programme emphasizing leg exercises was combined with an education programme (31). In those with neuromuscular disorders, scoliosis and a patient with a thoracoplasty, the 6-min walking distance increased, but there was no difference in the forced expiratory volume in 1 s (FEV_1)/forced vital capacity (FVC), maximum inspiratory mouth pressure, arterial PO_2 or PCO_2.

Exercise training programmes have been used extensively in scoliosis, particularly adolescent idiopathic scoliosis, in order to improve exercise performance and in general have shown most benefit in those with the more severe deformities and progressively less effect when the condition is milder (32, 33). Exercise ability increases more than FEV_1, FVC or maximum voluntary ventilation (MVV) (34). Most of these studies were carried out in adolescents and the improvements due to growth have to be taken into account.

Exercise and physiotherapy programmes have also been devised to prevent deterioration in the scoliotic deformity (35) since, if the scoliosis can be stabilized, it would be anticipated that deterioration in respiratory function would be prevented.

Respiratory muscle training

Several studies of respiratory muscle training in tetraplegia have shown improvements in indices such as peak expiratory flow rates when the muscles that are unaffected by the spinal cord lesion are specifically trained (36–38). There have been very few studies in thoracic wall deformities without any underlying neuromuscular disorder. Patients with sequelae of pulmonary tuberculosis and its treatment underwent a rehabilitation programme which included respiratory muscle training as well as relaxation and exercise training (39). Improvements were seen in FEV_1, FVC, PO_2, maximal inspiratory mouth pressure, 6-min walking distance and quality of life. The degree of benefit from respiratory muscle training was, however, uncertain because of the complex nature of this rehabilitation programme. There have been no studies of arm muscle training, which might be value since some of these muscles are also accessory respiratory muscles.

The principle of specific respiratory muscle training is that skeletal muscle deconditioning is reversible and that the contractile properties of the muscles can be improved by training. This is probably correct for those with normal muscles, but when a skeletal muscle abnormality, as in Duchenne's muscular dystrophy, underlies the thoracic wall deformity, the muscle abnormalities may not be correctable by, for instance, exercise training (40). A study of 15 subjects with Duchenne's muscular dystrophy found that those with the least severely affected muscles benefited most. Those who were more severely affected, and to whom the training programme might have been of most benefit, improved least (40). In a separate study, the vital capacity and endurance ability increased slightly, but the clinical significance of these changes is uncertain (41).

SURGERY

Several surgical techniques have been developed that may improve respiratory function and promote rehabilitation in those with thoracic wall deformities.

Spinal surgery

There have been several studies of the effects of spinal fusion on respiratory function in adolescent idiopathic scoliosis (42–44). In general these have shown a slight improvement in vital capacity and maximal inspiratory mouth pressures, but this is not associated with any significant increase in exercise tolerance. When the scoliosis is due to a neuromuscular disorder, however, spinal surgery may be of benefit. In Duchenne's muscular dystrophy, surgery may not only improve the sitting posture, but may also delay the decline in vital capacity by improving the thoracic scoliosis (45). The same effect has been demonstrated in adults with scoliosis following previous poliomyelitis (46), but postoperative complications are common and usually outweigh any benefits from surgery (Fig. 27.2). In Duchenne's muscular dystrophy it is important to carry out spinal fusion at the correct stage, when the scoliosis has already developed but before the vital capacity falls below around 30 per cent of the predicted value (47).

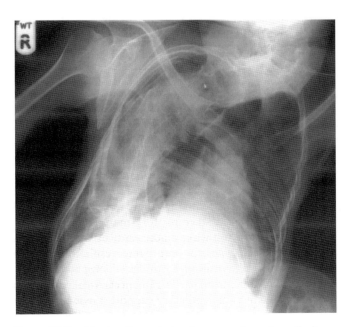

Figure 27.2 *Chest radiograph showing severe thoracic scoliosis following poliomyelitis with asymmetry of rib cage.*

Rib surgery

The cosmetic appearance of the thorax can be improved by costoplasty in thoracic scoliosis. In this operation the posterior aspects of the ribs which form the rib hump are resected. This is, in effect, a type of limited thoracoplasty, but does not significantly impair respiratory function (47).

Sternal surgery

Protrusion (pectus carinatum) and depression (pectus excavatum) deformities of the sternum often affect self-esteem and self-image. They rarely have any impact on respiratory function, but surgical correction may improve the cosmetic appearance (48).

NUTRITION

Adequate nutrition is important in order to optimize respiratory muscle strength and endurance (49). Malnutrition is common, however, particularly when thoracic wall deformities are associated with underlying neuromuscular disorders, such as amyotrophic lateral sclerosis (motor neuron disease). In this and similar conditions there may be difficulties in shopping for food, a physical inability to prepare or cook foods readily, weakness of the arms or hands so that food cannot be lifted to the mouth, difficulty in cutting it into sufficiently small pieces or chewing it satisfactorily as well an impairment of the swallowing mechanism. In thoracic wall deformities without a neuromuscular cause, some of these features may also be present. Swallowing is impaired when a tracheostomy tube is required to support ventilation because of difficulty in elevating the larynx and occasionally because of compression of the oesophagus (50). In addition, patients with thoracic wall deformities may feel breathless after meals, because of the increased intra-abdominal pressure which hinders diaphragmatic excursion. Many subjects eat progressively less rather than adapting to this difficulty by taking smaller meals more frequently.

Advice about the importance of maintaining adequate nutrition and providing food of an appropriate consistency is important. The composition of the food also has a bearing on respiratory function. A high-carbohydrate diet produces more carbon dioxide than a high-fat diet. In the presence of ventilatory failure this may be an important factor, although diets high in fat may cause diarrhoea. It is important for the diet to contain sufficient protein to increase muscle bulk. Food rich in protein is probably most effective in this respect if it is taken either immediately before or after exercise. If there is a persistent difficulty in swallowing, usually due to a neuromuscular disorder, nasogastric feeding is valuable in the short term, and insertion of a percutaneous endoscopic gastrostomy tube may enable adequate nutrition to be maintained in the long term (51, 52).

SLEEP DISTURBANCES

Respiratory-related arousals from sleep in thoracic wall deformities are common and are usually related to central sleep apnoeas (53). The arousals lead to fragmentation of sleep and excessive daytime sleepiness. This is often associated with loss of short-term memory, poor concentration, mood changes and social difficulties within the family and with friends, as well as problems with employment (54, 55). It is important to recognize the cause of the daytime sleepiness and to correct the respiratory abnormalities, e.g. with ventilatory support. Other causes may also be important. Patients may be afraid of falling asleep because of breathlessness at night and this fear needs to be addressed. Also, the limitation of physical activity and exposure to light during the day reduces the drive to remain alert during the day and to fall asleep at night. An increase in physical activity, particularly outdoors during the day, may be beneficial. Sleep at night may also be improved by reducing the intake of caffeine and alcohol, avoiding taking naps during the day, establishing regular patterns of going to bed and waking up in the morning, and ensuring that the sleep environment is as comfortable as possible.

DRUGS

Respiratory stimulants

A wide range of drugs have been used as respiratory stimulants. In the short term, doxapram is the most effective and it can be used as an alternative to mechanical ventilatory support in acute hypercapnic respiratory failure (56). There are few data regarding its effectiveness in thoracic wall deformities and it may cause tachycardias, agitation and epileptic seizures (57).

Drugs such as almitrine (58), theophyllines (59), acetazolamide (60) and progesterone (61) have been assessed for use in the long term but none significantly improves respiratory drive.

Inotropic agents

Digoxin (62) and salbutamol (63) have been proposed as inotropic agents, but have not been shown to have significant benefits. Theophyllines may improve respiratory muscle contractility (64). The effects are small, although it does also act as a bronchodilator and increases cardiac output.

Symptom control

The symptom of breathlessness can be improved by drugs acting on the central nervous system, such as benzodiazepines, opiates and buspirone (65). These are all respiratory depressants and increase the risk of hypercapnic ventilatory failure. There is little place for any of these in the treatment of thoracic wall deformities, except pre-terminally, when there is

an incurable underlying neuromuscular disorder, such as motor neuron disease, and when all other treatment options have been tried.

Drugs which improve airway function, such as bronchodilators and inhaled steroids, may improve exercise capacity and quality of life, as may those which improve right ventricular failure, including diuretics.

OXYGEN

Oxygen is often prescribed for breathlessness in thoracic wall deformities, but in general it is contraindicated at rest because of the risk that it will worsen hypercapnia by abolishing any residual hypoxic drive. It should only be prescribed after detailed studies of blood gas findings during the day and of oximetry and, ideally, transcutaneous $P\text{CO}_2$ recordings during sleep. Ventilatory support is preferable to oxygen in improving hypoxia associated with hypercapnia.

Oxygen may however be of value in relieving exertional breathlessness. Baseline walking tests without oxygen are required to assess the degree of hypoxia that occurs during exercise and identical tests with increasing oxygen flow rates will enable the optimum flow rate to be determined. Liquid oxygen is preferable to pressurized cylinders, although modern lightweight cylinders with a wide range of flow rates are now available. Oxygen can also be used briefly after exertion in order to hasten recovery and reduce the duration of breathlessness.

VENTILATORY SUPPORT

Hypercapnic respiratory failure occurs in many thoracic wall deformities, particularly scoliosis, kyphosis and following a thoracoplasty. Ventilatory failure occurs in sleep, primarily REM sleep, before wakefulness. Although the respiratory drive is intrinsically normal, the mechanical abnormalities of the thorax prevent it from being translated into a normal degree of lung inflation and deflation.

The mechanisms by which ventilatory support improves respiratory function are uncertain, but probably include a resetting of the respiratory drive, partly through relief of sleep deprivation and partly by reducing the cerebrospinal fluid bicarbonate concentration, thereby increasing the ventilatory response to hypercapnia (66). There may also be small changes in vital capacity due to improvement in chest wall and lung compliance and respiratory muscle function (67). Respiratory muscle rest while on the ventilator has been proposed as a mechanism for improving respiratory muscle function, but this may also lead to disuse atrophy (68). Any improvement comes from partial rather than total respiratory support. Non-invasive ventilatory support is associated with some residual muscle activity in triggering ventilator breaths or during the inspiratory or expiratory phases of the ventilator. The ventilator can be set to optimize the degree of inspiratory support and the timings of the inspiratory and expiratory phases so, in effect, it acts as a respiratory muscle training device.

Choice of ventilatory support

NON-INVASIVE POSITIVE PRESSURE VENTILATION

A nasal mask is usually preferable to a full facemask or mouthpiece, and while complications such as nasal ulcers, mask displacement, air leaks around the mask or through the mouth, upper airway symptoms, abdominal distension and upper airway obstruction may all occur, they are no more likely to do so in subjects with thoracic wall deformities than in other patients.

Either pressure- or volume-preset ventilators may be effective (69–71). An inspiratory time of 0.8–1.0 s with an expiratory time of around 2.0 s is often optimal. Sensitive pressure or flow triggering with a short response time is required in view of the rapid respiratory frequency that is adopted by these patients. A positive end-expiratory pressure of 1–3 cmH$_2$O may be of value in preventing closure of small airways, and is present in bilevel pressure support systems to flush the dead space to prevent carbon dioxide rebreathing. There is little difference between proportional assist ventilation (PAV) and pressure support ventilation (72). With volume-preset ventilators, the assist/control mode is preferable to controlled ventilation. Supplemental oxygen is rarely required unless there is an additional intrinsic disorder of the lungs.

INVASIVE POSITIVE PRESSURE VENTILATION

This is only required in acute episodes of ventilatory failure unless there is an underlying neuromuscular disorder, usually with poor cough or upper airway obstruction. The ventilatory requirements and settings are similar to non-invasive ventilation.

NEGATIVE PRESSURE VENTILATION

This is usually achieved using a cuirass or jacket (poncho), but tank ventilation (iron lung) is an alternative in the short term (73). These pressure-preset ventilators may cause upper airway obstruction, discomfort, pressure areas, and there may be air leaks and difficulties if the subject moves about while on the ventilator. Most negative pressure ventilators act in the control mode, but some can be triggered by pressure sensors placed in the nose (74).

The restricted range of movements during the night is particularly difficult for those with a kyphosis where the sharp angulation of the spine becomes uncomfortable, and occasionally with a scoliosis if it is severe. Upper airway obstruction is commonest if there is incoordination between the ventilator and patient. The inspiratory and expiratory times that are required are similar to those used for non-invasive positive pressure ventilation.

Patient selection

There have been no randomized control studies of ventilatory support in thoracic wall deformities, but it is usually used in the following situations.

ASYMPTOMATIC HIGH-RISK PATIENTS

Patients with a vital capacity of less than 1.0–1.5 L, a scoliosis developing before the age of 4–8 years, a high thoracic curve and those with an extensive thoracoplasty, especially if they have had a contralateral artificial pneumothorax, are particularly at risk of developing respiratory failure (75). These subjects should be followed up in the long term with sleep studies and arterial blood gas analysis and serial measurements of their vital capacity. Ventilatory failure may develop insidiously, but may also appear acutely, either during an illness such as a chest infection or even without any intercurrent illness.

ABNORMAL ARTERIAL BLOOD GAS TENSIONS

Ventilatory support should be considered even if there are no symptoms of ventilatory failure or complications such as polycythaemia or pulmonary hypertension. There is no evidence, however, to indicate whether it should be initiated if there is only nocturnal hypercapnia and hypoxia with normal arterial blood gas tensions while awake. Ventilatory support should be provided once symptoms appear in the presence of hypercapnia (76). The recommendation that this should be started when symptoms are present with a PCO$_2$ > 6 kPa or with more than 5 min spent asleep with an arterial oxygen saturation of less than 88 per cent is not based on any published data (77).

Symptom relief

Symptoms such as breathlessness on exertion, daytime sleepiness and fatigue, and early morning headaches can all be improved (78–80) and activities of daily living such as shopping, cleaning and cooking can be carried out more easily once ventilatory support has been started. Ventilatory support may enable education to proceed (9) and subjects to return to employment (81), as well as reducing the number of days spent in hospital (82–84), and improving psychosocial and mental function (82–85).

Physiological effects

Ventilatory support may improve sleep architecture (86) and oxygen saturation and transcutaneous PCO$_2$ during sleep as well as arterial blood gases during the day (Fig. 27.3) (87–90). Any effects on vital capacity, FEV$_1$ and maximum inspiratory and expiratory mouth pressures are smaller (82). Endurance times both on a bicycle and while walking improve once ventilatory support has been established (91).

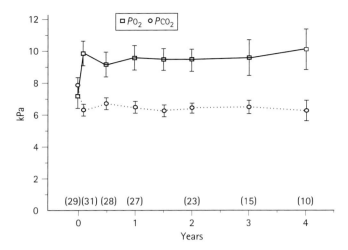

Figure 27.3 *Changes in arterial gas tensions in patients treated with non-invasive ventilation following a thoracoplasty (mean and 95 per cent confidence intervals are indicated; figures in brackets show the number of patients at each point) (89).*

Survival

Uncontrolled studies have shown 1-year survival figures of around 90 per cent in stable thoracic wall deformities such as scoliosis, with a 5-year survival of around 80 per cent (87, 92) with positive pressure ventilation. Similar results have been obtained with negative pressure ventilation (89). The survival following a thoracoplasty is similar (87, 89, 92), despite extensive pulmonary disease as well as the chest wall surgery. In thoracic wall deformities due to a progressive underlying neuromuscular disorder, the prognosis depends as much on this as on the scoliosis itself (82, 87).

Quality of life

The quality of life of patients with respiratory support is often underestimated by the care-givers (85, 86). In general it is greater with non-invasive than tracheostomy ventilation (88), but the latter may be preferred if there is a weak cough, a requirement for airway protection or when ventilation is required for more than 16 h each day, since it may enable the patients to return more readily to their everyday activities.

Key points

- Rehabilitation programmes should be constructed to meet each individual's needs.
- Psychological adjustments and coping strategies should be encouraged.
- Cough assistance and breathing techniques are most valuable if there is an underlying neuromuscular disorder.
- Exercise training may be useful, but evidence for this is limited.

- The value of nutritional advice is often underestimated.
- Oxygen is rarely indicated in chest wall deformities.
- Non-invasive ventilatory support can improve symptoms, quality of life, blood gases and survival, but careful patient selection is required.

REFERENCES

●1. Bradley TD, Chartrand DA, Fitting JW *et al.* The relation of inspiratory effort sensation to fatiguing patterns of the diaphragm. *Am Rev Respir Dis* 1986; **134**: 1119–24.

2. Loh L, Goldman M, Newsom-Davis J. The assessment of diaphragm function. *Medicine* 1977; **56**: 165–9.

3. Dowdell WT, Javaheri S, McGinnis W. Cheyne-Stokes respiration presenting as sleep apnea syndrome. *Am Rev Respir Dis* 1990; **141**: 871–8.

4. Trinder J, van Beveren JA, Smith P *et al.* Correlation between ventilation and EEG-defined arousal during sleep onset in young subjects. *J Appl Physiol* 1997; **83**: 2005–11.

◆5. Akerstedt T, Billiard M, Bonnet M *et al.* Awakening from sleep. *Sleep Med Rev* 2002; **6**: 267–86.

6. Dripps RD, Comroe JH Jr. The respiratory and circulatory response of normal man to inhalation of 7.6 and 10.4 per cent CO2 with a comparison of the maximal ventilation produced by severe muscular exercise, inhalation of CO2 and maximal voluntary hyperventilation. *Am J Physiol* 1947; **149**: 43–51.

7. Bach JR, Campagnolo DI, Hoeman S. Life satisfaction of individuals with Duchenne's muscular dystrophy using long-term mechanical ventilatory support. *Am J Phys Med Rehabil* 1991; **70**: 129–35.

8. Bach JR, Campagnolo DI. Psychosocial adjustment of post-poliomyelitis ventilator-assisted individuals. *Arch Phys Med Rehabil* 1992; **73**: 934–9.

9. Gilgoff IS, Kahlstrom E, MacLaughlin E, Keens TG. Long-term ventilatory support in spinal muscular atrophy. *J Pediatr* 1989; **115**: 904–9.

10. Sakuma T, Tatsumi K, Kumura H *et al.* Sleep oxygen desaturation in late sequelae of pulmonary tuberculosis. *Intern Med* 1996; **35**: 534–9.

●11. Bergofsky EH, Turino GM, Fishman AP. Cardio-respiratory failure in kyphoscoliosis. *Medicine* 1959; **38**: 263–317.

12. Smith IE, Laroche CM, Jamieson SA, Shneerson JM. Kyphosis secondary to tuberculous osteomyelitis as a cause of ventilatory failure. *Chest* 1996; **110**: 1105–10.

13. Franssen MJAM, van Herwaarden CLA, van de Putte LBA, Gribnau FWJ. Lung function in patients with ankylosing spondilitis. A study of the influence of disease activity and treatment with non-steroidal anti-inflammatory drugs. *J Rheumatol* 1986; **13**: 936–40.

14. Kafer ER. Idiopathic scoliosis. Mechanical properties of the respiratory system and the ventilatory response to carbon dioxide. *J Clin Invest* 1975; **55**: 1153–63.

15. Shneerson JM. The cardiorespiratory response to exercise in thoracic scoliosis. *Thorax* 1978; **33**: 457–63.

16. Shneerson JM. Pulmonary artery pressure in thoracic scoliosis during and after exercise while breathing air and pure oxygen. *Thorax* 1978; **33**: 747–54.

◆17. Shneerson J. Sleep in neuromuscular and thoracic cage disorders. *Eur Respir Mon* 1998; **10**: 324–44.

18. Tate D, Kirsch N, Maynard F *et al.* Coping with the late effects: differences between depressed and nondepressed polio survivors. *Am J Phys Med Rehabil* 1994; **73**: 27–35.

19. Kim T-S. Hope as a mode of coping in amyotrophic lateral sclerosis. *J Neurosci Nurs* 1989; **21**: 342–7.

20. Agre JC. Local muscle and total body fatigue. In: Halstead LS, Grimby G, eds. *Post-polio Syndrome*. Philadelphia: Hanley & Belfus, 1995; 35–67.

21. Siebens AA, Kirby NA, Poulos DA. Cough following transection of spinal cord at C-6. *Arch Phys Med Rehabil* 1964; **45**: 1–7.

22. Bach JR. Mechanical insufflation-exsufflation. Comparison of peak expiratory flows with manually assisted and unassisted coughing techniques. *Chest* 1993; **104**: 1553–62.

23. Bach JR, Smith WH, Michaels J *et al.* Airway secretion clearance by mechanical exsufflation for post-poliomyelitis ventilator-assisted individuals. *Arch Phys Med Rehabil* 1993; **74**: 170–6.

24. Sivasothy P, Brown L, Smith IE, Shneerson JM. Effect of manually assisted cough and mechanical insufflation on cough flow of normal subjects, patients with chronic obstructive pulmonary disease (COPD), and patients with respiratory muscle weakness. *Thorax* 2001; **56**: 438–44.

25. Ferris BG Jr, Pollard DS. Effect of deep and quiet breathing on pulmonary compliance in man. *J Clin Invest* 1960; **39**: 143–9.

26. Dail CW. Glossopharyngeal breathing by paralysed patients. A preliminary report. *Calif Med* 1951; **75**: 217–18.

27. Alvarez SE, Peterson M, Lunsford BR. Respiratory treatment of the adult patient with spinal cord injury. *Phys Ther* 1981; **61**: 1737–45.

28. Montero JC, Feldman DJ, Montero D. Effects of glossopharyngeal breathing on respiratory function after cervical cord transection. *Arch Phys Med Rehabil* 1967; **48**: 650–3.

29. Dail CW, Affeldt JE, Collier CR. Clinial aspects of glossopharyngeal breathing. Report of use by one hundred postpoliomyelitic patients. *J Am Med Assoc* 1955; **158**: 445–9.

30. Alexander MA, Johnson EW, Petty J, Stauch D. Mechanical ventilation of patients with late stage Duchenne muscular dystrophy: management in the home. *Arch Phys Med Rehabil* 1979; **60**: 289–92.

31. Foster S, Thomas HM. Pulmonary rehabilitation in lung disease other than chronic obstructive pulmonary disease. *Am Rev Respir Dis* 1990; **141**: 601–4.

32. Gotze HG, Sunram F, Scheele K, Munster IW. Die kardiopulmonale Belastbarkeit jugendlichen Skoliosepatienten. *Zeitschr Orthop* 1974; **112**: 832–6.

33. Shneerson JM, Madgwick R. The effect of physical training on exercise ability in adolescent idiopathic scoliosis. *Acta Orthop Scand* 1979; **50**: 303–6.

34. Athanasopoulos S, Paxinos T, Tsafantakis E *et al.* The effect of aerobic training in girls with idiopathic scoliosis. *Scand J Med Sci Sports* 1999; **9**: 36–40.

35. Weiss HR, Lohschmidt K, El-Obeidi N, Verres C. Preliminary results and worst-case analysis of in patient scoliosis rehabilitation. *Ped Rehabil* 1997; **1**: 35–40.

36. Gross D, Ladd HW, Riley EJ *et al.* The effect of training on strength and endurance of the diaphragm in quadriplegia. *Am J Med* 1980; **68**: 27–35.

37. Biering-Sorensen F, Knudsell JL, Schmidt A *et al.* Effect of respiratory training with a mouth-nose-mask in tetraplegics. *Paraplegia* 1991; **29**: 113–19.

38. Estenne M, van Muylem A, Gorini M *et al.* Evidence of dynamic airway compression during cough in tetraplegic patients. *Am J Respir Crit Care Med* 1994; **150**: 1081–5.

39. Tada A, Matsumoto H, Soda R *et al.* Effects of pulmonary rehabilitation in patients with pulmonary tuberculosis sequelae. *Nihon Kokyuki Gakkai Zasshi* 2002; **40**: 275–81.

40. Wanke T, Toifl K, Merkle M *et al.* Inspiratory muscle training in patients with Duchenne muscular Dystrophy. *Chest* 1994; **105**: 475–82.

41. Estrup C, Lyager S, Noeraa N, Olsen C. Effect of respiratory muscle training in patients with neuromuscular diseases and in normals. *Respiration* 1986; **50**: 36–43.

42. Gazioglu K. Pulmonary function before and after orthopaedic correction of idiopathic scoliosis. *Bull Physiopath Respir* 1973; **9**: 711–13.

43. Cooper CB, Waterhouse J, Howard P. Twelve year clinical study of patients with hypoxic cor pulmonale given long term domiciliary oxygen therapy. *Thorax* 1987; **42**: 105–10.

44. Shannon DC, Riseborough EJ, Kazemi H. Ventilation perfusion relationships following correction of kyphoscoliosis. *J Am Med Assoc* 1971; **217**: 579–84.

45. Jenkins JG, Bohn D, Edmonds JF *et al.* Evaluation of pulmonary function in muscular dystrophy patients requiring spinal surgery. *Crit Care Med* 1982; **10**: 645–9.

46. Gui L, Savini R, Vicenzi G, Ponzo L. Surgical treatment of poliomyelitic scoliosis. *Ital Orthop Traumatol* 1976; **2**: 191–205.

47. Geissele MAE, Ogilvie JW, Cohen M, Bradford DS. Thoracoplasty for the treatment of rib prominence in thoracic scoliosis. *Spine* 1994; **19**: 1636–42.

48. Nuss D, Kelly RE, Croitoru DP, Katz ME. A 10-year review of a minimally invasive technique for the correction of pectus excavatum. *J Pediatr Surg* 1998; **33**: 545–52.

49. Pingleton SK. Enteral nutrition in patients with respiratory disease. *Eur Respir J* 1996; **9**: 364–70.

50. Bonanno PC. Swallowing dysfunction after tracheostomy. *Ann Surg* 1971; **174**: 29–33.

51. Wicks C, Gimson A, Vlavianos P. Assessment of the percutaneous endoscopic gastrostomy feeding tube as part of an integral approach to enteral feeding. *Gut* 1992; **33**: 613–16.

52. Hull MA, Rawlings J, Murray FE *et al.* Audit of outcome of long-term enteral nutrition by percutaneous endoscopic gastrostomy. *Lancet* 1993; **341**: 869–72.

53. Martin SE, Engleman RM, Deary IJ, Douglas NJ. The effect of sleep fragmentation on daytime function. *Am J Respir Crit Care Med* 1996; **153**: 1328–32.

54. Martin SE, Wraith PK, Deary IJ, Douglas NJ. The effect of nonvisible sleep fragmentation on daytime function. *Am J Respir Crit Care Med* 1997; **155**: 1596–601.

55. Mendleson WB. Sleep fragmentation and daytime wakefulness. *Am J Respir Crit Care Med* 1997; **155**: 1499–500.

56. Canter HG, Luchsinger PC. The treatment of respiratory failure without mechanical assistance. *Am J Med Sci* 1964; **248**: 206–11.

57. Winnie AP. Chemical respirogenesis: a comparative study. *Acta Anaesthesiol Scan Supplement* 1973; **51**: 1–32.

58. Maxwell DL, Cover D, Hughes JMB. Almitrine increases the steady-state hypoxic ventilatory response in hypoxic chronic air-flow obstruction. *Am Rev Respir Dis* 1985; **132**: 1233–7.

59. Sanders JS, Berman TM, Bartlett MM, Kronenberg RS. Increased hypoxic ventilatory drive due to administration of aminophylline in normal men. *Chest* 1980; **78**: 279–82.

60. Galdston M, Geller J. Effects of aminophylline and diamox alone and together on respiration and acid-base balance and on

respiratory response to carbon dioxide in pulmonary emphysema. *Am J Med* 1957; **23**: 183–96.

61. Sutton FD Jr, Zwillich CW, Creagh CE *et al.* Progesterone for outpatient treatment of Pickwickian syndrome. *Ann Int Med* 1975; **83**: 476–9.

62. Aubier M, Viires N, Murciano D *et al.* Effects of digoxin on diaphragmatic strength generation. *J Appl Physiol* 1986; **61**: 1767–74.

63. Thompson PJ, Dhillon DP, Ledingham J, Turner-Warwick M. Shrinking lungs, diaphragmatic dysfunction, and systemic lupus erythematosus. *Am Rev Respir Dis* 1985; **132**: 926–8.

64. Sherman MS, Lang DM, Matityahu A, Campbell D. Theophylline improves measurements of respiratory muscle efficiency. *Chest* 1996; **110**: 1437–42.

65. Tooms McKenzie A, Gruy H. Nebulized morphine. *Lancet* 1993; **342**: 1123.

66. Annane D, Quera-Salva MA, Lofaso F *et al.* Mechanisms underlying effects of nocturnal ventilation on daytime blood gases in neuromuscular diseases. *Eur Respir J* 1999; **13**: 157–62.

67. Piper AJ, Sullivan CE. Effects of long-term nocturnal nasal ventilation on spontaneous breathing during sleep in neuromuscular and chest wall disorders. *Eur Respir J* 1996; **9**: 1515–22.

68. Sassoon CS, Caiozzo VJ, Manka A, Sieck GC. Altered diaphragm contractile properties with controlled mechanical ventilation. *J Appl Physiol* 2002; **92**: 2585–95.

69. Schonhofer B, Sonneborn M, Haidl P *et al.* Comparison of two different modes for noninvasive mechanical ventilation in chronic respiratory failure: volume versus pressure controlled device. *Eur Respir J* 1997; **109**: 184–91.

70. Tejeda M, Boix JH, Alvarez F *et al.* Comparison of pressure support ventilation and assist-control ventilation in the treatment of respiratory failure. *Chest* 1997; **111**: 1322–5.

71. Elliott MW, Aquilina R, Green M *et al.* A comparison of different modes of non-invasive ventilatory support: effects on ventilation and inspiratory muscle effort. *Anaesthesia* 1994; **49**: 279–83.

72. Hart N, Hunt A, Polkey MI *et al.* Comparison of proportional assist ventilation and pressure support ventilation in chronic respiratory failure due to neuromuscular and chest wall deformity. *Thorax* 2002; **57**: 979–81.

73. Shneerson JM. Non-invasive and domiciliary ventilation: negative pressure techniques. *Thorax* 1991; **46**: 131–5.

74. Smith IE, King MA, Shneerson JM. Choosing a negative pressure ventilation pump: are there any important differences? *Eur Respir J* 1995; **8**: 1792–5.

75. Branthwaite MA. Cardiorespiratory consequences of unfused idiopathic scoliosis. *Br J Dis Chest* 1986; **80**: 360–9.

◆76. Shneerson JM, Simonds AK. Noninvasive ventilation for chest wall and neuromuscular disorders. *Eur Respir J* 2002; **20**: 480–7.

◆77. Consensus Conference. Clinical indications for non-invasive positive pressure ventilation in chronic respiratory failure due to restrictive lung disease, COPD, and nocturnal hypoventilation – a Consensus conference report. *Chest* 1999; **116**: 521–34.

78. Leger P, Jennequin J, Gerard M *et al.* Home positive pressure ventilation via nasal mask for patients with neuromusculoskeletal disorders. *Eur Respir J* 1989; **2**(Suppl. 7): 640s–5.

79. Hill NS, Eveloff SE, Carlisle CC, Goff SG. Efficacy of nocturnal nasal ventilation in patients with restrictive thoracic disease. *Am Rev Respir Dis* 1992; **145**: 365–71.

80. Schiavina M, Fabiani A. Intermittent negative pressure ventilation in patients with restrictive respiratory failure. *Monaldi Arch Chest Dis* 1993; **48**: 169–75.

81. Sawicka EH, Loh L, Branthwaite MA. Domiciliary ventilatory support; an analysis of outcome. *Thorax* 1988; **43**: 31–5.

82. Kinnear W, Hockley S, Harvey J, Shneerson J. The effects of one year of nocturnal cuirass-assisted ventilation in chest wall disease. *Eur Respir J* 1988; **1**: 204–8.

83. Zaccaria S, Ioli F, Lusuardi M *et al.* Long-term nocturnal mechanical ventilation in patients with kyphoscoliosis. *Monaldi Arch Chest Dis* 1995; **50**: 433–7.

84. Ferris G, Servera-Pieras E, Vergara P *et al.* Kyphoscoliosis ventilatory insufficiency: non-invasive management outcomes. *Am J Phys Med Rehabil* 2000; **70**: 24–9.

85. Pehrsson K, Olofson J, Larsson S, Sullivan M. Quality of life in patients treated by home mechanical ventilation due to restrictive ventilatory disorders. *Respir Med* 1994; **88**: 21–6.

86. Ellis ER, Grunstein RR, Chan S *et al.* Noninvasive ventilatory support during sleep improves respiratory failure in kyphoscoliosis. *Chest* 1988; **94**: 811–15.

87. Simonds AK, Elliott MW. Outcome of domiciliary nasal intermittent positive pressure ventilation in restrictive and obstructive disorders. *Thorax* 1995; **50**: 604–9.

88. Schonhofer B, Kohler D. Effect of non-invasive mechanical ventilation on sleep and nocturnal ventilation in patients with chronic respiratory failure. *Thorax* 2000; **55**: 308–13.

89. Jackson M, Smith I, King M, Shneerson J. Long term non-invasive domiciliary assisted ventilation for respiratory failure following thoracoplasty. *Thorax* 1994; **49**: 915–19.

90. Zaccaria S, Zaccaria E, Zanaboni S *et al.* Home mechanical ventilation in kyphoscoliosis. *Monaldi Arch Chest Dis* 1993; **48**: 161–4.

91. Schonhofer B, Wallstein S, Wiese C, Kohler D. Noninvasive mechanical ventilation improves endurance performance in patients with chronic respiratory failure due to thoracic restriction. *Chest* 2001; **119**: 1371–8.

92. Leger P, Bedicam JM, Cornette A *et al.* Nasal intermittent positive pressure ventilation. Long term follow-up in patients with severe chronic respiratory insufficiency. *Chest* 1994; **105**: 100–5.

28

Physical medicine interventions and rehabilitation of patients with neuromuscular disease

JOHN R. BACH

INTRODUCTION

> People who want to make a living from the treatment of nervous patients must clearly be able to do something to help them. (Sigmund Freud MD, 1909) (1)

For the prevention of respiratory complications, three muscle groups must be considered: the inspiratory, expiratory and bulbar muscles. While inspiratory and expiratory muscle aids can fully support alveolar ventilation and eliminate airway secretions without the need to resort to tracheostomy, once bulbar muscle dysfunction results in an irreversible decrease in baseline oxyhaemoglobin saturation (S_pO_2), tracheostomy becomes necessary to prolong survival. Fortunately, this rarely becomes necessary for any patients with neuromuscular disease other than severely advanced patients with bulbar amyotrophic lateral sclerosis (ALS) and a small minority of patients with spinal muscular atrophy type 1.

CONVENTIONAL MANAGEMENT

Eighty to 90 per cent of conventionally managed people with Duchenne muscular dystrophy (DMD) without tracheostomy tubes die from respiratory failure between 16 and 19 years of age and rarely after age 25 (2–4). Ninety per cent of spinal muscular atrophy (SMA) type 1 children die by 12 months of age and 100 per cent by the age of 2 years (5). Patients with ALS die a mean of 15–20 months from the time of diagnosis (6, 7). In the great majority of cases for these diagnoses and for all others with neuromuscular disease, the causes of death are respiratory, although myopathy patients sometimes die from complications related to cardiomyopathy. Likewise, in virtually all cases, morbidity and mortality from respiratory causes can be prevented (Box 28.1).

Box 28.1 Neuromusculoskeletal conditions for which respiratory muscle aids can be used to avert respiratory failure and tracheostomy

---

Myopathies

- Muscular dystrophies
  - dystrophinopathies: Duchenne and Becker dystrophies
  - other muscular dystrophies: limb-girdle, Emery–Dreifuss, facioscapulohumeral, congenital, childhood autosomal recessive, and myotonic dystrophy
- Non-Duchenne myopathies
  - congenital and metabolic myopathies like acid maltase deficiency
  - inflammatory myopathies such as polymyositis
  - diseases of the myoneural junction such as myasthenia gravis, mixed connective tissue disease
  - myopathies of systemic disease such as carcinomatous myopathy, cachexia/anorexia nervosa, medication associated

Neurological disorders

- Spinal muscular atrophies
- Motor neuron diseases
- Spinal cord injuries

custom-moulded interface designs (14). Since everyone's face, and especially nose, has a different anatomy, one cannot predict which interface will provide the best seal with least insufflation leakage, or which interface any particular patient will find most comfortable. Therefore, no patient should be offered and expected to use only one nasal interface any more than one should be offered only lipseal or a single oronasal interface. Alternating interfaces nightly alternates skin pressure sites, minimizes discomfort, and is to be encouraged.

Excessive insufflation leakage via the mouth is prevented by keeping ventilatory drive intact by maintaining normal daytime CO_2 and avoiding supplemental O_2 and sedatives. However, in the presence of daytime hypercapnia and excessive nocturnal dS_pO_2s and bothersome arousals, for patients not wishing to switch to lipseal IPPV, a chin strap or plugged lipseal without mouthpiece can be used to decrease oral leakage. In the presence of nasal congestion, patients use decongestants to permit nasal IPPV, switch to lipseal ventilation or, on rare occasions, use a body ventilator. Most often the patient continues nasal IPPV using decongestants.

Oronasal interfaces

Oronasal interfaces can have strap-retention systems like those for mouthpiece or nasal IPPV or can be strapless and retained by a bite-plate. Since effective ventilatory support can usually be provided by either nasal or mouthpiece/lipseal IPPV, oronasal interfaces have been used for long-term ventilatory assistance in few centres. They are being used more frequently in the intensive care setting.

Although mouthpiece and nasal IPPV are usually used as open systems and the user relies on central nervous system (CNS) reflexes to prevent excessive insufflation leakage during sleep, (11) essentially closed non-invasive IPPV systems include lipseal with nasal pledgets, strap-retained and strapless oronasal interfaces.

Interface choice

Patients should be offered a variety of interfaces and, to a large degree, allowed to choose. In a study that demonstrated no differences in tolerance to ventilation, blood gases or breathing patterns whether using assist control or pressure-assist modes, it was concluded that, irrespective of the underlying pathology, the type of interface affects the non-invasive ventilation outcomes more than the ventilatory mode (15).

Benefits

While non-invasive ventilation is often used for continuous long-term ventilatory support, the benefits derived from its part-time, usually nocturnal, use appear to be due to some combination of respiratory muscle rest, increasing tidal volumes, alveolar ventilation and blood gases, improving lung compliance and chemotaxic sensitivity, and possibly by improving ventilation/perfusion matching by reducing atelectasis and small airway closure.

DAYTIME INSPIRATORY MUSCLE AIDS

The intermittent abdominal pressure ventilator (IAPV) involves the intermittent inflation of an elastic air sac that is contained

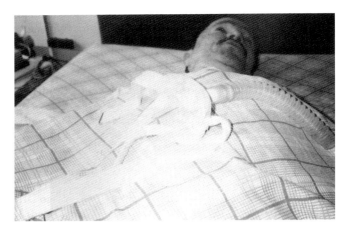

Figure 28.3 *The girdle of the intermittent abdominal pressure ventilator (IAPV) with the air sac connected to the tubing of a volume-cycled ventilator. This patient with no measurable vital capacity uses the IAPV for daytime ventilatory support.*

in a corset or belt worn beneath the patient's outer clothing (Fig. 28.3) (Exsufflation Belt, Respironics Inc., Murrysville, PA). The sac is cyclically inflated by a positive pressure ventilator. Bladder inflation moves the diaphragm upwards. During bladder deflation, gravity causes the abdominal contents and diaphragm to return to the resting position and inspiration occurs passively. A trunk angle of 30° or more from the horizontal is necessary for it to be effective. It requires a powerful ventilator (pump) to fill the air sac. Currently, the best portable pump on the market for this purpose appears to be the Achieva series (Tyco-Puritan-Bennett, Pleasanton, CA) (see Chapter 8). If patients have any inspiratory capacity or are capable of GPB, they can autonomously add volumes of air to those taken in mechanically. The IAPV generally augments tidal volumes by about 300 mL, but volumes as high as 1200 mL can be obtained (16). Patients with less than 1 h of breathing tolerance usually prefer to use the IAPV rather than non-invasive IPPV during daytime hours (16). The IAPV is less effective in the presence of scoliosis or obesity.

Mouthpiece IPPV

Mouthpiece IPPV is the most important method of daytime ventilatory support. Most commonly, simple, flexed mouthpieces are grabbed by the patient's lips and teeth for deep insufflations as needed (Fig. 28.1). Some patients keep the mouthpiece between their teeth all day. Most patients prefer to have the mouthpiece held near the mouth. A metal clamp attached to a wheelchair can be used for this purpose or the mouthpiece can be fixed onto motorized wheelchair controls, most often sip and puff, chin or tongue (Fig. 28.1) controls. The ventilator is set for large tidal volumes, often 1000–2000 mL. The patient grabs the mouthpiece with the mouth, thereby supplementing or substituting for inadequate autonomous breath volumes. Some patients prefer the comfort of custom orthotic mouthpieces (14). The patient varies the volume of air taken from ventilator cycle to ventilator cycle and breath to breath to vary tidal volume, speech volume and cough flows, as well as to air-stack to fully expand the lungs to maintain lung and chest wall compliance. To use mouthpiece IPPV effectively and conveniently, adequate neck rotation and oral motor function are necessary to grab the mouthpiece and receive IPPV without insufflation leakage. In addition, the patient must open the glottis and vocal cords, dilate the hypopharynx, and maintain airway patency to receive the air. These normally reflex movements may require a few minutes to re-learn for patients who have been receiving IPPV via an indwelling tube, especially one with an inflated cuff, because reflex abduction of the hypopharynx and glottis is lost during invasive IPPV. Often patients are thought to have tracheal stenosis or other reasons for upper airway obstruction before they learn to re-open the glottis to permit IPPV.

Since the low-pressure alarms of volume-cycled ventilators often cannot be turned off, to prevent their sounding during routine daytime IPPV when not every delivered volume is received by the patient, a flexed 15 mm mouthpiece (Fig. 28.1) for IPPV or an in-line regenerative humidifier can be used. These create 2–3 cmH$_2$O back pressure which is adequate to prevent low-pressure alarm sounding.

Nasal IPPV

Because patients prefer to use mouthpiece IPPV or the IAPV for daytime use, nasal IPPV is most practical only for nocturnal use. Daytime nasal ventilation, and usually high-span BiPAP since infants cannot air-stack, is indicated for infants and for those who cannot grab or retain a mouthpiece because of oral muscle weakness, inadequate jaw opening or insufficient neck movement. Twenty-four-hour nasal IPPV is a viable and desirable alternative to tracheostomy for some patients with severe lip and oropharyngeal muscle weakness (13).

WHY DOES NON-INVASIVE IPPV WORK DURING SLEEP FOR PEOPLE WITH NO BREATHING TOLERANCE?

Although most physicians continue mistakenly to think that intubation or tracheostomy is needed when patients have no ability to breathe, open systems of non-invasive IPPV have been used for continuous ventilatory support since 1964 by patients with little or no measurable VC or breathing tolerance. When using mouthpiece IPPV during sleep, why doesn't the insufflated air leak out of the nose to the extent that the patient asphyxiates? Likewise, when a patient with no inspiratory muscle function uses nasal IPPV, why doesn't too much air leak out of the mouth during sleep? 'Excessive oral leak (insufflation leakage) limiting the effectiveness of non-invasive IPPV was surprisingly uncommon' for patients with primarily neuromuscular ventilatory failure (13). However, the following have been described as required to effectively sustain long-term use of non-invasive IPPV for patients with little or no breathing tolerance: absence of a history of substance abuse, absence of acute pulmonary or intrinsic lung disease that warrants oxygen therapy, and absence of seizure activity (13). Narcotics, sedatives and oxygen administration depress ventilatory drive, leading the sleeping brain of patients with inspiratory muscle dysfunction to permit excessive insufflation leakage and hypercapnia (11, 17, 18). Seizure activity and post-ictal CNS depression also interfere with ventilatory drive,

with volitional access to a mouthpiece for non-invasive IPPV, and with the movements required to limit insufflation leakage during sleep (11). Indeed, apparently only users with no breathing tolerance and who either are under-ventilated during daytime hours, receive narcotics, sedatives, supplemental oxygen or consume excessive alcohol die from excessive insufflation leakage. All such deaths have in common the suppression of ventilatory drive.

COMPLICATIONS OF NON-INVASIVE IPPV AND BAROTRAUMA

Besides orthodontic deformities and skin pressure from the interface, other potential difficulties include allergy to the plastic lipseal or silicone interfaces (13 vs. 5 per cent for non-silicone interfaces), dry mouth (65 per cent), eye irritation from air leakage (about 24 per cent), nasal congestion (25 per cent) and dripping (35 per cent), sinusitis (8 per cent), nose bleeding (4–19 per cent), gum discomfort (20 per cent) and receding from nasal interface or lipseal pressure, maxillary flattening in children, aerophagia (19, 20) and, as for invasive ventilation, barotrauma. In addition, occasional patients express claustrophobia. Proper interface selection eliminates or minimizes discomfort. RoEzit™ is a petroleum-free moisturizer that can be applied to the nasal passages and to the face when skin becomes dry due to mask usage (LouSal Enterprises, Inc. www.roezit.com).

Pressure drop-off through the narrow air passages of the nose is normally between 2 and 3 cmH$_2$O. Suboptimal humidification dries out and irritates nasal mucus membranes, causes sore throat, and results in vasodilatation and nasal congestion. Increased airflow resistance to 8 cmH$_2$O can be caused by the loss of humidity due to unidirectional airflow with expiration via the mouth during nasal CPAP or IPPV (21). This problem cannot be ameliorated by using a cold passover humidifier but the increase in airway resistance can be reduced by 50 per cent by warming the inspired air to body temperature and humidifying it with the use of a hot water bath humidifier (21). Decongestants can also relieve sinus irritation and nasal congestion. Switching to lipseal IPPV can relieve most, if not all, difficulties associated with nasal IPPV. Lipseal IPPV also necessitates use of a hot water bath humidifier.

Abdominal distension tends to occur sporadically in non-invasive IPPV users. Normally the gastro-oesophageal sphincter can withstand peak airway pressures up to 25 cmH$_2$O without stomach dilatation. Aerophagia can occur when ventilator-delivered volumes meet with airway obstruction and this results in peak pressures over 25 cm H$_2$O. It may occur or be exacerbated when patients assume the supine position, especially when the patient reclines in the hour or so following meals (22). Gastric insufflation can often be decreased or eliminated by decreasing the inspiratory pressure delivery of pressure-cycled ventilators or by pressure-limiting volume-cycled ventilators, or at times by switching from one ventilator style to the other (23). If gastric insufflation persists, the air usually passes as flatus once the patient gets up or is placed into a wheelchair in the morning. When severe it can present as intestinal pseudo-obstruction with diminished bowel sounds and increased ventilator dependence. Although we have never had to discontinue non-invasive IPPV for any patient because of aerophagia first observed after beginning non-invasive ventilation, patients with aerophagia and severe abdominal distension before ever requiring ventilatory assistance will usually have the distension exacerbated by non-invasive IPPV, and for that reason will not tolerate it unless a gastrostomy tube is placed to alleviate the problem. Patients with lower intestinal distension may require colostomy or be better off with a tracheostomy.

Barotrauma is essentially volutrauma. It is lung damage due to over-expansion of lung units. It can occur with invasive or non-invasive ventilation. While its incidence has been cited as 4–15 per cent for ICU invasive ventilation users with primarily respiratory impairment (24), in 139 patients it has been reported to occur in 60 per cent of those with acute respiratory distress syndrome but was absent for those with heart failure or neurological disease (25).

It appears that high pressures might also present little or no risk if exposures are very short, as with air-stacking, and lung tissues essentially normal. We have had no barotrauma in hundreds of patients practising this technique at pressures of 40–70 cmH_2O. On the other hand, the risk of barotrauma is greatly increased by tissue fragility, secretion retention that leads to overexpansion of unobstructed lung units, and surfactant depletion (24).

Inspissated secretions are often considered a 'life-threatening' complication of non-invasive ventilation (26, 27). However, except for patients with ineffective assisted CPF less than 160 L/min and who have essentially respiratory rather than ventilatory impairment, secretion encumberment for patients with primarily ventilatory impairment is more a complication of the clinician's failure to teach assisted coughing than it is a complication of non-invasive ventilation. It might be recalled that there are 10^{12}–10^{17} bacteria/mL of saliva (28). Chronic aspiration of saliva to the extent of lowering baseline S_pO_2 can overwhelm normally sterile airways and lead to pneumonia (29), tracheitis, bronchitis (30) and chronic lung disease (31). Thus, the only respiratory indication for tracheostomy is assisted CPF less than 160 L/m and S_pO_2 baseline less than 95 per cent due to chronic airway secretion aspiration (32).

Goal 3: facilitate airway clearance

FACILITATION OF PERIPHERAL MUCUS CLEARANCE

Approaches to preventing peripheral airway secretion retention for patients with NMD include the use of medications to reduce mucus hypersecretion or to liquefy secretions, and facilitation of mucus mobilization. The latter can include manual or mechanical chest percussion or vibration, direct oscillation of the air column and postural drainage. The goal is to transport mucus from the peripheral to the central airways from where it can more easily be eliminated by assisted coughing and mechanical insufflation-exsufflation (MIE). Use of chest vibrators, such as the Jeannie Rub Percussor (Morfan Inc., Mishawaka,

IN) (Fig. 28.4) or Neo-Cussor (General Physical Therapy, St Louis, MO), may be the most practical and effective method of chest percussion. They vibrate the chest at optimal frequencies. They are small, light, very easy to use and inexpensive.

FACILITATION OF CENTRAL AIRWAY CLEARANCE BY PROVIDING FUNCTIONAL COUGHS BY ASSISTING EXPIRATORY MUSCLES

Manually assisted coughing

The importance of the use of manually assisted coughing to permit effective long-term use of non-invasive ventilation is being increasingly recognized by NMD clinic physicians and others (Fig. 28.5) (33, 34). CPF are increased by manually assisted coughing (35). If the VC is under 1.5 L, insufflating the patient to the MIC is especially important to optimize cough flows (36). Once the patient takes a breath to at least 1.5 L, maximally air-stacks or is maximally insufflated, an abdominal thrust is timed to glottic opening as the patient initiates the cough. It was recognized as early as 1966 that assisted CPF could be doubled and readily exceed 6 L/s in patients receiving

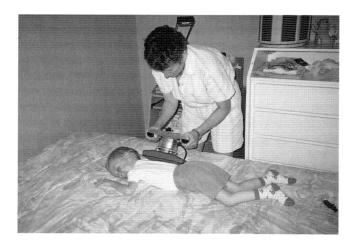

Figure 28.4 *A 7-year-old with spinal muscular atrophy type 2 using a portable chest vibrator to mobilize airway secretions.*

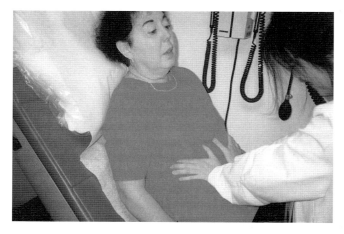

Figure 28.5 *Hand placement (below the rib cage) for manual cough assist.*

maximal insufflations prior to manual thrusts (37). In 364 evaluations of our NMD patients able to air-stack, the mean VC in the sitting position was 996.9 mL, the mean MIC was 1647.6 mL, and while CPF were 2.3 L/s (<2.7 L/s or the minimum needed to eliminate airway secretions) mean assisted CPF were 3.9 L/s.

Although an optimal insufflation followed by an abdominal thrust provides the greatest increase in CPF, this can also be significantly increased by providing only a maximal insufflation or providing only an abdominal thrust without a preceding maximal insufflation. Interestingly, CPF are increased significantly more by the maximal insufflation than by the abdominal thrust. In data from Dr Ishikawa's centre in Hokkaido, 21 DMD patients had unassisted CPF of 160 ± 88 L/min, CPF with an abdominal thrust of 242 ± 92 L/min, CPF from the MIC of 274 ± 80 L/min, and CPF from the MIC with an abdominal thrust (assisted CPF) of 356 ± 88 L/min (personal communication).

Techniques of manually assisted coughing involve different hand and arm placements for expiratory cycle thrusts. An epigastric thrust with one hand while applying counterpressure across the chest to avoid paradoxical chest expansion with the other arm and hand further increases assisted CPF for 20 per cent of patients (36).

Manually assisted coughing requires a cooperative patient, good coordination between the patient and care-giver, and adequate physical effort and often frequent application by the care-giver. It is usually ineffective in the presence of severe scoliosis because of a combination of restricted lung capacity and the inability to effect diaphragm movement by abdominal thrusting because of severe rib cage and diaphragm deformity.

Abdominal compressions should not be used aggressively for 1–1.5 h following a meal; however, chest compressions can be used to augment CPF. Chest thrusting techniques must be performed with caution in the presence of an osteoporotic rib cage.

Unfortunately, since it is not widely taught to health care professionals (38), manually assisted coughing is under-utilized (39). When inadequate, and especially when inadequacy is due to difficult air-stacking, the most effective alternative for generating optimal CPF and clearing airway secretions is the use of MIE.

The inability to generate over 2.7 L/s or 160 L/min of assisted CPF despite having a VC or MIC greater than 1 L usually indicates fixed upper airway obstruction or severe bulbar muscle weakness and hypopharyngeal collapse during coughing attempts. Vocal cord adhesions or paralysis may have resulted from a previous translaryngeal intubation or tracheostomy (40). Since some lesions, especially the presence of obstructing granulation tissue, can be corrected surgically, laryngoscopic examination is warranted.

MECHANICAL INSUFFLATION–EXSUFFLATION

Mechanical insufflator-exsufflators (Cough-Assist, JH Emerson Co., Cambridge, MA) (Fig. 28.6) deliver deep insufflations followed immediately by deep exsufflations. The insufflation and exsufflation pressures and delivery times are independently adjustable. Insufflation to exsufflation pressures of +40 to −40 cmH$_2$O delivered via oronasal interface or normal adult tracheostomy tubes are usually the most effective and preferred by most patients. Lungs are insufflated until fully expanded and then immediately exsufflated until the lungs are fully emptied and the chest wall retracted. Normal cough and exsufflation volumes exceed 2 L in adults. The combination of MIE with an abdominal thrust is a mechanically assisted cough (MAC). Mechanical in-exsufflation can be provided via an oronasal mask, a simple mouthpiece, or a translaryngeal or tracheostomy tube. When delivered via the latter, the cuff, when present, should be inflated.

The Cough-Assist can be manually or automatically cycled. Manual cycling facilitates care-giver–patient coordination of inspiration and expiration with insufflation and exsufflation, respectively, but it requires hands to deliver an abdominal thrust, to hold the mask on the patient, and to cycle the machine.

One treatment consists of about five cycles of MIE or MAC followed by a short period of normal breathing or ventilator use to avoid hyperventilation. While insufflation and exsufflation pressures when used via the upper airway are almost always from +35 to +60 cmH$_2$O to −35 to −60 cmH$_2$O, it must be kept in mind that the goal is for rapid maximal chest expansion followed immediately by rapid lung emptying, both in about 2–3 s. Thus, the use of MIE via narrow-gauge tubes may necessitate the application of pressures to 70 cmH$_2$O until the endpoints are clinically observed. Most patients use 35–45 cmH$_2$O pressures for insufflations and exsufflations via the upper airway or via wide-gauge adult size tracheostomy or translaryngeal tubes. In experimental models, +40 to −40 cmH$_2$O

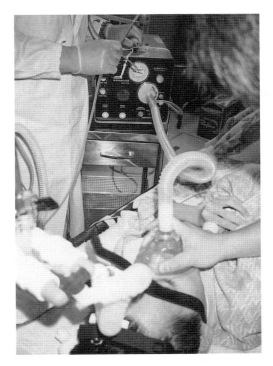

Figure 28.6   *Patient using mechanical insufflation-exsufflation (Cough-Assist™) via an oronasal interface.*

pressures have been shown to provide maximum forced defla-tion VCs and flows (41).

Multiple treatments are given in one sitting until no further secretions are expulsed and any secretion or mucus-induced dS_pO_2s are reversed. Use can be required as frequently as every few minutes around the clock during chest infections. Although no medications are usually required for effective MIE in neuro-muscular ventilator users, liquefaction of sputum using heated aerosol treatments may facilitate exsufflation when secretions are inspissated.

We routinely use MIE via oronasal interfaces (especially in the immediate post-extubation period for respiratory failure) or via translaryngeal and tracheostomy tubes in children with SMA under 1 year of age. For infants and others who use MIE via narrow-gauge paediatric tubes, even the maximum flow–pressure capabilities of the Cough-Assist are often inadequate to rapidly expand and empty the lungs. The severe pressure–flow drop-off across the narrow tubes greatly diminishes the efficacy of MIE for expelling airway secretions and more powerful units need to be developed for use through narrow tubes. The import-ance of using the Cough-Assist for the regular provision of full chest expansion should not be underestimated.

Whether via the upper airway or via indwelling airway tubes, routine airway suctioning misses the left main stem bronchus about 90 per cent of the time. MIE, on the other hand, pro-vides the same exsufflation flows in both left and right airways without the discomfort or airway trauma of tracheal suctioning and it can be effective when suctioning is not. Patients almost invariably prefer MIE to suctioning for comfort and effective-ness and they find it less tiring (42).

Indications for MIE

Since MIE has only been on the market since February 1993, there continues to be misinformation and confusion regarding its indications. Of the three muscle groups required for effect-ive coughing, MIE can only take the place of the inspiratory and expiratory muscles. Thus, it cannot be used to avert trache-ostomy for very long if bulbar function is inadequate to prevent airway collapse, as is often the case in advanced bul-bar ALS. On the other hand, patients with completely intact bulbar muscle function, such as most ventilator users with traumatic tetraplegia, can usually air-stack to volumes of 3 L or more and, unless very scoliotic or obese, a properly delivered abdominal thrust can often result in assisted CPF of 6–9 L/s. These flows should be more than adequate to clear the air-ways and prevent pneumonia and respiratory failure without the need for MIE. Thus, the patients who need MIE the most are those whose bulbar muscle function can maintain adequate airway patency but is insufficient to permit optimal air-stacking for assisted CPF over 250–300 L/min. This is typical of most patients with NMD except for those with no measur-able CPF due to bulbar ALS/MND (motor neuron disease). The most typical examples of patients who can consistently avoid hospitalization and respiratory failure by using MIE during intercurrent chest infections are DMD patients. Patients with respiratory muscle weakness complicated by scoliosis and inability to capture the asymmetric diaphragm by abdominal

thrusting also greatly benefit from MIE. A recent study of 21 SMA, DMD, post-polio and congenital muscular dystrophy patients confirmed an earlier study (36), which demonstrated a significantly greater increase in cough flows by MIE in com-parison with unassisted coughing, manually assisted cough-ing, and coughing following chest physiotherapy or with use of non-invasive IPPV alone (43).

Efficacy of MIE

The efficacy of MIE was demonstrated both clinically and on animal models (44). Flow generation can be adequate in both proximal and distal airways to effectively eliminate respiratory tract debris (45, 46). VC, pulmonary flow rates, and S_pO_2 when abnormal, improve immediately with clearing of airway secre-tions and mucus by MIE (38, 47). An increase in VC of 15–42 per cent was noted immediately following treatment in 67 patients with 'obstructive dyspnoea', and a 55 per cent increase in VC was noted following MIE in patients with NMDs (48). We have observed 15–400 per cent (200–800 mL) improve-ments in VC and normalization of S_pO_2 as MIE eliminates air-way mucus for ventilator-assisted NMD patients during chest infections (36).

No serious complications of the use of MIE have ever been reported, despite thousands of applications for hundreds of patients mostly with neuromuscular weakness, many of whom have regularly used MIE for over 50 years, either with the Cof-flators, available since 1952, or with the in-exsufflators that came onto the market in February 1993. Interestingly, prior to 1993, patients unable to procure Cof-flators often air-stacked then used their vacuum cleaners for exsufflation. We have a number of patients who have depended on continuous non-invasive IPPV at inspiratory positive airway pressures of over 40 cmH_2O for over 45 years. Thus, the use of equivalent pres-sures for brief periods of MIE would be very unlikely to cause any harm. A recent study using these pressures on baby mon-keys also demonstrated no barotrauma (49). The use of high insufflation pressures can cause acute rib cage muscle pulls for patients with low VCs, especially those with severe scoliosis who have not routinely been receiving maximal insufflations. Insufflation pressures are increased gradually for these patients.

THE OXIMETRY FEEDBACK RESPIRATORY AID PROTOCOL

Since supplemental oxygen is avoided for NMD patients in order to avoid exacerbation of hypercapnia and to facilitate use of oximetry, the patient and care providers are instructed that, once artifacts are ruled out (32), S_pO_2 <95 per cent is due to one of three causes: hypercapnia (hypoventilation), airway encumberment (secretions), and, if these are not man-aged properly, intrinsic lung disease, usually gross atelectasis or pneumonia. The oximetry respiratory muscle aid protocol consists of using an oximeter for feedback to maintain S_pO_2 greater than 94 per cent by maintaining effective alveolar ven-tilation and airway secretion elimination.

The protocol is most important during respiratory tract infections and when extubating patients with little or no breathing tolerance. Because respiratory muscles are weakened and bronchial secretions are profuse during chest infections and post-surgical general anaesthesia, patients often need to use non-invasive IPPV continuously at these times both to maintain alveolar ventilation and for air-stacking to increase CPF. If, when using non-invasive IPPV at adequate delivered volumes, the S_pO_2 is not above 94 per cent, the desaturation is not due to hypoventilation but to airway mucus accumulation. Indeed, sudden dS_pO_2s for ventilator users during chest infections are almost always due to mucus accumulation. Manually assisted coughing with air-stacking as needed and MAC are then used until the mucus is expulsed and S_pO_2 returns to normal or to baseline levels.

If the baseline S_pO_2 decreases and remains below 95 per cent despite ventilatory support and MAC, patients then present for a formal evaluation. A clear radiograph in the presence of a baseline S_pO_2 of 92–94 per cent often denotes microscopic atelectasis. Radiographic evidence of pneumonia accompanied by dS_pO_2 and ventilator dependence warrants admission and, when there is respiratory distress, possible intubation. Despite hyperpyrexia and elevated white blood cell counts, baseline S_pO_2 to 92 per cent often returns to normal and hospitalization can be avoided when patients use respiratory muscle aids with oximetry feedback (47). As the S_pO_2 baseline returns to normal, most patients gradually wean to nocturnal-only non-invasive IPPV or, at times, to no daily use of respiratory muscle aids until the next chest infection.

In the event of hospitalization, the patient's primary care providers are asked to continue to use MAC with oximetry feedback to eliminate airway secretions and avoid intubation. This is done because we have found it impossible to expect nursing and respiratory therapy staff to do this as often as needed either to avoid intubation, during intubation or post-extubation. It is most practical and efficacious to let the family and care providers administer the respiratory muscle aids up to every 5 min if necessary to expulse secretions and return S_pO_2 to normal, even when the patient is in intensive care. Overnight, provided that sedatives, narcotics and oxygen therapy are avoided, heavy mucus accumulation will arouse patients and they will request MAC. The family or primary care providers quickly learn that, since they are doing most of the work anyway, the patients can most often be best and most safely cared for at home as long as baseline S_pO_2 remains greater than 94 per cent.

NON-INVASIVE vs. TRACHEOSTOMY

Non-invasive respiratory muscle aids are most effective for patients with sufficient oropharyngeal muscle function to speak. Both inspiratory and expiratory muscle aids are usually necessary to avoid pulmonary complications, intubation and tracheostomy, and prolong survival (32, 35, 50). Non-invasive IPPV is also overwhelmingly preferred over tracheostomy for speech, sleep, swallowing, comfort, appearance, security, use

of GPB, and overall (42). Another study demonstrated 200 per cent cost savings by using non-invasive ventilatory support methods for patients with no ventilator-free time by facilitating community placement with personal care attendants rather than nursing care or long-term institutionalization (51). As noted, infants with NMD, in particular those with SMA type 1 who undergo tracheostomy, lose all ability to breathe unaided and do not develop the ability to speak, whereas infants with the same disease severity who are maintained by non-invasive methods require only nocturnal high-span BiPAP and usually develop the ability to verbalize (35). Despite the benefits of non-invasive interventions, such aids continue to be used in few centres and few clinicians are familiar with all the techniques available (33). As the difficulties in invasive endotracheal approaches become increasingly appreciated and patient preferences are taken into account, interest in exploring non-invasive alternatives can only increase.

GLOSSOPHARYNGEAL BREATHING

Both inspiratory and, indirectly, expiratory muscle activity can be assisted by GPB (9). This technique involves the glottis capturing air and propelling it downwards into the lungs with every 'gulp'. One breath usually consists of six to nine gulps of 60–100 mL each. During the training period the efficiency of GPB can be monitored by spirometrically measuring the mL of air per gulp, gulps per breath, and breaths/min. Excellent instructional material is available (52).

GPB can provide an individual with weak inspiratory muscles and little or no measurable VC or ventilator-free breathing time with normal lung ventilation for hours and perfect safety when not using a ventilator or in the event of ventilator failure day or night (9). Although potentially extremely useful, GPB is rarely taught since there are few health care professionals familiar with the technique. GPB is also rarely useful in the presence of an indwelling tracheostomy tube. It cannot be used when the tube is uncapped, as it is during tracheostomy IPPV, and even when capped, the gulped air tends to leak around the outer walls of the tube and out of the tracheostomy site as airway volumes and pressures increase during the air-stacking process of GPB. The safety and versatility afforded by effective GPB are key reasons to eliminate tracheostomy in favour of non-invasive aids.

Key points

● Three respiratory muscle groups must be considered: the inspiratory, expiratory, and bulbar muscles. While the inspiratory and expiratory muscles can almost always be assisted, supported or substituted for without resort to tracheostomy, once bulbar muscle dysfunction results in irreversible decrease in baseline oxyhaemoglobin saturation (S_pO_2), tracheostomy becomes necessary to prolong survival.

- The most objective measure of bulbar muscle function for patients with neuromuscular disease is the maximum insufflation capacity, vital capacity difference and the extent of assisted peak cough flows.
- Non-invasive ventilation and insufflation-exsufflation are preferred by patients and care providers over tracheostromy for speech, sleep, swallowing, comfort, appearance, safety, use of glossopharyngeal breathing, and overall.
- No one having S_pO_2 greater than 94 per cent in ambient air can develop respiratory failure, and S_pO_2 can be kept greater than 94 per cent by non-invasive ventilation and mechanically assisted coughing for neuromuscular disease patients other than those with bulbar amyotrophic lateral sclerosis and inability to 'air stack'.
- Outpatient and intensive care protocols that employ oximetry as feedback for use of non-invasive ventilation and assisted coughing can permit greatly prolonged survival without resort to tracheostomy for all except bulbar ALS patients.

REFERENCES

1. Kraft GH. Multiple sclerosis: future directions in the care and the cure. *J Neurol Rehabil* 1989; **3**: 61–4.
2. Bach JR, ed. *Noninvasive Mechanical Ventilation*. Philadelphia: Hanley & Belfus, 2002.
3. Emery AEH. Duchenne muscular dystrophy: genetic aspects, carrier detection and antenatal diagnosis. *Br Med Bull* 1980; **36**: 117–22.
4. Rideau Y, Gatin G, Bach J, Gines G. Prolongation of life in Duchenne muscular dystrophy. *Acta Neurol* 1983; **5**: 118–24.
5. Dubowitz V. Very severe spinal muscular atrophy (SMA type 0): an expanding clinical phenotype. *Eur J Paediatr Neurol* 1999; **3**: 49–51.
6. Norris F, Shepherd R, Denys E. Natural history and outcome in idiopathic adult motor neuron disease. *J Neurol Sci* 1993; **118**: 48–55.
7. Cazzoli PA. The use of noninvasive and tracheostomy positive pressure ventilation in amyotrophic lateral sclerosis survival, long-term outcomes, factors for success and failure, and quality of life. *8th Journées Internationales de Ventilation a Domicile (abstract 120), March 7, 2001, Hôpital de la Croix-Rousse, Lyon, France.*
8. *Conference on Respiratory Problems in Poliomyelitis, March 12–14 1952, Ann Arbor, National Foundation for Infantile Paralysis –* March of Dimes, White Plains, NY.
9. Bach JR, Alba AS, Bodofsky E *et al.* Glossopharyngeal breathing and non-invasive aids in the management of post-polio respiratory insufficiency. *Birth Defects* 1987; **23**: 99–113.
●10. Kang SW, Bach JR. Maximum insufflation capacity. *Chest* 2000; **118**: 61–5.
11. Bach JR. Noninvasive ventilation: mechanisms for inspiratory muscle substitution. In: Bach JR, ed. *Noninvasive Mechanical Ventilation*. Philadelphia: Hanley & Belfus, 2002; 83–102.
●12. Bach JR, Alba AS, Saporito LR. Intermittent positive pressure ventilation via the mouth as an alternative to tracheostomy for 257 ventilator users. *Chest* 1993; **103**: 174–82.
●13. Bach JR, Alba AS. Management of chronic alveolar hypoventilation by nasal ventilation. *Chest* 1990; **97**: 52–7.
14. Bach JR. Noninvasive respiratory muscle aids and intervention goals. In: Bach JR, ed. *Noninvasive Mechanical Ventilation*. Philadelphia: Hanley & Belfus, 2002; 129–64.
15. Navalesi P, Fanfulla F, Frigerio P *et al.* Physiologic evaluation of noninvasive mechanical ventilation delivered with three types of masks in patients with chronic hypercapnic respiratory failure. *Crit Care Med* 2000; **28**: 1785–90.
●16. Bach JR, Alba AS. Total ventilatory support by the intermittent abdominal pressure ventilator. *Chest* 1991; **99**: 630–6.
●17. Bach JR. Alternative methods of ventilatory support for the patient with ventilatory failure due to spinal cord injury. *J Am Paraplegia Soc* 1991; **14**: 158–74.
●18. Bach JR, Robert D, Leger P, Langevin B. Sleep fragmentation in kyphoscoliotic individuals with alveolar hypoventilation treated by nasal IPPV. *Chest* 1995; **107**: 1552–8.
19. Leger SS, Leger P. The art of interface: tools for administering noninvasive ventilation. *Med Klin* 1999; **94**: 35–9.
20. Pepin JL, Leger P, Veale D. Side effects of nasal continuous positive airway pressure in sleep apnea syndrome. Study of 193 patients in two French sleep centers. *Chest* 1995; **107**: 375–81.
21. Richards GN, Cistulli PA, Gunnar UR *et al.* Mouth leak with nasal continuous positive airway pressure increases nasal airway resistance. *Am J Respir Crit Care Med* 1996; **154**: 182–6.
22. Yamada S, Nishimiya J, Kurokawa K *et al.* Bilevel nasal positive airway pressure and ballooning of the stomach. *Chest* 2001; **119**: 1965–6.
23. Diaz Lobato S, Garcia-Tejero MT, Ruiz-Cobos A, Villasante C. Changing ventilator: an option to take into account in the treatment of persistent vomiting during nasal ventilation. *Respiration* 1998; **65**: 481–2.
24. Marcy TW. Barotrauma: detection, recognition, and management. *Chest* 1993; **104**: 578–84.
25. Gammon RB, Shin MS, Buchalter SE. Pulmonary barotrauma in mechanical ventilation. *Chest* 1992; **102**: 568–72.
26. Wood KE, Flaten AL, Backes WJ. Inspissated secretions: a life-threatening complication of prolonged noninvasive ventilation. *Respir Care* 2000; **45**: 491–3.
27. Hill NS. Complications of noninvasive ventilation. *Respir Care* 2000; **45**: 480–1.
28. Laraya-Cuasay L, Mikkilimeni S. Respiratory conditions and care. In: Rosenthal SR, Sheppard JJ, Lotze M, eds. *Dysphagia and the Child with Developmental Disabilities*. San Diego: Singular Publishing, 1995; 227–52.
29. Arvedson J, Rogers B, Buck G *et al.* Silent aspiration prominent in children with dysphagia. *Int J Pediatr Otorhinolaryngol* 1994; **28**: 173–81.
30. Loughlin GM. Respiratory consequences of dysfunctional swallowing and aspiration. *Dysphagia* 1989; **3**: 126–30.
31. Hess DR. The evidence for secretion clearance techniques. *Respir Care* 2001; **46**: 1276–92.
●32. Bach JR. Amyotrophic lateral sclerosis: prolongation of life by noninvasive respiratory aids. *Chest* 2002; **122**: 92–8.
33. Chaudhry SS, Bach JR. Management approaches in muscular dystrophy association clinics. *Am J Phys Med Rehabil* 2000; **79**: 193–6.
34. Ishikawa Y, Ishikawa Y, Minami R. The effect of nasal IPPV on patients with respiratory failure during sleep due to Duchenne muscular dystrophy. *Clin Neurol* 1993; **33**: 856–61.

●35. Bach JR, Baird JS, Plosky D *et al*. Spinal muscular atrophy type 1: management and outcomes. *Pediatr Pulmonol* 2002; **34**: 16–22.

36. Bach JR. Mechanical insufflation-exsufflation: comparison of peak expiratory flows with manually assisted and unassisted coughing techniques. *Chest* 1993; **104**: 1553–62.

37. Kirby NA, Barnerias MJ, Siebens AA. An evaluation of assisted cough in quadriparetic patients. *Arch Phys Med Rehabil* 1966; **47**: 705–10.

38. Bach JR, Smith WH, Michaels J *et al*. Airway secretion clearance by mechanical exsufflation for post-poliomyelitis ventilator assisted individuals. *Arch Phys Med Rehabil* 1993; **74**: 170–7.

39. Sortor S, McKenzie M. *Toward Independence: Assisted Cough* (video). Bioscience Communications of Dallas Inc, 1986.

40. Richard I, Giraud M, Perrouin-Verbe B. Laryngo-tracheal stenosis after intubation or tracheostomy in neurological patients. *Arch Phys Med Rehabil* 1996; **77**: 493–7.

41. Newth CJL, Asmler B, Anderson GP, Morley J. The effects of varying inflation and deflation pressures on the maximal expiratory deflation flow-volume relationship in anesthetized Rhesus monkeys. *Am Rev Respir Dis* 1991; **144**: 807–13.

42. Garstang SV, Kirshblum SC, Wood KE. Patient preference for in-exsufflation for secretion management with spinal cord injury. *J Spinal Cord Med* 2000; **23**: 80–5.

43. Chatwin M, Ross E, Hart N *et al*. Cough augmentation with mechanical insufflation/exsufflation in patients with neuromuscular weakness. *Eur Respir J* 2003; **21**: 502–8.

44. Bickerman HA. Exsufflation with negative pressure: elimination of radiopaque material and foreign bodies from bronchi of anesthetized dogs. *Arch Int Med* 1954; **93**: 698–704.

45. Leiner GC, Abramowitz S, Small MJ *et al*. Expiratory peak flow rate. Standard values for normal subjects. *Am Rev Respir Dis* 1963; **88**: 644.

46. Siebens AA, Kirby NA, Poulos DA. Cough following transection of spinal cord at C-6. *Arch Phys Med Rehabil* 1964; **45**: 1–8.

47. Bach JR, Ishikawa Y, Kim H. Prevention of pulmonary morbidity for patients with Duchenne muscular dystrophy. *Chest* 1997; **112**: 1024–8.

48. Barach AL, Beck GJ. Exsufflation with negative pressure. physiologic and clinical studies in poliomyelitis, bronchial asthma, pulmonary emphysema and bronchiectasis. *Arch Int Med* 1954; **93**: 825–41.

●49. Gomez-Merino E, Bach JR. Duchenne muscular dystrophy: prolongation of life by noninvasive respiratory muscle aids. *Am J Phys Med Rehabil* 2002; **81**: 411–15.

50. Bach JR, Intintola P, Alba AS, Holland I. The ventilator individual: cost analysis of institutionalization versus rehabilitation and in-home management. *Chest* 1992; **101**: 26–30.

51. Dail CW, Affeldt JE. *Glossopharyngeal Breathing* (video). Los Angeles: Department of Visual Education, College of Medical Evangelists, 1954.

52. Dail C, Rodgers M, Guess V, Adkins HV. *Glossopharyngeal Breathing Manual*. Downey, CA: Professional Staff Association of Rancho Los Amigos Hospital Inc, 1979.

29

Rehabilitation of patients with cystic fibrosis

MARGARET E. HODSON, KHIN M. GYI, SARAH L. ELKIN

INTRODUCTION

Rehabilitation has been defined as the development of the individual to the fullest physical, psychological, social, vocational, avocational and educational potential, consistent with his or her physiological or anatomical impairment and environmental limitations. Rehabilitation programmes include early recognition, in-patient, outpatient and extended care. The anticipated patient outcomes of a comprehensive, integrated rehabilitation programme include increased independence, fewer hospitalizations or shorter lengths of stay and improved quality of life (1). The whole of modern cystic fibrosis (CF) care could be included in this definition of rehabilitation. The dedication of a multidisciplinary team is essential. In the context of CF the key disciplines are shown in Box 29.1.

Box 29.1 Multidisciplinary skills for the comprehensive management of patients with cystic fibrosis (core team)

- Physician (paediatric or adult)
- Clinical nurse specialist
- Home care nurse
- Physiotherapist
- Dietician
- Social worker
- Occupational therapist
- Respiratory therapist
- Pharmacist
- Spiritual advisor
- Psychologist
- Educational advisor

Various organizations have defined staffing levels, appropriate for different patient numbers and ages (2). If good care and quality of life are to be obtained, a clear understanding of the disease, available treatments and the role of the multidisciplinary team, are essential.

CYSTIC FIBROSIS

Cystic fibrosis is the most common lethal inherited condition in the Caucasian population. It is inherited as a Mendelian recessive gene and 1 in 25 of the population are carriers. It therefore affects about 1 in 2500 births. Although it is a multisystem disease, it affects mainly the respiratory and alimentary systems.

Epidemiology

Cystic fibrosis used to be a disease of children but with improved care there are now almost as many patients over 16 years old as there are children. In 1938, 70 per cent of babies with CF died within the first year of life (3). Survival to over 30 years is now reported from many countries (Fig. 29.1). The estimated survival for patients born in 2000 is over 40 years (4). The improved survival is probably due to rising living standards, specialist centres, improved methods of physiotherapy, new antibiotics and improved nutrition (5). With improved survival, good quality of care needs to be available for paediatric and adult patients. This can best be provided by a multidisciplinary team (6–8).

Pathology

Cystic fibrosis is caused by a mutation in the CF transmembrane conductance regulator (CFTR) gene, situated on

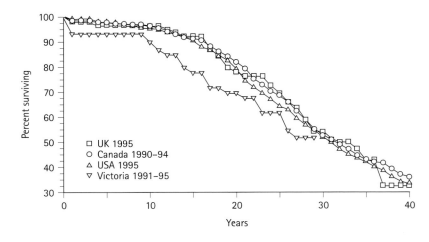

Figure 29.1 *Percentage of surviving cystic fibrosis patients from different countries. Reproduced with permission from Lewis (87).*

chromosome 7. Over 1000 mutations have been identified in that gene (9–11). The most common, affecting about 70 per cent of the patients in Western Europe and North America, is the phenylalanine deletion of amino acid position 508. This abnormality affects epithelial cells, which influence the transport of ions and water mainly in the respiratory, gastrointestinal, hepatobiliary and reproductive tracts. This leads to relative dehydration of the airway. Mutations in CFTR also lead to increased bacterial adherence in the airway (12). Both these factors result in increased airway infections. The major cause of morbidity and mortality is respiratory disease (13).

Microbiology

The bacteria most commonly isolated from the sputum of patients with CF are *Pseudomonas aeruginosa*, *Staphylococcus aureus* and *Haemophilus influenzae* (13). *Burkholderia cepacia* and *Stenotrophomonas maltophilia* have become a concern in recent years (14). Some patients are colonized with *Aspergillus fumigatus* and non-tuberculous mycobacteria. Others are infected with organisms such as mycobacterium tuberculosis. There is increasing colonization with methicillin-resistant *Staphylococcus aureus* (MRSA) (15). Viral and mycoplasma infection are also associated with exacerbations of pulmonary disease.

Cross-infection

Pseudomonas aeruginosa and *B. cepacia* are found in the environment, although there is some evidence of occasional patient-to-patient transfer. In view of this, good hygiene should be practised (16) not only to reduce the risks of cross-infection but also for the patient's peace of mind.

PRESENTATION

Some infants present at birth with meconium ileus, but the majority are diagnosed in infancy with failure to thrive,

malabsorption or chest infections, with up to 10 per cent being diagnosed after 16 years of age. The clinical diagnosis is based on the presence of one or more characteristic phenotypic features, a history of CF, an affected sibling or a positive sweat test, plus laboratory evidence of CFTR abnormalities, as documented by an elevated sweat chloride concentration, or identification of two known CF mutations (17).

PREVENTION

Genetic screening should be offered to all family members of a CF patient who are of reproductive age. There is increasing evidence that early diagnosis and institution of treatment may improve survival. Early diagnosis at least allows the parents to make reproductive choices about future pregnancies (18).

TREATMENT

Pulmonary rehabilitation

There is a growing consensus among CF care workers, that exercise training programmes have a therapeutic role by increasing exercise capacity, reducing breathlessness and enhancing sputum clearance (19, 20). Bilton *et al.* (19) compared the impact of exercise, physiotherapy and combinations of exercise and physiotherapy on sputum expectoration. Treatments that included physiotherapy produced a significantly higher sputum weight than exercise alone. However, the treatment option most preferred by patients was exercise followed by physiotherapy (Fig. 29.2), which the authors concluded should be the recommended daily regimen. Although the exact role of pulmonary rehabilitation for patients with cystic fibrosis remains to be defined, it seems logical that pulmonary rehabilitation programmes could also benefit this patient group, given their effectiveness in the management of severe dyspnoea, reduced exercise tolerance and multiple hospitalizations. Programmes might also influence pulmonary function, nutrition and peak oxygen consumption, all of

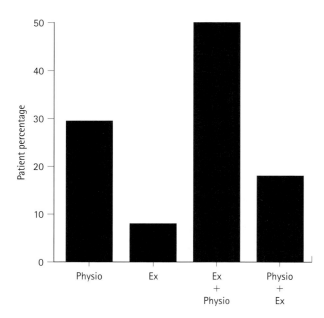

Figure 29.2   *Treatment modalities preferred by patients (n = 18) (19). Ex, exercise; Physio, physiotherapy.*

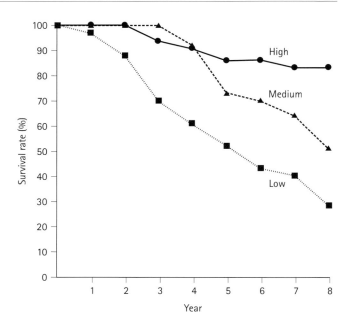

Figure 29.3   *Survival in 109 cystic fibrosis patients according to fitness level (22).*

which are associated with a better prognosis in CF. However, to date, research has concentrated on the benefits of exercise for CF patients, with little published evidence regarding the efficacy of a full pulmonary rehabilitation programme.

REASONS WHY PULMONARY REHABILITATION MIGHT BENEFIT PATIENTS WITH CF

Improved airways clearance (19).

Improved exercise capacity (21). Ten adolescent CF patients aged 21 ± 6.5 years underwent home exercise training for 3 months, consisting of daily, constant power, submaximal cycle exercise. After training there were significant improvements in maximal exercise capacity (W_{max} = 126 ± 10 W before and 146 ± 11 W after, P = 0.004), maximal oxygen uptake ($\dot{V}_{O_2,max}$ = 31.4 ± 2.1 mL/kg per min before and 36.5 ± 2.5 mL/kg per min after, P = 0.008), and degree of limitation in activities of daily living. Exercise capacity has been found to be an independent determinant of prognosis in patients with CF (22). In a prospective study of 109 CF patients, those with the highest levels of aerobic fitness ($\dot{V}_{O_2,max}$ >82 per cent of predicted) had a survival rate of 83 per cent at 8 years, compared with 51 and 28 per cent, respectively, for patients with middle ($\dot{V}_{O_2,max}$ = 59–81 per cent predicted) and lowest levels ($\dot{V}_{O_2,max}$ <59 per cent predicted), respectively. After adjustment for other risk factors, patients with higher levels of fitness were more than three times as likely to survive than were patients with lower levels of fitness. Although better aerobic fitness may just be a marker of disease severity, measurement of $\dot{V}_{O_2,max}$ may be valuable for predicting prognosis (Fig. 29.3). Studies in CF patients have shown activity programmes to improve exercise capacity due to a training effect on skeletal muscles, resulting in increased endurance time and increased cardiovascular fitness as well as reduced breathlessness (23).

Increased muscle mass and strength. A general exercise programme can be used to train peripheral muscles. Strauss *et al.* (24) noted that in 12 adolescent CF patients with moderately severe disease, 6 months of variable-weight training was associated with a significant increase in weight (>2.88 kg, P < 0.02), muscle size (1.6–1.8 cm upper arm, P < 0.01) and strength (increase from 16–32 muscle groups at normal strength, P < 0.05). Even moderately ill CF patients could engage in variable-weight training, resulting in desired weight gains and improvements in strength (24).

Enhanced coping mechanisms. The psychosocial support that is part of a comprehensive pulmonary rehabilitation programme may help certain patients and their families, with stress management, issues of sexuality and end-of-life issues.

Correct physiotherapy techniques, for chest drainage and exercise endurance.

Education of patients and families, regarding the underlying condition, indications and side-effects of medications, management of exacerbations and other components of the disease.

Maintenance of bone density. Published reports of low bone density occurring in both children and adults with CF (25–28) have led to recommendations of weight-bearing and impact exercises for promotion and maintenance of bone density. Lack of exercise is one of the causal negative factors, and activity is a positive factor for bone accretion and retention (29).

Promotion of adequate nutrition. Nutritional deficiencies contribute to the reduction in exercise capacity and respiratory muscle strength (30). High-calorie meals and compliance with pancreatic supplementation are a part of the rehabilitative approach.

An improved sense of well-being. A rehabilitative environment, together with exercise, education and psychological and social support, is associated with improved self-esteem, self-efficacy and health-related quality of life. Although some patients with CF have co-morbidities, such as severe hepatic dysfunction, that may contraindicate exercise training, and although some patients may lack motivation, rehabilitation is often possible even when the disease is advanced. Patients awaiting transplantation maintain better fitness and morale when engaged in an exercise programme (31). Oxygen-assisted training may also be necessary for those with resting or exercise hypoxaemia. In a report by Heijerman et al. (32), 16 CF patients with a mean FEV_1 (forced expiratory volume in 1 s) of 30 per cent of predicted underwent 3 weeks of exercise training, during which time oxygen was provided to maintain adequate exercise saturation. The authors reported improvements in maximal work, oxygen consumption, minute ventilation, resting P_aCO_2 and body weight (32).

Infection control. This is an issue that separates the rehabilitation of CF patients from those with other chronic respiratory conditions such as chronic obstructive pulmonary disease (COPD). Most clinicians actively discourage social activity between patients with CF, in order to reduce the chances of inter-patient cross-infection with resistant organisms. Therefore, individualized or home exercise sessions may be preferred to a close group environment. Summer camps can provide an excellent rehabilitative experience, with both exercise and psychosocial support. Blau et al. (33) reported on the benefit of a summer camp in 13 CF patients with mild-to-moderate disease. The campers received chest physiotherapy in separate rooms. Regular activities included mountain climbing, swimming, trampolining and ball games for 2 hours, three times a week. A high-calorie diet was provided. After 4 weeks all patients reported an improvement in well-being, with less dyspnoea, less fatigue, an increased sense of well-being and an increased appetite. In addition, maximum work capacity increased by 12.7 per cent, $\dot{V}O_{2,max}$ increased from 84 ± 5 to 93 ± 6 per cent of predicted ($P < 0.01$) and maximum ventilation increased by 18.5 per cent ($P < 0.0005$) (33). The intensive activity programme improved exercise capacity likely related to increased cardiovascular fitness and improved skeletal muscle function.

More gradual decline in pulmonary function. Schneiderman-Walker et al. (34) reported that a 3-year home exercise programme, involving 20 min of aerobic exercise three times a week, decreased the rate of decline of pulmonary function in children and teenagers with mild-to-moderate lung disease. Seventy-two patients aged 7–19 years were randomized to receive 20 min of aerobic exercise three times per week, or usual care. The control group demonstrated a decline in FVC (forced vital capacity) of -2.42 ± 4.15 compared with the study group decline of -0.25 ± 2.81 ($P = 0.02$), with a similar trend for the FEV_1. Issues of adherence and motivation remain. To promote adherence, the authors encouraged patients to choose aerobic activities according to their own interests.

In 14 patients with mild-to-moderate lung function impairment, Gulmans et al. (35) measured changes in fitness during a 6-month period of exercise cycle training, five times a week for 20 min each. Statistically significant improvements were noted for muscle strength in knee extensors (Fig. 29.4) and ankle dorsiflexors, with improvements in maximal oxygen

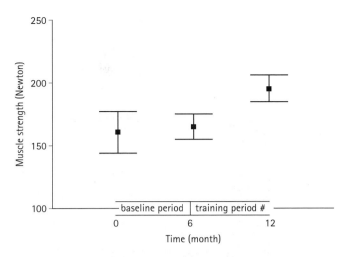

Figure 29.4   *Mean scores for muscle strength of knee extensors over time; significant differences between baseline period and training period (35).*

consumption. Indices of perceived well-being and efficacy also improved. Although scores reflecting programme acceptability were low, patients reported that they did wish to continue with another type of training (35).

FUTURE RESEARCH INTO THE BENEFITS OF PULMONARY REHABILITATION

A recent Cochrane review on the value of physical training in CF evaluated six studies that met the inclusion criteria out of 19 studies identified. These studies included 184 participants. Exercise tolerance in the short term was improved with physical training. In a 3-year study period there was no significant improvement in exercise at the end of the study. Conclusions regarding the efficacy of physical training were limited by the small size, short duration and incomplete reporting of outcome measures. Further research is needed, to comprehensively assess the added benefit of exercise to the care of patients with CF (36).

Therefore, those clinicians with access to exercise rehabilitation programmes have an opportunity to contribute outcomes research in this field. Information on health-related quality of life, pulmonary function, exercise ability and mortality would all be highly relevant. It would also be valuable to identify those most likely to benefit, as well as the key components to include in a rehabilitation programme for CF patients (37). Whereas children with mild-to-moderate disease can participate in sporting activities with their friends, their lifestyle often becomes more sedentary upon reaching adulthood, as their respiratory condition worsens. A combination of aerobic and anaerobic exercises is recommended (38, 39). Physical training is often part of the management of patients with CF, but there is a need for evidence-based clinical trials before this approach can become widespread. The rest of this chapter addresses other components of care for patients with CF.

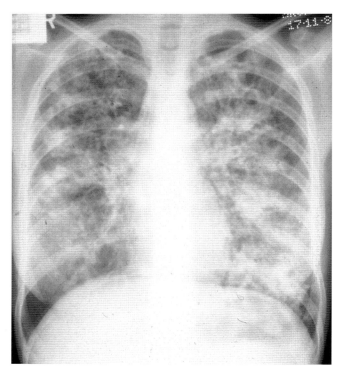

Figure 29.5 *Chest radiograph of cystic fibrosis patient with severe pulmonary disease.*

Lung disease

The age and natural history of pulmonary disease vary between patients, with some developing symptoms in childhood and others not until their teens. At the age of 15 years, approximately 50 per cent of patients are producing sputum every day (13). Haemoptysis, chest pain and wheezing are common. As the disease progresses, dyspnoea limits exercise tolerance. Some patients become oxygen-dependent and wheelchair-bound. Finger clubbing is almost universal. On auscultation, crepitations over areas of retained secretions and rhonchi over narrowed airways are heard (40, 41).

INVESTIGATIONS

These include chest radiology (Fig. 29.5), lung function tests, arterial blood gases, sputum microbiology or cough swabs. Special cultures should be set up for *B. cepacia* and the sputum should be examined for mycobacteria annually.

PREVENTION

Early diagnosis and prompt treatment of colonization with *P. aeruginosa* are important. Contact with individuals who have MRSA, *B. cepacia*, colds or influenza should be avoided. Routine immunization against pertussis, measles and influenza should be given. CF patients should avoid a smoking environment (42).

PHYSIOTHERAPY

This is a vital part of daily treatment (43) and will be reviewed later.

ANTIMICROBIALS

Patients known to be colonized with *S. aureus* are treated with oral antimicrobials (44). Similarly, *H. influenzae* can usually be eradicated. Given that the pulmonary function of patients with *Pseudomonas* infection deteriorates more rapidly than in those without, eradication is attempted with nebulized, oral and intravenous antibiotics (45–52), using repeat courses as required and monitoring drug levels to avoid toxicity. *B. cepacia* is treated according to its sensitivities, and other bacteria such as *Chlamydia* respond well to tetracycline.

DORNASE ALFA

This medication reduces the viscoelasticity of airway secretions and aids pulmonary clearance. It improves lung function in mild, moderate and severe disease and is given by nebulizer at a dose of 2.5 mg daily (53–55).

BRONCHODILATORS

Most patients have reduced airflow, with at least partial reversibility. Therefore, pulmonary function should be monitored and bronchodilators prescribed as appropriate (56–58).

CORTICOSTEROIDS

The use of inhaled steroids for patients with CF remains unclear. Oral prednisone is used to treat allergic bronchopulmonary aspergillosis (59).

ANTI-INFLAMMATORY AGENTS

Prednisone has unacceptable side-effects (60). Although ibuprofen showed some initial promise (61), there is increasing evidence that daily azithromycin will improve lung function, increase body mass index and reduce exacerbations (62).

TRANSPLANTATION

Transplantation can be life-saving for patients with end-stage disease (63–66), with 1-year survival rates of 70–80 per cent and many survivors of more than 10 years. Lung transplantation saves some patients and encourages others (Box 29.2). An exercise rehabilitation programme might well better prepare patients for transplantation as well as aiding post-transplant recovery. However, there is no available literature in this area.

Pulmonary complications

Pulmonary complications include atelectasis, haemoptysis, pneumothorax, empyema and allergic aspergillosis. For this reason it is very helpful for patients with CF to have prompt access to respiratory specialists (67). Management depends on the immediate cause and on the extent of symptoms. Pneumothorax occurs in 19 per cent of adults (68). Small pneumothoraces are treated conservatively but most require insertion of an intercostal tube. Allergic bronchopulmonary

Box 29.2   Selection criteria for lung transplantation in cystic fibrosis patients

Indication

- Severe respiratory failure despite optimal medical therapy
- Severely impaired quality of life
- Patient positively wants a transplant

Strong contraindications

- Active aspergillus or mycobacterium infection
- Non-compliance with treatment
- Negative psychological state
- Regular steroid therapy ($>10\,$mg/day prednisone)
- Other end-organ failure
- Gross malnutrition

Risk factors

- Pre-operative ventilation
- Previous thoracic surgery
- Severe liver disease necessitating combined heart–lung–liver transplantation

aspergillosis occurs in 11 per cent of patients with CF, diagnosed by transient parenchymal shadows, blood eosinophilia and a positive skin-prick test to *A. fumigatus* as well as serological markers (59). Hypoxia is treated with oxygen, but when a patient develops respiratory failure or cor pulmonale, a decision on transplantation should be made, as patients with acute exacerbations and those awaiting transplantation can be successfully treated using non-invasive ventilation (69, 70).

The digestive system

Malabsorption from pancreatic insufficiency requires pancreatic enzymes, taken with meals, as well as fat soluble vitamins (A, D, E, K) and a high calorie diet. Some patients may require gastrostomy feeding (71, 72). Small bowel obstruction is a common complication in adults, presenting with abdominal pain, constipation, nausea and vomiting. Other complications include pancreatitis, gastro-oesophageal reflux, peptic ulcer disease and malignancy of the gastrointestinal tract.

Other systems

Management of CF requires an appreciation that it is a multi-system disease, with both primary and secondary impairments. Other system involvement includes osteoporosis, for which patients are treated with bisphosphonates or hormone therapy (73), sinus disease, which is almost universal (74), diabetes mellitus, present in 25 per cent of patients over 30 years of age, liver and biliary disease, which is often asymptomatic (75), and joint disease in some adult patients (76).

PSYCHOLOGICAL AND SOCIAL ISSUES

Given that CF affects young people, rehabilitative aspects of psychological support are often centred around relationships (77–79), adolescent adjustments, poor body image and issues regarding fertility. Economic issues, relating to education and paid employment, promote autonomy, which is a key part of rehabilitation. Travel should be encouraged, provided that adequate health insurance is obtained. Another focus for psychological and social support relates to end-of-life decision-making and terminal care, as despite the very marked improvements in management, patients with CF still die prematurely (80).

Comprehensive care

Comprehensive management includes both hospital and home-based care, with good communication between team members. A specialized CF centre provides substantial expertise from a multidisciplinary team. CF centres can also provide leadership in professional education and clinical research. Comprehensive care also involves regular follow-up by the multidisciplinary team, in person or by telephone or telemedicine contact for patients who live a long way from the hospital (81). Regular reviews provide an opportunity for capturing important information regarding lung function, oxygenation, exercise tolerance and quality of life.

THE MULTIDISCIPLINARY TEAM

Medical staff

The physician responsible for patient care works closely with the multidisciplinary team. Patients must know and have access to whoever is medically responsible for their health.

Nursing staff

Cystic fibrosis centres include nurse specialists as well as home care nurses (81), who can liaise with school and work and help coordinate the activities of other members of the multidisciplinary team.

Physiotherapists and respiratory therapists

Physiotherapists teach and supervise a variety of drainage procedures, including active cycle of breathing techniques, autogenic drainage, high-frequency chest wall compression, high-frequency oscillation, flutter valves, positive expiratory pressure and postural drainage with percussion (82, 83).

As mentioned above, physiotherapists also supervise the exercise rehabilitation programme. When available, respiratory therapists are invaluable team members, with special responsibility for assessing oxygen, teaching medication administration and initiating non-invasive ventilation.

Dieticians

Many CF patients are malnourished and require supplementation, sometimes by nasogastric tube or by a percutaneous endoscopic gastrostomy. The dietician monitors their nutritional state, enzyme intake and caloric and salt requirements, especially when diabetes mellitus is present (71).

Social workers, educationalists and mental health workers

These members of the team provide support and information regarding education, accommodation, social security and employment (84). Most patients cope remarkably well but others have difficulty adjusting to life with a limited life expectancy. Some may develop eating problems and others may have difficulty in relationships. Some patients benefit from seeing a psychiatrist and being treated for clinical depression or anxiety. Psychological support is an important part of long-term management (85).

Occupational therapists

Occupational therapy enables patients to maintain independence. The therapist provides advice regarding home equipment for activities of daily living and teaches the skills for energy conservation (86).

Spiritual support

Patients tackling issues of disability, prolonged illness and transplantation often benefit from spiritual support, as do their families, during times of stress and bereavement.

CONCLUSIONS

For patients with CF, rehabilitation takes the form of lifelong care, aimed at maintaining autonomy and health-related quality of life. An adequately trained multidisciplinary team provides the best approach for patients. Although exercise rehabilitation programmes are likely to benefit CF patients, more research is needed in this field before firm recommendations can be given. There is therefore an opportunity to evaluate the application of rehabilitation more precisely, using well designed randomized controlled trials with valid, reproducible and interpretable outcome measures.

Key points

- Cystic fibrosis is a multisystem inherited disease.
- The mortality and morbidity are high.
- Life expectancy is now over 40 years for those born in the 1990s.
- A multidisciplinary team is essential.
- An ongoing rehabilitative approach will maintain the best quality of life.

REFERENCES

1. Delisa JA, Martin GM, Currie DM. Rehabilitation medicine: past, present and future. *Rehabilitation Medicine Principles and Practice.* Philadelphia: JB Lippincott, 1993; 3–25.
2. Cystic Fibrosis Trust. Standards for the clinical care of children and adults with cystic fibrosis in the UK. Bromley, Kent: Cystic Fibrosis Trust, 2001.
3. Andersen DH. A clinical and pathological study. *Am J Dis Child* 1938; **56**: 344–99.
4. Elborn JS, Shale DJ, Britton JR. Cystic fibrosis: current survival and population estimates to the year. *Thorax 1991*, 2000; **46**: 881–5.
5. Hodson ME. Treatment of cystic fibrosis in the adult. *Respiration* 2000; **67**: 595–607.
6. Neilsen OH, Schoits PO. Cystic fibrosis in Denmark in the period 1945–81; evaluation of centralised treatment. *Acta Paed Scand (Suppl.)* 1982; **301**: 107–19.
7. Mahadeva R, Webb K, Westerbeek RC *et al.* Clinical outcome in relation to care in centres specialising in cystic fibrosis: cross-sectional study. *Br Med J* 1998; **316**: 1771–5.
8. Walters S, Britton J, Hodson ME. Hospital care for adults with cystic fibrosis: an overview and comparison between special cystic fibrosis clinics and general clinics using a patient questionnaire. *Thorax* 1994; **49**: 300–6.
9. Rommens JM, Iannuzzi MC, Kerem B *et al.* Identification of the cystic fibrosis gene: chromosome walking and jumping. *Science* 1989; **245**: 1059–65.
10. Riordan JR, Rommens JM, Kerem B *et al.* Identification of the cystic fibrosis gene: cloning and characterization of complementary DNA. *Science* 1989; **245**: 1066–73.
11. Kerem B, Rommens JM, Buchanan JA *et al.* Identification of the cystic fibrosis gene: genetic analysis. *Science* 1989; **245**: 1073–80.
12. Davies J, Dewar A, Bush A *et al.* Reduction in the adherence of *Pseudomonas aeruginosa* to native cystic fibrosis epithelium with anti-asialoGM1 antibody and neuraminidase inhibition. *Eur Respir J* 1999; **13**: 565–70.
13. Penketh AR, Wise A, Mearns MB *et al.* Cystic fibrosis in adolescents and adults. *Thorax* 1987; **42**: 526–32.
14. Govan JR, Nelson JW. Microbiology of lung infection in cystic fibrosis. *Br Med Bull* 1992; **48**: 912–30.
15. Thomas SR, Gyi KM, Gaya H, Hodson ME. Methicillin-resistant *Staphylococcus aureus*: impact at a national cystic fibrosis centre. *J Hosp Infect* 1998; **40**: 203–9.
16. Cystic Fibrosis Trust. *Pseudomonas aeruginosa* infection in people with cystic fibrosis; suggestions for prevention and infection control. Bromley, Kent: Cystic Fibrosis Trust, 2001.

17. Rosenstein BJ. Diagnostic methods. In: Hodson ME, Geddes DM, eds. *Cystic Fibrosis*. London: Arnold, 2000; 177–88.

18. Brook DJH. *Diagnostic Methods*. In: Hodson ME, Geddes DM, eds. *Cystic Fibrosis*. London: Arnold, 2000; 189–202.

19. Bilton D, Dodd ME, Abbot JV, Webb AK. The benefits of exercise combined with physiotherapy in the treatment of adults with cystic fibrosis. *Respir Med* 1992; **86**: 507–11.

20. Andreasson B, Jonson B, Kornfalt R *et al.* Long-term effects of physical exercise on working capacity and pulmonary function in cystic fibrosis. *Acta Paediatr Scand* 1987; **76**: 70–5.

21. de Jong W, Grevink RG, Roorda RJ *et al.* Effect of a home exercise training program in patients with cystic fibrosis. *Chest* 1994; **105**: 463–8.

22. Nixon PA, Orenstein DM, Kelsey SF, Doershuk CF. The prognostic value of exercise testing in patients with cystic fibrosis. *N Engl J Med* 1992; **327**: 1785–8.

23. O'Neill PA, Dodds M, Phillips B *et al.* Regular exercise and reduction of breathlessness in patients with cystic fibrosis. *Br J Dis Chest* 1987; **81**: 62–9.

24. Strauss GD, Osher A, Wang CI *et al.* Variable weight training in cystic fibrosis. *Chest* 1987; **92**: 273–6.

25. Haworth CS, Selby PL, Webb AK *et al.* Low bone mineral density in adults with cystic fibrosis. *Thorax* 1999; **54**: 961–7.

26. Gibbens DT, Gilsanz V, Boechat MI *et al.* Osteoporosis in cystic fibrosis. *J Pediatr* 1988; **113**: 295–300.

27. Aris RM, Renner JB, Winders AD *et al.* Increased rate of fractures and severe kyphosis: sequelae of living into adulthood with cystic fibrosis. *Ann Intern Med* 1998; **128**: 186–93.

28. Elkin SL, Fairney A, Burnett S *et al.* Vertebral deformities and low bone mineral density in adults with cystic fibrosis: a cross-sectional study. *Osteoporos Int* 2001; **12**: 366–72.

29. Bachrach LK. Acquisition of optimal bone mass in childhood and adolescence. *Trends Endocrinol Metab* 2001; **12**: 22–8.

30. Lands L, Desmond KJ, Demizio D *et al.* The effects of nutritional status and hyperinflation on respiratory muscle strength in children and young adults. *Am Rev Respir Dis* 1990; **141**: 1506–9.

31. Webb AK, Egan TM, Dodd ME. Clinical management of CF patient awaiting and immediately following lung transplantation. In: Dodge JA, Brock DJH, Widdicombe JH, eds. *Cystic Fibrosis: Current Topics*. Chichester: Wiley, 1996.

32. Heijerman HG, Bakker W, Sterk PJ, Dijkman JH. Oxygen-assisted exercise training in adult cystic fibrosis patients with pulmonary limitation to exercise. *Int J Rehabil Res* 1991; **14**: 101–15.

33. Blau H, Mussaffi-Georgy H, Fink G *et al.* Effects of an intensive 4-week summer camp on cystic fibrosis: pulmonary function, exercise tolerance, and nutrition. *Chest*, 2002; **121**: 1117–22.

34. Schneiderman-Walker J, Pollock SL, Corey M *et al.* A randomized controlled trial of a 3-year home exercise program in cystic fibrosis. *J Pediatr* 2000; **136**: 304–10.

35. Gulmans VA, de Meer K, Brackel HJ *et al.* Outpatient exercise training in children with cystic fibrosis: physiological effects, perceived competence, and acceptability. *Pediatr Pulmonol* 1999; **28**: 39–46.

36. Bradley J, Moran F. Physical training for cystic fibrosis. *Cochrane Database Syst Rev* 2002; **2**: CD002768.

37. Turchetta A, Salerno T, Lucidi V *et al.* Usefulness of a program of hospital-supervised physical training in patients with cystic fibrosis. *Pediatr Pulmonol* 2004; **38**: 115–18.

38. Klijn PH, Oudshoorn A, van der Ent CKNJ *et al.* Effects of anaerobic training in children with cystic fibrosis: a randomized controlled study. *Chest* 2004; **125**: 1299–305.

39. Selvadurai HC, Blimkie CJ, Meyers N *et al.* Randomized controlled study of in-hospital exercise training programs in children with cystic fibrosis. *Pediatr Pulmonol* 2002; **33**: 194–200.

40. Marshall SG, Rosenfeld M, Ramsey BW. Respiratory system. In: Hodson ME, Geddes DM, eds. *Cystic Fibrosis*. London: Arnold, 2000; 204–17.

41. Hodson ME. Respiratory system. In: Hodson ME, Geddes DM, eds. *Cystic Fibrosis*. London: Arnold, 2000; 218–42.

42. Gilljam H, Stenlund C, Ericsson-Hollsing A, Strandvik B. Passive smoking in cystic fibrosis. *Respir Med* 1990; **84**: 289–91.

43. Pryor JA, Webber BA. Paramedical issues – physiotherapy. In: Hodson ME, Geddes DM, eds. *Cystic Fibrosis*. London: Arnold, 2000; 376–83.

44. Weaver LT, Green MR, Nicholson K *et al.* Prognosis in cystic fibrosis treated with continuous flucloxacillin from the neonatal period. *Arch Dis Child* 1994; **70**: 84–9.

45. Pamukcu A, Bush A, Buchdahl R. Effects of *Pseudomonas aeruginosa* colonization on lung function and anthropometric variables in children with cystic fibrosis. *Pediatr Pulmonol* 1995; **19**: 10–15.

46. Valerius NH, Koch C, Hoiby N. Prevention of chronic *Pseudomonas aeruginosa* colonisation in cystic fibrosis by early treatment. *Lancet* 1991; **338**: 725–6.

47. Cystic Fibrosis Foundation. *Consensus Conferences – Concepts in Care*, 5th edn. Bethesda, USA: Cystic Fibrosis Foundation, 1994.

48. Stead RJ, Davidson TI, Duncan FR *et al.* Use of a totally implantable system for venous access in cystic fibrosis. *Thorax* 1987; **42**: 149–50.

49. Touw DJ, Brimicombe RW, Hodson ME *et al.* Inhalation of antibiotics in cystic fibrosis. *Eur Respir J* 1995; **8**: 1594–604.

50. Mukhopadhyay S, Singh M, Cater JI *et al.* Nebulised antipseudomonal antibiotic therapy in cystic fibrosis: a meta-analysis of benefits and risks. *Thorax* 1996; **51**: 364–8.

51. Ramsey BW, Dorkin HL, Eisenberg JD *et al.* Efficacy of aerosolized tobramycin in patients with cystic fibrosis. *N Engl J Med* 1993; **328**: 1740–6.

52. Ramsey BW, Pepe MS, Quan JM *et al.* Intermittent administration of inhaled tobramycin in patients with cystic fibrosis. Cystic Fibrosis Inhaled Tobramycin Study Group. *N Engl J Med* 1999; **340**: 23–30.

53. Fuchs HJ, Borowitz DS, Christiansen DH *et al.* Effect of aerosolized recombinant human DNase on exacerbations of respiratory symptoms and on pulmonary function in patients with cystic fibrosis. The Pulmozyme Study Group. *N Engl J Med* 1994; **331**: 637–42.

54. Shah PL, Scott SF, Geddes DM, Hodson ME. Two years experience with recombinant human DNase I in the treatment of pulmonary disease in cystic fibrosis. *Respir Med* 1995; **89**: 499–502.

55. Quan JM, Tiddens HA, Sy JP *et al.* A two-year randomized, placebo-controlled trial of dornase alfa in young patients with cystic fibrosis with mild lung function abnormalities. *J Pediatr* 2001; **139**: 813–20.

56. Eggleston PA, Rosenstein BJ, Stackhouse CM, Alexander MF. Airway hyperreactivity in cystic fibrosis. Clinical correlates and possible effects on the course of the disease. *Chest* 1988; **94**: 360–5.

57. Avital A, Sanchez I, Chernick V. Efficacy of salbutamol and ipratropium bromide in decreasing bronchial hyperreactivity in children with cystic fibrosis. *Pediatr Pulmonol* 1992; **13**: 34–7.

58. Finnegan MJ, Hughes DV, Hodson ME. Comparison of nebulized and intravenous terbutaline during exacerbations of pulmonary infection in patients with cystic fibrosis. *Eur Respir J* 1992; **5**: 1089–91.

59. Hiller EJ. Pathogenesis and management of aspergillosis in cystic fibrosis. *Arch Dis Child* 1990; **65**: 397–8.

60. Auerbach HS, Williams M, Kirkpatrick JA, Colten HR. Alternate-day prednisone reduces morbidity and improves pulmonary function in cystic fibrosis. *Lancet* 1985; **2**: 686–8.

61. Konstan MW, Byard PJ, Hoppel CL, Davis PB. Effect of high-dose ibuprofen in patients with cystic fibrosis. *N Engl J Med* 1995; **332**: 848–54.

62. Pirzada OM, McGaw J, Taylor CJ, Everard ML. Improved lung function and body mass index associated with long-term use of macolide antibiotics. *J Cystic Fibrosis* 2003; **2**: 69–71.
63. Madden BM. Lung transplantation. In: Hodson ME, Geddes DM, eds. *Cystic Fibrosis*. London: Arnold, 2000; 376–83.
64. Vricella LA, Karamichalis JM, Ahmad S *et al.* Lung and heart-lung transplantation in patients with end-stage cystic fibrosis: the Stanford experience. *Ann Thorac Surg* 2002; **74**: 13–7.
65. Egan TM, Detterbeck FC, Mill MR *et al.* Long term results of lung transplantation for cystic fibrosis. *Eur J Cardiothorac Surg* 2002; **22**: 602–9.
66. Starnes VA, Barr ML, Cohen RG *et al.* Living-donor lobar lung transplantation experience: intermediate results. *J Thorac Cardiovasc Surg* 1996; **112**: 1284–90.
67. Stern RC, Wood RE, Boat TF *et al.* Treatment and prognosis of massive hemoptysis in cystic fibrosis. *Am Rev Respir Dis* 1978; **117**: 825–8.
68. Penketh AR, Knight RK, Hodson ME, Batten JC. Management of pneumothorax in adults with cystic fibrosis. *Thorax* 1982; **37**: 850–3.
69. Madden BM, Kariyawasam H, Siddiqi AJ *et al.* Noninvasive ventilation in cystic fibrosis patients with acute or chronic respiratory failure. *Eur Respir J* 2002; **19**: 310–3.
70. Stern RC, Borkat G, Hirschfeld SS *et al.* Heart failure in cystic fibrosis. Treatment and prognosis of cor pulmonale with failure of the right side of the heart. *Am J Dis Child* 1980; **134**: 267–72.
71. Poole S, McAlweenie A, Ashworth F. Paramedial issues – dietary treatment in CF. In: Hodson ME, Geddes DM, eds. *Cystic Fibrosis*. London: Arnold, 2000; 384–95.
72. Davidson AGF. Gastrointestinal and pancreatic disease in cystic fibrosis. In: Hodson ME, Geddes DM, eds. *Cystic Fibrosis*. London: Arnold, 2000; 261–88.
73. Elkin SL. Other organ systems. In: Hodson ME, Geddes DM, eds. *Cystic Fibrosis*. London: Arnold, 2000; 329–38.
74. Koch C, Lanng S. Other organ systems. In: Hodson ME, Geddes DM, eds. *Cystic Fibrosis*. London: Arnold, 2000; 314–28.
75. Westaby D. Liver and biliary disease in cystic fibrosis. In: Hodson ME, Geddes DM, eds. *Cystic Fibrosis*. London: Arnold, 2000; 289–300.
76. Hodson ME. Vasculitis and arthropathy in cystic fibrosis. *J Roy Soc Med* 1999; **85**(Suppl. 9): 38–40.
77. Cystic Fibrosis Foundation Patient Registry. *1998 Annual Data Report*. Bethesda, USA: Cystic Fibrosis Foundation, 1999.
78. Walters S, Britton J, Hodson ME. Demographic and social characteristics of adults with cystic fibrosis in the United Kingdom. *Br Med J* 1993; **306**: 549–52.
79. Sawyer SM. Reproductive and sexual health. In: Hodson ME, Geddes DM, eds. *Cystic Fibrosis*. London: Arnold, 2000; 301–12.
80. Saunders C. *The Management of Terminal Disease*. London: Edward Arnold, 1978.
81. Duncan-Skingle F, Bramwell E. Paramedical issues. In: Hodson ME, Geddes DM, eds. *Cystic Fibrosis*. London: Arnold, 2000; 413–8.
82. Thomas J, Cook DJ, Brooks D. Chest physical therapy management of patients with cystic fibrosis. A meta-analysis. *Am J Respir Crit Care Med* 1995; **151**: 846–50.
83. Heijerman HG, Bakker W, Sterk PJ, Dijkman JH. Long-term effects of exercise training and hyperalimentation in adult cystic fibrosis patients with severe pulmonary dysfunction. *Int J Rehabil Res* 1992; **15**: 252–7.
84. Cloutman N. Paramedical issues - social work. In: Hodson ME, Geddes DM, eds. *Cystic Fibrosis*. London: Arnold, 2000; 413–8.
85. Lask B. Psychological aspects of cystic fibrosis. In: Hodson ME, Geddes DM, eds. *Cystic Fibrosis*. London: Arnold, 2000; 339–48.
86. Groom V. Paramedical issues – occupational therapy. In: Hodson ME, Geddes DM, eds. *Cystic Fibrosis*. London: Arnold, 2000; 419–32.
87. Lewis PA. The epidemiology of cystic fibrosis. In: Hodson ME, Geddes DM, eds. *Cystic Fibrosis*, 2nd edn. London: Arnold, 2000, chapter 1b.

30

Pulmonary rehabilitation and lung volume reduction surgery

BARRY MAKE

INTRODUCTION

Lung volume reduction surgery (LVRS) is most commonly performed only for patients with severe symptomatic emphysema. The underlying lung disease and associated physiological abnormalities in candidates for LVRS are often so severe that these patients are at high risk for increased morbidity and mortality from elective surgical procedures, particularly thoracic surgery. It is a testament to modern respiratory care and the benefits of LVRS that patients with severe emphysema can successfully withstand and benefit from this surgical therapy.

One of the likely reasons that LVRS has been successful is the almost universal application of pulmonary rehabilitation prior to surgery (1–11). Improving physical conditioning, optimizing weight, assuring an adequate diet and smoking cessation are likely to contribute to the benefits of pulmonary rehabilitation prior to LVRS. Similarly, employing pulmonary rehabilitation following surgery may hasten postoperative recovery and more rapidly return the patient to functional activities.

This chapter will outline the rationale for and the role of pulmonary rehabilitation in association with lung volume reduction surgery.

RATIONALE FOR PULMONARY REHABILITATION IN ASSOCIATION WITH LVRS

Pulmonary rehabilitation prior to LVRS

BENEFITS OF PREOPERATIVE PULMONARY REHABILITATION

Box 30.1 lists several features encountered in patients with emphysema that may be expected to adversely impact the

---

Box 30.1 Features of emphysema that may adversely impact the outcome of lung volume reduction surgery

- Severity of airflow limitation
- Impaired physical function (e.g. walking, physical conditioning)
- Lower airway secretions
  - inability to effectively clear secretions spontaneously with cough
  - excessive secretions
- Body weight
  - low body weight
  - low muscle mass
  - poor cough strength
  - obesity
- Malnutrition
  - low caloric intake
  - low protein intake
- Psychological
  - depression
  - anxiety

---

outcomes of surgery. Each of these factors may be addressed and modified by pulmonary rehabilitation using the pulmonary rehabilitation programme components listed in Box 30.2. Controlled randomized clinical trials of the effectiveness and outcomes of pulmonary rehabilitation prior to LVRS are not available. However, based upon the available original investigations and evidence-based reviews and guidelines of pulmonary rehabilitation for patients with chronic obstructive pulmonary disease (COPD) (4, 12–20), it can reasonably be expected that comprehensive pulmonary rehabilitation

---

Box 30.2 Pulmonary rehabilitation components that may be of benefit in association with lung volume reduction surgery

- Medical evaluation and management
- Initial assessment and goal-setting
- Therapeutic modalities
  - smoking cessation
  - exercise training
  - education
  - psychosocial counselling
  - breathing retraining
  - daily activity performance and energy management
  - nutritional counselling
- Outcome evaluation
- Long-term continuation

---

applied prior to LVRS will decrease complications and hasten recovery.

One of the most important factors associated with mortality, morbidity, health care utilization and hospitalizations in patients with COPD is the physiological decrement in FEV_1 (forced expired volume in 1 s). The importance of FEV_1 in this regard is emphasized by its use as a criteria for staging COPD severity (1). In addition, patients with poorer lung function are at greater risk for complications following thoracic surgery for lung cancer. Factors associated with increased complications include worse airflow limitation (21, 22), greater hyperinflation (23), hypoxaemia (23), lower exercise capacity (24–27) and decreased diffusing capacity (28, 29). The National Emphysema Treatment Trial found that patients with a very low FEV_1 ($\leqslant 20$ per cent of predicted) and either homogeneous distribution of emphysema on CT scan or a low diffusing capacity ($\leqslant 20$ per cent of predicted) were at increased risk for 30-day mortality following LVRS (30). The National Emphysema Treatment Trial (NETT) also identified a second subgroup (patients with high exercise capacity and non-upper lobe predominant emphysema) that was at higher risk for death following LVRS compared with patients receiving medical therapy (31). A recent publication has found that a multidimensional score (BODE score) is superior to FEV_1 alone as a predictor of mortality in COPD (32). The BODE score combines **b**ody mass index, airflow **o**bstruction as measured by the FEV_1, **d**yspnoea assessed by the Modified Medical Research Council dyspnoea scale, and **e**xercise tolerance measured by the 6-min walk distance. The utility of this score to predict mortality following LVRS has not been tested but clinicians might consider this scale in evaluating patients for such surgery. Although exercise training does not directly lead to an improvement in the physiological function of the lungs (4, 12–20), pulmonary function can be increased with the appropriate use of regular bronchodilators and inhaled corticosteroids (33, 34). The medical management accompanying pulmonary rehabilitation can be expected to result in appropriate prescription of bronchodilators by pulmonary specialist physicians. The patient education

component of pulmonary rehabilitation includes patient incorporation of health-enhancing behaviours, including timely administration of medications and bronchodilators, thereby resulting in improved lung function. Bronchodilators and associated improvement in airflow limitation can also be expected to:

- reduce dyspnoea
- improve exercise capacity with a resultant increase in general activity level and better physical conditioning
- enhance secretion clearance.

Impaired physical function, as measured by a low formally tested 6-min walk distance or cardiopulmonary exercise test, has been shown to adversely impact the outcome of patients with COPD. Decreased exercise capacity is associated with increased mortality in COPD (32). Impaired quality of life is also associated with increased mortality in COPD (35, 36). Pulmonary rehabilitation improves exercise capacity, physical function and quality of life and might thus be expected to improve mortality. Additionally, pulmonary rehabilitation may decrease mortality and morbidity following LVRS, although this potential outcome has not been subject to rigorous clinical trials.

Although secretion clearance techniques, including postural drainage and percussion, as well as newer devices such as the flutter valve, Acapella and TheraVest, are included in the rehabilitation programme, extensive sputum production is a relative contraindication to LVRS. In some patients, 'huff' coughing, with an open glottis, avoids excessive airway collapse and is more effective than the typical closed-glottis technique. Cough and secretion clearance are enhanced by the use of bronchodilators. Improved respiratory muscle function may enhance coughing, and improved secretion clearance will reduce the potential for respiratory compromise following LVRS. Smoking cessation will also reduce respiratory secretions. Self-management techniques enable patients to assist in their care (37). Early recognition and management of respiratory exacerbations, prior to or after LVRS, will improve outcomes.

Many patients with emphysema have low body weight, which is a marker for increased mortality in COPD. Loss of lean body mass and loss of muscle from protein malnutrition should be addressed during pulmonary rehabilitation prior to LVRS. As weight loss is commonly associated with major surgery, patients should not be malnourished prior to this elective surgical procedure. Nutritional assessment, recommendations and monitoring should be part of the rehabilitation programme. In severely underweight patients, who fail to increase body mass with dietary manipulation, consideration may be given to the use of anabolic steroids, in conjunction with exercise training (38).

Since obesity is also a risk factor for postoperative complications, thoracic surgeons may delay surgery until adequate weight loss has been achieved. The dietary and exercise components of pulmonary rehabilitation may be used to foster weight reduction.

Patients with significant clinical depression or excessive anxiety may be poor candidates for major elective surgery.

Depressed patients may be unable comply with the pre and postoperative instructions required in order to achieve the best benefits from LVRS, and excessive anxiety may aggravate dyspnoea. Pulmonary rehabilitation and exercise training reduce depressive symptoms. Dyspnoea control, including pursed lips breathing, pacing and planning of activities, will help reduce anxiety. The psychosocial component of pulmonary rehabilitation can address depression and anxiety, using both pharmacological and non-pharmacological approaches.

Results of studies of pulmonary rehabilitation prior to other types of surgery suggest that pulmonary rehabilitation may also be effective prior to LVRS. Rajendran et al. (39) randomized 45 patients, prior to coronary artery bypass graft, to either short-term pulmonary rehabilitation or usual care. Patients of both groups were evenly matched with respect to age, sex, body surface area, duration and severity of COPD and coronary artery disease. Pulmonary rehabilitation decreased the number of postoperative pulmonary complications (4 vs. 11, $P < 0.01$), ventilator hours (24 vs. 35 h, $P < 0.01$) and length of hospital stay (12 vs. 18 days, $P < 0.01$). In a large cancer referral centre, Wilson (40) reported better lung resection outcomes after including 3 weeks of preoperative pulmonary rehabilitation for patients with COPD undergoing lung resection. Recent studies have noted the lack of preoperative physiotherapy as an independent predictor of postoperative pulmonary complications (41) and the protective effect of pulmonary rehabilitation for postoperative pulmonary complications in moderate- and high-risk patients (42).

ROLE OF PULMONARY REHABILITATION IN PATIENT SELECTION FOR LVRS

The overriding symptom that limits the function of patients with emphysema is dyspnoea. The goal of LVRS is to ameliorate the life-altering symptom of shortness of breath. Because LVRS is an expensive, major procedure with a small but definite risk of postoperative mortality and morbidity, it should not be undertaken unless the procedure is deemed necessary to control symptoms, improve health-related quality of life, or extend survival. Prior to considering LVRS it is important to be sure that symptoms of dyspnoea persist despite maximal pharmacotherapy, oxygen and pulmonary rehabilitation. The effect of pulmonary rehabilitation on dyspnoea reduction and quality of life is such that it is considered the prevailing standard in the recent COPD international clinical practice guidelines (43). Therefore, LVRS should only be considered after maximal medical therapy, including pulmonary rehabilitation. Some patients may defer LVRS based upon their response to rehabilitation. One author's experience is that 10–15 per cent of patients who consider LVRS choose not to proceed with it after they have experienced the benefits of pulmonary rehabilitation (44).

Markedly impaired functional capacity has been suggested as a risk factor for a poor outcome from LVRS. Szekely et al. (45) reviewed results of the first 47 subjects who had LVRS in a single institution. They found FEV_1, vital capacity, maximal inspiratory pressure, resting room air P_aCO_2, P_aCO_2 at maximum

exercise and pre- and post-pulmonary rehabilitation 6-min walk distance correlated with length of hospitalization. Walk distance of less than 200 m either before or after pulmonary rehabilitation and resting P_aCO_2 of >45 mmHg were the best predictors of poor outcomes. These investigators suggested that a minimal level of functioning is required for a successful outcome from LVRS. In the 16 subjects who had one or more of these limiting characteristics, six died, and 11 had a hospital stay of >21 days. In this report, pulmonary rehabilitation was not mandated prior to LVRS and rehabilitation could be completed at community centres. Moreover, 14 subjects (30 per cent) did not have supervised pulmonary rehabilitation prior to surgery. As patients completed pulmonary rehabilitation within 3 months of surgery, some may have subsequently deteriorated in the long period between rehabilitation and LVRS. Patients who did complete rehabilitation spent fewer days in hospital, required mechanical ventilation on fewer days, and had fewer chest tube days. They experienced a similar mortality, prolonged hospital course (>21 days) and postoperative complications as patients who did not complete rehabilitation.

Pulmonary rehabilitation following LVRS

The goals of pulmonary rehabilitation are to restore the patient to the highest functional capacity and allow optimal functioning within the community (46). Prior to discharge, patients must not only be medically stable, but also be able to manage their self-care and basic activities of daily living, such as safely getting in and out of bed, eating, toileting and taking medications. Pulmonary rehabilitation assists in rapidly mobilizing patients following LVRS. Exercise and activity in the home are encouraged and further assisted by the pulmonary rehabilitation team, until the patient has achieved maximal benefit. Patient participation in rehabilitation prior to LVRS and development of a rapport between staff and patients enhance the ability of rehabilitation staff to assist in postoperative rehabilitation. The most important components of postoperative pulmonary rehabilitation are exercise to achieve mobility and education about postoperative management.

PULMONARY REHABILITATION VS. LVRS

Several studies have compared the effects of pulmonary rehabilitation with those of LVRS (8–10, 47). Mineo et al. (47) randomized 60 patients to either LVRS or pulmonary rehabilitation. Follow-up was complicated by the cross-over of six rehabilitation subjects to LVRS and deaths (two in the LVRS arm and one in the rehabilitation group). Rehabilitation resulted in improved health status (measured by the Short Form-36 [SF-36] and St George's Respiratory Questionnaire [SGRQ]) at 6 and 12 months and improved walk distance at 6 months. However, at 6 months, LVRS subjects had greater improvements in health status than subjects randomized to rehabilitation. Goldstein et al. (8) reported on the results of a randomized study of LVRS following rehabilitation, compared with rehabilitation alone, in 55 subjects. They found LVRS resulted in greater improvement in health status as measured by the Chronic Respiratory Disease Questionnaire (CDRQ) at 12 months. LVRS patients had also sustained improvements in lung volumes and exercise at 12 months. Criner et al. (9) compared LVRS following 8 weeks of preoperative pulmonary rehabilitation to 3 months of additional pulmonary rehabilitation in 37 patients. Patients receiving LVRS had greater improvements in physiological parameters, exercise and health-related quality of life than patients receiving continued pulmonary rehabilitation.

PULMONARY REHABILITATION IN ASSOCIATION WITH LVRS

Unfortunately, controlled trials of preoperative pulmonary rehabilitation prior to lung volume surgery are not available. However, the majority of reported investigations of LVRS have routinely employed pulmonary rehabilitation prior to surgery (1–11). The duration of pulmonary rehabilitation has most commonly been 6 weeks (8, 31) but some investigators have used more prolonged rehabilitation (9). Exercise training, education and psychosocial support have been commonly incorporated in preoperative pulmonary rehabilitation.

Pulmonary rehabilitation in the National Emphysema Treatment Trial

The NETT is a randomized study comparing LVRS plus maximal medical therapy including pulmonary rehabilitation with maximal medical therapy (2). During the development of the protocol, the study investigators, including thoracic surgeons and pulmonologists, at the 17 NETT centres agreed that pulmonary rehabilitation was a standard part of maximal medical therapy for patients with emphysema. This was particularly notable since some of the NETT centres did not have formal pulmonary rehabilitation programmes in place prior to the start of this clinical trial. In the NETT, pulmonary re-habilitation was performed before randomization to prepare patients for LVRS, after surgery to speed recovery and return to the highest functional capacity, and periodically thereafter when needed. Patients were encouraged to incorporate life-long regular exercise into their daily routines.

Pulmonary rehabilitation as part of a programme of maximal medical therapy along with bronchodilators and oxygen therapy when appropriate was applied to all patients who met the inclusion criteria for NETT. Successful completion of pulmonary rehabilitation was required of all patients prior to randomization to LVRS or continued medical management. The outcomes (exercise capacity, health status, walk distance, pulmonary function) following LVRS were compared with the assessments performed *after* the completion of pulmonary rehabilitation.

APPLICATION OF PULMONARY REHABILITATION IN NETT

Pulmonary rehabilitation in NETT was designed to effectively apply this therapy in the face of several key issues related to the overall goals and conduct of the larger clinical trial:

- *Pulmonary rehabilitation was not the intervention under study but was an adjunct to maximal medical management.* Therefore, pulmonary rehabilitation had to be conducted within a reasonable amount of time. The investigators chose a 6-week duration of pulmonary rehabilitation. In the event of an intervening medical problem such as a COPD exacerbation, or in patients who were deemed by the rehabilitation team to need additional time and therapy to achieve maximal medical benefit, pulmonary rehabilitation could be extended up to 12 weeks at the discretion of the NETT investigators.

- *In order to enrol the largest number of patients with emphysema in the trial, the investigators needed to evaluate patients who, in some cases, resided at great distances from the clinical centres.* Such patients often had to travel by car to reach the centres for evaluation and therapy prior to and following LVRS. Pulmonary rehabilitation had to be designed to minimize the travel and expense for individuals who lived at sites remote from the clinical centres so that patients would not be excluded due to socioeconomic issues and their lack of ability to pay for travel expenses. Thus it was impractical to require that all patients reside near the clinical centres for the extended period of time necessary to ensure successful completion of pulmonary rehabilitation. Satellite rehabilitation centres in areas closer to the patients' homes were recruited and personnel trained to provide continuing pulmonary rehabilitation. Rehabilitation at satellites was monitored with training logs and telephone communication with the NETT clinical centres.

- *Pulmonary rehabilitation needed to be standardized* so that all NETT centres and rehabilitation satellites provided a similar programme. A manual of operations was developed and all NETT personnel were trained in the pulmonary rehabilitation procedures. NETT satellite rehabilitation personnel received initial training and certification, and periodic re-training and yearly re-certification to ensure consistency of application of pulmonary rehabilitation. The first four pulmonary rehabilitation sessions were conducted at the NETT centre in an attempt to standardize the initial evaluation and training. Another issue affecting standard application of pulmonary rehabilitation was that some of the NETT enrollees had pulmonary rehabilitation prior to the trial. Since the time period between completion of prior pulmonary rehabilitation and enrolment in NETT was variable and could not be controlled for, the investigators decided to apply pulmonary rehabilitation to all trial enrollees, including those who had had prior pulmonary rehabilitation.

Table 30.1 *Characteristics of the first 761 National Emphysema Treatment Trial (NETT) patients*

Age	67 ± 6 (SD) years
Gender	61% male/39% female
Forced expired volume in 1 s (FEV_1)	0.76 ± 0.24 L (26 ± 7% predicted)
FEV_1/FVC	0.32 ± 0.07
Total lung capacity	129 ± 14% predicted
Single breath diffusing capacity	28 ± 10% predicted
Work max (cycle ergometry)	36 ± 21 watts
6-min walk distance	358 ± 96 m

Table 30.2 *Pulmonary rehabilitation outcomes of the first 761 National Emphysema Treatment Trial (NETT) patients (% change from baseline)*

Work max	$+8.1$%*
Dyspnoea[a]	-4%*
Quality of life	
SGRQ[b]	-6%*
Quality of Well-Being Scale	$+6$%*
SF-36	$+4$ units (34%)*
6-min walk distance	6.1%*

*$P < 0.0001$.
[a]University of San Diego Shortness of Breath Questionnaire.
[b]St George's Respiratory Questionnaire Total Score. Reduction in score indicates improvement in quality of life.

- *The investigators needed to ensure that all patients successfully completed pulmonary rehabilitation.* Using pre-defined goals for pulmonary rehabilitation, such as a pre-specified percentage or degree of improvement in functional capacity or decrease in dyspnoea, was felt to be impractical for the entire range of patients in the trial. Thus, the investigators determined that patient attendance at the rehabilitation sessions and adherence with the rehabilitation programme were required of all patients. The pre-randomization pulmonary rehabilitation programme consisted of 20 sessions of exercise supervised by NETT rehabilitation personnel and 20 education/psychosocial sessions. Patients who completed 16 or more exercise sessions, 16 or more education/psychosocial sessions, and were adherent with therapy were deemed to have successfully completed pulmonary rehabilitation. In addition to supervised sessions, patients were encouraged to continue training sessions in the home and community, and the philosophy that pulmonary rehabilitation and continued exercise are part of a daily, lifelong programme was emphasized to all subjects.

PRELIMINARY OUTCOMES OF PULMONARY REHABILITATION IN NETT

The results of pulmonary rehabilitation in NETT should be viewed within the context noted above. For the purposes of this chapter, however, the results of pulmonary rehabilitation

as a part of maximal medical therapy in NETT may also be viewed as a model that can be used to plan the preoperative and postoperative management of patients who have LVRS outside the trial. Pulmonary rehabilitation outcomes in NETT do not reflect the results of a controlled clinical trial of the efficacy of this therapy, but rather can be viewed as an example of the clinical effectiveness of this therapy in a real-world setting in multiple centres. In addition, in order to enrol patients who lived at a distance from the NETT clinical centres, a portion of the rehabilitation was permitted at selected rehabilitation satellites closer to their residence. The outcomes of pulmonary rehabilitation prior to LVRS in the first group of NETT subjects have been presented in abstract form (48), but results in the entire cohort of over 1200 patients have not yet been published.

Table 30.1 shows the characteristics of the first 761 patients in the NETT who had pulmonary rehabilitation. The results of pulmonary rehabilitation in NETT (Table 30.2) are consistent with the outcomes of clinical trials. Patients in NETT had improvements in exercise capacity as assessed with incremental cycle ergometry in the laboratory and increased 6-min walk distance. Shortness of breath assessed by a self-administered questionnaire (University of California, San Diego, Shortness of Breath Questionnaire) decreased, and health status (SGRQ) improved. Improvements were greater in patients who had not had prior pulmonary rehabilitation. Individuals who had their entire 6 weeks of rehabilitation at a NETT clinical centre had slightly greater improvement in exercise tolerance but similar improvements in symptoms and health status compared with patients receiving a portion of their rehabilitation at satellite centres.

Key points

- Pulmonary rehabilitation is an important adjunct to standard medical care and results in improvements in exercise, respiratory symptoms and health status in patients with COPD.
- Patients and physicians may best assess their symptoms in relation to the risks and benefits of LVRS after maximal medical treatment and pulmonary rehabilitation.
- Pulmonary rehabilitation is beneficial in patients with severe emphysema and should routinely be considered part of the preoperative treatment for patients scheduled for LVRS.
- Pulmonary rehabilitation should be considered part of the postoperative treatment following LVRS.

REFERENCES

1. Cooper JD, Trulock EP, Triantafillou AN *et al.* Bilateral pneumectomy (volume reduction) for chronic obstructive pulmonary disease. *J Thor Cardiovasc Surg* 1995; **109**: 106–19.

2. National Emphysema Treatment Trial Research Group. Rationale and design of the National Emphysema Treatment Trial: a prospective randomized trial of lung volume reduction surgery. *Chest* 1999; **116**: 1750–61.

3. Moy ML, Ingenito EP, Mentzer SJ *et al.* Health-related quality of life improves following pulmonary rehabilitation and lung volume reduction surgery. *Chest* 1999; **115**: 383–9.

4. Miller JD, Malthaner RA, Godsmith CH *et al.* Lung volume reduction for emphysema and the Canadian Lung Volume Reduction Surgery (CLVR) Project. *Can Respir J* 1999; **6**: 26–32.

5. Benditt JO, Lewis S, Wood DE *et al.* Lung volume reduction surgery improves maximal O₂ consumption, maximal minute ventilation, O₂ pulse, and dead-space-to-tidal volume ratio during leg cycle ergometry. *Am J Respir Crit Care Med* 1997; **156**: 561–6.

6. Ferguson G, Fernandez E, Zamora MR *et al.* Improved exercise tolerance following lung volume reduction surgery for emphysema. *Am J Respir Crit Care Med* 1998; **157**: 1195–203.

7. Szekely LA, Oelberg DA, Wright C *et al.* Preoperative predictors of operative morbidity and mortality in COPD patients undergoing bilateral lung volume reduction surgery. *Chest* 1997; **111**: 550–8.

8. Goldstein RS, Todd T, Guyatt GH *et al.* Influence of lung volume reduction surgery on health related quality of life in patients with chronic obstructive pulmonary disease. *Thorax* 2003; **58**: 405–10.

9. Criner GJ, Cordova FC, Furukawa S *et al.* Prospective randomized trial comparing bilateral lung volume reduction surgery to pulmonary rehabilitation in severe chronic obstructive pulmonary disease. *Am J Resp Crit Care Med* 1999; **160**: 2018–27.

10. Geddes D, Davies M, Koyama H *et al.* Effect of lung volume reduction surgery in patients with severe emphysema. *N Engl J Med* 2004; **343**: 239–45.

11. Pompeo E, Marino M, Matteucci G *et al.* Reduction pneumoplasty versus respiratory rehabilitation in severe emphysema: a randomized trial. *Ann Thorac Surg* 2000; **70**: 948–53.

12. Güell R, Casan P, Belda J *et al.* Long-term effects of outpatient rehabilitation of COPD: a randomized trial. *Chest* 2000; **117**: 976–83.

13. Troosters T, Gosselink R, Decramer M. Short- and long-term effects of outpatient rehabilitation in patients with chronic obstructive pulmonary disease: a randomized trial. *Am J Med* 2000; **109**: 207–12.

14. Ries AL, Carlin BW, Carrieri-Kohlman V *et al.* Pulmonary rehabilitation: evidence-based guidelines. *Chest* 1997; **112**: 1363–96.

◆15. Lacasse Y, Wong E, Guyatt GH *et al.* Meta-analysis of respiratory rehabilitation in chronic obstructive pulmonary disease. *Lancet* 1996; **348**: 1115–19.

◆16. British Thoracic Society Standards of Care Subcommittee on Pulmonary Rehabilitation. Pulmonary rehabilitation. *Thorax* 2001; **56**: 827–34.

17. Lareau SC, Zuwallack R, Carlin B *et al.* Pulmonary rehabilitation – 1999. *Am J Respir Crit Care Med* 1999; **159**: 1666–82.

18. Enström C-P, Persson L-O, Larsson S *et al.* Long-term effects of a pulmonary rehabilitation programme in outpatients with chronic obstructive pulmonary disease: a randomized controlled study. *Scand J Rehab Med* 1999; **31**: 207–13.

19. Ries AL, Kaplan RM, Limberg TM *et al.* Effects of pulmonary rehabilitation on physiologic and psychological outcomes in patients with chronic obstructive pulmonary disease. *Ann Intern Med* 1995; **122**: 823–32.

20. Wedzicha JA, Bestall JC, Garrod R *et al.* Randomized controlled trial of pulmonary rehabilitation in severe chronic obstructive pulmonary disease patients, stratified with the MRC dyspnoea scale. *Eur Respir J* 1998; **12**: 363–9.

21. Mitsudomi T, Mizoue T, Yoshimatsu T. Postoperative complications after pneumonectomy for treatment of lung cancer: a multivariate analysis. *J Surg Oncol* 1996; **61**: 218–22.

22. Sekine Y, Behnia M, Fujisawa T. Impact of COPD on pulmonary complications and on long-term survival of patients undergoing surgery for NSCLC. *Lun Cancer* 2002; **37**: 95–101.

23. Uramoto H, Nakanishi R, Fujino Y. Prediction of pulmonary complications after a lobectomy in patients with non-small cell lung cancer. *Thorax* 2001; **56**: 59–61.

24. Smith TP, Kinasewitz GT, Tucker WY *et al.* Exercise capacity as a predictor of post-thoracotomy morbidity. *Am Rev Respir Dis* 1984; **129**: 730–4.

25. Brutsche MH, Spiliopoulos A, Bolliger CT *et al.* Exercise capacity and extent of resection as predictors of surgical risk in lung cancer. *Eur Respir J* 2000; **15**: 828–35.

26. Sciurba FC. Preoperative predictors of outcome following lung volume reduction surgery. *Thorax* 2002; **57**(Suppl. 2): II47–52.

27. Bolliger CT, Jordan P, Soler M *et al.* Exercise capacity as a predictor of postoperative complications in lung resection candidates. *Am J Resp Crit Care Med* 1995; **151**: 1472–80.

28. Vaporciyan AA, Merriman KW, Ece F *et al.* Incidence of major pulmonary morbidity after pneumonectomy: association with timing of smoking cessation. *Ann Thorac Surg* 1999; **73**: 420–5.

29. Melendez JA, Barrera R. Predictive respiratory complication quotient predicts pulmonary complications in thoracic surgical patients. *Ann Thorac Surg* 1998; **66**: 220–4.

30. National Emphysema Treatment Trial Research Group. Patients at high risk of death after lung-volume-reduction surgery. *N Engl J Med* 2001; **345**: 1075–83.

●31. National Emphysema Treatment Trial Research Group. A randomized trial comparing lung volume reduction surgery with medical therapy for severe emphysema. *N Engl J Med* 2003; **348**: 2059–73.

32. Celli BR, Cote CG, Marin JM *et al.* The body-mass index, airflow obstruction, dyspnea, and exercise capacity index in chronic obstructive pulmonary disease. *N Engl J Med* 2004; **350**: 1005–12.

33. Calverley P, Pauwels RA, Vestbo J *et al.* Combined salmeterol and fluticasone in the treatment of chronic obstructive pulmonary disease: a randomised controlled trial. *Lancet* 2003; **361**: 449–56.

34. Donohue JF, van Noord JA, Bateman ED *et al.* A 6-month, placebo-controlled study comparing lung function and health status changes in COPD patients treated with tiotropium or salmeterol. *Chest* 2002; **122**: 47–55.

35. Nishimura K, Izumi T, Tsukino M, Oga T. Dyspnea is a better predictor of 5-year survival than airway obstruction in patients with COPD. *Chest* 2002; **121**: 1434–40.

36. Domingo-Salvany A, Lamarca R, Ferrer M *et al.* Health-related quality of life and mortality in male patients with chronic obstructive pulmonary disease. *Am J Resp Crit Care Med* 2002; **166**: 680–5.

37. Make B. COPD: developing comprehensive management. *Respir Care* 2003; **48**: 1225–37.

38. Schols AMW, Soeters PB, Mosteret RM *et al.* Physiological effects of nutritional support and anabolic steroids in COPD patients. *Am J Respir Crit Care Med* 1995; **152**: 1268–74.

39. Rajendran AJ, Pandurangi UM, Murali R. Pre-operative short-term pulmonary rehabilitation for patients of chronic obstructive pulmonary disease undergoing coronary artery bypass graft surgery. *Indian Heart J* 1998; **50**: 531–4.

40. Wilson DJ. Pulmonary rehabilitation exercise program for high-risk thoracic surgical patients. *Chest Surg Clin N Am* 1997; **7**: 697–706.

Derby Hospitals NHS Foundation Trust
Library and Knowledge Service

41. Algar FJ, Alvarez A, Salvatierra A *et al.* Predicting pulmonary complications after pneumonectomy for lung cancer. *Eur J Cardiothorac Surg* 2003; **23**: 201–8.

42. Chumillas S, Ponce JL, Delgado F *et al.* Prevention of postoperative pulmonary complications through respiratory rehabilitation: a controlled clinical study. *Arch Phys Med Rehabil* 1998; **79**: 5–9.

43. Pauwels RA, Anthonisen N, Bailey WC *et al. Global Strategy for the Diagnosis, Management, and Prevention of Chronic Obstructive Pulmonary Disease: NHLBI/WHO, Workshop.* Online. http://www.goldcopd.com, updated August 2003.

44. Ries AL. Pulmonary rehabilitation and lung volume reduction surgery. In: Fessler HE, Reilly JJ, Sugarbaker DJ, eds. *Lung Volume Reduction Surgery for Emphysema.* New York: Marcel Dekker, 2003; 123–48.

45. Szekely LA, Oelberg DA, Wright C *et al.* Preoperative predictors of operative morbidity and mortality in COPD patients undergoing bilateral lung volume reduction surgery. *Chest* 1997; **111**: 550–8.

46. Fishman AP. Pulmonary rehabilitation research: NIH workshop summary. *Am J Respir Crit Care Med* 1994; **149**: 825–33.

47. Mineo TC, Ambrogi V, Pompeo E *et al.* Impact of lung volume reduction surgery versus rehabilitation on quality of life. *Eur Respir J* 2004; **23**: 275–80.

●48. Ries A, Christensen P, Kalra S *et al.* Pulmonary rehabilitation in the National Emphysema Treatment Trial (NETT): effect of prior rehab experience and use of satellite centers. *Am J Resp Crit Care Med* 2002; **163**: A13.

31

Pulmonary rehabilitation and transplantation

STEVEN E. GAY, FERNANDO J. MARTINEZ

INTRODUCTION

Lung transplantation is a viable and useful therapeutic intervention for patients with end-stage lung disease (1, 2). Although this text addresses the utility of pulmonary rehabilitation for chronic lung diseases, of the type and severity associated with referral to a transplant centre, the post-transplant patient is still affected by diminished exercise capacity when compared with healthy individuals or control patients (3). In this chapter, we discuss issues related to this diminished exercise capacity and how pulmonary rehabilitation may be used to improve patient function.

FUNCTIONAL CHANGES AFTER LUNG TRANSPLANTATION

Pulmonary function

Improvements in pulmonary function are well established following single lung (SLT) or double lung (DLT) transplantation (3). In patients with chronic obstructive pulmonary disease (COPD), there is little functional difference in outcomes between patients who undergo a left versus a right SLT (4). In a study of 14 patients with COPD who underwent SLT, 11 survived for at least 1 year; three received left-sided SLTs while eight received right-sided transplants (4). Although there was radiographic evidence that the native right lung might compress the transplanted lung, there were no significant differences in FEV_1 (forced expiratory volume in 1 s) between groups (0.64 ± 0.20 vs. 0.48 ± 0.15 L, left versus right lung transplant, respectively). The improvements at 3 and 12 months post-transplantation were similar between the groups, with the only statistically significant difference being a mild reduction in total lung capacity among the left lung transplant group compared with the right lung transplant group. Quantitative ventilation and perfusion were greater to the graft in patients receiving a right lung transplant.

Patients who undergo SLT for COPD improve in all indices of pulmonary function immediately post-transplant. In one study, the FEV_1 significantly increased at 3 months and remained stable for 12–24 months post-transplant (5). The forced vital capacity (FVC) followed a similar course. The mean FEV_1/FVC ratio improved at 3 and 6 months but then deteriorated at 12 and 24 months, primarily due to the development of obliterative bronchiolitis.

Exercise response

Although patients who undergo lung transplantation experience marked improvements in pulmonary function, they still experience a limitation in exercise capacity, not defined by one specific mechanism. A summary of published studies (3, 6) is presented in Table 31.1. In one study, the response to incremental exercise, using a cycle ergometer, was compared between lung transplant recipients (11 HLT [heart–lung transplant], six DLT, 16 SLT) and control subjects. Within the first year of transplantation, at peak exercise, the transplant recipients reached maximum oxygen uptakes ($\dot{V}O_{2,max}$) in the range of 40–60 per cent, irrespective of whether they were HLT, DLT or SLT recipients. No patients had a ventilatory limitation to exercise. Instead, their response to exercise was characterized by a reduced aerobic capacity and diminished oxygen pulse which the authors interpreted as suggesting an abnormal cardiovascular response (7). In a separate comparison of COPD patients who received either a right or left SLT, both groups exhibited comparable aerobic capacity, maximum heart rate (HR), anaerobic threshold and maximum minute ventilation ($\dot{V}_{E,max}$) (4). In another study, patients experienced improvement in $\dot{V}O_{2,max}$, $\dot{V}_{E,max}$ and HR_{max},

Table 31.1 Studies of cardiopulmonary exercise training post-transplantation

Author	Intervention	Changes in exercise
Cassivi et al. 1991 (1)	SLT, DLT in COPD	↑ 6-min walk
Gibbons et al. 1991 (8)	SLT in COPD	↓ HR_{max}, ↑ $\dot{V}o_{2max}$, ↑ $work_{max}$, ↑ ventilatory equivalents, ↑MVV
Levy et al. 1993 (7)	HLT, DLT and SLT in obstructive and restrictive lung diseases	↓ Aerobic capacity
Ross et al. 1993 (14)	SLT and DLT in obstructive and interstitial lung disease	↓ Oxygen pulse, compared with controls; ↑ $\dot{V}o_{2,max}$, ↑ stroke volume index and ↑ mean PAP at rest and exercise; ↓ anaerobic thresholds compared with controls
Orens et al. 1995 (9)	Lung transplants in patients with chronic airflow obstruction, idiopathic pulmonary fibrosis and pulmonary vascular disease	No difference in HRR, $\dot{V}_E$, RR or V_T between disease states, $\dot{V}o_{2,max}$, work rate, O_2 pulse and AT lower in pulmonary fibrosis group
Ambrosino et al. 1996 (62)	HLT recipients (n = 11) post-rehabilitation	Improved but persistently abnormal peak work rate, $\dot{V}o_2$ up to 18 months after transplant
Evans et al. 1997 (44)	Lung transplant recipients (SLT, n = 7; DLT, n = 2) contrasted to healthy controls	Decreased peak $\dot{V}o_2$, $\dot{V}_E$ in recipients compared with controls
Systrom et al. 1998 (11)	SLT with COPD (n = 12) pre- and post-transplant	Increased maximum workload achieved after transplantation although maximum $\dot{V}o_2$ remains decreased (46.6% of predicted)
Tirdel et al. 1998 (45)	4 SLT and 2 DLT recipients and age-matched controls	Decreased peak $\dot{V}o_2$ in recipients (45% of predicted) contrasted to controls (101% of predicted). 'Circulatory limitation' in recipients
Oelberg et al. 1998 (64)	10 cystic fibrosis patients undergoing DLT	Improved peak $\dot{V}o_2$ after transplant but still reduced; reduced systemic O_2 extraction remained after transplantation
Lands et al. 1999 (42)	SLT, DLT for obstructive and interstitial lung disease	Improved maximum exercise performance, improved peripheral and respiratory muscle strength, improved $\dot{V}o_{2,max}$, improved W_{max}
Pantoja et al. 1999 (65)	SLT, DLT for obstructive lung disease, pulmonary fibrosis and primary pulmonary hypertension	Reduced maximal expiratory pressures in transplant recipients with maximal inspiratory pressures that did not exhibit change from pre- to post-transplant
Vachiery et al. 1999 (18)	HLT in patients with primary pulmonary hypertension, cystic fibrosis, alpha-1-antitrypsin deficiency and coalminer's pneumoconiosis 12–55 months post transplant	Chronotrophic incompetence, reduced increase in cardiac index and stroke volume index, increased left ventricular filling pressures from immediately post-transplant
Wang et al. 1999 (46)	Transplant recipients, 3 SLT, 1 HLT, 4 DLT and age-matched controls	Lower peak work rate, $\dot{V}o_{2,peak}$ lactate threshold, in transplant recipients compared with controls
Schwaiblamair et al. 1999 (10)	Pre- and post-transplant exercise testing in 103 recipients (46 SLT, 25 HLT, 32 DLT)	Improved aerobic capacity, anaerobic threshold and ventilatory response after transplantation
Murciano et al. 2000 (20)	Eight SLT recipients	X Peak work load (72% of predicted) and $\dot{V}o_2$ (65% of predicted). Seven patients exhibit flow limitation during maximal exercise
McKenna et al. 2003 (47)	Lung transplant recipients and one HLT recipient	Higher Po_2 in post-transplant recipients as compared with controls. Lower peak exercise work rates and markedly lower $\dot{V}o_{2,peak}$
Tegtbur et al. (13)	27 bilateral lung transplant recipients and 30 controls	X Peak work load and $\dot{V}o_2$; quality of life similar between lung transplant recipients and controls

AT, anaerobic threshold; COPD, chronic obstructive pulmonary disease; DLT, double lung transplant; HLT, heart–lung transplant; HR, heart rate; HRR, heart rate reserve; MVV, maximal voluntary ventilation; PAP, pulmonary arterial pressure; RR, respiratory rate; SLT, single lung transplant; $\dot{V}_E$, minute ventilation; $\dot{V}o_2$, oxygen uptake; V_T, tidal volume.

that were sustained at 12 and 24 months, although the $\dot{V}O_{2,max}$ remained below that of control subjects at exercise iso-time (5).

After SLT, patients with obstructive or restrictive lung diseases do not differ in their lung function or their response to cardiopulmonary exercise testing, the oxygen consumption being similarly reduced in both circumstances (8). In patients with chronic airflow obstruction, idiopathic pulmonary fibrosis or pulmonary vascular disease no statistically significant differences in many exercise measures after transplantation were noted; the maximum oxygen consumption, work rate and anaerobic threshold were lower among patients with pulmonary fibrosis (9). The $\dot{V}O_{2,max}$ increased 3–6 months post-transplantation and then gradually fell over the subsequent 6–9 months such that there were no differences in $\dot{V}O_{2,max}$ between 3 and 9 months after transplantation. Work rates improved at 3–6 months and remained stable thereafter. Aerobic capacity was reduced in all groups throughout the study, irrespective of the underlying disease or type of transplant procedure performed (9).

Schwaiblmair et al. (10) reported on the results of incremental exercise in 103 consecutive recipients of SLT ($n = 46$), DLT ($n = 32$) and HLT ($n = 25$) before and shortly after surgery. All patients were severely impaired before transplantation. After transplantation (mean 55 days), the $\dot{V}O_{2,max}$ improved to 22–71 per cent of predicted. Maximum work capacity, oxygen pulse, tidal volume and peak ventilation did not differ between those with SLT compared with DLT or HLT. In a previous, smaller study Systrom et al. (11) also confirmed a doubling of maximum workload before and after SLT in 12 patients with COPD (11). In 10 cystic fibrosis (CF) patients undergoing DLT, Oelberg et al. (12) confirmed improved peak $\dot{V}O_2$ after transplantation (31–45 per cent of predicted); the post-transplantation result was still much lower than an age-matched control group (12). It is evident that improvement in exercise capacity occurs after transplantation, although a persistent aerobic limitation persists, which appears to be independent of underlying disease state or type of transplant procedure. One group has noted that despite a decreased peak workload and $\dot{V}O_2$ in 27 lung transplant recipients compared with 30 controls, quality of life was remarkably similar between the two groups (13).

POTENTIAL MECHANISMS FOR EXERCISE LIMITATION

Numerous authors have examined the potential mechanisms for the persistent exercise limitation noted after transplantation. Reports have evaluated cardiovascular and respiratory function as well as peripheral muscle function and the effects of medications.

Cardiac limitation

Several groups have examined the cardiovascular response to exercise after lung transplantation. A prospective study reported on the haemodynamic responses to incremental cycle ergometry in eight patients who underwent 6 weeks of supervised exercise training (14). The patients experienced increases in $\dot{V}O_{2,max}$ post-transplant compared with pre-transplant, 13.4 ± 0.8 vs. 9.2 ± 0.8 mL/min per kg ($P < 0.01$). Increased maximum stroke volume index was also noted in six out of seven patients. The mean pulmonary arterial pressure at rest was increased, and increased further with exercise. After transplantation, pulmonary vascular resistance remained slightly elevated but decreased appropriately during incremental exercise and was associated with a normal cardiac output response. Patients did not achieve their anaerobic threshold prior to lung transplant, but post-transplant thresholds were found to be abnormally low: $\dot{V}O_2 = 9.4 \pm 0.6$ mL/min per kg or 35 ± 3 per cent of predicted $\dot{V}O_{2,max}$ (14). Other investigators have suggested that in some patients right ventricular impairment may contribute to exercise limitation after transplantation (15–17).

More recently, nine stable HLT recipients 12–55 months post-transplant were studied (18). At baseline, their heart rate was slightly increased and their stroke volume index was slightly decreased. Stroke volume index and cardiac index increased at the onset of exercise, but did not change significantly at 40–80 per cent of maximal workload. The authors suggested that HLT recipients exhibited chronotropic insufficiency during dynamic exercise (18). Although subtle cardiovascular limitations may be present in some lung transplant recipients, this may be more evident in HLT recipients.

Ventilatory limitation

The majority of investigators have not documented evidence of ventilatory limitation among lung transplant recipients. Two groups have confirmed flow limitation in SLT recipients with COPD. Martinez et al. (19), using tidal flow–volume studies, confirmed expiratory flow limitation during exercise in SLT recipients with COPD. Similarly, Murciano et al. (20) confirmed flow limitation in seven out of eight SLT recipients with COPD, utilizing the negative expiratory pressure method (20). Despite these results, ventilatory limitation is unlikely to be a major contributor to exercise limitation in most lung transplant recipients.

Peripheral muscle dysfunction

Most reports support peripheral muscle dysfunction as the predominant cause of exercise limitation after lung transplantation (6, 21). Peripheral muscle dysfunction is quite prevalent in patients awaiting lung transplantation (22), particularly those patients with COPD (23, 24). In 184 consecutive lung transplant candidates (COPD, $n = 66$; alpha-1-antitrypsin deficiency, $n = 30$; CF, $n = 35$; lung fibrosis, $n = 25$; primary pulmonary hypertension, $n = 28$), quadriceps muscle force was lower than reference values (22). This was particularly evident in CF patients, who demonstrated a significant correlation between body mass index and quadriceps muscle force.

Several reports have addressed peripheral muscle function in COPD (23–26). Leg fatigue is common in COPD patients during exercise (24, 27, 28). Reduced muscle mass, strength, endurance and enzymatic activity have also been described (29–35). Goskers *et al.* (36) recently confirmed a shift in the relative composition of type I and type IIX fibres in stable patients with COPD (FEV_1 = 42 per cent of predicted) (36). Type IIX fibre atrophy was also noted to be present (37).

Inflammatory mediators are released during bouts of rejection and infection, common in the post-transplant course. These inflammatory mediators, together with the chronic inflammatory processes that develop, contribute to muscle injury (38, 39). Immunosuppressive therapy for maintenance of the transplant organ also contributes to the development of a myopathic process (40, 41). Both inflammatory mediators and administered medications act on peripheral muscle that is already deconditioned from the decreased activity and poor nutrition associated with chronic illness.

Several reports have evaluated the contribution of peripheral muscles to the diminished exercise capacity of post-lung transplant patients. Lands *et al.* (42) studied 10 SLT and nine DLT recipients 37.5 months after transplantation. Both groups exhibited limited exercise capacity (W_{max} = 38.0 [30.0–65.0] and 37.5 [30.0–44.0] per cent of predicted in SLT and DLT, respectively), diminished leg power and leg work capacity. Respiratory muscle strength was normal in both groups. Maximal exercise capacity, peripheral muscle strength and endurance were reduced 18 months post-transplant in both SLT and DLT groups. The investigators postulated that most of the peripheral muscle dysfunction was attributable to detraining (42).

Pantoja *et al.* (43) examined nine lung transplant recipients (eight SLT, one DLT) 5–102 months after transplantation. In a subset of six patients, the contractile properties and fatigue characteristics of the tibialis anterior muscle were measured using electrical stimulation. Maximal voluntary contraction was decreased by 39 per cent ($P < 0.05$). The force and fatigue characteristics of the tibialis anterior muscles were not different from controls. Although the maximal inspiratory pressures did not differ from control values, the maximal expiratory pressures were diminished by 30 per cent relative to control ($P < 0.05$). The authors concluded that peripheral and expiratory muscle weakness, atrophy and reduction in muscular function with exercise were present in patients up to 3 years post-transplant (43).

Evans *et al.* (44) studied nine lung transplant recipients, 5–38 months post-transplant, as well as eight healthy controls, as they performed incremental quadriceps exercise to exhaustion. In addition to measures of gas exchange, minute ventilation and serum lactate, quadriceps muscle pH as well as phosphorylation potential were measured using ^{31}P magnetic resonance spectroscopy. Quadriceps muscle intracellular pH was more acidic at rest and fell during exercise at a lower metabolic rate in transplant recipients versus the healthy controls. The decrease in aerobic capacity could not be explained by ventilatory limitation, arterial oxygen desaturation or the presence of mild anaemia. The persistent decrease in $\dot{V}_{O_2,max}$

correlated closely with the metabolic rate at which muscle pH fell. The authors concluded that impaired aerobic capacity after lung transplantation could be related to abnormalities of skeletal muscle oxidative capacity.

Systrom *et al.* (11) examined 12 SLT recipients with COPD before and 3–6 months after transplantation. Although maximum workload doubled after surgery, $\dot{V}_{O_2,max}$ remained markedly reduced. Although cardiac output during peak exercise was normal, the arterial–mixed venous oxygen content difference was reduced to half of normal, as mixed venous oxygen saturation did not fall normally, reflecting reduced systemic oxygen extraction. These observations were confirmed in 10 CF patients who underwent DLT (12).

Using a non-invasive optical technique for the analysis of oxygen delivery and utilization in exercising muscle, Tirdel *et al.* (45) reported that six post-lung transplant patients had a reduced maximum oxygen consumption and an earlier onset of anaerobic threshold compared with six matched healthy controls. Transplant patients also demonstrated a smaller change in the optical density in the spectrum of absorption characteristics of haemoglobin and myoglobin at maximal exercise, suggesting an alteration in peripheral oxygen utilization by the muscle cell.

Wang *et al.* (46) analysed vastus lateralis muscle biopsies in post-lung transplant patients following exercise. Patients had a mean peak $\dot{V}_{O_2}$ of 52 per cent of that of controls. Biopsies showed a lower mitochondrial adenosine triphosphate (ATP) production rate, lower activity of mitochondrial enzymes, a lower proportion of type 1 fibres and a higher lactate and inosine monophosphate content in the transplant recipients versus controls. In addition, a higher lactate and inosine monophosphate and lower ATP content at rest were noted, suggesting greater reliance on anaerobic metabolism. These authors have previously reported reduced muscle calcium regulation and impaired potassium regulation after lung transplantation (47, 48), contributing to impaired muscular performance during exercise.

The cause of peripheral muscle dysfunction post-transplantation remains unclear. Chronic disease, drug therapy, disuse and poor nutrition have all been invoked. Skeletal muscle is altered in chronic disease (49), with more type II fibres and decreased oxidative enzymes, which increase after transplantation. Immunosuppressive medications, such as corticosteroids, are recognized to contribute to myopathy of both peripheral and respiratory muscles (50). Variation in fibre diameter, fibre atrophy, necrosis and basophilic infiltrates have been reported, as has increased connective tissue between fibres. Fibre atrophy affects mainly the fast fibres (51).

Cyclosporine A, a common component in the post-transplantation immunosuppressive regimen, has well defined effects on mitochondrial respiration. Cyclosporine A inhibits maximal coupled and uncoupled skeletal muscle mitochondrial respiration *in vitro*. It is believed to exert its toxic effects on the enzyme complexes of the electron transfer chain or on the inner mitochondrial membrane integrity (52). In rats, cyclosporine has been found to have clear effects on mitochondrial respiration and endurance time *in vivo* after a short

(14 day) course of administration. In one study, there were significant decreases in submaximal endurance exercise time and lower state 3 and uncoupled mitochondrial respiration as compared with control rats (53). Although the mechanism remains unclear, it may relate to diminished mitochondrial calcium efflux and subsequent mitochondrial dysfunction (52, 54). In addition, cyclosporine may functionally and anatomically reduce the microcirculatory network within the muscle (53).

REHABILITATION NEEDS AND RESULTS IN THE LUNG TRANSPLANT POPULATION

In a patient population with a chronic debilitating illness, severe enough to warrant lung transplantation, rehabilitation improves functional exercise capacity and health-related quality of life prior to transplantation. An early pilot study in nine transplant recipients was reported (55). Four patients were randomized to a 6-week programme of health maintenance education, while five were randomized to education plus exercise. In both groups quality of well-being and 6-min walk distance significantly improved (Fig. 31.1) (55). Given the acute deconditioning associated with a major surgical procedure, superimposed on the general deconditioning of chronic illness, pulmonary rehabilitation should be an ideal therapeutic modality for post-transplant patients.

Support for the potential benefit of pulmonary rehabilitation on peripheral muscle function in this patient group is found in the results of exercise among healthy subjects, in whom it has been documented to improve mitochondrial ATP production. Muscle biopsies before and after 6 weeks of

endurance training and after 3 weeks of detraining in nine healthy men showed a 70 per cent increase in mitochondrial ATP production rate as well as mitochondrial and glycolytic enzymes following 6 weeks of endurance training, diminishing by 12–28 per cent after 3 weeks of detraining. $\dot{V}O_{2,max}$ increased by 9.6 per cent following training and fell by 6.0 per cent after detraining (56). Intense exercise training will increase the proportion of type I fibres, the number of mitochondria, muscle capillarization and muscle oxidative enzyme activity in patients with COPD (57–59). Finally, in patients with primary defects of mitochondrial function, 8 weeks of exercise training was associated with a 30 per cent increase in aerobic capacity, a reduction in blood lactic acid and an improvement in ADP recovery (60). Following 8 weeks of exercise training, patients with a mitochondrial myopathy improved their aerobic capacity by 30 per cent, whereas patients with a non-metabolic myopathy improved by 16 per cent and healthy volunteers by only 10 per cent (61).

There have been few reports of pulmonary rehabilitation post-transplantation. In one study, 11 HLT recipients underwent in-patient pulmonary rehabilitation immediately post-transplant (62). Respiratory and peripheral muscle function, functional exercise capacity and maximum oxygen uptake

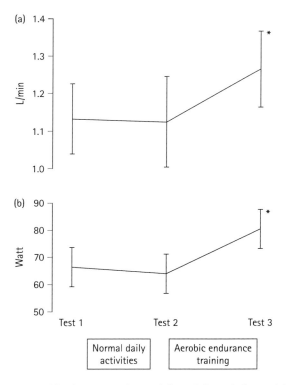

Figure 31.2 *Nine lung transplant recipients followed after an initial 11-week period of normal activity and after a 6-week period of aerobic endurance training. Peak oxygen uptake ($\dot{V}O_2$) (a) and peak physical work capacity (b) of all nine patients over the study period. The period of normal daily activities did not change peak $\dot{V}O_2$ or peak workload, whereas after the 6-week endurance training, both parameters increased significantly. Values are mean ± 1 SEM. *P < 0.05. Reproduced with permission from Stiebellehner et al. (63).*

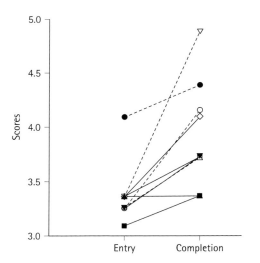

Figure 31.1 *Change in quality of well-being in nine patients randomized to a 6-week programme of health education (n = 4; dotted lines) or education plus exercise (n = 5; solid lines). Improvement was noted in both groups. Reproduced with permission from Manzetti et al. (55).*

increased only slightly, although small increases continued in the absence of further rehabilitation (62).

Stiebellehner *et al.* (63) enrolled nine lung transplant recipients (mean 12 months after transplantation) in a 6-week aerobic endurance training programme of cycle ergometer exercise three to five times per week. Training intensity was defined by the training heart rate, calculated as 60 per cent of the maximum heart rate reserve. Exercise capacity was evaluated after an initial 11-week period of usual daily activities and again after the 6-week training programme. Peak oxygen uptake and maximum power output remained unchanged following normal daily activities but significant improvements were noted after the training program (Fig. 31.2). Post-training, resting ventilation decreased from 14 ± 5 to 11 ± 3 L/min, and at an identical submaximal level of exercise (isowork), significant decreases in minute ventilation (from 47 ± 14 to 39 ± 13 L/min) and heart rate (from 144 ± 12 to 133 ± 17 beats/min) were noted.

CONCLUSION

Exercise limitation is very severe prior to lung transplantation. Post-transplantation, exercise improves, but remains below predicted values. Peripheral muscle dysfunction is the most likely cause of this exercise limitation, caused by a combination of poor conditioning and the use of immunosuppressive medications, especially corticosteroids and cyclosporine. Pulmonary rehabilitation is an important adjunctive therapy among patients who require lung transplantation. Exercise training prior to transplantation will be of benefit, although training will be limited by their ventilatory impairment. Post-transplantation, rehabilitation has the potential to improve functional exercise capacity and health-related quality of life. It is likely that these benefits will be sustained in both the short and long term after successful lung transplantation, provided that the patient adheres to an exercise regimen.

Key points

- Pulmonary function generally improves after lung transplantation, although exercise capacity remains impaired.
- Cardiac limitation does not appear to limit exercise after lung transplantation.
- Ventilatory limitation may be present in selected patients after single lung transplantation.
- A peripheral myopathic process is the most likely source of exercise limitation after lung transplantation.
- Mitochondrial oxygen utilization may be impaired due to the deconditioning and immunosuppressive medications.
- Pulmonary rehabilitation can ameliorate the exercise limitation noted after transplantation.

REFERENCES

● 1. Cassivi SD, Meyers BF, Battafarano RJ *et al.* Thirteen-year experience in lung transplantation for emphysema. *Ann Thorac Surg* 2002; **74**: 1663–9 (discussion 1669–70).

◆ 2. Meyers BF, Patterson GA. Chronic obstructive pulmonary disease. 10: Bullectomy, lung volume reduction surgery, and transplantation for patients with chronic obstructive pulmonary disease. *Thorax* 2003; **58**: 634–8.

◆ 3. Williams TJ, Snell GI. Early and long-term functional outcomes in unilateral, bilateral, and living-related transplant recipients. *Clin Chest Med* 1997; **18**: 245–57.

4. Levine SM, Anzueto A, Gibbbons WJ *et al.* Graft position and pulmonary function after single lung transplantation for obstructive lung disease. *Chest* 1993; **103**: 444–8.

5. Levine SM, Anzueto A, Peters JI *et al.* Medium term functional results of single-lung transplantation for endstage obstructive lung disease. *Am J Respir Crit Care Med* 1994; **150**: 398–402.

6. Williams TJ, Slater WR. Role of cardiopulmonary exercise testing in lung and heart-lung transplantation. In: Weisman I, Zeballos R, eds. *Clinical Exercise Testing. Progress in Respiratory Research.* Basel: Karger, 2002; 254–63.

7. Levy RD, Ernst P, Levine SM *et al.* Exercise performance after lung transplantation. *J Heart Lung Transplant* 1993; **12**: 27–33.

8. Gibbons WJ, Levine SM, Bryan CL *et al.* Cardiopulmonary exercise responses after single lung transplantation for severe obstructive lung disease. *Chest* 1991; **100**: 106–11.

9. Orens JB, Becker FS, Lynch JP *et al.* Cardiopulmonary exercise testing following allogeneic lung transplantation for different underlying disease states. *Chest* 1995; **107**: 144–9.

● 10. Schwaiblmair M, Reichenspurner H, Muller C *et al.* Cardiopulmonary exercise testing before and after lung and heart lung transplantation. *Am J Respir Crit Care Med* 1999; **159**: 1277–83.

11. Systrom DM, Pappagianopoulos P, Fishman RS *et al.* Determinants of abnormal maximum oxygen uptake after lung transplantation for chronic obstructive pulmonary disease. *J Heart Lung Transplant* 1998; **17**: 1220–30.

12. Oelberg DA, Systrom DM, Markowitz DH *et al.* Exercise performance in cystic fibrosis before and after bilateral lung transplantation. *J Heart Lung Transplant* 1998; **17**: 1104–12.

13. Tegtbur U, Sievers C, Busse MW *et al.* [Quality of life and exercise capacity in lung transplant recipients]. *Pneumologie* 2004; **58**: 72–8.

14. Ross DJ, Waters PF, Mohsenifar Z *et al.* Hemodynamic responses to exercise after lung transplantation. *Chest* 1993; **103**: 46–53.

15. Carerem R, Patterson GA, Liu P *et al.* Right and left ventricular performance after single and double lung transplantation. The Toronto Lung Transplant Group. *J Thorac Cardiovasc Surg* 1991; **102**: 115–22.

16. Globits S, Burghuber OC, Koller J *et al.* Effect of lung transplantation on right and left ventricular volumes and function measured by magnetic resonance imaging. *Am J Respir Crit Care Med* 1994; **149**: 1000–4.

17. Katz WE, Gasior TA, Quinlan JJ *et al.* Immediate effects of lung transplantation on right ventricular morphology and function in patients with variable degrees of pulmonary hypertension. *J Am Coll Cardiol* 1996; **27**: 384–91.

18. Vachiery J-L, Niset G, Antoine M *et al.* Haemodynamic response to dynamic exercise after heart-lung transplantation. *Eur Respir J* 1999; **14**: 1131–5.

19. Martinez FJ, Orens JB, Whyte RI *et al.* Lung mechanics and dyspnea after lung transplantation for chronic airflow obstruction. *Am J Respir Crit Care Med* 1996; **153**: 1536–43.

20. Murciano D, Ferretti A, Boxzkowski J *et al.* Flow limitation and dynamic hyperinflation during exercise in COPD patients after single lung transplantation. *Chest* 2000; **118**: 1248–54.

◆21. Kerber AC, Szidon P, Kesten S. Skeletal muscle dysfunction in lung transplantation. *J Heart Lung Transplant* 2000; **19**: 392–400.

22. van der Woude BT, Kropmans TJB, Douma KW *et al.* Peripheral muscle force and exercise capacity in lung transplant candidates. *Int J Rehabil Res* 2002; **25**: 351–5.

23. Mador MJ, Bozkanat E. Skeletal muscle dysfunction in chronic obstructive pulmonary disease. *Respir Res* 2001; **2**: 216–24.

24. American Thoracic Society, European Respiratory Society. Skeletal muscle dysfunction in chronic obstructive pulmonary disease. A statement of the American Thoracic Society and European Respiratory Society. *Am J Respir Crit Care Med* 1999; **159**: S1–40.

25. Krieger AC, Szidon P, Kesten S. Skeletal muscle dysfunction in lung transplantation. *J Heart Lung Transplant* 2000; **19**: 392–400.

26. Wouters EFM. Chronic obstructive pulmonary disease. 5: Systemic effects of COPD. *Thorax* 2002; **57**: 1067–70.

27. Killian KJ, Leblanc P, Martin DH *et al.* Exercise capacity and ventilatory, circulatory and symptoms limitation in patients with chronic airflow limitation. *Am Rev Respir Dis* 1992; **146**: 935–40.

28. Gosselink R, Troosters T, DeCramer M. Peripheral muscle weakness contributes to exercise limitation in COPD. *Am J Respir Crit Care Med* 1996; **153**: 976–80.

29. Maltais F, Jobin J, Sullivan MJ. Metabolic and hemodynamic responses of lower limb exercise in patients with COPD. *J Appl Physiol* 1998; **84**: 1573–80.

30. Bernard S, Leblanc P, Whittom F *et al.* Peripheral muscle weakness in patients with chronic obstructive pulmonary disease. *Am J Respir Crit Care Med* 1998; **158**: 629–34.

31. Maltais F, Simard A, Simard C *et al.* Oxidative capacity of the skeletal muscle and lactic acid kinetics during exercise in normal subjects and in patients with COPD. *Am J Respir Crit Care Med* 1996; **153**: 288–93.

32. Pouw EM, Schols AMWJ, van der Vusse GJ *et al.* Elevated inosine monophosphate levels in resting muscle of patients with stable chronic obstructive pulmonary disease. *Am J Respir Crit Care Med* 1998; **157**: 453–7.

33. Saey D, Debigare R, Leblanc P *et al.* Contractile leg fatigue after cycle exercise: a factor limiting exercise in patients with chronic obstructive pulmonary disease. *Am J Respir Crit Care Med* 2003; **168**: 425–30.

34. Couillard A, Maltais F, Saey D *et al.* Exercise-induced quadriceps oxidative stress and peripheral muscle dysfunction in patients with chronic obstructive pulmonary disease. *Am J Respir Crit Care Med* 2003; **167**: 1664–9.

35. Goskers HR, van Mamaren H, van Dijk PJ *et al.* Skeletal muscle fibre-type shifting and metabolic profile in patients with chronic obstructive pulmonary disease. *Eur Respir J* 2002; **19**: 617–25.

36. Goskers HR, Kubat B, Schaarf G *et al.* Myopathological features in skeletal muscle of patients with chronic obstructive pulmonary disease. *Eur Respir J* 2003; **22**: 280–5.

37. Goskers HR, Engelen MP, van Mamaren H *et al.* Muscle fiber type IIX atrophy is involved in the loss of fat-free mass in chronic obstructive pulmonary disease. *Am J Clin Nutr* 2002; **76**: 113–19.

38. Wilcox PG, Wakai Y, Walley KR *et al.* Tumor necrosis factor alpha decreases *in vivo* diaphragm contractility in dogs. *Am J Respir Crit Care Med* 1994; **150**: 1368–73.

39. Noguchi Y, Yoshikawa T, Matsumoto A *et al.* Are cytokines possible mediators of cancer cachexia? *Surg Today* 1996; **26**: 467–75.

40. Goy JJ, Stauffer JC, Deruaz JP *et al.* Myopathy as possible side-effect of cyclosporin. *Lancet* 1989; **1**: 1446–7.

41. Arellano F, Krupp P. Muscular disorders associated with cyclosporin. *Lancet* 1991; **337**: 915.

42. Lands LC, Smountas AA, Mesiano G *et al.* Maximal exercise capacity and peripheral skeletal muscle function following lung transplantation. *J Heart Lung Transplant* 1999; **18**: 113–20.

43. Pantoja JG, Andrade FJ, Stokic DS *et al.* Respiratory and limb muscle function in lung allograft recipients. *Am J Respir Crit Care Med* 1999; **160**: 1205–1211.

44. Evans AB, Al-Himyary AJ, Hrovat MI *et al.* Abnormal skeletal muscle oxidative capacity after lung transplantation by ^{31}P-MRS. *Am J Respir Crit Care Med* 1997; **155**: 615–21.

45. Tirdel GB, Girgis R, Fishman RS, Theodore J. Metabolic myopathy as a cause of the exercise limitation in lung transplant recipients. *J Heart Lung Transplant* 1998; **17**: 1231–7.

46. Wang XN, Williams TJ, McKenna MJ *et al.* Skeletal muscle oxidative capacity, fiber type and metabolites after lung transplantation. *Am J Respir Crit Care Med* 1999; **160**: 57–63.

●47. McKenna MJ, Fraser SF, Li JL *et al.* Impaired muscle Ca^{2+} and K^+ regulation contribute to poor exercise performance post-lung transplantation. *J Appl Physiol* 2003; **95**: 1606–16.

48. Hall MJ, Snell GI, Side EA *et al.* Exercise, potassium, and muscle deconditioning post-thoracic organ transplantation. *J Appl Physiol* 1994; **77**: 2784–90.

49. Bussieres LM, Pflugfelder PW, Taylor AW *et al.* Changes in skeletal muscle morphology and biochemistry after cardiac transplantation. *Am J Cardiol* 1997; **78**: 630–4.

50. DeCramer M, Stas KJ. Corticosteroid-induced myopathy involving respiratory muscles in patients with chronic obstructive pulmonary disease or asthma. *Am Rev Respir Dis* 1992; **146**: 800–2.

51. DeCramer M, de Bock V, Dom R. Functional and histologic picture of steroid-induced myopathy in chronic obstructive pulmonary disease. *Am J Respir Crit Care Med* 1996; **153**: 1958–64.

52. Hokanson JF, Mercier JG, Brooks GA. Cyclosporine A decreases rat skeletal muscle mitochondiral respiration *in vitro*. *Am J Respir Crit Care Med* 1995; **151**: 1848–51.

53. Mercier JG, Hokanson JF, Brooks GA. Effects of cyclosporine A on skeletal muscle mitochondrial respiration and endurance time in rats. *Am J Respir Crit Care Med* 1995; **151**: 1532–6.

54. Biring MS, Fournier M, Ross DJ, Lewis MI. Cellular adaptations of skeletal muscles to cyclosporin. *J Appl Physiol* 1998; **84**: 1967–75.

55. Manzetti JD, Hoffman LA, Sereika *et al.* Exercise, education and quality of life in lung transplant candidates. *J Heart Lung Transplant* 1994; **13**: 297–305.

56. Wibom R, Hultman E, Johansson M *et al.* Adaptation of mitochondrial ATP production in human skeletal muscle to endurance training and detraining. *J Appl Physiol* 1992; **73**: 2004–10.

57. Howard H, Hoppeler H, Claassen H *et al.* Influences of endurance training on the ultrastructural composition of the different muscle fiber types in humans. *Pflugers Arch* 1985; **403**: 369–76.

58. Maltais F, Leblanc P, Simard C *et al.* Skeletal muscle adaptation to endurance training in patients with chronic obstructive pulmonary disease. *Am J Respir Crit Care Med* 1996; **154**: 442–7.

59. Puente-Maestu L, Tena T, Trascasa C *et al.* Training improves muscle oxidative capacity and oxygenation recovery kinetics in patients with chronic obstructive pulmonary disease. *Eur J Appl Physiol* 2003; **88**: 580–7.

60. Taivassalo T, DeStefano N, Argov Z *et al.* Effects of aerobic training in patients with mitochondrial myopathies. *Neurology* 1998; **50**: 1055–60.

61. Taivassalo T, DeStefano N, Chen J *et al.* Short-term aerobic training response in chronic myopathies. *Muscle Nerve* 1999; **22**: 1239–43.

62. Ambrosino N, Bruschi C, Callegari G *et al.* Time course of exercise capacity, skeletal and respiratory muscle performance after heart-lung transplantation. *Eur Respir J* 1996; **9**: 1508–14.

63. Stiebellehner J, Wuittan M, End A *et al.* Aerobic endurance training program improves exercise performance in lung transplant recipients. *Chest* 1998; **113**: 906–12.

64. Oelberg DA, Systrom DM, Markowitz DH *et al.* Exercise performance in cystic fibrosis before and after bilateral lung transplantation. *J Heart Lung Transplant* 1998; **17**: 1104–12.

65. Pantoja JG, Andrade FH, Stoki DS *et al.* Respiratory and limb muscle function in lung allograft recipients. *Am J Respir Crit Care Med* 1999; **160**: 1205–11.

32

Long-term oxygen therapy

BRIAN TIEP, RICK CARTER

Long-term oxygen therapy (LTOT) is prescribed to patients with chronic lung disease to protect them from the destructive ravages of tissue hypoxia, empower their ability to function, and enhance their survival. Amidst this positivism by the clinician, introducing oxygen into the life of patients can conjure up glimpses of their own mortality. Tied to oxygen, it is now undeniable that this grave illness will take their life in the foreseeable future. This negative perspective impedes the restorative thrust of rehabilitation by dampening any optimism that life will get better. In fact, implementation of LTOT can be enabling and contribute to years of quality and active living.

In pulmonary rehabilitation, oxygen therapy, quality medical care, the proper use of medications and exercise training work in unison to maximize oxygen transport. Both require effort and commitment – thus, oxygen transport must be paralleled by 'behavioural transport'. Patients must accept both as being integral to one another as they assume an active lifestyle (1).

PHYSIOLOGICAL EXPECTATIONS

The rationale for the clinical implementation of LTOT is founded in the physiology of gas exchange and oxygen transport to the tissues as well as an understanding of the destructive nature of tissue hypoxia and the protective impact of supplemental oxygen. Arterial partial pressure of oxygen (P_aO_2) is determined by the fraction of inspired oxygen (F_IO_2), alveolar ventilation, ventilation/perfusion matching, and diffusion of gases across the alveolar–capillary membrane. Oxygen transport to the tissues is determined by the foregoing plus the oxygen-carrying and -releasing capacity of haemoglobin, cardiac output, capillary distribution and the uptake and utilization of oxygen by the mitochondria. A deficiency in any of these physiological links in oxygen transport is likely to impede the oxygen from reaching its final destination, the living cell.

Chronic hypoxia impairs cellular function and may progress to necrosis. Initially, cell survival will be prolonged through anaerobic glycolysis, which causes the build-up of lactate in the cell. Cells can function temporarily in this anaerobic environment, albeit inefficiently and uncomfortably. A return to oxidative metabolism must occur in short order if the cell is to survive and function optimally.

The clinician must be vigilant for signs of tissue hypoxia. The clinical hallmarks depend on the affected tissue. Brain tissue hypoxia begins with a loss of short-term memory, then euphoria, followed by impaired judgment (2). Psychomotor function falters and more severe cerebral hypoxia induces cerebral oedema, a life-threatening event (3).

Cardiac muscle hypoxia is manifested by tachycardia, a reduction in stroke volume or cardiac contractility, atrial or ventricular arrhythmias and congestive heart failure. Hypoxaemia promotes pulmonary vasoconstriction that may manifest as right heart failure, bronchospasm, respiratory muscle dysfunction and eventual respiratory failure (4).

The science of oxygen therapy is rooted in the late 1700s with its discovery by Joseph Priestly and/or Karl Wilhelm Scheele. Both 'oxygen discoverers' conceived medicinal applications for this 'pure air'. Oxygen has sought a clinical role ever since. Proof that LTOT for hypoxaemic patients was beneficial

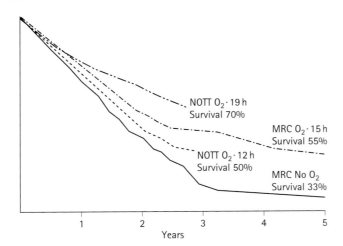

Figure 32.1 *Combined results of the Medical Research Council (MRC) and Nocturnal Oxygen Therapy Trial (NOTT) studies. This demonstrates the dose-related benefit of using oxygen for an increasing number of hours per day.*

appeared in 1980 with results from the United Kingdom Medical Research Council (MRC) study and the National Heart, Lung, and Blood Institute's Nocturnal Oxygen Therapy Trial (NOTT) (5, 6). These controlled multi-centre trials clearly demonstrated increased survival from oxygen in a time–dose-dependent relationship (Fig. 32.1).

The British MRC study randomly assigned hypoxaemic patients to receive LTOT 15 h/day (including the hours of sleep) versus no oxygen. After 4 years, 19 out of 42 oxygen therapy patients died as compared with 30 out of 45 control patients, who received no oxygen (5).

The NOTT study, performed in North America on a similar population of 203 hypoxaemic COPD patients, randomly assigned them to receive oxygen 12 h/day (including the hours of sleep) or 24 h/day. The data demonstrated that the 12-h/day nocturnal group fully complied whereas the continuous group averaged 18 h/day. Survival was 1.94 times better for the continuous versus the nocturnal oxygen therapy group, with a significant survival difference noted at 12 months (6).

Composite results of both studies demonstrated poor survival in patients receiving no oxygen, better survival when patients received oxygen part of the time and best survival when they approached continuous oxygen usage. Survival was correlated with the number of hours per day of oxygen usage (Fig. 32.1).

These results were particularly profound in patients with CO_2 retention and acidotic tendencies. There was a significant fall in haematocrit and pulmonary vascular resistance (PVR) in the continuous oxygen group. However, these changes were not sufficient to explain the survival difference. An autopsy study on 15 patients in each group of the NOTT study showed no differences in pathology, supporting the concept that the survival difference was due to the difference in hours of oxygen therapy (7). Pulmonary haemodynamics appears to play an important role in survival (8).

Whether the survival benefits demonstrated in the NOTT were partly due to receiving oxygen during exertion is unclear. It is known that oxygen enables patients to perform better during exercise. When oxygen is administered to moderately hypoxaemic patients (P_aO_2 55–65 mmHg), there appears to be no survival benefit (9). Younger age, pulmonary function and a higher body mass index (BMI) were predictors of survival. Importantly, oxygen is not only life-saving, but also improves quality of life, decreases hospitalizations and enhances neuropsychological performance (10).

HAZARDS OF OXYGEN THERAPY

While oxygen therapy is generally considered to be safe, clinicians must be aware of the potential hazards associated with oxygen and equipment used to store it. These include absorptive atelectasis, oxygen toxicity, CO_2 retention, and the possibility of accidents or fires relating to the storage, handling and use of oxygen.

Absorptive atelectasis

High oxygen concentrations replace nitrogen in the alveoli; as that oxygen becomes absorbed into the bloodstream, alveolar collapse may occur. Further, high oxygen concentrations may increase pulmonary vasodilatation, thereby exacerbating $\dot{V}/\dot{Q}$ mismatch and promoting arterial hypoxaemia. Yet, clinicians must remain focused on reversal of hypoxaemia and then be prepared to address other clinically relevant issues.

Oxygen toxicity on LTOT

Long-term oxygen therapy patients breathe mostly atmospheric air – with a summated F_IO_2 typically <32 per cent. Patients who receive prolonged oxygen with an F_IO_2 >50 per cent may experience oxygen toxicity (11). Oxygen toxicity results from free radical generation and cell injury. While the major end-product of normal oxygen metabolism is water, some oxygen molecules are converted into cytotoxic free radicals, including superoxide anions, perhydroxy radicals, hydroxyl radicals and hydrogen peroxide.

Normally, antioxidant enzymes, including metalloproteins (superoxide dismutase), catalase and glutathione peroxidase, protect cells by scavenging oxygen radicals. During prolonged hyperoxic exposure, antioxidant systems become overwhelmed and oxidative destruction of lung tissue ensues. Acute changes may include tracheobronchial irritation, impaired mucociliary clearance, and diminished vital capacity secondary to oedema and reabsorption atelectasis (12). Exudative and proliferative changes consistent with oxygen toxicity have been observed at autopsy in chronic low-flow oxygen COPD users. However, these changes had no apparent impact on survival (13).

CO$_2$ retention

Some clinicians, being concerned that oxygen suppresses the respiratory drive, causing hypercapnia, may be overly timid in prescribing it. This creates a bigger risk of tissue hypoxia. Oxygen-induced hypercapnia does occasionally occur, but it rarely leads to respiratory acidosis. The prevailing mechanism may not be respiratory drive suppression. Aubier *et al.* (14) and later Sassoon *et al.* (15) demonstrated that minute ventilation did not decrease, but CO$_2$ retainers had an increase in the ratio of dead space to tidal volume (V_D/V_T). Accordingly the conclusion was that CO$_2$ retention occurred due to a widening of $\dot{V}/\dot{Q}$ mismatch.

Later, Dunn *et al.* (16) found evidence for respiratory drive depression. Ventilator patients receiving hyperoxic mixtures had an increase in the CO$_2$ recruitment threshold. V_D/V_T increased but $\dot{V}CO_2$ remained constant. Robinson *et al.* (17) found that a reduction in ventilation occurs in some patients undergoing an exacerbation. Patients with lower room air S_aO_2 (haemoglobin oxygen saturation) tended to be retainers, and hyperoxic concentrations decreased hypoxic vasoconstriction leading to an increase in perfusion. This, combined with a reduction in ventilation, caused a redistribution in $\dot{V}/\dot{Q}$. Hence, several effects probably come into play. In most cases, titrating oxygen flow so as to maintain P_aO_2 between 60 and 65 mmHg minimizes the likelihood of hypercapnia and respiratory acidosis. When hypercapnia is present, initial oxygen delivery settings should be titrated via arterial blood gases (ABGs).

Chronic hypercapnia is tolerable for patients with an intact renal system that can maintain their acid–base balance. Accordingly, CO$_2$ retention can actually be an adaptive mechanism that relieves the patient from excessive work of breathing. Chronic hypercapnia need not be an ominous prognostic sign in patients receiving LTOT (18). Any adverse consequences of hypercapnia are related to acute acidaemia. Acute changes in acid–base balance can be detected by ABG monitoring and attention to changes in mentation such as decreased alertness, sleepiness or stupor. In all cases, *correction of hypoxaemia takes precedence over concerns about CO$_2$ retention.*

Physical hazards

The major physical hazards of oxygen therapy are fires or explosions. A dangerous situation occurs when patients light up a cigarette when oxygen is flowing (19). Although nasal cannulae are made of fire-retardant plastic, both the cannula and the patient's nose will burn vigorously in the presence of oxygen. Patients, family members and other care-givers must be warned not to smoke near oxygen.

GAS OXYGEN

Compressed gas oxygen containers should not be stored near water heaters, furnaces or other sources of heat or flame. A pressurized oxygen cylinder may be accidentally knocked over, causing explosive disconnection of the regulator and rendering the cylinder a dangerous missile.

LIQUID OXYGEN

Serious freeze burns can occur while transfilling liquid oxygen. In general, major accidents associated with liquid oxygen are rare and can be avoided by common sense and good patient and family training.

OPTIMAL MEDICAL REGIMEN

One of the goals of any medical regimen is to optimize $\dot{V}/\dot{Q}$ matching as a means of correcting hypoxaemia. This is particularly important during an acute exacerbation. If there is evidence of congestive heart failure due to cor pulmonale, diuretic therapy may be advisable. The clinician ought to be mindful that alterations in electrolyte balance from diuretics may actually worsen cor pulmonale (20).

The adequacy of oxygen delivery to the tissues may be improved by correcting anaemia or polycythaemia. An exercise programme may improve oxygen transport to muscles through central and peripheral adaptation. If the patient nevertheless remains hypoxaemic, LTOT is warranted.

One aspect of good medical management is the oxygen therapy itself. Oxygen may have a reparative effect in the lung by reducing pulmonary artery vasoconstriction and improving $\dot{V}/\dot{Q}$ matching (21, 22). Continuation of oxygen therapy may stabilize improvement in $\dot{V}/\dot{Q}$ matching. If this is the case, withdrawal of oxygen because of improved P_aO_2 may be detrimental.

OXYGEN THERAPY DURING SLEEP

People with no sign of cardiorespiratory disease commonly undergo transient mild desaturations, particularly during REM (rapid eye movement) sleep. Patients with chronic lung disease may start from a lower S_aO_2 and dip below 90 per cent for longer periods. Some patients may spend more than 30 per cent of the night with an S_aO_2 <90 per cent (23). COPD patients with no sign of obstructive sleep apnoea (OSA) may undergo desaturations of 9–21 per cent (24). Some patients have the confluence of both COPD and OSA, sometimes called overlap syndrome (25). Either COPD or OSA predisposes patients to fragmented sleep and impaired quality of life.

The mechanism of nocturnal oxygen desaturation has been attributed to ventilatory drive suppression. Desaturations are common during REM sleep but may occur during any sleep stage. Other mechanisms for nocturnal oxygen desaturation include alveolar hypoventilation, increased V_D/V_T or exaggerated $\dot{V}/\dot{Q}$ mismatch. The tendency to desaturate at night is not always predictable by daytime blood gases, suggesting involvement of sleep dynamics (24). Fifty per cent of COPD patients on LTOT with corrected daytime saturation require an increase in oxygen flow during sleep. Patients with both hypercapnia and hypoxaemia are most likely to desaturate at night (26).

The consequences of nocturnal oxygen desaturation (NOD) include ventricular ectopy, elevated pulmonary artery pressure (PAP), increased PVR and shortened survival (27). In a subgroup of COPD patients with nocturnal oxygen desaturation, oxygen therapy can prevent or reverse complications (28).

Mild daytime hypoxaemia and NOD

Chaouat et al. (29) studied COPD patients with mild daytime hypoxaemia (P_aO_2 >55 mmHg), who were nocturnal desaturators versus non-desaturators over 2 years. Desaturators had a slightly higher P_aCO_2 and PAP. Non-desaturators did not increase their P_aCO_2 or PAP. Further, non-desaturators did not become sleep desaturators. It therefore appears that NOD is a characteristic for a specific COPD cohort experiencing CO_2 retention and not a step towards requiring LTOT (29). Disease severity, CO_2 retention, and high BMI are predictive of NOD (30). Fletcher et al. (31) determined that patients who desaturate during sleep tend to have severely impaired pulmonary mechanics along with hypercarbia.

In a large multi-centre trial that studied patients with mild daytime hypoxaemia (P_aO_2 >55 mmHg), nocturnal oxygen therapy did not modify the evolution of pulmonary hypertension or delay patients from meeting criteria for LTOT. A survival difference was not detected, albeit their study population was small and of insufficient length to draw a definite conclusion (32).

Overlap syndrome

Weitzenblum et al. (33) found that 11 per cent of his OSA patients had coexisting COPD. Patients with overlap syndrome may have an abnormally high rise in PAP during exercise (34). The primary treatment for these patients is to perform polysomnography and address the OSA component with nasal continuous positive airways pressure (CPAP) or non-invasive positive pressure ventilation (NIPPV) (35). It is doubtful whether the occurrence of OSA is higher in COPD patients.

OXYGEN DURING EXERCISE

Exercise hypoxaemia

Daily exercise and an active lifestyle are essential to health maintenance. The normal response to submaximal exercise is to maintain or increase arterial oxygenation while maintaining or lowering P_aCO_2. The lung and cardiovascular system are well suited to meeting the $\dot{V}O_2$ demands of exercising muscles. Lung diffusion (D_L) and capillary blood flow can more than double (36).

At rest, patients with severe lung impairment are generally not limited by D_L or red cell transit time (37). Yet during exercise these factors may limit exertion (38), along with accentuation of $\dot{V}/\dot{Q}$ mismatch, progressive hyperinflation (39), a demanding oxygen cost, an oppressive work of breathing (40)

and a compromised respiratory muscle length–tension relationship.

Immediate benefits of oxygen

Oxygen therapy enables patients to exercise longer, at higher workloads, with less dyspnoea (41, 42). There is less dynamic hyperinflation, which provides a greater mechanical advantage with a reduced energy demand (39, 43). One mechanism for greater exercise tolerance from oxygen is a reduction in minute ventilation, toleration of slightly higher P_aCO_2, obtunding the carotid and aortic body chemo-sensors (44).

Studies addressing the foregoing concepts demonstrated that oxygen administration during exercise can avert transient increases in PAP and PVR (45), reduce dyspnoea and improve exercise tolerance at submaximal workloads (46), and increase peak exercise capacity via a reduction in minute ventilation (47). Some of the exercise metabolic indices remain abnormal, possibly indicating cellular damage from chronic hypoxaemia or a chronically stressed system that has undergone compensatory changes (48).

Oxygen to prevent exercise oxygen desaturation

Eaton et al. (49) showed that ambulatory oxygen can improve quality of life in a randomized trial. McDonald et al. (50) supplied patients with portable oxygen and compared delivery of oxygen versus compressed air using a portable cylinder with an oxygen conserving device (50). They demonstrated immediate improvements in exercise performance, but no long-term benefit in exercise performance or quality of life. Survival benefits have not been demonstrated nor have functional improvements over time (44, 50–53).

Rooyackers et al. (52) compared training with oxygen versus room air. There was no statistical or clinical difference in exercise capacity between groups, although the oxygen group experienced a greater reduction in exercise dyspnoea. Garrod et al. (54) found no exercise training benefit from ambulatory oxygen therapy in a rehabilitation programme, even though there was a reduction in dyspnoea. Definitive studies combining pulmonary rehabilitation or disease management with oxygen to prevent exercise desaturation have yet to be performed. Clinical judgment would lean towards protecting patients from exercise desaturation.

Hyperoxia to enhance exercise benefits

Several investigations have addressed the possible benefits of administering hyperoxic oxygen concentrations to boost oxygen uptake and utilization at peripheral muscle and improve exercise and/or functional performance (44). Somfay et al. (43) demonstrated a dose-dependent reduction in hyperinflation and improvement in endurance with F_IO_2 up to 50 per cent, with no further benefit at higher F_IO_2. These studies lend elegant support to the early findings by Cotes and Gilson (41)

Derby Hospitals NHS Foundation Trust Library and Knowledge Service

in 1956, who found progressive improvement in exercise performance up to an F_IO_2 of 50 per cent. O'Donnell *et al.* (39) determined that oxygen ameliorated exercise dyspnoea by lowering ventilatory demand, reducing hyperinflation and decreasing lactate levels. Dean *et al.* (55) discovered a positive correlation between exercise performance and decreased dyspnoea, but not minute ventilation, heart rate or right ventricular pressure. Jolly *et al.* (42) found that, although oxygen administered to non-desaturators led to a substantial reduction in dyspnoea, it did not necessarily enhance exercise performance. Mannix *et al.* (53) determined that 30 per cent oxygen lowered the oxygen cost of ventilation.

Exercise oxygen seems to improve muscle performance without altering muscle kinetics (49, 56). The immediate effect of exercise oxygen is to reduce minute ventilation by slowing breath rate. This has a salutary impact on hyperinflation which is a major contributor to dyspnoea (39). The overall effect is to decrease the work of breathing by lowering minute ventilation at the cost of minimal CO_2 retention. The mechanism appears to be a blunting of the chemoreceptor response (57). Maltais *et al.* (56), administering an F_IO_2 of 75 per cent, demonstrated improvement in blood flow to the lower limb muscles. In essence, oxygen with activity prevents exertional desaturation and relieves breathlessness, which enables patients to be more active. At this point, hyperoxic F_IO_2 makes clinical sense in specific instances, particularly for patients who are disabled by their dyspnoea where oxygen can be symptomatically enabling.

PHYSIOLOGICAL CRITERIA FOR PRESCRIBING LTOT

Both GOLD (Global Initiative for Chronic Obstructive Lung Diseases) guidelines and ATS (American Thoracic Society) standards qualify a patient for LTOT with the diagnosis of COPD and $P_aO_2 \leq 7.3$ kPa (55 mmHg) or $S_aO_2 \leq 88$ per cent. Patients may also qualify with P_aO_2 between 7.3 kPa (55 mmHg) and 8.0 kPa (60 mmHg) or S_aO_2 of 89 per cent, if there is evidence of pulmonary hypertension, peripheral oedema suggesting congestive heart failure, or polycythaemia (58, 59).

Arterial blood gas measurement

Arterial blood gas measurement rather than pulse oximetry is recommended to initially qualify patients for LTOT. The ABG is more accurate and provides information about the ventilatory status, P_aCO_2, and acid–base status (pH). ABG is recommended by GOLD for patients with $FEV_1 <40$ per cent of predicted and/or with clinical signs suggestive of respiratory failure or right heart failure (59).

Pulse oximetry

Arterial blood gas measurement is the gold standard for determining arterial oxygenation. However, S_pO_2 (saturation of oxygen measured by pulse oximetry) usually tracks the

arterial S_aO_2; it is non-invasive and provides continuous tracking of arterial oxygenation. During exercise the S_pO_2 determines the extent and rapidity of exercise desaturation. When the accuracy of exercise S_pO_2 is in question, it can be corroborated by ABG before and after exercise (60).

PRESCRIBING LTOT

Initial qualification for oxygen therapy is best accomplished by ABG, while the patient is breathing room air. Concomitant pulse oximetry will establish a reliable baseline for further measurements and flow adjustments. The ATS-ERS Standards Algorithm adapted for this text (Fig. 32.2) is a guide to adjusting oxygen settings. The resting flow rate can be adjusted to $S_pO_2 \geq 90$ per cent. If hypercarbia is a concern, ABG should be utilized to make initial and major adjustments. With corroborating oximetry S_pO_2, the oxygen flow can be titrated to an $S_aO_2 >90$ per cent.

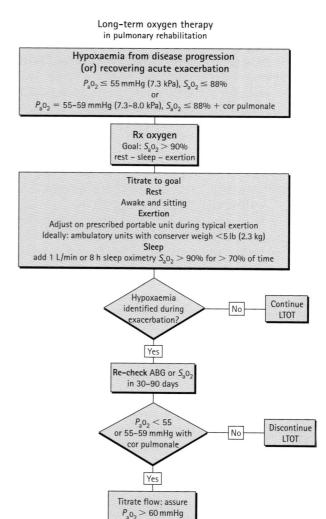

Figure 32.2 *Prescribing and adjusting the settings for long-term oxygen therapy. Adapted from (61) and modified.*

COPD patients are encouraged to be active and mobile. Hence, the home oxygen system should include a portable component and the patients tested on that system. As the patient performs a typical level of exertion, such as a hallway walk, the oxygen setting is titrated to S_pO_2 >90 per cent. If dyspnoea is especially prevalent during arm exertion, the patient may also be tested while performing arm tasks. The goal is to assure S_aO_2 >90 per cent. Oxygen during sleep is often set 1 L/min higher than the daytime setting. If there are signs of cor pulmonale despite adequate daytime oxygenation, an overnight oximetry should be considered.

OXYGEN SYSTEMS

Oxygen is furnished in three forms: compressed gas, liquid and oxygen concentrator. Each has advantages and drawbacks. The choice of system depends on the needs of the individual patient, and practical considerations such as availability, cost, ease of use and maintenance.

Compressed gas oxygen

Compressed gas oxygen is stored in pressurized cylinders at 2000 psi. The H cylinder stands as tall as some patients, weighs >200 lb, stores 6900 L and lasts for 2.4 days set at 2 L/min. As such, it is considered a stationary system. The E cylinder is a commonly used portable or backup system. It weighs 18 lb, stores 523 L and lasts 5 h at 2 L/min. The M-6 cylinder weighs 4 lb and lasts 1.2 h at 2 L/min. These cylinders are only practical if combined with an oxygen-conserving device, which extends the cylinder life threefold or more. Small cylinders may be transfilled from specialized oxygen concentrators.

Liquid oxygen

Liquid oxygen stores efficiently in small volumes. One liquid litre provides nearly 1000 gaseous litres of oxygen. Liquid oxygen is easily transfilled by the patient from larger reservoirs and provides hours of lightweight use. Hybrid portable systems come with a built-in oxygen-conserving device. Consequently, a portable liquid reservoir weighing 3.5 lb can provide up to 10 h of oxygen set at 2 L/min. Liquid oxygen systems do experience some loss over time due to venting, and occasionally some units will temporarily freeze up.

Oxygen concentrator

The oxygen concentrator is an electrically powered molecular sieve that extracts from room air. At the lowest flows, oxygen purity is 97 per cent; higher flows reduce the purity to <94 per cent. Most oxygen concentrators operate on wall current, but a new concentrator weighs <10 lb and has a battery of 50 min between charges. Noise can be a factor. It is not unusual for a concentrator to put out 60 dB (decibels) of sound. The greatest advantages of concentrators are low cost and high availability. Specialized concentrators that refill small 4.5 lb portable cylinders are now available. These represent the first fully self-contained oxygen delivery systems.

OXYGEN DELIVERY METHODS

Continuous-flow nasal cannulae

The standard continuous-flow nasal cannula is generally well tolerated and meets the needs of most patients on home oxygen. Continuous-flow oxygen delivery works well with an oxygen concentrator. For portable oxygen therapy, where weight and portability become critical factors, oxygen delivery is best targeted to early inspiration (62).

Oxygen-conserving devices

Continuous-flow delivery adds a small volume of oxygen to a much larger inhalation of room air (63, 64). A typical model of oxygen delivery is based on the patient breathing 20 breaths/min, where each breath lasts 3 s. For COPD patients, who exhale twice as long as they inhale, 1 s is spent inhaling. The last third of a 450 mL inhalation fills the dead space and requires about half of the inhalation time due to slowing at end-inhalation. This leaves 0.5 s for early inhalation of air that reaches the alveolar-capillary surface. For continuous flow of 2 L/min, 16.7 mL of oxygen will arrive during early inhalation. At 20 breaths/min that patient will receive 333.3 ml (20×16.7 mL) of oxygen per minute. Thus, 17 per cent (333.3 mL/2000 mL) of oxygen is available for oxygen transport to tissues – the rest is largely wasted (62).

RESERVOIR CANNULAE

Reservoir cannulae store oxygen during exhalation for delivery upon the next inhalation (65, 66). They are constructed with a membrane that cycles in order to create the 20 mL reservoir chamber for storage and delivery in response to the patient's ventilatory cycle. Because most oxygen is delivered during early inhalation, the litre-flow can be turned down while still maintaining adequate oxygen saturations. The gain in efficiency is between 2:1 and 4:1 over continuous-flow cannulae.

Reservoir cannulae are available in two configurations, Oxymizer and Pendant. The Oxymizer stores oxygen in a chamber located on the moustache area and the Pendant stores oxygen in a reservoir located at the mid-anterior chest wall and in the tubing leading to the nasal prongs (64–65). Reservoir cannulae are inexpensive and reliable but large and noticeable. They have been utilized as high-flow devices for patients who are difficult to oxygenate (67, 68).

TRANSTRACHEAL CATHETERS

Transtracheal oxygen delivery (TTO) requires the percutaneous insertion of a catheter between the second and third rings of the trachea (69, 70). Oxygen flows directly into the trachea, bypassing the dead space of the nose, throat and upper trachea. Oxygen is conserved through upper airway storage, with efficiencies of 2:1 to 3:1 over continuous flow (71, 72).

TTO has the cosmetic advantage of being off the face. TTO is associated with a reduction in dyspnoea, minute ventilation and tension-time index of the diaphragm. TTO reduces total respiratory dead space in volumes proportional to the flow setting (73).

Candidates for TTO have a strong desire to remain active, are not heavy sputum producers, do not experience frequent exacerbations, are willing and able to follow the care protocol, and live nearby. A team of clinicians evaluate, educate and monitor patients (71).

DEMAND DELIVERY DEVICES

Demand oxygen delivery devices sense the beginning of inhalation, whereupon they deliver a small bolus of oxygen. Efficiency of these devices improves as they deliver earlier in inhalation (74). Available in several configurations, these devices vary in efficiency from 2:1 to 7:1 (75–77). The most efficient devices have electronic sensors. Pneumatic devices sense and deliver pneumatically, and thereby never require a battery. Newer devices now combine the low-volume storage of liquid oxygen with oxygen conservation to create systems that are small and portable. More than a dozen oxygen-conserving devices are on the market, most of which have not been clinically tested. System failure may be the result of a late pulse or failure to sense inspiration. Demand systems sometimes fail to provide adequate oxygenation during exercise. This deficiency has been addressed with larger pulses and higher delivery settings (78). It is essential that patients be tested during rest and exercise on the device being contemplated.

Humidification

There is no evidence, either subjective or physiological, that humidification is beneficial for oxygen flows <5 L/min (79). This may be explained by the low water vapour output of bubble humidifiers and a proportionately small oxygen flow compared with inspiratory flow. Bubble humidifiers function at room temperature; when oxygen is raised to body temperature, the relative humidity falls.

In TTO, where the upper airway is bypassed, humidification is essential even at low flow rates (1 L/min). Some TTO patients may be at high risk for mucus ball formation and may benefit from a servocontrolled heated humidifier like Vapotherm, which delivers gas mixtures heated to body temperature and a relative humidity of nearly 100 per cent.

PATIENT EDUCATION AND TRAINING

The role of education and training is central to medical care. Education regarding oxygen therapy has the formidable task of convincing the patient of the benefits of a therapy that is inconvenient, burdensome and raises issues of impending disability and death. Patient training and encouragement are part of a continuing process that addresses understanding, acceptance and safe use of oxygen equipment. Patients who embrace an active lifestyle with their portable oxygen will benefit the most from good training.

FUTURE DEVELOPMENTS

Technological advances will continue to refine and shape our understanding of oxygen delivery for patients with cardiorespiratory disorders. The full scope of oxygen transport and utilization at the cellular level will obviate the need for oxygen in some individuals. Genetic engineering will generate new and functional lung tissue for many individuals. For those who still require supplemental oxygen, small, efficient and economical delivery methods will be developed to ensure adequate oxygenation while promoting an active lifestyle.

Key points

- LTOT improves survival, exercise, sleep and ability to function.
- Active patients require portable oxygen.
- Prevention of hypoxaemia takes precedence over CO_2 retention concerns.
- LTOT is delivered by cannula, pulse demand, reservoir cannula or transtracheal catheter.
- The goal of LTOT is to maintain S_pO_2 >92 per cent during rest, sleep and exertion.
- Patient education improves compliance.

REFERENCES

1. Tiep BL. Disease management of COPD with pulmonary rehabilitation. *Chest* 1997; **112**: 1630–56.
2. Fix AJ, Daughton D, Kass I et al. Cognitive functioning and survival among patients with chronic obstructive pulmonary disease. *Int J Neurosci* 1985; **27**: 13–17.
●3. Fix AJ, Golden CJ, Daughton D et al. Neuropsychological deficits among patients with chronic obstructive pulmonary disease. *Intern J Neurosci* 1982; **16**: 99–105.
4. Alpert JS. Pulmonary hypertension and cardiac function in chronic obstructive pulmonary disease. *Chest* 1979; **75**: 6–651.
●5. Medical Research Council Working Party. Long-term domiciliary oxygen therapy in chronic hypoxic cor pulmonale complicating chronic bronchitis and emphysema. *Lancet* 1981; **1**: 681–6.
●6. Nocturnal Oxygen Therapy Trial Group. Continuous or nocturnal oxygen therapy in hypoxemic chronic obstructive lung disease. *Ann Intern Med* 1980; **93**: 391–8.
7. Jacques J, Cooney TP, Silvers GW et al. The lungs and causes of death in the nocturnal oxygen therapy trial. *Chest* 1984; **86**: 230–3.

●8. Oswald-Mammosser M, Weitzenblum E, Quoix E *et al.* Prognostic factors in COPD patients receiving long-term oxygen therapy: importance of pulmonary artery pressure. *Chest* 1995; **107**: 1193–8.

●9. Gorecka D, Gorzelak K, Sliwinski P *et al.* Effect of long term oxygen therapy on survival in patients with chronic obstructive pulmonary disease with moderate hypoxaemia. *Thorax* 1997; **52**: 674.

●10. Heaton RK, Grant I, McSweeny AJ *et al.* Psychologic effects of continuous and nocturnal oxygen therapy in hypoxemic chronic obstructive pulmonary disease. *Arch Intern Med* 1983; **143**: 1941–7.

11. Jenkinson SG. Oxygen toxicity. *New Horiz Nov* 1993; **1**: 504–11.

12. Housset B, Hurbain I, Masliah J *et al.* Toxic effects of oxygen on cultured alveolar epithelial cells, lung fibroblasts and alveolar macrophages. *Eur Respir J* 1991; **4**: 1066–75.

●13. Petty TL, Stanford RE, Neff TA. Continuous oxygen therapy in chronic airway obstruction: observations on possible oxygen toxicity and survival. *Ann Intern Med* 1971; **75**: 361–7.

●14. Aubier M, Murciano D, Fournier M *et al.* Central respiratory drive in acute respiratory failure of patients with chronic obstructive pulmonary disease. *Am Rev Respir Dis* 1980; **122**: 191–9.

15. Sassoon CS, Hassell KT, Mahutte CK. Hyperoxic-induced hypercapnia in stable chronic obstructive pulmonary disease. *Am Rev Respir Dis* 1987; **135**: 907–11.

16. Dunn WF, Nelson SB, Hubmayr RD. Oxygen-induced hypercarbia in obstructive pulmonary disease. *Am Rev Respir Dis* 1991; **144**: 526–30.

●17. Robinson TD, Freiberg DB, Regnis JA, Young IH. The role of hypoventilation and ventilation-perfusion redistribution in oxygen-induced hypercapnia during acute exacerbations of chronic obstructive pulmonary disease. *Am J Respir Crit Care Med* 2000; **161**: 1524–9.

18. Aida A, Miyamoto K, Nishimura M *et al.* Prognostic value of hypercapnia in patients with chronic respiratory failure during long term oxygen therapy. *Am J Respir Crit Care Med* 1998; **158**: 188–93.

19. West GA, Primeau P. Nonmedical hazards of long-term oxygen therapy. *Respir Care* 1983; **28**: 906–12.

20. Kiely DG, Cargill RI, Lipworth BJ. Effects of furosemide and hypoxia on the pulmonary vascular bed in man. *Br J Clin Pharmacol* 1997; **43**: 309–13.

●21. Weitzenblum E, Sautegeau A, Ehrhart M *et al.* Long-term oxygen therapy can reverse the progression of pulmonary hypertension in patients with chronic obstructive pulmonary disease. *Am Rev Respir Dis* 1985; **131**: 493–8.

●22. O'Donohue WJ. Effect of oxygen therapy on increasing arterial oxygen tension in hypoxemic patients with stable chronic obstructive pulmonary disease while breathing ambient air. *Chest* 1991; **100**: 968–72.

23. Weitzenblum E, Chaouat A, Charpentier C *et al.* Sleep-related hypoxaemia in chronic obstructive pulmonary disease: causes, consequences and treatment. *Respiration* 1997; **64**: 187–93.

24. Mohsenin V, Guffanti EE, Hilbert J, Ferranti R. Daytime oxygen saturation does not predict nocturnal oxygen desaturation in patients with chronic obstructive pulmonary disease. *Arch Phys Med Rehabil* 1994; **75**: 285–9.

25. Flenley DC. Breathing during sleep. *Ann Acad Med Singapore* 1985; **14**: 479–84.

26. Plywaczewski R, Sliwinski P, Nowinski A *et al.* Incidence of nocturnal desaturation while breathing oxygen in COPD patients undergoing long-term oxygen therapy. *Chest* 2000; **117**: 679–83.

27. Kimura H, Suda A, Sakuma T *et al.* Nocturnal oxyhemoglobin desaturation and prognosis in chronic obstructive pulmonary disease and late sequelae of pulmonary tuberculosis. *Intern Med* 1998; **37**: 354–9.

●28. Fletcher EC, Luckett RA, Goodnight-White S *et al.* A double-blind trial of nocturnal supplemental oxygen for sleep desaturation in patients with chronic obstructive pulmonary disease and a daytime PaO2 above 60 mm Hg. *Am Rev Respir Dis* 1992; **145**: 1070–6.

●29. Chaouat A, Weitzenblum E, Kessler R *et al.* Outcome of COPD patients with mild daytime hypoxaemia with or without sleep-related oxygen desaturation. *Eur Respir J* 2001; **17**: 848–55.

30. De Angelis G, Sposato B, Mazzei L *et al.* Predictive indexes of nocturnal desaturation in COPD patients not treated with long term oxygen therapy. *Eur Rev Med Pharmacol Sci* 2001; **5**: 173–9.

31. Fletcher EC, Scott D, Qian W *et al.* Evolution of nocturnal oxyhemoglobin desaturation in patients with chronic obstructive pulmonary disease and a daytime PaO2 above 60 mm Hg. *Am Rev Respir Dis* 1991; **145**: 401–5.

●32. Chaouat A, Weitzenblum E, Kessler R *et al.* A randomized trial of nocturnal oxygen therapy in chronic obstructive pulmonary disease patients. *Eur Respir J* 1999; **14**: 997–9.

33. Weitzenblum E, Krieger J, Oswald M *et al.* Chronic obstructive pulmonary disease and sleep apnea syndrome. *Sleep* 1992; **15**: S33–5.

34. Hawrylkiewicz I, Palasiewicz G, Plywaczewski R *et al.* Effects of nocturnal desaturation on pulmonary hemodynamics in patients with overlap syndrome (chronic obstructive pulmonary disease and obstructive sleep apnea). *Pneumonol Alergol Pol* 2000; **68**: 28–36.

35. Nicholson D, Tiep B, Sadana G *et al.* Noninvasive positive pressure ventilation. *Curr Opin Pulmon Med* 1999; **4**: 66–75.

36. Hsia C. Recruitment of lung diffusing capacity – update of concept and application. *Chest* 2002; **122**: 1774–83.

37. Hadeli KO, Siegel EM, Sherril DL *et al.* Predictors of oxygen desaturation during sub-maximal exercise in 8000 patients. *Chest* 2001; **120**: 88–92.

38. Owens GR, Rogers RM, Pennock BE, Levin D. The diffusing capacity as a predictor of arterial oxygen desaturation during exercise in patients with COPD. *N Engl J Med* 1984; **310**: 1218–21.

●39. O'Donnell DE, D'Arsigny C, Fitzpatrick M, Webb KA. Exercise carbon dioxide retention in chronic obstructive pulmonary disease: a case for ventilation/perfusion mismatch combined with hyperinflation. *Am J Respir Crit Care Med* 2002; **166**: 663.

40. Alverti A, Macklem PT. How and why exercise is impaired in COPD. *Respiration* 2001; **68**: 229–39.

●41. Cotes JE, Gilson JC. Effect of oxygen on exercise ability in chronic respiratory insufficiency: use of portable apparatus. *Lancet* 1956; **1**: 872–6.

42. Jolly EC, Di Boscio V, Aguirre L *et al.* Effects of supplemental oxygen during activity in patients with advanced COPD without severe resting hypoxemia. *Chest* 2001; **120**: 437–43.

43. Somfay A, Porszasz J, Lee SM, Casaburi R. Dose-response effect of oxygen on hyperinflation and exercise endurance in non-hypoxemic COPD patients. *Eur Respir J* 2001; **18**: 77–84.

◆44. Snider GL. Enhancement of exercise performance in COPD patients by hyperoxia – a call for research. *Chest* 2002; **122**: 1830–6.

45. Cotes JE, Pisa Z, Thomas AJ. Effects of breathing oxygen upon cardiac output, heart rate, ventilation, systemic and pulmonary blood pressure in patients with chronic lung disease. *Clin Sci* 1963; **25**: 305–21.

●46. Lilker ES, Karnick A, Lerner L. Portable oxygen in chronic obstructive lung disease with hypoxemia and cor pulmonale. *Chest* 1975; **68**: 236.

●47. Carter R, Peavler M, Zinkgraf S *et al.* Predicting maximal exercise ventilation in patients with chronic obstructive pulmonary disease. *Chest* 1987; **92**: 253–9.

48. Payen JF, Wuyam B, Levy P et al. Muscular metabolism during oxygen supplementation in patients with chronic hypoxemia. Am Rev Respir Dis 1993; 147: 592–8.

49. Eaton T, Garrett JE, Young P et al. Ambulatory oxygen improves quality of life of COPD patients: a randomised controlled study. Eur Respir J 2002; 20: 306–12.

50. McDonald CF, Blyth CM, Lazarus MD et al. Exertional oxygen of limited benefit in patients with chronic obstructive pulmonary disease and mild hypoxemia. Am J Respir Crit Care Med 1995; 152: 1616–19.

51. Ram FS, Wedzicha JA. Ambulatory oxygen for chronic obstructive pulmonary disease. Cochrane Database Syst Rev 2002; 2: CD000238.

52. Rooyackers JM, Dekhuijzen PN, Van Herwaarden CL, Folgering HT. Training with supplemental oxygen in patients with COPD and hypoxaemia at peak exercise. Eur Respir J 1997; 10: 1278–84.

53. Mannix ET, Manfredi F, Palange P et al. Oxygen may lower the O_2 cost of breathing in chronic obstructive lung disease. Chest 1992; 101: 910–15.

54. Garrod R, Paul EA, Wedzicha JA. Supplemental oxygen during pulmonary rehabilitation in patients with COPD with exercise hypoxaemia. Thorax 2000; 55: 539–43.

55. Dean NC, Brown JK, Himelman RB et al. Oxygen may improve dyspnea and endurance in patients with chronic obstructive pulmonary disease and only mild hypoxemia. Am Rev Respir Dis 1992; 146: 941–5.

56. Maltais F, Simon M, Jobin J et al. Effects of oxygen on lower limb blood flow and O_2 uptake during exercise in COPD. Med Sci Sports Exerc 2001; 33: 916–22.

57. Somfay A, Pórszász J, Lee S, Casaburi R. Effect of hyperoxia on gas exchange and lactate kinetics following exercise onset in nonhypoxemic COPD Patients. Chest 2002; 121: 393–400.

◆58. Celli BR, Snider GL, Heffner J et al. Standards for the diagnosis and care of patients with chronic obstructive pulmonary disease. ATS statement. Am J Respir Crit Care Med 1995; 152: S77.

◆59. Hurd S, Pauwels R. Global Initiative for Chronic Obstructive Lung Diseases (GOLD). Pulm Pharmacol Ther 2002; 15: 353–5.

60. Webb RK, Ralston C, Runciman WB. Potential errors in pulse oximetry. Part II: effects of changes in saturation and signal quality. Anesthesia 1991; 46: 207–12.

61. Celli BR, MacNee W and committee members. Standards for the diagnosis and treatment of patients with COPD: a summary of the ATS/ERS position paper. Eur Respir J 2004; 23: 932–46.

◆62. Tiep BL. Continuous flow oxygen therapy and basis for improving the efficiency of oxygen delivery. In: Tiep BL, ed. Portable Oxygen Therapy: Including Oxygen Conserving Methodology. Mt Kisco, New York: Futura Publishing, 1991; 205–31.

63. Kory RC, Bergmann JC, Sweet RD et al. Comparative evaluation of oxygen therapy techniques. J Am Med Assoc 1962; 179: 123–8.

●64. Gibson RL, Comer PB, Beckman RW et al. Actual tracheal oxygen concentration with commonly used therapy. Anesthesiology 1976; 44: 71–3.

65. Soffer M, Tashkin DP, Shapiro BJ et al. Conservation of oxygen supply using a reservoir nasal cannula in hypoxemic patients at rest and during exercise. Chest 1985; 89: 806–10.

66. Carter R, Williams JS, Berry J et al. Evaluation of the pendant oxygen-conserving nasal cannula during exercise. Chest 1986; 89: 806–10.

67. Sheehan JC, O'Donohue WJ. Use of a reservoir nasal cannula in hospitalized patients with refractory hypoxemia. Chest 1996; 110: 1s.

68. Dumont CP, Tiep BL. Using a reservoir nasal cannula in acute care. Crit Care Nurse 2002; 22: 41–6.

●69. Heimlich HJ, Carr GC. The Micro-Trach: a seven-year experience with transtracheal oxygen therapy. Chest 1989; 95: 1008–12.

●70. Hoffman LA, Johnson JT, Wesmiller SW et al. Transtracheal delivery of oxygen: efficacy and safety for long-term continuous therapy. Ann Otolol Rhinol Laryngol 1991; 100: 108–15.

●71. Christopher KL, Spofford BT, Petrun MD et al. A program for transtracheal oxygen delivery: Assessment of safety and efficacy. Ann Int Med 1987; 107: 802–8.

72. Kampelmacher MJ, Deenstra M, van Kesteren RG et al. Transtracheal oxygen therapy: An effective and safe alternative to nasal oxygen administration. Eur Respir J 1997; 10: 828–33.

73. Benditt JM, Pollock J, Roa, Celli B. Transtracheal delivery of gas decreases the oxygen cost of breathing. Am Rev Respir Dis 1993; 147: 1207–10.

74. Tiep BL, Christopher KL, Spofford BT et al. Pulsed nasal and transtracheal oxygen delivery. Chest 1990; 97: 364–8.

75. Bower JS, Brook CJ, Zimmer K, Davis D. Performance of a demand oxygen saver system during rest, exercise, and sleep in hypoxemic patients. Chest 1988; 94: 77.

76. Tiep BL, Nicotra MB, Carter R et al. Low-concentration oxygen therapy via a demand oxygen delivery system. Chest 1985; 87: 636–8.

77. Carter R, Tashkin D, Djahed B et al. Demand oxygen delivery for patients with restrictive lung disease. Chest 1989; 96: 1307.

78. Tiep BL, Barnett J, Schiffman G et al. Maintaining oxygenation via demand oxygen delivery during rest and exercise. Respir Care 2002; 47: 887–92.

●79. Campbell EJ, Baker D, Crites-Silver P. Subjective effects of humidification of oxygen for delivery by nasal cannula. Chest 1988; 93: 289–93.

33

Pulmonary rehabilitation in the intensive care unit (ICU) and transition from the ICU to home

GERARD J. CRINER, UBALDO MARTIN, STEFANO NAVA

INTRODUCTION

The intensive care unit is an extremely different environment from those in which pulmonary rehabilitation services are usually performed. The latter usually involves patients who have chronic stable diseases, who most often are treated as outpatients, while the ICU is a chaotic environment comprising critically ill patients who have multiple ongoing dynamic medical and/or surgical problems. However, patients admitted to the ICU also suffer from severe manifestations of deconditioning and immobility, and rehabilitative services are instrumental in facilitating and improving their outcome. This is especially true for patients in the ICU who receive prolonged ventilation, a patient population that is growing due to advances in medical and surgical therapy, and something that requires prolonged ICU stay and extensive ICU and hospital resources. Although only 5–10 per cent of patients in the ICU require ≥7 days of mechanical ventilation, this group consumes 35–55 per cent of all ICU patient days and resources (1). Recent data suggest that optimum treatment of these patients necessitates a well-honed multidisciplinary approach. The results from the Health Care Financing Administration (HCFA) in America, now known as the Center for Medicare/Medicaid Services (CMS), demonstrate that multidisciplinary rehabilitation of the ventilator-dependent patient is more likely to result in improved patient survival and less need for mechanical ventilation at discharge, and the patient is more likely to be discharged to home if ventilator support is required (2).

Patients who receive multidisciplinary care are also more likely to be independent in locomotion and require less assistance with feeding. Results such as these, although limited, illustrate that multidisciplinary care of the critically ill respiratory patient, even if mechanical ventilation is required, can have a salutary effect on patient outcome.

This chapter will review the care of the ventilator-dependent patient who requires rehabilitation in the ICU, so as to make the appropriate transition from the ICU to home.

NEED FOR PULMONARY REHABILITATION

The most common reason for an ICU admission is an episode of respiratory failure, due to either an exacerbation of chronic obstructive pulmonary disease (COPD), or an acute medical or surgical event, superimposed on some other underlying chronic lung disease. Weaning from mechanical ventilation therefore becomes an obstacle in these patients, because:

- the underlying disease contributes to immobility and deconditioning prior to the current episode of respiratory failure
- substantial airflow obstruction requires treatment with systemic corticosteroids or neuromuscular blocking agents, which leads to further immobility and disuse atrophy
- under-nutrition exists due to the underlying disease compounded by the new disease process
- there are gas exchange abnormalities present.

In aggregate, all of these abnormalities compound the process of mechanical ventilation and lead to further immobility, deconditioning and the requirement for comprehensive multidisciplinary rehabilitation in order to restore the patient's pre-existing level of health. These interventions include nutritional and psychological support, whole-body rehabilitation and respiratory muscle reconditioning.

WHAT IS PULMONARY REHABILITATION?

There is general agreement that the term 'rehabilitation' refers to a multidisciplinary intervention that includes physicians along with respiratory, physical and occupational therapists, as well as a primary care nurse, speech and swallowing therapist, psychologist, dietician and social worker. The key element to any rehabilitation programme is that each patient's care is individualized, and geared towards restoration of optimum functional status. A recent official definition of rehabilitation given by the European Respiratory Society Task Force Physician paper states that (3):

> pulmonary rehabilitation is a process which systematically uses scientifically based diagnostic management and evaluation options to achieve optimum daily functioning, and health-related quality of life in individual patients suffering from impairment and disability due to chronic respiratory disease, as measured by clinically, and/or physiologically relevant outcome measures.

The American Thoracic Society adopted the following definition of pulmonary rehabilitation: 'multidisciplinary programme of care for patients with chronic respiratory impairment that is individually tailored and designed to optimize physical and social performance, and autonomy' (4). These broad definitions give a panoramic overview of what should be achieved, but do not give specific details on how to accomplish the rehabilitation of any patient, let alone those who are critically ill or ventilator-dependent in the ICU. Rehabilitation, therefore, varies according to the patient's individual needs and may range from simple mobilization of a patient to more complex interventions, such as weaning from mechanical ventilation or ambulating the patient who remains on chronic, continuous ventilator support. Whatever the difference between the objectives for individual patients, however, these statements do convey the notion that restoration of functional status is key, and dispels the nihilistic notion that little can be done to improve the patient's performance.

IMPACT OF MULTIDISCIPLINARY UNITS ON OUTCOME IN CHRONIC VENTILATED PATIENTS

Several reports have demonstrated that patients receiving chronic ventilation have an improvement in outcome when they are appropriately selected and receive aggressive multidisciplinary rehabilitation. Two HCFA chronic ventilator demonstration sites have reported that survival in selected patients requiring long-term invasive ventilation is much better than previously reported. Gracey *et al.* (5) reported outcomes in 206 patients admitted to the Mayo Clinic chronic ventilator-dependent unit during a 5-year study period. In 206 patients who received mechanical ventilation for at least 6 h/day, for 21 consecutive days, 92 per cent (190) survived to hospital discharge, of whom 77 per cent returned to their homes; 153 of these patients were totally weaned from mechanical ventilation, whereas 37 remained completely or partially dependent. Of the patients receiving mechanical ventilation at discharge, the majority received it only at night (73 per cent); 4-year survival in these patients was 53 per cent. A significant percentage of these patients, however, received chronic ventilation for postoperative conditions (60 per cent), which may have skewed the results to be more optimistic than other studies reporting a greater concentration of medical patients. In a separate report from another HCFA chronic ventilator demonstration unit, Criner *et al.* (6) reported on 77 patients receiving long-term ventilation, 74 per cent of whom had underlying medical causes (29 per cent, advanced lung disease; 26 per cent, neuromuscular disease; 5 per cent, congestive heart failure; and 40 per cent, various other disorders): 93 per cent of patients were discharged alive, 82 per cent were alive at 6 months, and 61 per cent were alive at 1 year follow-up; 86 per cent of patients were totally weaned from mechanical ventilation, 11 per cent required continuous ventilation and 10 per cent required nocturnal ventilation at discharge. In those patients who were discharged alive, a significant improvement in functional status was observed at 6 and 12 months follow-up. Overall, both studies suggest that in patients receiving chronic ventilation, when appropriately selected, and following correction of the underlying process causing respiratory failure, aggressive multidisciplinary rehabilitation results in an acceptable clinical outcome and successful home discharge can be realized.

Recent data also suggest that the quality of life in patients who survive chronic ventilation and multidisciplinary rehabilitation is acceptable. Chatila *et al.* (7) recently reported on 25 consecutive patients who received long-term invasive mechanical ventilation and solicited their quality of life 23 ± 18 months post-discharge (7). Overall, using the Short Form-36 (SF-36) impact scores as a measure of quality of life, these patients were comparable to patients suffering from hypothyroidism or rheumatoid arthritis, as well as being substantially better than those who had chronic diseases such as COPD (Fig. 33.1). These long-term survivors had satisfactory performance in all the physiological SF-36 measures. These data, although limited, suggest that patients who survive chronic invasive ventilation can achieve a good quality of life, thereby making worthwhile the extraordinary rehabilitative efforts that their families and hospital staff have made in relation to their care during their period of prolonged ventilation.

LOCATION OF CARE

Patients receiving long-term ventilation benefit when that care is provided in non-ICU locations and is geared towards

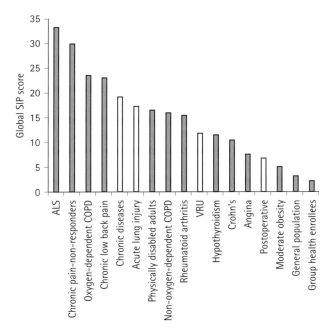

Figure 33.1 *Quality of life in survivors of prolonged mechanical ventilation in contrast to patients with other chronic diseases. ALS, amyotrophic lateral sclerosis; SIP, Sickness Impact Profile; VRU, ventilation rehabilitation unit. Reproduced with permission from Chatila et al. (7).*

Box 33.1   Criteria for transfer of ventilator-dependent patients from intensive care unit to ventilation rehabilitation unit

---

Respiratory stability

- Airway – tracheostomy for invasive ventilation, minimal aspiration
- Secretions – manageable with infrequent suctioning
- Oxygen – adequate oxygenation with F_IO_2 <60%, PEEP <10 cmH$_2$O (S$_p$O$_2$ >92%); ventilator settings: stable, no sophisticated modes
- Patient assessment – comfortable, no increased WOB or dyspnoea
- Weaning technique – tracheal collar or T-piece
- NIPPV – tolerates breaks off, stable settings

Non-respiratory medical stability

- Sepsis controlled
- No uncontrolled haemorrhage
- No arrhythmias, CHF, unstable angina
- No coma
- Secure intravenous access
- Secure alimentation route

CHF, congestive heart failure; F_IO_2, functional inspired oxygen concentration; NIPPV, non-invasive positive pressure ventilation; PEEP, positive end-expiratory pressure; S$_p$O$_2$, saturation of oxygen by pulse oximetry; VRU, ventilator rehabilitation unit; WOB, work of breathing.

---

multidisciplinary rehabilitation. A non-invasive respiratory care unit has some advantages over ICU care, because it is housed in a less expensive environment. It makes for a more efficient transition from the hospital setting to eventual home care, or discharge to a non-acute care setting, and the emphasis is placed on rehabilitation by the staff rather than on minute-to-minute details of stabilization of cardiac or pulmonary parameters. Before patients are transferred to a non-ICU location for ventilator care, certain requirements for respiratory and non-respiratory medical stability must be met. Some of these criteria shown in Box 33.1. In all cases, however, patients must have a stable airway in place established by a tracheostomy. They must have manageable secretions and should not be on sophisticated modes of ventilatory support. They should have only modest requirements for supplemental oxygen, or positive end-expiratory pressure to oxygenate the patient. In addition, they must not have uncontrolled cardiac arrhythmias, ischaemia or instabilities in haematological fluids or electrolyte status. They should also have secure routes for alimentation, as well as access for intravenous medications. If they require non-invasive ventilation, then they should be stable for short periods of time off non-invasive ventilatory support.

ORGANIZATION OF REHABILITATION IN THE ICU

The complex and diverse problems of chronic ventilator patients require treatment by a multidisciplinary team of specialists comprising, among others, pulmonary and critical care physicians, respiratory nurses, nutritionists, respiratory and physical speech therapists, psychologists and a social worker (Fig. 33.2). The daily care of each patient is divided among different disciplines, such that the medical, nursing, respiratory and rehabilitation components all have clearly defined responsibilities. Weekly meetings are attended by all team members, and lead by the medical director of the unit. The emphasis of the treatment plan is placed on restoration of functional status, despite requirements for prolonged ventilation. In the United States, pulmonary rehabilitation almost always includes both respiratory therapists and physiotherapists, but most European institutions have only one of these two professional groups. Norremberg and Vincent (8) recently reported that 29 per cent of physiotherapists working in an ICU have postgraduate specialization in critical care, and 43 per cent in respiratory therapy, while 28 per cent do not belong to any specific categories. In addition, most, if not all, ICUs lack, for the most part, an autonomous physiotherapy service, and therefore have to depend upon the resources of the hospital's physical therapy department. There is a need currently in Europe to define the tasks of physical therapists mainly involved in non-specific rehabilitation programmes (i.e. ambulation, limb muscle strengthening, posture, and torso control) and the delineation of respiratory therapists mainly involved in specific objectives (e.g. respiratory muscle training, secretion removal, breathing exercises, utilization of ventilatory equipment, and weaning from mechanical ventilation).

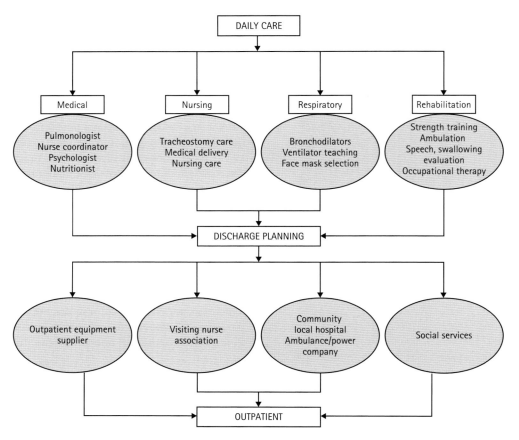

Figure 33.2 *Multidisciplinary care of the chronic ventilator-dependent patient. Patients' daily care is divided into four components: medical, nursing, respiratory and rehabilitative. All four groups deliver care daily, as indicated. Additionally, team members meet weekly for discharge planning.*

REHABILITATIVE NEEDS OF THE PATIENT REQUIRING CHRONIC VENTILATION

Patients who are receiving chronic ventilation have special needs which include a requirement to be evaluated for the optimum form of ventilatory support that enables optimization of functional status; the risk of swallowing dysfunction; impaired communication skills; psychological dysfunction; under-nutrition; respiratory and whole-body deconditioning; and the possibility of developing new medical conditions, which requires close attention (Box 33.2). In an effort to improve patients' portability and facilitate whole-body reconditioning, they are transitioned to portable and/or intermittent mechanical ventilation as soon as possible, based on their underlying medical condition (Fig. 33.3). This not only enables them to maximize their functional capabilities, and more actively participate in rehabilitative efforts, but also allows them to be acclimatized to the ventilator settings, in case long-term ventilation, and even home discharge with mechanical ventilation, is required. Moreover, the transitioning of patients from a large stationary ventilator to a more portable, smaller ventilatory device signals to the patients and their families that clear-cut progress has been made in relation to their condition, and usually fosters greater patient 'buy-in' to the rehabilitation programme. The types of mechanical ventilation

> **Box 33.2** Special needs of chronically ventilated patients
>
> - Ventilatory augmentation
> - Swallowing dysfunction
> - Impaired communication skills
> - Psychological dysfunction
> - Renutrition
> - Respiratory and whole-body reconditioning
> - Close attention to new or changing medical conditions

used and the strategies for the different modes for various types of disease causing respiratory failure are beyond the scope of this chapter, but have recently been reviewed by others (9).

In patients who are critically ill, and especially those who require mechanical ventilation, psychological dysfunction is a common problem (Box 33.3). A host of factors contribute to the development of psychological dysfunction in these patients, including the ICU environment (e.g. continuous input of meaningless monotonous sensory input from multiple patient alarms); sensory deprivation afforded by a sterile visual environment; and, finally, sleep deprivation, a common finding in any ICU environment. Prior studies have demonstrated that critically ill patients are susceptible to sleep deprivation because of the severity of the underlying disease, the

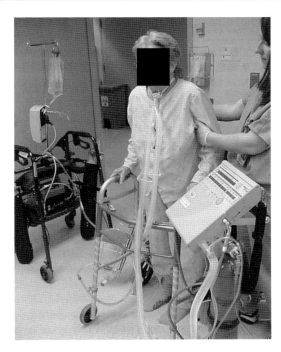

Figure 33.3   *Priority is given to use of portable home positive pressure ventilators to facilitate whole-body reconditioning and ambulation.*

Box 33.3   Psychological dysfunction in ventilator-dependent patients

Environmental factors

- Monotonous, meaningless sensory input (i.e. alarms)
- Sensory deprivation
- Sleep deprivation

Factors associated with chronic ventilation

- Hypoxaemia, illness, medication-induced short-term memory loss
- Inability to communicate
- Lack of normal bodily function (e.g. eating, social interaction, ambulation)

---

medications used to treat it, and staff activity required to treat and stabilize the underlying process. Noise levels in the ICU are greater in magnitude and more sustained throughout a 24-h period, a potentially important factor that leads to a perpetual state of sleep deprivation in ICU patients (10). Psychological dysfunction may also be contributed by the patient's inability to speak, a factor that most patients describe as the most disturbing aspect of the experience of receiving ventilatory support. Finally, a lack of ability to perform bodily functions normally, such as social interaction, eating and ambulation, can also markedly contribute to a state of despair, apathy and a sense of disorientation, and further contribute to social withdrawal and psychological dysfunction. Previous studies reported by our group (11) commonly found cognitive deficits in patients receiving ventilatory support. Figure 33.4 shows

that a number of these patients have problems with orientation, long-term memory recall, processing and reasoning. In fact, it is rare that patients have no cognitive deficit, and most patients have multiple cognitive deficits that contribute to their abnormalities.

Several techniques may be useful in reversing the disorientation that accompanies the process of mechanical ventilation, as well as environmental issues as a result of care in the ICU. Orientation aids, including large clocks and calendars, with an outlined daily care plan, and prominent display of personal effects of patients and family members may help to reorient patients and encourage them to participate more actively in the rehabilitation plan (Fig. 33.5). Re-instituting a regular schedule of daily tasks, such as weaning and physical and occupational therapy sessions, may also enable patients to be more aware of their treatment plan, and gives structure to their lives by avoiding the more chaotic experience of the ICU that results from the seriousness of their condition. Finally, placing patients in rooms with windows to the exterior allows them to better orientate themselves to the time of day and season, something that Wilson (12) showed decreased the incidence of delirium by two-thirds in critically ill patients. In order to improve patient orientation and sense of well-being, attempts should be made to restore verbal communication in chronic ventilated patients as soon as possible.

In the ventilated patient, several techniques are available to restore verbal communication. A buccal resonator, electrolarynx or the use of one-way valves worn over a deflated tracheostomy tube in line with the ventilator circuit (e.g. Passy-Muir valve) while patients spontaneously breathe can enable self-initiated speech (Fig. 33.6). Manzano *et al.* (13) reported that the use of the Passy-Muir unidirectional valve in chronic ventilator patients is effective in improving communication, has no significant adverse cardiorespiratory effects, can lead to a decrease in secretions by facilitating expectoration, and results in considerable improvement in patient well-being. They found that patients felt better, and were therefore more motivated to participate in their own care.

The mode of ventilation chosen may also be important in facilitating speech in patients with chronic tracheostomy who receive invasive ventilation. Prigent *et al.* (14) reported that speech may be improved when patients use bilevel positive pressure ventilation as opposed to assist-controlled ventilation. They found that speech duration was longer during inspiration with bilevel positive pressure ventilation and that speech production extended into expiration in contrast to assist-controlled ventilation. In addition, some patients could speak continuously during several respiratory cycles while receiving bilevel positive pressure ventilation, but not with assist-controlled ventilation. Whatever the modality chosen, however, chronic ventilated patients with enhanced verbal communication are less likely to be anxious and more likely to require minimal sedation, and these effects are responsible for fostering greater participation in rehabilitative efforts, perhaps hastening the weaning and rehabilitation process.

Swallowing impairment is another major abnormality which faces patients who receive chronic invasive ventilation

COPD and those suffering from chronic inflammatory polyneuropathy (CIP). COPD patients frequently have systemic complications of diseases, including depression, osteoporosis and peripheral muscle dysfunction, that may even predate the period of chronic ventilation. Peripheral muscle wasting is estimated to be prevalent in about 30 per cent of COPD patients, and these patients exhibit a decrease in muscle mass, even though total body weight may be preserved. Recent studies using computed tomography (CT) have shown that thigh muscle cross-sectional area is reduced by 30 per cent in patients with moderate to severe COPD (17). In these patients, loss of muscle mass is associated with muscle weakness (18) and poor exercise intolerance. A host of factors may be responsible for this, including inactivity and disuse atrophy, poor nutritional intake, systemic inflammation causing myositis, the presence of hypoxaemia or electrolyte disturbances, and the use of systemic steroids to treat the underlying lung disease.

Chronic inflammatory polyneuropathy patients also warrant special attention. We recently reported, in 11 chronic ventilated patients with electromyography-proven CIP admitted to our non-invasive respiratory care unit, that swallowing dysfunction was commonly present, and patients were liberated from mechanical ventilation before it resolved and before they were able to ambulate (19). Substantial morbidities from immobility were present in these patients, including deep venous thrombosis, sacral decubitus and the presence of pneumonia, all signifying that immobility is a major complication in this disease, and perhaps that aggressive and early rehabilitation may help to rectify the high mortality (e.g. 36 per cent) found in this group of patients.

RESPIRATORY AND NON–RESPIRATORY RECONDITIONING

The physiological changes caused by inactivity involve skeletal muscle, cardiovascular and respiratory function, body and blood composition, and the central nervous and endocrine systems. During a period of inactivity, muscle mass decreases and its effectiveness to perform aerobic exercise diminishes. The skeletal muscles, overall, are composed of two major muscle fibre types: type I fibres are involved mainly in aerobic activities, while type II fibres have a lower capacity to perform this function. Deconditioning causes a distinct transformation of type II fibre subtypes, such that type IIa fibres convert to type IIb, the former having a higher aerobic capacity (20). The overall number and density of mitochondria decrease with this transformation. The cardiovascular response to exercise is dramatically reduced after a period of bed rest, causing a decrease in cardiac output and stroke volume during exercise, and an increase in heart rate during submaximal exercise (21–25). Importantly, in critically ill bedridden patients, the ability of the cardiovascular system to adjust to a change in posture, such as moving from a supine to a seated position, or from seated to standing, is impaired (26, 27). Moreover, in patients with underlying pulmonary processes,

if early rehabilitation is not started, including changes in body posture and the more upright posture, functional residual capacity and lung compliance may be reduced, leading to problems with atelectasis, the retention of secretions and, in some cases, the development of lower respiratory tract infections ranging from tracheobronchitis to pneumonia, factors which may increase markedly the patient's risk of death. Immobility also leads to bone demineralization, an increase in protein wastage (26) and a decrease in total body water and sodium (28). Abnormalities in central nervous system function may contribute to a decreased capacity to maintain the standing and ambulatory postures, and perform ambulatory tasks, resulting in a further decline in intellectual function, and contributing to disorientation and lack of cooperation in the rehabilitative programme (29).

The initial goals in respiratory and non-respiratory reconditioning are targeted towards early mobilization. Maintenance of the upright posture and passive mobilization of legs and arms are preliminary steps, followed by sitting out of bed on a chair. Correction of electrolyte disturbances, optimum nutrition and psychological support as previously described are also important to improve the clinical condition. Specific training of the upper and lower limbs with classical rehabilitative techniques, such as arm cycling and lower extremity ergometry, is very seldom performed in the ICU because of the critical nature of the illnesses afflicting these patients. In addition to training as an important aspect of the recovery phase of these patients, the restoration of normal basic daily activities, such as eating, speaking, performing daily hygiene and ambulating independently, is also important.

Exercise training is a critical feature of pulmonary rehabilitation programmes, and several studies in COPD patients, in particular, have demonstrated the effectiveness of rehabilitation programmes geared towards arm and leg exercise. Successful completion of rehabilitation programmes in these patients has shown improvements in maximum oxygen uptake, enhanced muscle strength and improved coordination. Exercise programmes are also effective in reducing dyspnoea, improving ambulatory function and improving quality of life in patients who have substantial underlying lung disease.

Besides the effects of skeletal limb muscle retraining on improving patients' positioning and hastening the return of cardiovascular performance, special emphasis should be placed on the benefits of arm exercise in patients who have respiratory compromise. The muscles of the upper torso and shoulder serve a dual purpose: a postural action for the arms, and a respiratory action when the arms are aligned in certain postures and stabilized. When the arms are externally rotated and elevated, the pectoralis muscles apply an inspiratory vector to the thorax; with the arms medially rotated and at the side, contraction of the pectoralis muscles applies an expiratory action to the thorax. It has previously been shown in patients with severe underlying COPD that arm exercise can result in dyssynchronous thoraco-abdominal excursions, not related to diaphragmatic fatigue, but rather related to derecruitment of the pectoralis muscles to perform respiratory tasks, as opposed to upper arm positioning (30). Criner and

Celli (31) and Celli *et al.* (32) reported that upper unsupported arm exercise altered ventilatory recruitment in both normal subjects and patients with severe COPD. They found that during upper extremity exercise, the inspiratory contribution of the pectoralis muscles is lost, thereby placing a greater demand on the diaphragm, a muscle group already impaired by severe underlying hyperinflation in this patient group.

Three studies have shown the importance of upper extremity exercise, as part of a rehabilitation programme, in improving respiratory muscle strength and endurance. Keens *et al.* (33) studied seven cystic fibrosis patients and found a 57 per cent increase in ventilatory muscle endurance at the end of a summer camp rowing programme. Clanton *et al.* (34) demonstrated that isometric upper extremity training in 16 female varsity swimmers, resulted in a 25 per cent improvement in maximum inspiratory pressure, and a 100 per cent increase in ventilatory endurance time in comparison to a control group. Estenne *et al.* (35) studied 12 patients suffering from low tetraplegia, and found that training of the pectoralis muscles resulted in a significant increase in expiratory reserve volume after 6 weeks of isometric training. Several studies have also recently shown that the use of arm exercise in rehabilitative programmes may result in a decrease in metabolic costs and an improvement in endurance while performing arm exercise (36–39).

Although these studies were not conducted in ventilator-dependent patients, it is reasonable to expect that such patients who have deranged ventilatory mechanics and disuse atrophy may realize similar gains. Because of the large variability in the rehabilitative needs of patients who have been critically ill, the prescription for exercise should be broad-based, but should also be individualized to provide each patient with a tailored comprehensive treatment plan. Training programmes for respiratory and non-respiratory skeletal muscle groups must be specifically targeted for strength training and also for endurance. Individual goals for muscle strength endurance and mobility for each patient must be set. As patients progress, increments in their task performance should be added to further foster improvements in strength and endurance recovery.

In our institution, physical therapy is conducted at least once daily, as patients become stronger and realize these gains and spend less time on ventilatory support. Patients undergo at least two sessions of physical therapy daily, and eventually an additional treatment session of occupational therapy. In those patients who are ventilator-dependent but ambulatory, the use of newer, more portable ventilators while performing physical therapy increases their exercise tolerance during sessions and hastens the achievement of their rehabilitative goals.

RESPIRATORY MUSCLE TRAINING

As for other skeletal muscles, the ventilatory pump, which is composed of respiratory skeletal muscle, may be profoundly affected by bed rest and/or the underlying disease or co-morbid conditions. In addition, the use of controlled mechanical ventilation may lead to the development of selected diaphragmatic atrophy, after only 24 h, as shown in laboratory studies performed in rats (40), or after 11 days or longer in primates (41). Respiratory muscle weakness, and particularly an imbalance between the imposed load to breathe in light of ventilatory pump capacity, is the major determinant causing weaning failure in ventilated patients. Despite this, however, there are few data examining respiratory muscle training in patients recovering from respiratory failure. This topic is important, because some degree of respiratory muscle weakness may be present as a result of the process of mechanical ventilation, and further compounded by the fact that some who require long-term ventilation suffer hyperinflation, airways resistance and increased dead-space ventilation due to underlying COPD, all factors which simultaneously increase the work of breathing and energy expenditure.

In reported trials, two methods of ventilatory muscle training have been used. Hyperpnoeic training requires patients to rebreathe at high minute ventilations for prolonged periods of time and improves ventilatory muscle endurance. The second method employs resistive training in which patients breathe through inspiratory resistance of varying magnitudes, usually at normal breathing frequencies. Most studies showing benefit support the use of inspiratory muscle training in normal subjects, tetraplegics and patients suffering from COPD. In a prospective study by Levine *et al.* (42), COPD patients who underwent respiratory muscle endurance training using isocapnic hyperventilation showed significant increases in maximum sustainable ventilation, exercise time and peak oxygen uptake ($\dot{V}o_2$) during progressive increments in work. These patients also showed a significant improvement in the ability to perform the activities of daily living. Studies showing inspiratory resistive training in patients with COPD have reported improvements in inspiratory muscle strength, increases in lower extremity cycle endurance time, and increases in maximum work and maximum oxygen uptake (43–45). Others, however, have not been able to show similar improvements in exercise performance. Currently, there is very little experience with ventilatory muscle training in patients recovering from respiratory failure. In a small study by Belman (46), two patients recovering from acute respiratory failure were ultimately weaned from mechanical ventilation after the implementation of inspiratory muscle training. In a larger, uncontrolled trial, Aldrich *et al.* (47) provided inspiratory muscle training to 30 subjects who suffered from prolonged respiratory failure, who had previously failed multiple weaning attempts. Patients were intermittently trained by breathing through a resistive inspiratory device for periods ranging from 10 to 46 days. Twelve out of 30 patients (40 per cent) were finally successfully weaned from mechanical ventilation. No prospective randomized controlled trials have demonstrated the role of inspiratory muscle training in patients weaning from prolonged ventilatory support.

Currently in our practice, chronic ventilated patients undergo inspiratory muscle training with an inspiratory threshold device set at approximately one-third of the patient's maximum inspiratory pressure. They undergo two daily 15-min sessions, supervised by a respiratory therapist, after they are able to spontaneously breathe for 1–2 h early on in the weaning process. Threshold levels are adjusted on a weekly basis, based on the patients' maximum inspiratory pressure, until they are ventilator-independent.

OTHER THERAPIES

Occupational therapy

Occupational therapists assess patients' ability to optimally perform their activities of daily living. They also instruct patients in energy conservation techniques and provide them with assisted devices to improve functional performance. Patients are taught how to use wheelchairs or walkers to make themselves more independent. Adaptive aids are used in providing daily care, such as toileting, bathing, dressing and also preparing meals and articles of clothing.

Secretion clearance

Clearance of secretions and airway humidification are primary goals of respiratory therapists working in the ICU. Insufficient cough and accumulation of secretions are important factors that increase the respiratory complication rate. Principal techniques of secretion removal are directed cough, postural drainage, forced expiratory techniques and the use of chest physiotherapy devices. The use of mucolytics and expectorants is also evaluated on an individual basis, but hard data showing superiority of one agent over another are currently lacking. Newer devices, such as a cufflator that applies inspiratory and positive negative pressures to the airway, an external jacket that applies external chest wall percussion (ABI Vest), positive expiratory pressure (PEP) valves, or flutter valve devices that facilitate cough and clearance of secretions, can be tried on an individual basis.

SUMMARY

Advances in critical medicine and the art of medical ventilation have improved the long-term survival of critically ill patients, some of whom require prolonged ventilatory support and substantial whole-body deconditioning, and have lost the ability to be independent in the performance of routine daily activities, such as sitting, speaking, eating and ambulation. To accomplish the goal of restoring patients to an optimum quality of life, rehabilitation programmes require a multidisciplinary approach by physicians, respiratory therapists, nurses, physical and occupational therapists, speech therapists, nutritionists and social services working in a concerted effort. Special attention must be paid to aggressive respiratory and non-respiratory muscle rehabilitation, early ambulation, re-nutrition, psychological support and ventilatory strategies geared to support spontaneous ventilation and foster patient independence, thereby resulting in an overall improvement in quality of life.

Key points

● A growing number of patients require long-term ventilation support because of advances in medical and surgical care.
● Multidisciplinary rehabilitation in ventilator-dependent patients is most likely to improve patient survival, and facilitate successful weaning from mechanical ventilation and discharge to the home environment.
● Multidisciplinary care of ventilator-dependent patients requires the expertise of many specialities, including pulmonary medicine, respiratory therapy, physical therapy, psychology, and speech and swallowing specialist evaluation, complemented by nurses skilled in the management of patients with airway and ventilator care needs.
● The use of multidisciplinary care improves the quality of life of patients receiving chronic ventilation; a combination of respiratory and non-respiratory whole-body reconditioning is required to optimize patients' respiratory and whole-body function.

REFERENCES

1. Wagner DP. Economics of prolonged mechanical ventilation. *Am Rev Respir Dis* 1989; **140** (Suppl.): S14–18.
◆2. Criner GJ. Long-term ventilation. Introduction and perspectives. *Respir Care Clinics* 2002; **8**: 345–53.
◆3. Donner CF, Muir JF and the Rehabilitation and Chronic Care Scientific Group of the European Respiratory Society. Position paper. Selection criteria and programmes for pulmonary rehabilitation in COPD patients. *Eur Respir J* 1997; **10**: 744–57.
◆4. American Thoracic Society. Pulmonary rehabilitation – 1999. *Am J Respir Crit Care Med* 1999; **159**: 1666–82.
5. Gracey DR, Hardy DC, Naessens JM *et al.* The Mayo Ventilator-Dependent Rehabilitation Unit: a 5 year experience. *Mayo Clin Proc* 1997; **72**: 13–9.
6. Criner GJ, Kreimer DT, Pidlaoan L. Patient outcome following prolonged mechanical ventilation (MV) via tracheostomy. *Am Rev Respir Dis* 1993; **147**: A874.
●7. Chatila w Kreimer DT, Criner GJ. Quality of life in survivors of prolonged mechanical ventilation. *Crit Care Med* 2001; **29**: 737–42.
8. Norrenberg M, Vincent JL. A profile of European intensive care unit physiotherapists. *Intensive Care Med* 2000; **26**: 841–4.
◆9. Schonhofer B. Choice of ventilator types, modes and settings for long-term ventilation. *Resp Care Clinics* 2002; **8**: 419–49.
10. Bentley S, Murphy F, Dudley H. Perceived noises in surgical wards and an intensive care area. An objective analysis. *Br Med J* 1977; **2**: 1503–6.
11. Criner GJ, Isaac L. Psychological problems in the ventilator-dependent patient. In: Tobin M, ed. *Principles and Practice of Mechanical Ventilation*. New York: McGraw-Hill, 1994; 1163–75.
12. Wilson M. Intensive care delirium. *Arch Intern Med* 1972; **130**: 225–6.

13. Manzano J, Lubillo S, Henriquez D et al. Verbal communication of ventilator dependent patients. Crit Care Med 1993; 21: 512–17.

14. Prigent H, Samuel C, Rouis B et al. Comparative effects of two ventilatory modes on speech in tracheostomized patients with neuromuscular disease. Am J Respir Crit Care Med 2003; 167: 114–19.

●15. Tolep K, Getch KL, Criner GJ. Swallowing dysfunction in patients requiring prolonged mechanical ventilation. Chest 1996; 109: 167–72.

16. Martin UJ, Hincapie L, Gilmartin ME et al. Impact of whole body rehabilitation on functional status in chronic ventilator-dependent patients (Abstract). Am J Respir Crit Care Med 1999; 159: 374.

17. Schols AMWJ, Soeters PB, Dingemans MC et al. Prevalence and characteristics of nutritional depletion in patients with stable COPD eligible for pulmonary rehabilitation. Am J Respir Crit Care Med 1993; 147: 1151.

●18. Bernard S, Le Blanc P, Witton F et al. Peripheral muscle weakness in patients with COPD. Am J Respir Crit Care Med 1998; 158: 629.

19. Marchetti N, Cordova FC, Criner GJ. Patterns of neurologic recovery and clinical outcome in patients with critical illness neuropathy. Am J Respir Crit Care Med 2002; 165: A688.

20. Coyle EF, Martin WH, Bloomfield SA et al. Effects of detraining on response to submaximal exercise. J Appl Physiol 1985; 59: 853–9.

21. Debusk RF, Convertino VA, Hung J, Goldwater D. Exercise conditioning in middle-aged men after 10 days of bed rest. Circulation 1983; 58: 245–50.

22. Hung J, Goldwater D, Concertino VA et al. Mechanism for decreased exercise capacity after bed rest in normal middle-aged men. Am J Cardiol 1983; 51: 344–8.

23. Saltin B, Blomqvist G, Mitchell JH et al. Response to exercise after bed rest and after training. Circulation 1968; 38 (Suppl. 7): 1–78.

24. Martin WH, Coyle EF, Bloomfield SA, Eshani AA. Effects of physical deconditioning after intense endurance training on left ventricular dimension and stroke volume. J Am Coll Cardiol 1986; 7: 982–9.

25. Ehsani AA, Hagberg JM, Hiskson RC. Rapid changes in left ventricular dimensions and mass in response to physical conditioning and deconditioning. Am J Cardiol 1978; 42: 52–6.

26. Deitrick JE, Whedon GD, Shorr E. Effects of immobilization upon various metabolic and physiologic functions of normal men. Am J Med 1948; 4: 3–36.

27. Fareeduddin K, Abelmann WH. Impaired orthostatic tolerance after bed rest in patients with myocardial infarction. N Engl J Med 1969; 280: 345–50.

28. Bortz WM. Disuse and aging. J Am Med Assoc 1982; 248: 1203–8.

29. Downs F. Bed rest and sensory disturbances. Am J Nurs 1974; 74: 434–8.

●30. Celli BR, Rassulo J, Make B. Dyssynchronous breathing associated with arm, but not with leg exercise in patients with COPD. N Engl J Med 1986; 314: 1485.

31. Criner GJ, Celli BR. Effect of unsupported arm exercise on ventilatory muscle recruitment in patients with severe chronic airflow obstruction. Am Rev Respir Dis 1988; 138: 856–61.

32. Celli BR, Criner GJ, Rassulo J. Ventilatory muscle recruitment during unsupported arm exercise in normal subjects. J Appl Physiol 1988; 64: 1936–40.

33. Keens TG, Krastens IRB, Wanamaker JM et al. Ventilatory muscle endurance training in normal subjects and patient with cystic fibrosis. Am Rev Respir Dis 1977; 116: 853–60.

34. Clanton T, Dixon G, Drake J, Gadek J. Effects of swim training on lung volumes and inspiratory muscle condition. J App Physiol 1987; 62: 39–46.

●35. Estenne M, Kroop C, Van Vaerehnbergj J et al. The effect of pectoralis muscle training in tetraplegia patients. Am Rev Respir Dis 1989; 139: 1218–22.

36. Lake FR, Henderson K, Briffa T et al. Upper limb and lower limb exercise training in patients with chronic airflow obstruction. Chest 1990; 97: 1077–82.

37. Couser JI, Martinez FJ, Celli BR. Pulmonary rehabilitation that includes arm exercise reduces metabolic and ventilatory requirements for simple arm elevation. Chest 1993; 103: 37–41.

●38. Martinez FJ, Vogel PD, Dupont DN et al. Supported arm exercise vs. unsupported arm exercise in the rehabilitation of patients with severe chronic airflow limitation. Chest 1993; 103: 1397–402.

39. Ries AL, Ellis BE, Hawkins RW. Upper extremity training in chronic obstructive pulmonary disease. Chest 1988; 93: 688–92.

40. Lebourdelle G, Vires N, Bockzowki J et al. Effects of mechanical ventilation on diaphragmatic contractile properties in rats. Am J Respir Crit Care Med 1994; 149: 1539–44.

41. Anzueto A, Peters JI, Tobin MJ et al. Effects of prolonged controlled mechanical ventilation on diaphragmatic function in healthy adult baboons. Crit Care Med 1997; 25: 1187–90.

42. Levine S, Weiser P, Gillen J. Evaluation of a ventilatory muscle endurance training program in the rehabilitation of patients with chronic obstructive pulmonary disease. Am Rev Respir Dis 1986; 133: 400–6.

43. Belman MJ, Shadmehr R. Targeted resistive ventilatory muscle training in chronic obstructive pulmonary disease. J Appl Physiol 1988; 65: 2726–35.

44. Pardy RL, Rivington RN, Despas PJ et al. The effects of inspiratory muscle training on exercise performance in chronic airflow limitation. Am Rev Respir Dis 1981; 123: 426–33.

45. Chen H, Dukes R, Martin GJ. Inspiratory muscle training in patients with chronic obstructive pulmonary disease. Am Rev Respir Dis 1985; 131: 251–5.

46. Belman MJ. Respiratory failure treated by ventilatory muscle training: a report of two cases. Eur J Respir Dis 1981; 62: 391–3.

●47. Aldrich TK, Karpel JP, Uhrlass RM et al. Weaning from mechanical ventilation adjunctive use of inspiratory muscle resistive training. Crit Care Med 1989; 17: 143–7.

34

Chronic ventilatory assistance in the hospital

MONICA AVENDAÑO, PETER WIJKSTRA

INTRODUCTION

Chronic respiratory failure secondary to neuromuscular diseases (NMDs) has been recognized for many decades. However, it was not actively managed until Emerson and Drinker developed the iron lung, mainly for treating patients with severe respiratory muscle involvement due to poliomyelitis (1).

Mechanical ventilation was originally delivered through an endotracheal tube to allow control of the respiratory system during general anaesthesia. Subsequently, ventilation through a tracheostomy tube was used for the treatment of acutely ill patients in the intensive care unit (ICU). A number of these patients cannot be weaned from the ventilator and remain on mechanical support after achieving medical stability. These patients are subject to sleep deprivation, sensory deprivation, immobility, isolation, inability to speak, external regulation of the body clock and uncertainty. Therefore, the resource-intensive ICU is not the most appropriate place to keep patients who are no longer critically ill. It is better for them to leave the ICU.

More than 20 years ago it was recognized that patients with chronic respiratory diseases or complications could be cared for outside the ICU with reasonable outcomes and at a considerably lower cost. In 1982, Indihar and Forsberg (2) reported an 18-month experience with a prolonged respiratory care unit. This unit was staffed by a multidisciplinary team, including physicians, nurses, respiratory therapists, social services, dietary services, volunteer and chaplaincy services, plus available consultations by physical therapists and occupational therapists. Initially, the unit was thought to be the permanent residence for these chronic patients; however, a significant number were discharged home or to a long-term care facility. Forty-three per cent of the patients admitted to this unit required chronic ventilatory assistance (CVA) but the authors did not specify if the ventilator-assisted individuals (VAIs) were among those discharged into the community.

In this chapter we review a number of specific issues concerning patients requiring CVA in the hospital setting. First, we discuss the types of patient who require CVA in the hospital; second, we describe the different settings where patients can be ventilated chronically; and finally, we focus on different issues of our own 15-year experience with a chronic assisted ventilatory care unit (CAVC).

Definition of chronic ventilatory assistance (long-term mechanical ventilation)

Make (3) suggested an acceptable working definition of long-term ventilation, as follows:

> A long-term VAI is a person who requires mechanical ventilatory assistance for more than 6 hours a day for more than 3 weeks after all acute illnesses have been maximally treated and in whom multiple weaning attempts by an experienced respiratory care team have been unsuccessful.

This definition refers mainly to patients who are 'ICU survivors' and does not include those in whom disease progresses and ventilatory support is electively initiated. Elective initiation of ventilation is most commonly done in patients with neuromuscular and thoracic cage disorders. Lately, elective ventilation has been increasingly implemented in patients with chronic obstructive pulmonary disease (COPD); however, the effects have not been clearly established (4–6).

WHO REQUIRES CVA?

We can distinguish two different groups of patients:

- The ICU 'survivors' in whom mechanical ventilation has been initiated during a critical, life-threatening illness. In these patients CVA is usually invasive and continuous (24 h/day). It replaces spontaneous ventilatory efforts and allows the patient to achieve medical stability, and/or maintain life. In some of these patients, ventilatory support will change over time to non-invasive and might become necessary only at night.
- Patients in whom CVA has been electively initiated to augment spontaneous ventilation. In these patients, CVA is usually non-invasive and mostly nocturnal (7).

The underlying diagnosis of patients requiring CVA might be the same in both groups, especially those with neuromuscular disorders whose impending ventilatory failure is not recognized in a timely manner, and who progress to acute respiratory failure requiring intensive care management.

Patients that require CVA in the hospital have in common that the return to their pre-morbid, usual environment is no longer possible.

DIFFERENT SETTINGS FOR VAIs

The VAI's definitive placement does not depend on medical needs alone, but more on the availability of a safe environment that optimizes the individual's potential to achieve a maximal level of function, enhances quality of life, prolongs life and is cost-effective (8).

For the majority of VAIs, home ventilation offers the best option for the rehabilitative potential and it allows better psychosocial functioning and enhances social integration and quality of life (9, 10). Most medically stable VAIs reside in the community, in private homes, in attendant care facilities or in group homes. For some VAIs community placement is not an option, mainly due to psychosocial factors, e.g. lack of family/friends who can provide the care; not enough health care resources (home care); breakdown of home care support (death or serious illness of the care providers); or lack of financial resources. Very few patients cannot be discharged from the acute care setting due to protracted medical instability. For these patients, different settings where chronic ventilatory support can be provided are possible.

Intensive care unit

In the ICU we find two types of patients:

- Patients who stay alive with CVA while medical stability cannot be achieved – they require ongoing continuous invasive monitoring and might be in the ICU for months; the majority of these patients will eventually die in the ICU.

- Patients who have achieved medical stability but cannot be weaned from the ventilator and there is no appropriate discharge setting outside the ICU – these patients might reside in the ICU for months or years awaiting placement in another facility. In these patients CVA may sustain and extend life while morbidity might not necessarily be reduced. Most often their quality of life is poor while care is extremely expensive. In this group, a rehabilitative approach in the ICU must be attempted to facilitate the eventual discharge to a more appropriate setting.

Subacute care unit

These are sometimes referred as 'step-down units'. Most of these centres originated as an increasing number of patients survived catastrophic illnesses but remained ventilator-dependent. Caring for them in the ICU was no longer necessary and became increasingly more expensive.

They are usually considered 'weaning centres', depending on highly selective admission criteria in order to ensure success with the weaning (11–14). Some of these centres have evolved from a purely custodial care facility for VAIs to a regional centre where patients can be weaned or trained to continue CVA outside the hospital. Bagley and Cooney (15) report on a community-based regional ventilator weaning unit located in a long-term acute-care facility. This centre accepted patients who were tracheostomized, had a feeding gastrostomy or jejunostomy tube to ensure reliable enteral feeding, were haemodynamically stable and did not require dialysis. Patients with terminal malignancies or in a severe and persistent vegetative state following hypoxic brain injury were not excluded from admission. The focus in this centre was to maximize the level of function and improve nutrition rather than exclusively weaning from the ventilator. This has been reported to be the best approach to weaning (16–18). These weaning centres apply a rehabilitative approach to the VAIs that appears to be beneficial even though weaning is not possible. They prepare patients and families for the eventual discharge to home ventilation and offer a lower-cost venue for VAIs who cannot be discharged to their home or to an extended care facility (19).

General medical ward in an acute care hospital

Latriano et al. (20) reported on a 4.5-year experience caring for haemodynamically stable mechanically ventilated patients on a nine-bed non-monitored respiratory care floor located on a 22-bed general medical ward in a tertiary care hospital. A team of intensivists, respiratory therapists and nurses at a nurse/patient ratio of 1:3 staffed this unit. Patients had been on mechanical ventilation for a mean of 23 days (range 0–126) prior to admission to the unit and were ventilated for 49 days (range 1–535) in the unit. Slightly over 50 per cent of the patients survived and, of those, over 93 per cent were successfully weaned from mechanical ventilation. Survival was higher in patients with trauma (mostly transferred from the surgical ICU) and lower in those with multisystem failure (transferred from the medical ICU). More than one-third of the survivor patients were discharged home, another third went to a rehabilitation unit, and the remaining patients went to a skilled nursing facility. The authors advocate that caring for these patients in a general medical floor allows acceptable outcomes with a considerable reduction in costs. Gracey *et al.* (21) concluded from their experience that the management of stable ventilator-dependent patients outside the ICU is rewarding and educational, as 91 (77 per cent) of the 132 patients admitted to their ventilator-dependent unit were eventually discharged home and 22 (18 per cent) were discharged to a nursing home.

Chronic assisted ventilatory care units (CAVC units)

These units might be attached to or associated with an acute care facility, a rehabilitation hospital or a chronic hospital. They require skilled health care workers familiar with ventilators, as well as trained personnel who will provide a 'rehabilitative' approach and not just custodial care.

The authors of this chapter have been associated with a CAVC located in a rehabilitation and complex continuing care hospital. Most of the issues addressed in this section reflect the authors' opinions and are strongly influenced by their personal experience. We later summarize the outcome of such a unit after 15 years of experience (22).

The transition from the acute care setting to a CAVC must be as smooth as possible. Patients and families are usually fearful of the lack of 'intensive nursing care and monitoring'. A visit by the patient and family to the unit prior to transfer helps to develop confidence and trust. It is advisable that patients referred to a CAVC unit from an ICU are initially assessed by the multidisciplinary team while still in the ICU. Patients' ventilation and the physiological effects of mechanical ventilation must be well established. Patients must have a stable airway (tracheostomy) and cannot require suctioning more often than every 2 h, they must be haemodynamically stable and must understand and be motivated to be moved outside the ICU. In a CAVC unit, the health care providers must keep in mind that patients have significant issues related to their need for long-term ventilation. Their life is prolonged but they become more dependent on third-party care as well as on highly developed technology and electrical devices. As a consequence, patients lose control over their lives and this might lead to depression and behavioural problems. Patients resent the fact that they must abide by hospital rules and the routine of life in an institution (i.e. when to get up, when to go back to bed, when to eat, sleep, etc.).

Most of the families of the VAIs who reside in a chronic care facility are under stress and some are plagued by feelings of guilt. The relationships change when family interactions occur within the hospital setting. Therefore it is important to provide as much privacy as possible in order to regain the spontaneity which was lost outside the home environment. The team must be alert as to indications of family 'dysfunction' and be supportive and understanding. In addition, the team members need to be supportive of each other as it is not unusual for patients and families to turn their frustrations, arising from their lack of control over the illness and situation, against the staff.

Patients must be encouraged to play an active part in care decisions. It is important to show the patient respect, a positive attitude and to individualize the care as much as possible. Patients must be helped to enjoy simple pleasures. Nurses caring for these patients have an important role as they can promote conversations toward positive themes that interest them (family, past working history and achievements, hobbies, etc.).

Assessment of the communication abilities and needs of the patients must be addressed as soon as possible and the communication requirements should always be incorporated into the nursing care plan.

In a CAVC unit, the approach is a multidisciplinary one with a team of skilled and experienced staff to look after the medical aspects, the physical needs, and the psychosocial needs, always maintaining a rehabilitative approach to the care of the patients.

THE MULTIDISCIPLINARY TEAM WORKING IN A CAVC UNIT

PHYSICIAN

The physician provides medical leadership to the rest of the team and is responsible for the medical assessment and management of the patients. He or she is responsible for the prescription of the most appropriate treatment, including medical therapies and oxygen as well as, in conjunction with the respiratory therapist, the selection of an adequate and effective ventilator system, including settings and interfaces.

NURSE

Nurses must be skilled in the care of VAIs and are responsible for the daily care of patients in relation to their physical needs.

On admission, in addition to the customary nursing assessment, the nurse explores patients' impressions of the unit and their expectations. Patients transferred from the ICU might present with 'ICU syndrome' (23), characterized by a wide range of symptoms including fear, anxiety, fatigue, confusion, delusions and disorientation. It is therefore important to reassure patients and allow them to express these feelings. The health care team, particularly the nurses, must try to detect these symptoms. Patients admitted from the ICU need to be reassured regarding safety and especially regarding prompt response to their calls in spite of the much lower nurse:patient ratio. At night the nurse is frequently the only health care professional in the unit and the patients and their families need to be reassured of their safety.

We agree with Ecklund (24), who reported on the design of a unit for ventilator-dependent patients called the progressive pulmonary care unit (PPCU), located in a tertiary care institution, and stated that the success of such a unit depends on proper staffing. Ecklund advised on an advanced practice nurse (APN), who directly manages the plan of care for each of the patients in collaboration with the attending physician and the multidisciplinary team, and a director of nursing who manages the unit and is responsible for the daily operations, staffing and budget.

RESPIRATORY THERAPIST

The respiratory therapist (RT), who has knowledge and experience of assessing the ventilatory needs of the patients, is responsible, in concert with the physician's direction, for establishing the most appropriate ventilatory support system and interface. Patients who come from the ICU frequently need to have the interface and settings changed to a more 'long-term ventilation-friendly' mode.

Tracheobronchial ruptures have been reported as long-term complications of tracheostomy. Fortunately these are rare events (25, 26). The RT does have special care to avoid excessive cuff inflation in all patients with permanent tracheostomies when they require cuffed tubes. The RT is also responsible for establishing the ideal degree of humidification in the ventilator circuit. This will benefit the clearance of airway secretions. In some patients, the instillation of normal saline together with endotracheal suctioning will help in removing thick, tenacious secretions. The RT will also assess the need for using an in-exsufflator (27) to facilitate bronchial hygiene. The RT performs the tracheostomy routine care: stoma and tube cleaning, tube changing, dressing and tie changes. In addition, the RT provides training to patients and families in the management of oxygen, ventilator equipment, as well as suctioning and manual ventilation. This is important as it will allow the patients to go out of the unit accompanied by their significant others, and, in some cases, to be discharged back to the community.

PHYSICAL THERAPIST

The physical therapist (PT) performs a functional assessment at baseline to set goals for activity and assists in maintaining muscle strength and avoiding contractures. The initial assessment includes not only establishing the baseline functional status, but also the cough effectiveness. The PT is responsible for designing an exercise routine that will depend on the patient's mobility, going from passive range-of-motion or simple bed exercises to a comprehensive interval training programme.

OCCUPATIONAL THERAPIST

The occupational therapist (OT) establishes patients' goals relative to activities of daily living and provides the necessary assistive devices to enhance functional independence. In addition, the OT assesses patients' needs to achieve maximum functional mobility. When indicated, the OT advises on the most appropriate wheelchair and provides the training for patients in the safe operation of the power (electric/battery-operated) wheelchair. These power wheelchairs are customized, they have a portable ventilator mounted in a special tray and are provided with pressure-relief cushions in order to avoid tissue trauma. The OT also assists patients in the use of computers.

SPEECH LANGUAGE PATHOLOGIST

The speech language pathologist (SLP) assesses and assists patients in maintaining the ability to communicate, as this is very important for all individuals. Tracheostomized patients with an inflated cuff cannot speak. Some patients will be able to tolerate and use a one-way speaking valve (28), while in others, communication can be facilitated by a variety of methods customized to the patient's ability, e.g. letter board, written communication, electrolarynx or computer. The SLP, whenever possible, trains some patients in lip reading.

The SLP will also assess the effectiveness and safety of swallowing. Swallowing dysfunction in patients on prolonged mechanical ventilation is multifactorial, including the effect of the tracheostomy on laryngeal movement and the presence of an underlying neuromuscular illness. The recognition of this swallowing dysfunction permits the identification of patients at high risk for pulmonary aspiration (29). In addition, the majority of patients with neuromuscular disorders (Duchenne muscular dystrophy, amyotrophic lateral sclerosis, spinal muscular atrophy, myotonic dystrophy) will have severe dysphagia and all phases of swallowing can be affected (30). The SLP assesses every patient on admission and on an ongoing basis. In some patients, oral intake can be preserved or restored; in others, swallowing deteriorates and enteral feeding becomes necessary.

SOCIAL WORKER

The social worker determines the family dynamics and the cultural and religious influences that might have an impact on the care of the patient. The social worker also assists the family in exploring community support agencies as well as funding access for equipment as necessary.

PSYCHOLOGIST

The psychologist performs a psychological assessment and assists the team in designing and applying the appropriate approach in conflict situations among patients, between patients and their families, and between patients and staff. The psychologist also assesses mental competency, especially in patients who sometimes pose unreasonable and unrealistic demands. If necessary, a consulting psychiatrist is involved in the assessment and care plan. This is especially necessary if a patient wants to have the mechanical ventilation discontinued. The psychiatrist must assess the patient in order to determine mental competency to make such a decision (31). Although this is not common, it might happen and the attending team must be prepared to assist and support the patient and the family.

The elective discontinuation of life-sustaining mechanical ventilation on a ventilator-dependent individual is addressed on page 337.

RECREATIONAL THERAPIST

The recreational therapist assesses the patient's goals for leisure activities and designs a plan for diverse activities and structured group work. The recreational therapist is also involved in the organization of outings for groups of patients (field trips).

CHAPLAIN

The chaplain functions as a consultant, assessing the wishes of patients and their families and assisting in fulfilling their spiritual needs.

CLINICAL DIETICIANS

They assess the baseline nutritional status of all patients and advice in the maximization of the caloric intake, either oral or enteral. This professional frequently works in conjunction with the SLP in order to maintain ideal body weight and nutrition in the VAIs.

ONGOING CARE

Once the assessment of patients is completed and their goals have been defined, the multidisciplinary team formulates a plan of care. The team will meet the patient, the family and significant others (family conferences) to discuss the care plan. Patients are subsequently reviewed by the team on a weekly basis. The goals have a set time limit and are reassessed on an annual basis, or more frequently if necessary. The family conferences are held at annual intervals, or earlier if the patient's condition changes.

Special considerations

NUTRITION

It is necessary to determine the nutritional status of the patient. Nutritional status has been reported to affect the possibility of weaning, survival and the predisposition to respiratory tract infections in VAIs. It is known that the majority of patients with neuromuscular disorders (Duchenne muscular dystrophy, amyotrophic lateral sclerosis, spinal muscular atrophy, myotonic dystrophy) will have severe dysphagia, as all phases of their swallowing can be affected (30). Weight loss correlates with swallowing impairment. If the oral route can no longer maintain nutrition and hydration, gastrostomy or jejunostomy must be considered. In most patients, however, after bedside assessment and advice by the SLP, it is possible to continue some oral feeding in small amounts with special food consistencies, mostly to enhance quality of life. Aspiration is a serious complication of tube feedings, even in patients without compromise of the level of consciousness, and therefore the SLP routinely assesses patients on tube feeding for the possibility of aspiration by adding dye to the feeding formula and observing for it in tracheobronchial secretions. In some

cases the SLP will use reagents to detect the presence of enteral formula in the tracheobronchial secretions (32). In some patients videofluoroscopy is necessary.

On the other hand, it has been our experience that some patients who conserve an intact swallowing mechanism become grossly overweight. This is difficult to avoid and will usually lead to alterations of the ventilatory mechanics and disruption of the routine care. Transfers become difficult, with increasing risk of injury to both the patient and the health care staff. In addition, mobility might be affected, as the wheelchair (always customized) might no longer be comfortable to the patient. Therefore a dietician is an important member of the team for both underweight and overweight patients.

TISSUE TRAUMA (PRESSURE ULCERS)

Some patients transferred from the ICU will have different degrees of tissue trauma. It has been reported that pressure ulcers are associated with substantial and significant increases in hospital costs and length of stay, and the potential for the development of serious nosocomial infections (33). An advance practical nurse with special expertise assesses and advises in the proper care necessary to minimize or cure these conditions. We have not encountered serious ongoing problems with tissue trauma. The patient care plan is detailed enough to include the frequency of turning, as well as the need for special mattresses and other pressure relief devices.

PERMANENT TRACHEOSTOMY

It is necessary to avoid bacterial colonization, trauma to the tracheal mucosa, trauma to the vocal cords and its effect on speech and swallowing. The RT and the nurse are mainly responsible for the safe care of the tracheostomy (34).

PNEUMONIA

Establishing the diagnosis of pneumonia, especially to differentiate between lower respiratory tract colonization and infection, is sometimes difficult in VAIs. The clinical symptoms, the chest radiograph, the white blood cell count and the bacteriology studies of tracheobronchial secretions lack specificity. For an accurate diagnosis, bronchoscopy with bronchoalveolar lavage or a protected specimen brush, might be necessary. Special considerations must be given to avoid cross-infection from other patients and staff, as many VAIs will be colonized with hospital pathogens, most commonly Gram-negative bacilli and *Staphylococcus aureus*, by the time they leave the ICU and are transferred to a CAVC unit. Staff education, proper isolation techniques and effective infection-control practices are extremely important in such a unit. The use of sedatives must be carefully assessed as they may increase the risk of aspiration and subsequent pneumonia as well as decrease the clearance of lower respiratory tract secretions (35).

TREATMENT OF DIFFERENT PATIENT GROUPS IN A CAVC

Patients with progressive degenerative NMDs

The care of patients with amyotrophic lateral sclerosis (ALS) and other progressive degenerative NMDs poses a special challenge, as patients' cognitive function is not impaired. Survival is the primary factor in the management of patients in general; however, in patients with a chronic, progressive disabling condition, decision-making might need to be modified, as survival is no longer the issue, but rather patients' comfort is the main goal (36, 37). In this group of patients it is important to focus on ways to maximize the level of functioning and overall quality of life.

As it is sometimes difficult to communicate with these patients, it is difficult to assess their quality of life as shown by Gelinas et al. (38). They concluded that it was difficult to assess quality of life in these patients as everyday functions and activities by which healthy people can assess quality of life no longer apply. In spite of the extreme limitations imposed by their disease, the authors found that no patient regretted the decision to go on a ventilator and most felt contented and satisfied for most of the time. In addition, all patients found that the ability to communicate was essential for their happiness. These ALS patients were residing at home. On the other hand, their care-givers reported frustration and unhappiness and felt the burden to be excessive, overall expressing significant dissatisfaction with the ventilator decision. Moss et al. (39) studied 58 ALS patients able to communicate and participate in structured interviews. Thirty-six lived at home and 14 in an institution. Those living at home rated their quality of life on a 10-point scale better than those living in an institution.

Patients with Duchenne muscular dystrophy

Mechanical ventilation is a therapeutic option for the respiratory failure associated with Duchenne muscular dystrophy (DMD) (40–42). In our experience (unpublished data), most patients will remain in the community, most commonly the family home. However, there are some in whom home ventilation is not possible, especially if there is more than one affected individual or if the family breaks down under the stress of caring for one such patient. In 1979, Buchanan et al. (43) showed that 76 per cent of the families of patients with DMD identified psychological issues as the major problem. In 1984 Botvin Madorskyalso highlighted psychosocial issues, especially related to death and dying, and lack of education and support as disease progresses (44). These issues do not resolve when mechanical ventilation is implemented. The care of young males with DMD in a CAVC unit therefore represents a major challenge to the staff, as they present with problems related to depression, loss of control, increasing disability, loss of the ability to swallow, separation from family and friends, and anger at not being able to remain at home. This is often reflected in behavioural issues.

In 1991 Bach et al. (45) reported on the quality of life of individuals with DMD using long-term ventilation. In this study patients residing at home were compared with those residing in an institution. Forty-three patients residing in the home environment were slightly more satisfied with their families than the 33 patients residing in chronic care facilities. They concluded that, overall, the vast majority of these patients 'have a positive affect and are satisfied with life despite the physical dependence which precludes many of the activities most commonly associated with perceived quality of life for physically intact individuals'.

Patients with spinal cord injury

Historically, the majority of individuals who presented with apnoea after suffering spinal cord injury (SCI) died at the scene of the accident or the acute trauma centre. A spinal cord injury is a traumatic event causing many unanticipated and irreversible physical changes that immediately affect the individual's capability of meeting life demands. Usually these patients are young, previously healthy and active. These individuals are suddenly confronted with a totally new experience of their body in relation to the physical, psychological and social environments. Pain is reported frequently after spinal cord injury. The physician needs to assess the patient to elucidate the aetiology of the pain, identify a pain generator and implement medical treatment as indicated. Acetaminophen and non-steroidal anti-inflammatory drugs are first-line therapy for pain relief. Anti-depressants have been found to be effective and may assist with sleep and relieve depression. Narcotic analgesics are usually avoided because of the risks of tolerance and escalating dosage, addiction, sedating effects and the possibility of deliberate drug-seeking. Substance abuse has been reported as a significant risk after spinal cord injury (46). The health care team must be supportive and must try to understand the patients and their families. Frequently, following admission to the CAVC unit, these patients are quiet, depressed and do not actively seek communication with the staff, keeping their eyes closed while receiving care. In our experience, it sometimes takes years for these patients to accept their devastating situation and begin to participate in individual and group activities.

Elective discontinuation of mechanical ventilation

Although physicians feel their professional duty is to preserve life, it can be argued that a physician's duty is also to ensure an acceptable quality of life and, in certain cases, to ensure a comfortable and dignified death (47). Terminal weaning (TW) provides patients with the option of electively discontinuing mechanical ventilation and accepting death. It allows for more precise titration of narcotics and sedatives to accomplish the goal of therapy, which is alleviating patient suffering while discontinuing ventilation. Campbell et al. (48) define

TW as the removal of ventilatory support while an artificial airway remains in place, as contrasted with extubation, which is the removal of the artificial airway with the removal of the ventilatory support.

Most of the published literature on this subject has discussed the withdrawal of mechanical ventilation in hospital ICUs. On a chronic ventilator unit, as opposed to an ICU, the decision to discontinue life-sustaining mechanical ventilation is made, in many cases, by patients who are medically stable and able to make decisions. The decision to discontinue mechanical ventilation is difficult for many physicians, patients and families. Christakis and Asch (49) found that physicians consider mechanical ventilation the most difficult treatment to withdraw. The decision to terminally wean has been a very rare occurrence in our CAVC unit. In fact, only one patient with high spinal cord injury and intractable pain in spite of aggressive therapy opted for TW. Campbell and Carlson (50) discussed the indications for TW. The three common reasons identified by them were patient's informed request, medical futility and reduction of patient's pain and suffering. The usual protocol for this procedure involves the use of morphine and a benzodiazepine; however, guidelines for optimal use of these medications are lacking and are usually based on physicians' preferences (51).

The decision to allow TW in our unit was made after the patient was fully assessed in order to determine mental integrity to make such a decision and to rule out depression. Both the patient and his family were cared for by the physicians and members of the team with the aim of giving as much comfort as possible under the circumstances. Caring continued even as the patient died. Words, human touch and the compassionate use of narcotics were the focus of the withdrawal rather than the 'pulling out of the tube'. It is crucially important that the physician should focus on the comfort needs of the patient rather than on the patient's likely death.

EXPERIENCE OF 15 YEARS WITH A CAVC UNIT

Recently, we reviewed all patients who were admitted to our CAVC unit between 1986 and 2000 (22). Fifty patients with different diagnoses were admitted to the unit (Table 34.1). During their stay, ventilation time increased from 16 h (SD 5.6) to 22.9 h (SD 3.0) per 24 h ($P < 0.05$) in patients with COPD and from 18.9 h (SD 6.1) to 22.9 h (SD 4.5) in those with thoracic restriction (TR) (not significant). In contrast, the need for ventilatory support decreased in the three other groups. Five out of 10 patients with SCI were decannulated, two were switched to non-invasive positive pressure ventilation (NIPPV) and one remains dependent on a diaphragmatic pacer (see Case Study 34.1). Two patients with SCI below C4 became completely ventilator-free. The level of functional mobility decreased in patients with COPD and patients with TR, whereas it remained stable in patients with NMD and parenchymal restriction (PR). Functional mobility improved among patients with SCI. The complication rate was generally low, except for depression, which occurred in 50 per cent of the patients, mainly in the early stages. Severe urinary tract infections occurred in nine patients (18 per cent), of whom four required transfer to the ICU. Eighteen patients (36 per cent) were discharged to the community, either home or an attendant care facility. Eleven patients (22 per cent) died while residing in the CAVC unit and seven others were transferred back to the ICU, and subsequently died there (Table 34.2). The average cost per patient is around Canadian $700/day

Table 34.1 *Demographics of patients admitted between 1986 and 2000*

Diagnosis	Number	Age (years [SD])	Sex (M/F)	Time ventilated at home (months)	Time ventilated in hospital[a] (months)	Admitted from (n):
Obstructive (chronic obstructive pulmonary disease)	7	66.5 (8.5)	4/3	3.4 (2.5–111)[b]	5.6 (0.5–9)	ICU (7)
Non–obstructive Neuromuscular diseases	24	40.1 (17.1)	16/8	23.4 (54–180)[c]	16.3 (0–132)	ICU (15) Home (3) Rehabilitation unit (3) Children's hospital (3)
Spinal cord injury	10	39.2 (19.2)	7/3	0	11.7 (2–36)	ICU (10)
Thoracic restriction	7	61.4 (10.9)	4/3	25.9 (12–83)[d]	64.5 (0–420)	ICU (5) Home (1) Rehabilitation unit (1)
Parenchymal restricition	2	46.5 (4.9)	1/1	0	5.3 (0–10)	ICU (1) Rehabilitation unit (1)

[a]Time ventilated in hospital, ICU or rehabilitation unit prior to chronic assisted ventilatory care unit.
[b]$n = 4$.
[c]$n = 5$.
[d]$n = 4$.

Table 34.2 *Chronic assisted ventilatory care unit (CAVC) outcomes*

Diagnosis	Complications (*n*)	Length of stay (mean months [range])[a]	Discharge
Obstructive (COPD)	Depression (4)	27.2 (2–56)	Died (6) (disease progression) Home (1)
Non–obstructive			
Neuromuscular disease	Arrhythmia (1) Urinary tract infection (2) Urinary sepsis (2) → ICU Ischial pressure sore → surgery Gastrointestinal (GI) bleeding (1) → ICU[b] Haemoptysis (1) → ICU[b] Gastric atony, vomiting (1) → ICU Obesity (1) Renal cell carcinoma (1) Thymoma (1) → surgery Depression (5)	26 (1.5–120)	CAVC (10) (current) Home (6) Rehabilitation (4) Died ICU (3) (sepsis 2, abdominal pain 1) Died CAVC (1) (disease progression)
Spinal cord injury	Seizures (2) Urinary tract infection (2) Urinary sepsis (2) → ICU[c] Central line (1) → ICU[b] Depression (5) Instability of DM → ICU	26.4 (0.5–96)	CAVC (2) (current) Home (2) Died (1) (disease progression) Transitional community living (3) Died ICU (3) (sepsis 1, diabetes 1)
Thoracic restriction	Cirrhosis (1) GI bleeding (1) Cardiovascular accident (1) Glaucoma (1) Coronary artery disease (1) Prostatic cancer (1) Haemoptysis (1) → ICU Depression (4)	84.6 (1–186)	CAVC (2) current Died CAVC (3) (disease progression) Died ICU (2) (haemoptysis)
Parenchymal restriction	None	9 (2–16)	Home (2)

[a]Mean (range) of patients who were discharged from CAVC (excluding patients who are still on CAVC).
[b]Returned to CAVC.
[c]One remained, one returned.

(1999 figure), which is about half of the cost of residing in the ICU.

This retrospective analysis showed that the CAVC unit is a good environment for the severely impaired VAI. The complication rate has been low and 36 per cent of those admitted for chronic care were able to leave the unit for a more independent community-based environment. The best outcomes were seen among those with SCI and NMD.

Case Study 34.1 'Samuel': returning to living in the community

'Samuel' is a 40-year old man who was injured in a diving accident in a pool in 1982, at age 19. He sustained complete spinal cord transection at the level C1–2, became immediately quadriplegic and developed respiratory distress. A nurse present at the pool initiated immediate cardiorespiratory resuscitation (CPR) and the patient was taken to a trauma centre. He was intubated and started on mechanical ventilation. A tracheostomy was inserted 3 weeks after the accident. Four months later, a diaphragmatic pacer (52) was inserted and the patient was slowly moved to diaphragmatic pacer ventilation. He was admitted to the CAVC unit 4 years after the accident. His parents were divorced and neither of them could care for him at home.

Initially, 'Samuel' was very depressed and withdrawn. After 2.5 years in the unit, he became receptive to a more rehabilitative approach. He was repeatedly assessed regarding the maximization of his functional ability. He was trained in glossopharyngeal breathing (GPB) (53, 54). Once he was able to maintain adequate gas exchange for over 1 h with GPB alone (the pacers being disconnected), he was allowed to leave the unit without an escort. He was also trained in the use of environmental control devices, including a power wheelchair. Clinically he was very stable other than urinary tract infections which responded promptly to the right antibiotic.

Subsequently Samuel became very interested in exploring alternative residence in the community. Once a place and the necessary support in an attendant care facility were identified, more than 7 years after his admission to the CAVC unit, he was transferred to our home ventilation training programme in preparation for his return to the community. He admitted to a very hectic period when first transferred to the attendant care facility, although he was very confident that safety was never an issue. He recognized that he had forgotten the demands of daily life in the community.

Samuel still resides in his own apartment at the attendant care facility. He was reassessed in our home ventilation reassessment programme initially at yearly intervals. For the past 6 years he calls only if he has a problem and is then readmitted, otherwise he comes mainly for 'social visits' and to see patients who are being considered for discharge into the community. He has been medically stable, still with a functioning diaphragmatic pacer. After 5 years of living in the community he had the tracheostomy tube removed (his choice). We facilitated the process and established a back-up system of non-invasive ventilation.

This patient is a founder member of a programme called 'Citizens for Independence in Living and Breathing', designed to support VAIs who wish to reside in the community.

SUMMARY

The challenges of working with VAIs in a specialized unit (CAVC) are many. A multidisciplinary team must design a plan of care unique to the patient's needs. It is necessary to provide an environment conducive to both the patient and the family to accept the situation. It is important to underline that the care of VAIs in the hospital must always have a rehabilitative approach as some patients have the possibility of being discharged back to the community. In our experience, more activity and independence correlate with greater psychological well-being for the patients.

Our retrospective analysis showed that a CAVC unit is a good option for VAIs who cannot reside in the community.

Key points

- Chronic ventilatory assistance (CVA) is defined as mechanical ventilation for more than 6 h/day for more than 3 weeks after all acute illnesses have been maximally treated in those in whom multiple weaning attempts by an experienced respiratory care team have been unsuccessful.
- Chronic respiratory failure, although recognized for many decades, was not actively managed until Emerson and Drinker developed the iron lung for patients with severe respiratory muscle involvement secondary to poliomyelitis.
- Mechanical ventilation was originally delivered through an endotracheal tube during general anaesthesia. Subsequently, mechanical ventilation was used for the treatment of acute respiratory failure in the intensive care unit (ICU).

- Some patients, after achieving clinical stability, cannot be weaned from the ventilator, but the resource-intensive ICU is not the appropriate placement for them.
- There are two groups of patients who require CVA: those who, having had an episode of acute respiratory failure, become clinically stable but cannot be weaned from the ventilator, and those in whom CVA has been electively initiated to augment spontaneous ventilation.
- Most patients who require CVA can, after adequate training and preparation, be discharged home. Others must remain in institutional settings due to the lack of support in the community.
- Different settings, outside the ICU, for these ventilator-assisted individuals (VAIs) have been explored. Some patients, however, remain in the ICU waiting for a more appropriate placement.
- Some other patients are transferred to subacute care units, sometimes referred as 'step-down units'. These units have evolved from a purely custodial care facility to centres where patients may be eventually weaned from the ventilatory support and reintegrated back into the community.
- A general medical ward in acute care hospitals is another option for VAIs. These units allow for acceptable outcomes with a considerable cost reduction.
- An option that appears to be the preferred one is a chronic assisted ventilatory care unit (CAVC). These units might be attached to an acute care facility, a rehabilitation hospital or a chronic care facility.
- In a CAVC unit the approach is multidisciplinary with a team of professionals experienced in the care of VAIs. The goal is to assist VAIs in achieving their maximum level of functional independence, even though they cannot be weaned from the ventilator.
- Special considerations for VAIs in a CAVC unit are nutrition and prevention of tissue trauma.
- Different diagnostics groupings pose different challenges for the multidisciplinary team in a CAVC. These include patients with progressive neuromuscular diseases, including patients with Duchenne's muscular dystrophy (young adult males), patients with spinal cord injury and patients with thoracic wall deformities.
- The management and the prognosis of these diagnostic groupings differ and the professionals looking after them must adapt their approach to these patients.
- An issue that must be considered and acknowledged in a CAVC unit is the elective discontinuation of mechanical ventilation. This is a difficult issue as health care professionals feel their duty is to preserve life. Although infrequent, VAIs might choose to become disconnected from the ventilator. After assessing the mental ability of the patient to make such a decision, the CAVC team must ensure a comfortable and dignified death for the patient.

REFERENCES

1. JH Emerson Company. *The Evolution of Iron Lungs.* 50th Anniversary Issue. Cambridge, MA: JH Emerson, 1978.

2. Indihar FJ, Forsberg DP. Experience with a prolonged respiratory care unit. *Chest* 1982; **81**: 189–92.

◆3. Make BJ. Epidemiology of long term ventilatory assistance. In: Hill NS, ed. *Long-Term Mechanical Ventilation. Lung Biology in Health and Disease, Vol. 152.* New York, NY: Marcel Dekker, 2001.

4. Clini E, Sturani C, Rossi A *et al.* The Italian multicentre on noninvasive ventilation in chronic obstructive pulmonary disease patients. *Eur Respir J* 2002; **20**: 529–38.

5. Casanova C, Celli BR, Tost L *et al.* Long-term controlled trial of nocturnal nasal positive pressure ventilation in patients with severe COPD. *Chest* 2000; **118**: 1582–90.

●6. Wijkstra PJ, Lacasse Y, Guyatt G *et al.* A meta-analysis of nocturnal noninvasive positive pressure ventilation in patients with stable COPD. *Chest* 2003; **124**: 337–43.

●7. Goldstein RS. Hypoventilation: neuromuscular and chest wall disorders. Clin Chest Med 1992; **13**: 507–21.

◆8. Make BJ, Hill NS, Goldberg AI *et al.* Mechanical ventilation beyond the intensive care unit: report of a consensus conference of the American College of Chest Physicians. *Chest* 1998; **113**(Suppl.): 289S–344S.

9. Make BJ, Gilmartin ME. Mechanical ventilation in the home. *Crit Care Clinics* 1990; **6**: 785.

10. Goldstein RS, Psek JA, Gort EH. Home mechanical ventilation: Demographics and user perspectives. *Chest* 1995; **108**: 1581.

11. Criner GJ, Kreimer DT, Pidlaoan L. Patient outcome following prolonged mechanical ventilation via tracheostomy. *Am Rev Respir Dis* 1993: A874.

12. O'Donohue WJ, Jr. Chronic ventilator-dependent units in hospitals: attacking the front end of long-term problem. *Mayo Clin Proc* 1992; **67**: 198–200.

13. Niskanen M, Ruokonen E, Takala J *et al.* Quality of life after prolonged intensive care. *Crit Care Med* June 1999; **27**: 1132–9.

14. Scheinhorn DJ, Chao DC, Stear-Hassenpflug MS *et al.* Post-ICU mechanical ventilation. Treatment of 1,123 patients at a regional weaning center. *Chest* 1997; **111**: 1654–9.

15. Bagley PH, Cooney E. A community-based regional ventilator weaning unit. *Chest* 1997; **111**: 1024–9.

16. Scheinhorn DJ, Artinian BM, Catlin JL. Weaning from prolonged mechanical ventilation: the experience at a regional weaning center. *Chest* 1994; **105**: 534–9.

17. Gracey DR, Viggiano RW, Naessens JM *et al.* Outcome of patients admitted to a chronic ventilator-dependent unit in an acute-care hospital. *Mayo Clinic Proc* 1992; **67**: 131–6.

18. Indihar FJ. A 10-year report of patients in a prolonged respiratory care unit. *Minn Med* 1991; **74**: 23–7.

19. Dasgupta A, Rice R, Mascha E *et al.* Four year experience with a unit for long-term ventilation (respiratory special care unit) at the Cleveland Clinic Foundation. *Chest* 1999; **116**: 447–55.

20. Latriano B, McCauley P, Astiz ME *et al.* Non-ICU care of hemodynamically stable mechanically ventilated patients. *Chest* 1996; **109**: 1591–6.

21. Gracey DR, Naessens JM, Viggiano RW *et al.* Outcome of patients cared for in a ventilator-dependent unit in a general hospital. *Chest* 1995; **107**: 494–9.

◆22. Wijkstra PJ, Avendaño M, Goldstein RS. Inpatient chronic assisted ventilatory care. A 15-year experience. *Chest* 2003; **124**: 850–6.

23. McKegney FP. The intensive care syndrome. *Connecticut Med* 1966; **30**: 633–6.

24. Ecklund M. Successful outcome for the ventilator-dependent patient. *Crit Care Nursing Clinics North Am* 1999; **11**: 249–60.

25. Chew JY, Cantrell RW. Tracheostomy. Complications and their management. *Arch Otolaryng* 1972; **96**: 538–45.

26. Meyer M. Iatrogenic tracheobronchial lesions. A report on 13 cases. *Thorac Cardiov Surg* 2001; **49**: 115–19.

27. Bach JR. Prevention of morbidity and mortality with the use of physical medicine aids. In: Bach J, ed. *Pulmonary Rehabilitation: the Obstructive and Paralytic Conditions.* Philadelphia: Hanley, & Belfus, 1996.

28. Manzano JL, Lubillo S, Henriquez D *et al.* Verbal communication of ventilator- dependent patients. *Crit Care Med* 1992; **21**: 512.

29. Tolep K, Leonard Getch C, Criner GJ. Swallowing dysfunction in patients receiving prolonged mechanical ventilation. *Chest* 1996; **109**: 167–72.

30. Willig TN, Gilardeau C, Kazandjian MS *et al.* Dysphagia and nutrition in neuromuscular disorders. In: Bach J, ed. *Pulmonary Rehabilitation: the Obstructive and Paralytic Conditions.* Philadelphia: Hanley, & Belfus, 1996.

●31. Ankrom M, Zelesnick L, Barofsky I *et al.* Elective discontinuation of life-sustaining mechanical ventilation on a chronic ventilator unit. *J Am Geriatr Soc* 2001; **49**: 1549–54.

32. Metheny NA, Clouse RE. Bedside methods for detecting aspiration in tube-fed patients. *Chest* 1997; **111**: 724–31.

33. Allman RM, Goode PS, Burst N *et al.* Pressure ulcers, hospital complications and disease severity: Impact on hospital costs and length of stay. *Adv Wound Care* 1999; **12**: 22–30.

34. Special critical care considerations in tracheostomy management. *Clin Chest Med* 1991; **12**: 573.

35. Fleming CA, Balaguera HU, Craven DE. Risk factors for nosocomial pneumonia. focus on prophylaxis. *Med Clin N Am* 2001; **85**: 1545–63.

36. Baydur A, Gilgoff I, Prentice W *et al.* Decline in respiratory function and experience with long-term assisted ventilation in advanced Duchennes muscular dystrophy. *Chest* 1990; **97**: 884–9.

37. Pascuzzi RM. ALS, motor neuron disease and related disorders: a personal approach to diagnosis and management. *Semin Neurol* 2002; **22**: 75–87.

38. Gelinas DF, O'Connor P, Miller RG. Quality of life for ventilator-dependent ALS patients and their caregivers. *J Neurol Sci* 1998; **160**: s134–6.

39. Moss AH, Casey P, Stocking CB *et al.* Home ventilation for amyotrophic lateral sclerosis patients: outcomes, costs, and patient, family and physician attitudes. *Neurology* 1993; **43**: 438.

40. Newsom Davis J. The respiratory system in muscular dystrophy. *Br Med Bull* 1980; **36**: 135–8.

41. Gilroy J, Cahalan JL, Berman R *et al.* Cardiac and pulmonary complications in Duchenne's progressive muscular dystrophy. *Circulation* 1963; **27**: 484–93.

42. Inkley SR, Oldenburg FC, Vignos PJ. Pulmonary function in Duchenne's muscular dystrophy related to stage of disease. *Am J Med* 1974; **56**: 297–306.

43. Buchanan D, La Barbera C, Roelofs R *et al.* Reactions of families to children with Duchenne muscular dystrophy. *Gen Hosp Psychiatry* 1979; **1**: 262–9.

44. Botvin Madorsky JG, Radford LM, Neumann EM. Psychosocial aspects of death and dying in Duchenne's muscular dystrophy. *Arch Phys Med Rehabil* 1984; **64**: 79–82.

45. Bach JR, Campagnolo DI, Hoeman S. Life satisfaction of individuals with Duchenne muscular dystrophy using long-term ventilatory support. *Am J Phys Med Rehabil* 1991; **70**: 129–35.

46. Roth EJ, Lu A, Primack S et al. Ventilatory function in cervical and high thoracic spinal cord injury: relationship to level of injury and tone. Am J Phys Med Rehabil 1997; 76: 262–7.

47. President's Commission for the Study of Ethical Problems in Medicine and Biomedical and Behavioral Research . Deciding to Forego Life-sustaining Treatment. Washington, DC: US Government Printing Office, 1983.

48. Campbell ML, Bikek KS, Thrill M. Patient responses during rapid terminal weaning from mechanical ventilation: a prospective study. Crit Care Med 1999; 27: 73–7.

49. Chistakis NA, Asch DA. Biases in how physicians choose to withdraw life support. Lancet 1993; 342: 642–6.

50. Campbell ML, Carlson RW. Terminal weaning from mechanical ventilation: Ethical and practical considerations for patient management. Am J Crit Care 1992; 3: 52–6.

51. Citron ML, Johnson-Early A, Fossieck BE Jr et al. Safety and efficacy of continuous intravenous morphine for severe cancer pain. Am J Med 1984; 77: 199–204.

52. Chervin RD, Guilleminault C. Diaphragm pacing. Rev Reassessment Sleep 1994; 17: 176–87.

◆53. American College of Chest Physicians. Mechanical ventilation beyond the intensive care unit. Report of a consensus conference of the American College of Chest Physicians, chapter 3. Noninvasive and invasive mechanical ventilation. Chest 1998; 113: 305S.

54. Dail CW, Affeldt JE, Collier CR. Clinical aspects of glossopharyngeal breathing. J Am Med Assoc 1953; 158: 445–9.

35

Ventilatory assistance at home

DOMINIQUE ROBERT, MICHELE VITACCA

INTRODUCTION

As a consequence of modern, efficient, intensive care medicine, a number of patients with chronic respiratory insufficiency are dependent, for either their health status or their survival, on the long-term use of mechanical ventilation. After patients become clinically stable, the provision of nocturnal or, in some instances, continuous ventilation may make it possible for the patient to return to the community.

Long-term home mechanical ventilation (LTHMV) has numerous financial, social and psychological advantages. For the non-obstructive conditions, the results vary from excellent – for thoracic restriction (non-paralytic kyphoscoliosis, thoracoplasty for tuberculosis) and non-progressive neuromuscular diseases (post-polio) – to good, for other neuromuscular diseases with slow or intermediate progression (Duchenne's muscular dystrophy, dystrophia myotonica, various myopathies), to poor for rapidly progressive neurological conditions (amyotrophic lateral sclerosis, ALS). For patients with chronic obstructive pulmonary disease (COPD), as there has been only equivocal evidence of survival or benefits to health status associated with ventilating stable patients, LTHMV tends to be reserved for the management of acute respiratory failure associated with reversible circumstances such as an acute exacerbation.

A structured organization is needed to carry out LTHMV successfully. This includes a hospital team and a home team, cooperating closely. The hospital team is responsible for identifying the appropriate patients, organizing all aspects of ventilation (choice of equipment, ventilator settings, patient and family education etc.) and providing both medical regular follow-up as well as emergency medical support. The home team is responsible for providing home equipment and specialized nursing staff, who will attend at home, evaluating and reinforcing correct health care habits, and delivering community-based physician coverage.

Background

Long-term mechanical ventilation (LTMV) has existed for over 50 years, with polio survivors, predominantly children, of the mid-twentieth century representing the first generation of ventilator-assisted individuals (1, 2). LTMV was subsequently used as the major mode of treatment for patients (children and adults) with chronic ventilatory failure consequent upon neuromuscular conditions, who received ventilatory support via a tracheostomy (2–4). The advantages of living at home while receiving LTMV became apparent early in its use (5–7). More recently, the widespread application of non-invasive ventilation (NIV) has influenced the habits of physicians and patients towards increasing acceptance of LTMV without a tracheostomy (3, 4, 8–15).

The necessity for reducing the use of health care and social resources has been a motivating factor in the development of LTHMV as a less expensive approach compared with hospital-based patient care. The transfer of LTMV from the hospital to the home setting reduces staff costs, unless the level of the patient's disability necessitates permanent nurse attendance at home (16–18). The lowest costs associated with LTHMV are in relation to independent patients with minimal impairments, such as idiopathic kyphoscoliosis, and the highest costs are for patients with conditions such as ALS or high-level spinal cord lesions (19, 20).

In the 1980s, acute and chronic care hospitals remained the major sites for LTMV, with 20–25 per cent of patients requiring LTMV in the US being managed at home (21). Subsequently, recognizing that all the people concerned (patients, families, health care providers) regard the home as the first choice, where feasible, a great deal of effort has been expended to transform LTMV from a hospital-centred to a home-centred treatment. In consequence, increasing numbers of patients are being discharged from the hospital to the home (22, 23).

This chapter presents the indications, outcomes, technical considerations, home transfer and follow-up associated with LTHMV.

INDICATIONS FOR THE USE OF VENTILATORY ASSISTANCE AT HOME

Diseases which may potentially be treated with LTMV

The main conditions for which LTMV may be indicated are summarized in Box 35.1. All may be severe enough to cause alveolar hypoventilation, sufficient to result in morbidity or mortality. In selecting suitable patients for LTMV, it is important to be aware of:

- the relative contribution of the chest wall, neuromuscular and pulmonary mechanics to ventilatory failure, knowing that the latter remains a controversial indication

---

Box 35.1 Main diseases which can benefit from long-term mechanical ventilation (LTMV) classified according to clinical categories, pulmonary functional test profile and progressiveness[a]

Restrictive parietal disorders ($\Downarrow$ VC, $\Downarrow$ FEV$_1$, $\rightarrow$ FEV$_1$/VC, $\Downarrow$ RV, $\Downarrow$ TLC)

- Chest wall
  - slow worsening ($>$15 years): kyphoscoliosis
  - intermediate worsening (5–15 years): sequelae of tuberculosis
- Neuromuscular
  - no worsening ($>$30 years): polio
  - slow worsening ($>$15 years): spinal muscular atrophy, acid maltase deficit
  - intermediate worsening (5–15 years): Duchenne's muscular dystrophy, myotonic myopathy
  - rapid worsening (0–5 years): amyotrophic lateral sclerosis

Obstructive lung diseases ($\rightarrow$ or $\downarrow$ VC, $\Downarrow$ FEV$_1$, $\Downarrow$ FEV$_1$/VC, $\Uparrow$ RV, $\Uparrow$ TLC)

- COPD
- Bronchiectasis
- Cystic fibrosis

FEV$_1$, forced expiratory volume in 1 s; RV, respiratory volume; TLC, total lung capacity; VC, vital capacity.
[a]Symbols indicate actual compared with theoretical values.

- the natural history of the underlying condition, in order to anticipate future needs such as extending from nocturnal to diurnal ventilatory assistance
- the associated co-morbidities and level of impairment that might determine the success of maintaining the individual at home.

Signs and symptoms used to judge indications for LTMV

The presence of clinical and physiological markers of hypoventilation defines the severity of ventilatory failure in relation to consideration of LTMV. Clinical symptoms and signs of hypoventilation (Box 35.2) should be evaluated. Hypoventilation is defined by an increase in arterial carbon dioxide tension (P_aCO_2) with an associated reduction of arterial oxygen tension (P_aO_2). If the disease is slowly progressive, hypoventilation may first occur during rapid eye movement (REM) sleep, subsequently extending to non-REM sleep and eventually progressing to include daytime wakefulness (24–26). The combined clinical evaluation and measured carbon dioxide tension enable hypoventilation to be categorized as 'severe' (clinical symptoms and daytime awake hypoventilation), 'moderate' (limited to non-REM and REM sleep) or 'mild' (restricted to REM sleep).

Chronic daytime hypoventilation is an important indicator of a low respiratory reserve and should be considered as an unstable state, with a risk of life-threatening acute failure being triggered by minimal additional factors. Sleep-related hypoventilation is invariably present in patients with daytime hypoventilation, although the extent to which the P_aCO_2 will increase during sleep is difficult to predict. Measurements of S_pO_2 (saturation of oxygen measured by pulse oximetry) and $P_{Tc}CO_2$ (or capnography) during sleep, together with measures of rib cage and abdominal excursion (as part of full respiratory polysomnography) will facilitate the assessment of the mechanism of hypoventilation, i.e. central, obstructive or

---

Box 35.2 Clinical features of hypoventilation

- Shortness of breath during activities of daily living in the absence of paralysis
- Orthopnoea in disorders of diaphragmatic dysfunction
- Sleep disturbances – insomnia, nightmares, frequent arousals
- Nocturnal or early morning headaches
- Daytime fatigue and sleepiness, loss of energy
- Decrease in intellectual performance
- Loss of appetite
- Loss of weight
- Appearance of recurrent complications – respiratory infections, respiratory failure
- Cor pulmonale – ankle oedema, hepatomegaly with jugular reflux, electrocardiograph

---

mixed. Such measurements also allow for the assessment of the effects of sleep on respiration and gas exchange. As polysomnography is expensive and not always available, screening measures of S_pO_2 and transcutaneous PCO_2 are very helpful. In the absence of consensus statements addressing the duration and degree of hypoventilation, it seems reasonable to assume that hypoventilation present throughout sleep (non-REM + REM) will be more likely to be associated with clinical consequences than hypoventilation restricted to REM sleep.

Pulmonary function tests help confirm and quantify the underlying diagnosis, but correlate only weakly with PCO_2 such that they have very limited predictive value. Nevertheless, in neuromuscular disorders, an inspiratory vital capacity of less than 40 per cent of predicted, a peak inspiratory pressure of less than $-20\,cmH_2O$ and a daytime P_aCO_2 above 40 mmHg are good predictors of reduced oxygen saturation during sleep (26, 27).

Indications for LTMV and LTHMV

The patient's informed consent for LTMV is essential. Considerations to discuss include the level of impairment and handicap at the point of considering LTMV; the predicted rate of disease progression; and the current and future requirements for care-givers. In clinical practice, LTMV is initiated either electively or in the subsequent to acute ventilatory failure (28). In the latter circumstance the indications for LTMV should be ascertained after the acute episode has resolved, when the patient is clinically stable. Useful clinical indicators include the levels of hypoventilation and their aetiologies. For example, patients with neuromuscular conditions with an awake $P_aCO_2 >45$ mmHg and a $P_aO_2 <65$ mmHg, as well as those with hypoventilation at night plus daytime symptoms, are also usually considered to be good candidates. For patients with thoracic deformities, more profound daytime hypoventilation ($P_aCO_2 >55$ mmHg, $P_aO_2 <60$ mmHg) plus clinical symptoms are often noted when LTMV is commenced. As there is little evidence to support LTMV in COPD (29, 30), it might be restricted to patients in whom long-term oxygen therapy has already been optimized, who experience frequent episodes of acute respiratory failure or a stable $P_aCO_2 >70$ mmHg. In patients with rapidly progressive conditions, it is important to balance the need for earlier LTMV with the requirement of maximizing independence and mobility.

Although a non-invasive approach to ventilation is clearly preferred, tracheostomy remains an option for those requiring longer periods of ventilation (31–36). Patients with Duchenne's muscular dystrophy who have been using non-invasive ventilation for 16–20 h/day demonstrate weight gain and psychological improvements when converted to ventilation via a tracheostomy, probably because they are released from the obligation to repeatedly access the mouthpiece (37). The decision to convert to tracheostomy is dependent on the philosophy and experience of the clinical team as well as the views of the patient and the family environment. Such discussions should be started well before it becomes imperative to make a decision. The only compelling indication for tracheostomy is

to protect the airway in those with dysfunctional swallowing and aspiration (e.g. in ALS).

There is limited information regarding the use of non-invasive ventilation in patients who do not have chronic ventilatory failure. One study reported the absence of benefit in patients with muscular dystrophy (38).

OUTCOMES WITH LTMV

In this section we present the effects of assisted ventilation during ventilatory assistance, on daytime unassisted function, on subsequent days in hospital, on health status and on LTHMV, which is closely related to survival.

Effects of LTMV during ventilatory assistance

During ventilatory assistance, overnight recordings of S_pO_2 and $P_{Tc}CO_2$ have confirmed improvements in gas exchange, although episodic transient hypoventilation, related to leaks, may persist (39, 40). Respiratory muscles are rested during mechanical ventilation, an observation confirmed during wakefulness and presumed to occur during sleep (41). The effects on the quality and distribution of sleep have been inconsistent (42).

Effects on daytime (unassisted) function

For patients receiving nocturnal ventilation, daytime blood gases show improvements in both P_aO_2 and P_aCO_2 of 11–15 mmHg (42) in thoracic and neuromuscular conditions, with a smaller improvement (5 mmHg) in patients with COPD. Neither maximal inspiratory pressure nor vital capacity (VC) changed as a result of nocturnal NIV (42).

For patients with restrictive conditions, improvement in respiratory muscle function, resetting of chemoreceptors and a decrease in ventilatory load have all been suggested as contributing mechanisms to the clinical and physiological improvement. Ventilatory assistance may improve respiratory muscle dysfunction ('fatigue'). The observed change in ventilatory pattern characterized by lower frequencies and higher tidal volumes would enable the muscles to develop more force per breath (43). In response to chronic hypercapnia, the respiratory centres perpetuate hypoventilation by changing the set point rather than trying to generate a non-sustainable ventilatory muscle effort. Improvement in the P_aCO_2 during ventilation may reset the respiratory centres' 'central wisdom' (12, 44–46). Improved respiratory mechanics increases the efficiency of the respiratory muscles. One study reported transient improvements in dynamic compliance after mechanical hyperinflation among patients with kyphoscoliosis (47). The inconsistent modest improvement in vital capacity does not favour a major role for improved respiratory mechanics.

The minimum mandatory duration of ventilatory assistance is unknown, but clinical observations suggest that nocturnal ventilation during sleep is sufficient to improve daytime function (43).

Effects of LTMV on hospitalization

Comparison between the year before and the first and second years subsequent to initiating nocturnal ventilation revealed a significant reduction in the number of days of hospitalization (34 days vs. 6 and 5 days in years 1 and 2, respectively) for patients with scoliosis. This was also observed in patients who were post-tuberculosis (31 days vs. 10 and 9 days for years 1 and 2, respectively) and for those with Duchenne's muscular dystrophy (18 days vs. 7 and 2 days for years 1 and 2, respectively). In contrast, the number of hospital days for COPD patients decreased significantly only during the first year of ventilation (49 days vs. 17 and 25 days), and for patients with bronchiectasis there were no statistically significant changes in hospital days following ventilation (13).

Effect on health status

The quality of life among patients with severe chronic alveolar hypoventilation improves in all dimensions following the introduction of LTMV, although it remains below that of the general population. Quality of life with LTMV is better in patients with restrictive than in those with obstructive conditions. In thoracic restrictive conditions, the improvements in health status continue for long periods, but are influenced by the underlying disease progression in those with neuromuscular conditions (48–55).

Adherence and survival according to different aetiologies

There are similarities between the older reports in which ventilation was via tracheostomy and the more recent studies of non-invasive ventilation (2, 4, 13, 14). Survival is excellent in stable neuromuscular conditions (post-polio), good in thoracic cage disorder (kyphoscoliosis and sequelae of tuberculosis), relatively good for progressive neuromuscular conditions (Duchenne), poor in COPD and very poor in rapidly progressive neuromuscular conditions (ALS). Adherence with non-invasive ventilation varies with the underlying diagnosis, being best in post-tuberculosis, post-poliomyelitis and kyphoscoliosis and worst in COPD (4, 13).

PRACTICAL CONSIDERATIONS

Optimal achievement of LTHMV requires several steps in the hospital and at home (56). A team approach should be encouraged. The team usually comprises:

- physicians with experience in LTHMV – responsible for providing information about the disease, the degree of impairment, the burden as well as the benefit and the prescription (57, 58)
- nurses directly involved in LTHMV – responsible for the education of patients and care-givers in practical techniques such as application of the nasal mask, tracheal suctioning, tracheostomy care, skin care, general hygiene and emergency procedures (59)
- respiratory and physical therapists – for mobility devices, specific manoeuvres, such as assisted cough and postural drainage, and a home exercise programme; advice and information on social services, financial and human resources is also given
- organizations responsible for providing and maintaining the ventilatory equipment
- trained and confident attendants who assist the patients with self-care and activities of daily living.

Technical considerations

CHOICE OF VENTILATOR

The choice of ventilator depends on the disease process and the extent of ventilator dependency. Patients with neuromuscular diseases who are highly ventilator-dependent and tracheostomized will require the ventilator to function continuously with battery back-up, to deliver consistent volumes, as well as having an efficient alarm. Other conditions may be treated with either volume- or pressure-preset ventilator with minimal alarms. The trend is towards pressure-preset systems which are more comfortable (60, 61). The majority of 'home care' ventilators offer performances similar to those of the more expensive 'ICU' ventilators (62, 63). It should be noted that different ventilator models do have individual characteristics which should be checked regularly (64–66). Patient compliance may also be influenced by the selected ventilator (60). We compared the patient–ventilator interaction and the patient's comfort using five different commercial bilevel pressure home ventilators, all set on the basis of the maximal tolerated inspiratory positive airway pressure (67). These ventilators were used with 28 patients with chronic ventilatory failure (obstructive or restrictive). Despite intersubject variability in comfort, all these ventilators were well tolerated and produced similar physiological effects, fulfilling the aims of mechanical ventilation (28). It is important when prescribing a ventilator for LTHMV to test it specifically with the patient, in a setting in which various models can be tried.

There are several options for the circuits and valves: either without an expiratory valve (leaking circuit available with bilevel pressure ventilation) or with an expiratory valve (either close to the patient in a one-branch circuit or inside the ventilator as a two-branch circuit, to allow easy monitoring of expiratory volume). In tracheostomized patients, a circuit with an expiratory valve is preferable. A leaking circuit is responsible for a rebreathing effect which varies with the ventilator settings (68–70). Types of circuit are summarized in Table 35.1.

CHOICE OF MASK OR TRACHEOSTOMY CANNULA

For non-invasive ventilation, different masks should be tried, to minimize leaks and obtain the best comfort. One study reported the most comfort with nasal masks, but the best

Table 35.1 *Main characteristics of circuits and their application*

Expiratory valve	Mode	Branch	Monitoring of expiratory volume	Tracheostomy	NIV
Yes	Volume or pressure	One or two	+/−, yes	Yes	Yes
No	Pressure (bilevel)	One with leak	No	No	Yes

NIV, non-invasive ventilation.

minute ventilation and P_aCO_2 with a facial mask (71). A customized mask is an ideal solution (72–74). For patients with a tracheostomy, the fit of the cannula to the tracheal morphology is important. It is difficult to avoid a cuffed cannula in patients who cannot protect their airways. Speech remains an important goal, as does adequate humidification. An experienced team is necessary to tackle the above issues (35, 75–78).

DETERMINATION OF THE VENTILATOR SETTINGS

Figure 35.1 shows an example of settings recommended by those experienced in this area. There is an element of trial and error before the optimal settings are established. Both patient comfort and the physiological effects (during wakefulness and sleep) should be monitored. Improvements during ventilation may be measured directly with arterial blood gases, or indirectly using non-invasive measures. Full polysomnography enables the effects of ventilation on sleep quality and the patient–ventilator interaction to be measured. Overnight S_pO_2 and transcutaneous PCO_2, as well as arterial blood gases, are the basic requirements to confirm adequate ventilation. This stage of determining optimal settings for LTHMV requires a few days in hospital.

For tracheostomized patients, usually in volume-preset mode, it is relatively easy to establish adequate settings since there are usually only minimal air leaks (cuffed cannula) or the leaks are predictable and measurable (uncuffed cannula) (79).

During non-invasive ventilation, leaks are unavoidable and may change from breath to breath (39, 40, 80). In patients with COPD, nasal pressure support ventilation is set to achieve a decrease in P_aCO_2 and optimal comfort ('usual setting'). This does not provide information regarding respiratory muscle unloading or work of breathing related to the intrinsic positive end-expiratory pressure ($PEEP_i$). The best reduction in respiratory load occurs with the 'physiological setting' in which the application of extrinsic PEEP ($PEEP_e$) is required to unload the diaphragm (titrating to 80–90 per cent of intrinsic dynamic PEEP). An incorrect setting (e.g. in the case of over-assistance) may result in further hyperinflation (81). The 'usual setting' and the 'physiological setting' might have different implications in clinical practice. In a recent study among patients with stable COPD and chronic hypercapnia, non-invasive pressure support ventilation set by patient comfort or by physiological measurement provided similar improvements in arterial blood gases. However, the physiological setting with inspiratory assistance and $PEEP_e$ resulted in a reduction of ineffective inspiratory efforts related to patient–ventilator dyssynchrony (67).

Home set-up and discharge process

IDENTIFICATION OF CARE-GIVERS

Sufficient provision and training of care-givers are mandatory. Requirements for each patient will depend on disease severity, psychological profile, family availability, home location, mobility goals and financial circumstances. This process may actually be the rate-limiting step that prevents or enhances LTHMV.

EDUCATIONAL PROGRAMME

The education of patients and all other individuals involved with their care is a major component of the discharge process that greatly influences the effectiveness of care at home (58, 82–87). The education process should begin as soon as possible during the patient's hospital stay. The most appropriate method is bedside teaching, in small groups, for 30- to 60-min sessions (88). Education should include the description of the disease and its natural history, the principles of assisted ventilation and the goals of LTMV. Training should include routine and emergency care of all respiratory equipment (i.e. suctioning, tracheostomy care, emergency change of tracheostomy cannulae, etc.) as well as the administration of medications and any other care, as needed. Each learned task should be reinforced, repeated and periodically reviewed. Before transition home, all individuals involved should be well prepared, confident in their abilities, and able to demonstrate the necessary competencies for the specific patient. A short trial of 'home care' is often recommended before discharge. During this trial the home care team takes charge of the patient, but can receive help and advice from the hospital team.

HOME SET-UP

Prior to discharge it is important to verify that the home environment includes adequate space for the patient, the family and any additional care-givers, as well as having some storage facilities (85, 89–92). The home should be free of fire, health and safety hazards, provide adequate heating, cooling and ventilation, and have adequate electrical service (28). In addition, it is mandatory for the care-givers to have easy access (preferably via a 'hotline') to a designated medical team, for advice and readmission if necessary. Staff accessibility is often best through a telephone call centre, available 24 hours a day.

EQUIPMENT DELIVERY

The ventilator is selected on an individual basis according to the required modes and settings. For patients needing only

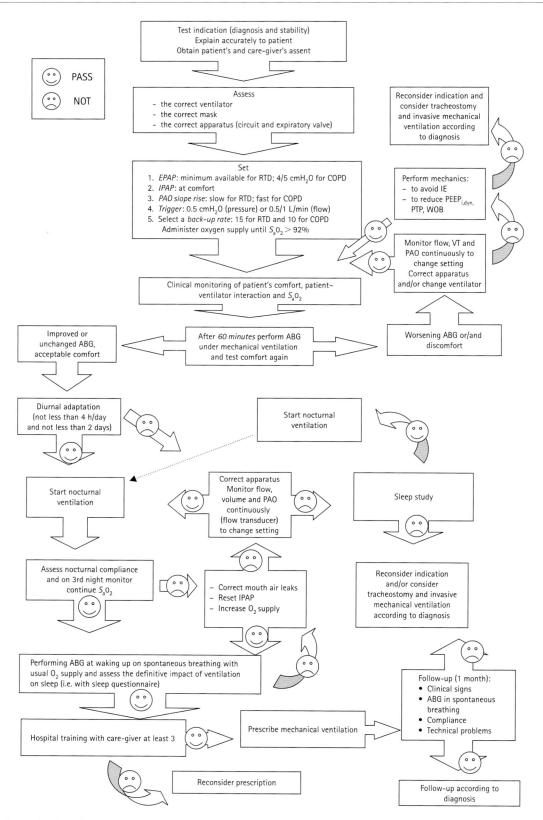

Figure 35.1 *Determination of ventilator settings. Abbreviations – ABG, arterial blood gases; EPAP, expiratory positive airway pressure; IE, ineffective efforts; IPAP, inspiratory positive airway pressure; PAO, airway pressure; PEEP$_{i,dyn}$, dynamic intrinsic positive end-expiratory pressure; PTP, pressure–time product; RTD, respiratory thoracic disease; S$_a$O$_2$, arterial saturation of oxygen; VT, tidal volume; WOB, work of breathing.*

nocturnal ventilation, simple alarms are sufficient. For tracheostomized patients who are entirely dependent on mechanical ventilation, a high level of security is required, including internal and external batteries, monitoring and alarms for pressure and volume, as well as back-up equipment, including a hand bag, ventilator and suction device.

HOME DISCHARGE

Home discharge requires appropriate medical support for urgent requirements as well as for scheduled follow-up. A trial home period often precedes the 'definitive' return home. The care-givers should receive a written care plan which clearly identifies the roles and responsibilities of the various team members with regard to daily care, describes the correct use (maintenance and troubleshooting) of all equipment, identifies the circumstances in which re-evaluation may be required, specifies the local hospital emergency department and the medical centre for re-evaluation and outlines emergency and contingency plans (21, 57, 85, 88, 89, 91, 93–97).

Follow-up

Follow-up requirements vary with the diagnosis, level of impairment and disability, model of care, available resources and local practice. LTHMV requires medical, nursing and technical resources (23, 98–101). Medical care is best given in collaboration between a family physician and a respiratory specialist. The goals include ensuring clinical stability, managing co-morbidities and addressing acute deteriorations. Specific questionnaires may be used to assess health-related quality of life (23). Regular monitoring of daytime and overnight gas exchange (arterial blood gases and overnight non-invasive monitoring of S_aO_2, P_{CO_2}) at 6-monthly or annual intervals is recommended. Changes that cannot be quickly addressed at home should trigger a prompt in-patient assessment. Nurses (or respiratory therapists) experienced in LTHMV are extremely valuable for regular home monitoring. In addition to a clinical and psychosocial assessment of the ventilator user, with a special emphasis on the ventilator–patient interface (masks, skin care, tracheostomy cannula, suctioning, humidification, etc.), their expertise provides important support for the many issues that challenge the care-givers. Technical support includes the regular maintenance checks of all devices, in keeping with the manufacturer's specifications. Advances in communication now enable improved home monitoring, especially for those who reside in more remote areas, linking professional support and data exchange through modalities such as telemedicine.

CONCLUSIONS

Long-term home mechanical ventilation is a very rewarding challenge for the clinically stable patient, the health care team and the care-givers, requiring good motivation and planning by all concerned. The main objectives are to enable ventilator users to remain clinically stable outside the hospital environment and to improve their health-related quality of life in a cost-effective way. The care requirements vary with the underlying diagnosis, the level of impairment and the natural history of the condition. The approach may also vary depending on whether mechanical ventilation was introduced electively or subsequent to an emergency situation. Patient selection, assessment and planning for LTHMV require close collaboration between the hospital and home care providers. Regular monitoring and follow-up, both in the home and periodically in the hospital (especially for the more impaired and disabled patients), is essential to the success of LTHMV. The experience that most ventilator users and their families prefer home care, in addition to the requirement to reduce health care costs, will probably drive increasing efforts to return individuals who require long-term ventilatory support to a community-based environment.

> ## Key points
>
> - Long-term use of mechanical ventilation (LTMV) is increasing.
> - When good stabilization is obtained, patients with LTMV could regularly stay at home.
> - The main goals of LTMV are to improve nocturnal hypoventilation and patient's quality of life, and reduce morbidity and mortality.
> - Results depends on the disorder concerned and its level of progression.
> - In COPD, no clear benefits in terms of survival have been obtained; LTMV may reduce exacerbations and hospital admissions.
> - A well structured organization is needed to carry out LTMV successfully.
> - The hospital team is responsible for indication, choice of ventilator, mode, setting and medical follow-up on a regular basis or in an emergency.
> - Specialized nurses visiting the home setting are involved in checking the correct practice and reinforcing training of the family doctor.
> - Health care professionals need to increase efforts to transform prolonged mechanical ventilation from a hospital-centred to a home-centred treatment.

REFERENCES

1. Engström CG. Treatment of devere cases of respiratory paralysis by the Engström universal respirator. Br Med J 1954: 666–9.
2. Robert D, Gerard M, Leger P et al. Permanent mechanical ventilation at home via a tracheotomy in chronic respiratory insufficiency. Rev Fr Mal Respir 1983; 11: 923–36.
3. Bach JR, Alba A, Mosher R, Delaubier A. Intermittent positive pressure ventilation via nasal access in the management of respiratory insufficiency. Chest 1987; 92: 168–70.
4. Simonds AK, Elliott MW. Outcome of domiciliary nasal intermittent positive pressure ventilation in restrictive and obstructive disorders. Thorax 1995; 50: 604–9.

5. Bertoye A, Garin JP, Vincent P et al. Le retour à domicile des insuffisants respiratoires chroniques appareillés. Lyon Med 1965; 38: 389–410.

6. Bolot JF, Robert D, Chemorin B et al. Assisted ventilation at home by tracheotomy in subjects with chronic respiratory insufficiency. Minerva Med 1977; 68: 409–14.

7. Alexander MA, Johnson EW, Petty J, Stauch D. Mechanical ventilation of patients with late stage Duchenne muscular dystrophy: management in the home. Arch Phys Med Rehabil 1979; 60: 289–92.

8. Ellis ER, McCauley B, Mellis C, Sullivan CE. Treatment of alveolar hypoventilation in a six-year-old girl with intermittent positive pressure ventilation through a nose mask. Am Rev Respir Dis 1987; 136: 188–91.

9. Carroll N, Branthwaite M. Control of nocturnal hypoventilation by nasal intermittent positive ventilation. Thorax 1988; 43: 349–53.

10. Leger P, Jennequin J, Gerard M, Robert D. Home positive-pressure ventilation via nasal mask for patients with neuromuscular weakness or restrictive lung or chest-wall disease. Respir Care 1989; 34: 73–7.

11. Bach J, Alba AS. Management of chronic alveolar hypoventilation by nasal ventilation. Chest 1990; 97: 52–7.

12. Elliott MW, Mulvey DA, Moxham J et al. Domiciliary nocturnal nasal intermittent positive pressure ventilation in COPD, mechanisms underlying changes in arterial blood gas tensions. Eur Respir J 1991; 4: 1044–52.

13. Leger P, Bedicam JM, Cornette A et al. Nasal intermittent positive pressure ventilation. Long-term follow-up in patients with severe chronic respiratory insufficiency. Chest 1994; 105: 100–5.

14. Simonds AK, Ward S, Heather S et al. Outcome of paediatric domiciliary mask ventilation in neuromuscular and skeletal disease. Eur Respir J 2000; 16: 476–81.

15. Annane D, Chevrolet JC, Chevret S, Raphael JC. Nocturnal mechanical ventilation for chronic hypoventilation in patients with neuromuscular and chest wall disorders. Cochrane Database Syst Rev 2000; 2: CD001941.

16. Fields AI, Rosenblatt A, Pollack MM, Kaufman J. Home care cost-effectiveness for respiratory technology-dependent children [see comments]. Am J Dis Child 1991; 145: 729–33.

17. Sivack ED, Cordasco EM, Gipson WT. Pulmonary mechanichal ventilation at home: a reasonable and less expensive alternative. Respir Care 1983; 28: 42–9.

18. Sevick MA, Kamlet MS, Hoffman LA, Rawson I. Economic cost of home-based care for ventilator-assisted individuals: a preliminary report. Chest 1996; 109: 1597–606.

19. Oppenheimer EA. Decision-making in the respiratory care of amyotrophic lateral sclerosis: should home mechanical ventilation be used? Palliat Med 1993; 7: 49–64.

20. Hayashi H, Oppenheimer EA. ALS patients on TPPV: totally locked-in state, neurologic findings and ethical implications. Neurology 2003; 61: 135–7.

21. Make BJ, Gilmartin ME. Rehabilitation and home care for ventilator-assisted individuals. Clin Chest Med 1986; 7: 679–91.

22. Muir JF, Voisin C, Ludot A. Organization of home respiratory care: the experience in France with ANTADIR. Monaldi Arch Chest Dis 1993; 48: 462–7.

23. Gasperini M, Clini E, Zaccaria S. Mechanical ventilation in chronic respiratory insufficiency: report on an Italian nationwide survey. The Italian Telethon Committee and the AIPO Study Group on Pulmonary Rehabilitation and Intensive Care. Monaldi Arch Chest Dis 1998; 53: 394–9.

24. Becker HF, Piper AJ, Flynn WE et al. Breathing during sleep in patients with nocturnal desaturation. Am J Respir Crit Care Med 1999; 159: 112–18.

25. Phillips MF, Smith PE, Carroll N et al. Nocturnal oxygenation and prognosis in Duchenne muscular dystrophy. Am J Respir Crit Care Med 1999; 160: 198–202.

26. Mellies U, Ragette R, Schwake C et al. Daytime predictors of sleep disordered breathing in children and adolescents with neuromuscular disorders. Neuromuscul Disord 2003; 13: 123–8.

27. Hukins CA, Hillman DR. Daytime predictors of sleep hypoventilation in Duchenne muscular dystrophy. Am J Respir Crit Care Med 2000; 161: 166–70.

28. Clinical indications for noninvasive positive pressure ventilation in chronic respiratory failure due to restrictive lung disease, COPD, and nocturnal hypoventilation – a consensus conference report. Chest 1999; 116: 521–34.

29. Casanova C, Celli BR, Tost L et al. Long-term controlled trial of nocturnal nasal positive pressure ventilation in patients with severe COPD. Chest 2000; 118: 1582–90.

30. Clini E, Sturani C, Rossi A et al. The Italian multicentre study on noninvasive ventilation in chronic obstructive pulmonary disease patients. Eur Respir J 2002; 20: 529–38.

31. Raphael JC. [Home mechanical ventilation in Duchenne de Boulogne muscular dystrophy. Mandatory ventilation and preventive ventilation]. Rev Mal Respir 1987; 4: 195–7.

32. Robert D, Willig TN, Paulus J, Leger P. Long-term nasal ventilation in neuromuscular disorders: report of a consensus conference. Eur Respir J 1993; 6: 599–606.

33. Curran FJ, Colbert AP. Ventilator management in Duchenne muscular dystrophy and postpoliomyelitis syndrome: twelve years' experience. Arch Phys Med Rehabil 1989; 70: 180–5.

34. Bach J. Noninvasive options for ventilatory support of the traumatic high level quadriplegic patient. Chest 1990; 98: 613–19.

35. Bach JR, Alba AS. Tracheostomy ventilation. A study of efficacy with deflated cuffs and cuffless tubes. Chest 1990; 97: 679–83.

36. Bach JR, Alba AS, Saporito LR. Intermittent positive pressure ventilation via the mouth as an alternative to tracheostomy for 257 ventilators users. Chest 1993; 103: 174–82.

37. Bach JR. Update and perspective on noninvasive respiratory muscle aids; Part 1: the inspiratory aids. Chest 1994; 105: 1230–40.

38. Raphael JC, Chevret S, Chastang C, Bouvet F. Randomised trial of preventive nasal ventilation in Duchenne muscular dystrophy. French Multicentre Cooperative Group on Home Mechanical Ventilation Assistance in Duchenne de Boulogne Muscular Dystrophy [see comments]. Lancet 1994; 343: 1600–4.

39. Bach JR, Robert D, Leger P, Langevin B. Sleep fragmentation in kyphoscoliotic individuals with alveolar hypoventilation treated by NIPPV. Chest 1995; 107: 1552–8.

40. Meyer TJ, Pressman MR, Benditt J et al. Air leaking through the mouth during nocturnal nasal ventilation: effect on sleep quality. Sleep 1997; 20: 561–9.

41. Carrey Z, Gottfried SB, Levy RD. Ventilatory muscle support in respiratory failure with nasal positive pressure ventilation. Chest 1990; 97: 150–8.

42. Robert D, Leger P. Noninvasive Ventilation for Sleep Breathing Disorders, 3rd edn. Philadelphia: WB Saunders; 2000.

43. Schonhofer B, Geibel M, Sonneborn M et al. Daytime mechanical ventilation in chronic respiratory insufficiency. Eur Respir J 1997; 10: 2840–6.

44. Fernandez E, Weinert P, Meltzer E et al. Sustained improvement in gas exchange after negative pressure ventilation for 8 hours per day on 2 successive days in chronic airflow limitation. Am Rev Respir Dis 1991; 144: 390–4.

45. Annane D, Quera-Salva MA, Lofaso F et al. Mechanisms underlying effects of nocturnal ventilation on daytime blood gases in neuromuscular diseases. Eur Respir J 1999; 13: 157–62.

46. Dellborg C, Olofson J, Hamnegard CH et al. Ventilatory response to CO_2 re-breathing before and after nocturnal nasal intermittent positive pressure ventilation in patients with chronic alveolar hypoventilation. Respir Med 2000; 94: 1154–60.

47. Sinha R, Bergowski EH. Prolonged alteration of lung mechanics in kyphoscoliosis by positive pressure hyperinflation. Am Rev Respir Dis 1972; 106: 47–57.

48. Pehrsson K, Olofson J, Larsson S, Sullivan M. Quality of life of patients treated by home mechanical ventilation due to restrictive ventilatory disorders. Respir Med 1994; 88: 21–6.

49. Janssens JP, Penalosa B, Degive C et al. Quality of life of patients under home mechanical ventilation for restrictive lung diseases: a comparative evaluation with COPD patients. Monaldi Arch Chest Dis 1996; 51: 178–84.

50. Perrin C, El Far Y, Vandenbos F et al. Domiciliary nasal intermittent positive pressure ventilation in severe COPD effects on lung function and quality of life. Eur Respir J 1997; 10: 2835–9.

51. Lyall RA, Donaldson N, Fleming T et al. A prospective study of quality of life in ALS patients treated with noninvasive ventilation. Neurology 2001; 57: 153–6.

52. Dellborg C, Olofson J, Midgren B et al. Quality of life in patients with chronic alveolar hypoventilation. Eur Respir J 2002; 19: 113–20.

53. Nauffal D, Domenech R, Martinez Garcia MA et al. Noninvasive positive pressure home ventilation in restrictive disorders outcome and impact on health-related quality of life. Respir Med 2002; 96: 777–83.

54. Windisch W, Freidel K, Schucher B et al. Evaluation of health-related quality of life using the MOS 36-Item Short-Form Health Status Survey in patients receiving noninvasive positive pressure ventilation. Intensive Care Med 2003; 29: 615–21.

55. Bourke SC, Bullock RE, Williams TL et al. Noninvasive ventilation in ALS: indications and effect on quality of life. Neurology 2003; 61: 171–7.

56. Leger P, Laier-Groeneveld G. Infrastructure, funding and follow-up in a programme of noninvasive ventilation. Eur Respir J 2002; 20: 1573–8.

57. Smith CE, Mayer LS, Parkhurst C et al. Adaptation in families with a member requiring mechanical ventilation at home. Heart Lung 1991; 20: 349–56.

58. Smith CE, Mayer LS, Perkins SB et al. Caregiver learning needs and reactions to managing home mechanical ventilation. Heart Lung 1994; 23: 157–63.

59. Donner CF, Lusuardi M. Advances in pulmonary rehabilitation and management of chronic respiratory failure. Monaldi Arch Chest Dis 1998; 53: 257–8.

60. Meecham Jones DJ, Wedzichia JA. Comparison of pressure and volume preset nasal ventilator systems in stable chronic respiratory failure. Eur Respir J 1993; 6: 1060–4.

61. Schonhofer B, Sonneborn M, Haidl P et al. Comparison of two different modes for noninvasive mechanical ventilation in chronic respiratory failure: volume-versus pressure-controlled device. Eur Respir J 1997; 10: 184–91.

62. Lofaso F, Brochard L, Hang T et al. Home versus intensive care pressure support devices. Experimental and clinical comparison. Am J Respir Crit Care Med 1996; 153: 1591–9.

63. Bunburaphong T, Imanaka H, Nishimura M et al. Performance characteristics of bilevel pressure ventilators: a lung model study. Chest 1997; 111: 1050–60.

64. Smith IE, Shneerson JM. A laboratory comparison of four positive pressure ventilators used in the home. Eur Respir J 1996; 9: 2410–15.

65. Mehta S, McCool FD, Hill NS. Leak compensation in positive pressure ventilators: a lung model study. Eur Respir J 2001; 17: 259–67.

66. Highcock MP, Shneerson JM, Smith IE. Functional differences in bi-level pressure preset ventilators. Eur Respir J 2001; 17: 268–73.

67. Vitacca M, Nava S, Confalonieri M et al. The appropriate setting of noninvasive pressure support ventilation in stable COPD patients. Chest 2000; 118: 1286–93.

68. Ferguson GT, Gilmartin M. CO_2 rebreathing during BiPAP ventilatory assistance. Am J Respir Crit Care Med 1995; 151: 1126–35.

69. Lofaso F, Brochard L, Touchard D et al. Evaluation of carbon dioxyde rebreathing during pressure support ventilation with airway management system (BiPAP) devices. Chest 1995; 108: 772–8.

70. Hill NS. Saving face: better interfaces for noninvasive ventilation. Intensive Care Med 2002; 28: 227–9.

71. Navalesi P, Fanfulla F, Frigerio P et al. Physiologic evaluation of noninvasive mechanical ventilation delivered with three types of masks in patients with chronic hypercapnic respiratory failure. Crit Care Med 2000; 28: 1785–90.

72. Cornette A, Mougel D. Ventilatory assistance via the nasal route: masks and fitting. Eur Respir Rev 1993; 3: 250–3.

73. Leger SS, Leger P. The art of interface. Tools for administering noninvasive ventilation. Med Klin 1999; 94: 35–9.

74. Tsuboi T, Ohi M, Kita H et al. The efficacy of a custom-fabricated nasal mask on gas exchange during nasal intermittent positive pressure ventilation. Eur Respir J 1999; 13: 152–6.

75. Sherman JM, Davis S, Albamonte-Petrick S et al. Care of the child with a chronic tracheostomy. This official statement of the American Thoracic Society was adopted by the ATS Board of Directors, July 1999. Am J Respir Crit Care Med 2000; 161: 297–308.

76. Estournet-Mathiaud B. Tracheostomy in chronic lung disease: care and follow-up. Pediatr Pulmonol Supplement 2001; 23: 135–6.

77. Heffner JE, Hess D. Tracheostomy management in the chronically ventilated patient. Clin Chest Med 2001; 22: 55–69.

78. Mirza S, Cameron DS. The tracheostomy tube change: a review of techniques. Hosp Med 2001; 62: 158–63.

79. Prigent H, Samuel C, Louis B et al. Comparative effects of two ventilatory modes on speech in tracheostomized patients with neuromuscular disease. Am J Respir Crit Care Med 2003; 167: 114–19.

80. Schettino GP, Tucci MR, Sousa R et al. Mask mechanics and leak dynamics during noninvasive pressure support ventilation: a bench study. Intensive Care Med 2001; 27: 1887–91.

81. Appendini L, Patessio A, Zanaboni S et al. Physiologic effects of positive end expiratory pressure and mask pressure support during exacerbation of chronic obstructive pulmonary disease. Am J Respir Crit Care Med 1994; 149: 1069–76.

82. Fischer DA. Long-term management of the ventilator-dependent patient: levels of disability and resocialization. Eur Respir J Suppl 1989; 7: 651s–4s.

83. Moss AH, Casey P, Stocking CB et al. Home ventilation for amyotrophic lateral sclerosis patients: outcomes, costs, and patient, family, and physician attitudes. Neurology 1993; 43: 438–43.

84. Sevick MA, Sereika S, Matthews JT et al. Home-based ventilator-dependent patients: measurement of the emotional aspects of home caregiving. Heart Lung 1994; 23: 269–78.

85. Findeis A, Larson JL, Gallo A, Shekleton M. Caring for individuals using home ventilators: an appraisal by family caregivers. Rehabil Nurs 1994; 19: 6–11.

86. Stuart M, Weinrich M. Protecting the most vulnerable: home mechanical ventilation as a case study in disability and medical care: report from an NIH conference. Neurorehabil Neural Repair 2001; 15: 159–66.

87. Rossi Ferrario S, Zotti AM, Zaccaria S et al. Caregiver strain associated with tracheostomy in chronic respiratory failure. Chest 2001; 119: 1498–502.

88. Thompson CL, Richmond M. Teaching home care for ventilator-dependent patients: the patients' perception. *Heart Lung* 1990; **19**: 79–83.

89. Make B, Gilmartin M, Brody JS, Snider GL. Rehabilitation of ventilator-dependent subjects with lung diseases. The concept and initial experience. *Chest* 1984; **86**: 358–65.

90. Goldberg AI, Noah Z, Fleming M *et al.* Quality of care for life-supported children who require prolonged mechanical ventilation at home. *QRB Qual Rev Bull* 1987; **13**: 81–8.

91. Miller MD, Steele NF, Nadell JM *et al.* Ventilator-assisted youth: appraisal and nursing care. *J Neurosci Nurs* 1993; **25**: 287–95.

92. Rozell BR, Newman KL. Extending a critical path for patients who are ventilator dependent: nursing case management in the home setting. *Home Healthc Nurse* 1994; **12**: 21–5.

93. Goldberg AI, Monahan CA. Home health care for children assisted by mechanical ventilation: the physician's perspective. *J Pediatr* 1989; **114**: 378–83.

94. Haynes N, Raine SF, Rushing P. Discharging ICU ventilator-dependent patients to home healthcare. *Crit Care Nurse* 1990; **10**: 39–47.

95. Dettenmeier PA. Planning for successful home mechanical ventilation. *AACN Clin Issues Crit Care Nurs* 1990; **1**: 267–79.

96. Clini E, Vitacca M. From intermediate intensive unit to home care. *Monaldi Arch Chest Dis* 1994; **49**: 533–6.

97. Spence A. Home ventilation: how to plan for discharge. *Nurs Stand* 1995; **9**: 38–40.

98. Hazlett DE. A study of pediatric home ventilator management: medical, psychosocial, and financial aspects. *J Pediatr Nurs* 1989; **4**: 284–94.

99. Fields AI, Coble DH, Pollack MM, Kaufman J. Outcome of home care for technology-dependent children: success of an independent, community-based case management model. *Pediatr Pulmonol* 1991; **11**: 310–17.

100. Nelson VS, Carroll JC, Hurvitz EA, Dean JM. Home mechanical ventilation of children. *Dev Med Child Neurol* 1996; **38**: 704–15.

101. Norregaard O. Noninvasive ventilation in children. *Eur Respir J* 2002; **20**: 1332–42.

36

The challenge of self-management

JEAN BOURBEAU, JUDITH SOICHER

INTRODUCTION

Chronic obstructive pulmonary disease (COPD) is a chronic illness for which no cure exists. However, health and illness can coexist. The meaning of health is in large part the patient's ability to manage and cope with the illness. In the trajectory of a chronic illness, the patient and family are in a constant process of learning new skilled behaviours that are needed for appropriate disease management.

Many interventions are known to be beneficial for the COPD patient (1, 2), including pulmonary rehabilitation. However, these interventions are too often used with the philosophy of an acute care approach, where the physician makes the diagnosis, provides treatment and reacts to medical complications. A chronic care approach is by far more appropriate to COPD, as it is for all chronic diseases. The patient and family must learn to engage in self-management activities that promote health and prevent complications, ensuring the patient's engagement in daily management decisions. As the disease progresses to different stages and complications, education based on self-management principles in the continuum of care will help the patient and family in adapting to COPD-related changes and maintaining healthy behaviours.

In this chapter, we review the definition of and the existing evidence for self-management effectiveness in COPD. We look at the features of a successful self-management programme, more specifically at the programme components and content, and what might be needed for enhancing behaviour modification. Finally, we look at the interrelationship between self-management, self-efficacy, and exercise behaviour modification.

DEFINITION OF SELF-MANAGEMENT

Self-management applies to any formalized patient education programme aimed at teaching skills needed to carry out a specific medical regimen and to achieve health behaviour modification. It refers to the various tasks that patients carry out for management of their condition.

More specifically, self-management refers to (3):

- engaging in activities that promote health, build physiological reserves and prevent adverse sequelae
- interacting with health care providers and adhering to recommended treatment protocols
- monitoring both physical and emotional status and making appropriate management decisions based on self-monitoring
- managing the effects of illness on the patient's self-esteem, self-efficacy and ability to function in important roles.

Patients' abilities to care for themselves are enhanced by services that provide education, guidance for health behaviour change, emotional support and the skills needed to carry out medical regimens specific to COPD. A continuum of self-management training can range from self-help to more intensive case-management approaches. Case management is a system of managing patients with complex disease that promotes continuity, communication and collaboration among the patient, the family, the physician and various health professionals within the health care system and the community. A case manager will coordinate the services required by the patient at different stages along the continuum of care.

SELF-MANAGEMENT EFFECTIVENESS

A recent Cochrane review (4) has systematically evaluated eight clinical trials of self-management education compared with usual care for patients with COPD. For most of the results presented, meta-analytical comparisons could not be made because both the outcomes and follow-up periods varied considerably between studies. Self-management education did reduce the need for rescue medication; however, this was measured in only one study (5). Self-management education led to an increase in use of oral corticosteroids and/or antibiotics as demonstrated in two studies (6, 7). These results could be due to patients' increased awareness of worsening symptoms, although no information is provided on the appropriateness of the medication use. On the other hand, the review (4) showed no effect of self-management on health service use, including hospitalization, and only a trend towards better quality of life when disease-specific questionnaires were used (5, 7).

Another review article with a comprehensive and critical evaluation of self-management in COPD has recently been published (8). This review included one additional randomized clinical trial (9) that was not published at the time of the Cochrane review. Table 36.1 shows an overview of the study results with respect to health status and health service outcomes. Of the 11 studies presented in Table 36.1, four (6, 9–11) showed an improvement in health status, and only one of the six studies that assessed hospitalization showed a reduction in hospital admission (9). Favourable findings are primarily driven by the results of a recent multicentre randomized clinical trial by Bourbeau et al. (9); this is the first study to show a reduction in hospital admissions and emergency room visits in COPD patients receiving self-management education compared with those receiving only usual care (Table 36.2). Table 36.2 shows a marked reduction (40–60 per cent) in emergency visits and hospitalizations. Furthermore, unscheduled visits to the physician were also reduced by 60 per cent in the self-management as compared to the usual care group. In this study, there is reason to believe that self-care was implemented by many patients. Patients in the self-management group made a total of 143 calls to the case manager due to changes in respiratory symptoms. The same group of patients, however, reported 299 exacerbations over the same time period. This difference suggests that patients in the self-management group were managing many exacerbations on their own, without the need for communication with the case manager.

The study by Bourbeau et al. (9), which included COPD patients with advanced disease, is the only study showing an impact of a disease-specific self-management programme on both health care resource utilization and health status. Figures 36.1 and 36.2 show that health-related quality of life improved after 4 and 12 months of a self-management programme, while it did not change in patients on usual care. There was a statistically significant treatment difference with respect to the St George's Respiratory Questionnaire (SGRQ) 'impact' subscale and total scores.

This difference reached the minimal clinically important difference of -4. By 12 months, however, the treatment difference was significant with a P-value of 0.05 only for the 'impact' score.

There may be several reasons why many studies have not been able to demonstrate that self-management is effective in COPD patients. Health-related quality of life has often been assessed using generic questionnaires (6, 10–12), which are known to be less sensitive to change than disease-specific questionnaires. Furthermore, some studies used non-validated questionnaires (13–15). Most of the studies on self-management in COPD have been done with a small sample size, making it more difficult to detect a statistically significant difference. However, two large studies (9, 16) that have recently been published produced different results and conclusions. Although they share similarities in their intervention and outcome measures, the differences are worth mentioning as they might help guide clinicians' practice. In the COPE study by Monninklhof et al. (16), patients were randomized to a self-management and a control group after taking part in a pharmacological trial. Additionally both control and intervention groups had standard pharmacological treatment and could report to the study staff in the case of exacerbation. This add-on therapy and additional care to the patients in the comparison group may have reduced the chance of showing a treatment effect. Furthermore, patients selected in the two studies were quite different. In the study by Monninklhof et al. (16), at baseline patients had less severe airflow obstruction ($FEV_1 = 57$ per cent of predicted) and a relatively good health status (SGRQ total score of 37–38/100) as compared with those in the study by Bourbeau et al. (9) ($FEV_1 = 40$ per cent of predicted; SGRQ total score of 54–56/100). Consequently, the response to improve health could have been limited. There is also the possibility that the SGRQ is less accurate than expected when it is used at the extremes of it scaling range.

Furthermore, in order to be eligible for the study by Bourbeau et al. (9), patients also had to be hospitalized for acute exacerbation at least once in the preceding year. Benefits of a self-management programme to the health care system were more likely to be observed and could potentially add to the patients' quality of life by avoiding hospitalization. In the study by Monninklhof et al. (16), the twofold increase of exacerbation rate in the self-management group is somehow difficult to explain. It is not known if the decreased proportion of exacerbations requiring hospital admission in the intervention group was driven by less severe exacerbations or if the intervention was able to prevent hospitalizations.

Until recently, the evidence of self-management effectiveness was based on experience with other chronic diseases, such as diabetes (17), congestive heart failure (18) and asthma (19). Important conclusions can still be drawn while we are awaiting further research in the emerging field of self-management in COPD. Self-management programmes should primarily target COPD patients with impaired health and exacerbations. There is now evidence that a multi-component self-management education programme

Table 36.1   *Overview of chronic obstructive pulmonary disease study results comparing self-management to usual care. Adapted from Bourbeau (8)*

Author	Health–related quality of life	Use of health resources	Other outcomes
Howland et al. (11)	SIP =, Multidimensional health locus of control scale =, except for health locus of control V*	Not reported	Not reported
Cockcroft et al. (13)	General health questionnaire =	Hospital admissions =, duration of hospitalization due to respiratory conditions V, duration of hospitalization due to non-respiratory conditions =	Knowledge on their condition/drugs required to treat their condition V
Blake et al. (10)	SIP total and physical scores V*, life-changes =, self-esteem =	Hospitalisation admissions =, physician visits =	Not reported
Littlejohns et al. (6)	SIP physical score V*, HAD =	Hospital admissions =, physician visits at home =	Nebulizer, ipratropium and antibiotics V, patient satisfaction with the programme V
Sassi-Dambron et al. (14)	Quality of well being =, STAI =, depression =	Not reported	Transitional dyspnoea index (TDI) V*, 6-min walking test and Borg scale =
Watson et al. (7)	SGRQ =	Not reported	Self-administration of antibiotics and prednisone for exacerbation V
Emery et al. (12)	SIP =, multidimensional health locus of control =, STAI =, depression =	Not reported	Knowledge of disease V but associated with greater distress
Gourley et al. (15), Solomon et al. (48)	Health state questionnaire =	Hospital admissions =, use of other health providers X*	Knowledge on medication V, patient satisfaction with the programme V
Gallefoss et al. (49), Gallefoss and Bakke (50)	Lung-specific quality-of-life questions =, SGRQ =	Duration of hospitalization =, physician visits (acute) X*	Need for rescue drug X, patient satisfaction V
Bourbeau et al. (9)	SGRQ impact and total score V	Hospital admissions X*, emergency room visits X*, physician visits (acute) X*	Lung function and 6-min walking test =, acute exacerbation X
Monninkhof et al. (16)	SGRQ =, X days with limitation post-exacerbation	Hospital admission =	Lung function and 6-min walking test =

* $P < 0.05$.
HAD, hospital anxiety and depression scale; SGRQ, St George's Respiratory Questionnaire; SIP, sickness impact profile; STAI, state-trait anxiety inventory.
V, indicates an improvement in the self-management group compared with the usual-care group; X indicates a decrease or deterioration in the self-management group compared with the usual-care group; = indicates no change in the self-management group compared with the usual-care group.

Table 36.2   *Health service use following a self-management programme in chronic obstructive pulmonary disease. Data from Bourbeau et al. (9)*

Variable	Usual care group (n = 95)	Self-management group (n = 96)	Treatment difference (%)	P-value
Hospital admissions				
For acute exacerbations	118	71	−39.8	0.01
For other health problems	49	21	−57.1	0.01
Emergency visits for acute exacerbations				
Emergency department	161	95	−41.0	0.02
Physician	112	46	−58.9	0.003

with the supervision and support of a case manager is effective (9) and should be an integral part of the care of patients with COPD. The benefits, especially those on health care utilization, are important and warrant serious consideration by both health care administrators and providers. In addition to diminishing the burden on the health care system, reduced hospitalization could also potentially enhance patients' quality of life.

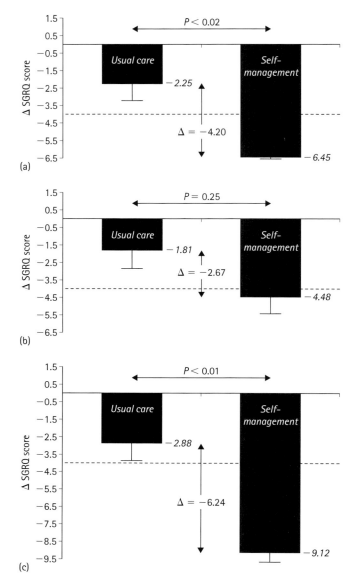

Figure 36.1 *Health-related quality of life (St George's Respiratory Questionnaire) changes and treatment difference at 4 months in patients receiving self-management education compared with those on usual care. (a) Total score; (b) subscale activity score; (c) subscale impact score.*

FEATURES OF A SUCCESSFUL SELF-MANAGEMENT PROGRAMME

In the study by Bourbeau *et al.* (9), the features that distinguish the strategies of care from current standard practice include the following:

- philosophy of care based on principles of patient empowerment and self-management specific to the disease
- continuity of care ensured by ongoing communication with a health professional
- patient education and follow-up carried out by a health professional with proper skills, using standardized

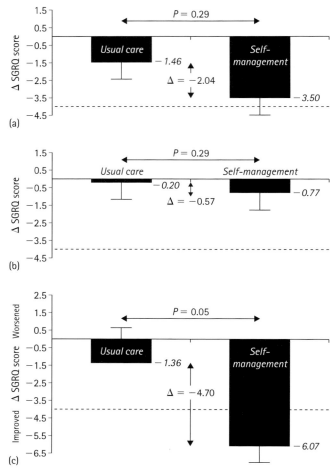

Figure 36.2 *Health-related quality of life (St George's Respiratory Questionnaire) changes and treatment difference at 12 months in patients receiving self-management education compared with those on usual care. (a) Total score; (b) subscale activity score; (c) subscale impact score.*

teaching and follow-up tools, to ensure consistency in clinical care and expertise.

Programme components and content

The teaching material *Living Well with COPD* consisted of a multi-component education programme with a flipchart designed for health educators, seven skill-oriented self-help patient workbook modules detailing COPD management of all facets of the disease, inhalation technique sheets, and a plan of action. All patient materials were written in clear, simple language with friendly, upbeat graphics. The programme promotes the physical and psychosocial health and quality of life of patients, and optimizes medical treatment. The components and contents of the *Living Well with COPD* programme are presented in Box 36.1.

The flipchart is used by the health professional for patient teaching. This learning tool can be adapted to the needs of each individual patient: it can be used in sequence, section-by-section or with a focus on selected topics. The self-help

Box 36.1   Components and content of a self-management programme, *Living Well with COPD*[a]

Flipchart

Provides simple images that help patients to gain a better understanding of their chronic obstructive pulmonary disease (COPD), learn more about strategies to stay well, and better manage their disease and exacerbations. Includes facilitator notes.

Patient workbooks

Seven comprehensive modules detailing management of all facets of disease.

Breathing, energy conservation and relaxation

- Anatomy and physiology of COPD
- Breathing techniques
- Positions to reduce shortness of breath
- Coughing techniques
- Energy conservation during day-to-day activities
- Anxiety–breathlessness cycle and how to break it

Preventing and controlling your symptoms

- COPD and symptoms
- Avoiding environmental factors that make your symptoms worse
- Medication and inhalation devices
- Relaxation exercise: progressive muscular relaxation

Your symptoms and plan of action

- Your plan of action
- Recognizing your symptoms in different situations
- Relaxation exercise: practising progressive muscular relaxation and deep breathing

Adopting a healthy lifestyle

- Health
- Compliance with therapy
- Nutrition
- Exercise
- Sleep
- Sexuality
- Managing emotions and stress
- Relaxation exercise: relaxation and positive thinking

Taking time to breathe in the good things in life

- Leisure activities
- Travelling
- Thinking positively
- Relaxation exercise: visualization

Home exercise programme

- The value of exercise
- The when, where, and how of exercise
- Too much and too little exercise

- The movement of your body
- Your exercise programme
- Exercising the muscles of your mind

Long-term oxygen therapy

- Learning to live with long-term home oxygen therapy
- Oxygen and oxygen equipment
- How to take care of your oxygen equipment

Inhalation technique sheets

Reference sheets for patients so that they can see and learn how to use inhalation devices

Plan of action

- Includes what the patients should be doing if their condition is stable: medication, exercise, diet
- Includes a medical prescription that helps patients to treat their COPD when symptoms become worse
- Also helps patients to recognize when their condition is not improving and when to call for help

[a]This material was developed by the team of D Bourbeau in collaboration with Boehringer Ingelheim Canada and the Respiratory Network of the Fonds de la Recherche en Santé du Québec (FRSQ).

patient workbooks include seven comprehensive modules detailing management of all facets of disease. They are presented in more detail in Box 36.1. The action plan for acute exacerbation is an important part of the programme. The action plan should not be seen only as a prescription to be self-administered when a patient has an exacerbation, but more like a life plan. It is customized for each patient and includes a contact list as well as a symptom-monitoring list for different situations (stress, environmental change and respiratory infection). Each item on the list is linked to the appropriate therapeutic action, such as filling a prescription from the treating physician in the event of an exacerbation. The action plan emphasizes healthy habits, such as regular exercise at home, breathing techniques and relaxation, increased used of a rescue bronchodilator, and the prompt initiation of an antibiotic and an oral corticosteroid for 10–14 days for exacerbation with infective symptoms. Infective symptoms are defined as at least two symptom changes (dyspnoea, sputum or sputum purulence) from the patient's baseline condition (20). The action plan also includes safeguards such as calling the case manager or treating physician if symptoms become worse despite the use of the antibiotics and corticosteroids.

A programme that addresses both the physical and psychosocial aspects of COPD will probably have the greatest impact on patients' health. However, some components of a programme may be more important than others in their effect on specific outcomes. It is unlikely that one component alone will suit the complex needs of patients with advanced disease. Furthermore, we know that patients' needs vary not only with respect to the stage of disease, but also from one individual to another. In order to achieve optimal outcomes, careful attention is needed to identify the specific clinical features of COPD in individual patients and their specific needs.

Many interventions, when implemented by the patient, are known to be effective on specific outcomes. Smoking cessation as an individual component is the only intervention that can prevent or slow down the progression of lung disease (21). Exercise training is another key component known to be effective in reducing dyspnoea and improving exercise capacity and health-related quality of life (2). Pulmonary rehabilitation should have an important place in the management of COPD patients. An action plan that emphasizes the prompt initiation of an antibiotic and/or prednisone for exacerbation has also been advocated. Patients can learn to recognize the onset of exacerbation of COPD and initiate early treatment at home (8). As part of a multi-faceted programme, an action plan has been shown to be effective with regard to patient health (9) and to reduce hospitalizations. A recent retrospective cohort study (22) has shown that in outpatient practice the use of an action plan was associated with a reduction in hospitalization. In this study, the action plan included a customized prescription of antibiotic and/or prednisone for 7–10 days for exacerbation with infective symptoms – types I and II of Anthonisen *et al.* (20). Physicians' involvement in self-management needs to be emphasized, as they are a key partner in the health care team. They will be essential to follow-up patient care, and in developing an effective exacerbation protocol with prescription.

There may be other programme components that are effective, although this has yet to be shown. Recently, the results of a qualitative study (26) provided preliminary information on how specific components of a self-management programme are perceived by patients as important to explain improvements in their well-being. When asked about which were the most useful strategies, patients answered as follows: 81 per cent responded 'to adopt energy conservation principles'; 69 per cent 'to use their action plan'; 62 per cent 'to use pursed lip breathing'; 58 per cent 'to implement regular home exercise'. These data of a qualitative study are very useful and help to provide descriptive findings that allow us to share the experience of COPD patients.

Enhancing behaviour modifications

Self-management requires the knowledge and skills to evaluate and implement one's own individual plan for health behaviour changes. Improving knowledge is necessary, but insufficient on its own (23). Education programmes often concentrate more on disease content, while they should also focus on how

to integrate the demands of the disease into daily activities. Patients may memorize information well, but are not necessarily able to put the information to use. Furthermore, skill training has to be incorporated in order to address specific skill deficits in activities of daily living. Studies in COPD have shown that disease-specific self-management programmes can increase knowledge (12, 15, 24, 25) and specific skills, e.g. the appropriate use of respiratory medication and breathing techniques such as pursed lip breathing (26). Successful self-management, however, requires a multi-faceted approach that incorporates not only disease information but also strategies to adopt and maintain healthy behaviour. Other studies in chronic disease, such as the meta-analysis by Mazzuca (23), have demonstrated that behaviour-oriented programmes were the most successful. The most effective interventions included regular contact with the same health professional, rewards for progress, implementation of a memory aid system and self-care rituals.

The real challenge of any self-management education programme is for patients to acquire new behaviour skills and to integrate these skills into their everyday life. The ability of a self-management programme to improve health status and optimize health service utilization will only be realized if we can achieve behaviour modification. Behaviour modification in turn is caused by enhancement of self-efficacy, knowledge and skill. This rather complex causal chain is illustrated in Fig. 36.3.

Self-efficacy, or the patient's confidence in his ability to perform a specific task, is an essential, if not the most important, component in the complex causal chain of behaviour modification. People build their confidence on success. Patients may have the intention to adopt a healthy behaviour, but they may doubt their ability to carry out the specific task (efficacy-based futility) or may believe that they cannot influence the outcome regardless of their ability (outcome-based futility) (27). In self-management programmes, interventions designed to enhance the patient's efficacy beliefs and confidence in outcomes should be considered as important as strategies to increase knowledge and skills. Self-efficacy plays an important role in determining whether a patient will perform or avoid a particular activity or behaviour.

As clinicians, we must ask ourselves how self-efficacy can be effectively increased through our practice. First, behavioural skills need to be practised by patients during the programme. Second, patients need to have feedback on their behavioural performance. Each visit or telephone call will become an opportunity for you to reassure them and reinforce appropriate behaviour. Third, negative experiences need to be addressed. Patients need to reattribute the perceived

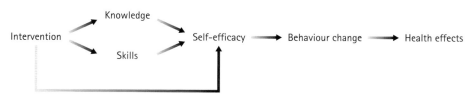

Figure 36.3 *Causal chain of behaviour modification. Reproduced with permission from Bourbeau et al. (51).*

causes of this failure. Fourth, role models are also important. Patients with positive experiences can provide a strong modelling effect in a group setting. Sharing experiences can be useful, as this will enhance self-efficacy expectations and may also discourage passivity.

Bandura and Adams (28) advised that self-efficacy should be tailored to the particular function of interest. We will use the example of the action plan for COPD exacerbation. The action plan will usually include a symptom-monitoring list for specific situations (stress, environmental change and respiratory infection) linked to appropriate actions. In the specific situation of an infection, the action plan includes a customized prescription for self-administration of an antibiotic and/or prednisone. First, patients must have a general sense of personal efficacy as well as a belief in a positive outcome. A belief in the outcome (or outcome expectation) will help patients to stay motivated and to make the effort needed to overcome perceived barriers. Task-specific efficacy (or confidence) is often low at first, but increases as patients persist, master new skills and achieve behaviour modification. As part of a self-management programme, the presence of a case manager as a contact person will help to ensure close follow-up and appropriate actions. You have to coach patients. When they call you about using their prescription as part of their action plan, you shouldn't tell them what to do but instead help them to think through their problem and come to a decision. You should reassure patients and reinforce appropriate action. If they have not used their action plan, or have used it inappropriately, you need to help them see the cause of the failure. If they were not adequately prepared, then you have to work with them so they know what to do next time. With time, patients will develop and strengthen their sense of self-efficacy, through past and present success in mastering specific tasks and achieving behaviour change.

Because COPD patients are often elderly, it is believed that they may have difficulty in understanding the issues presented in an education programme. However, even if some patients have difficulties with comprehension, this deficit does not appear to reduce their perceived ability or personal efficacy beliefs. Ferrini et al. (29) demonstrated that elderly people with positive beliefs similar to young people were more likely to report positive changes in health behaviour. In a review of behaviour change in the elderly, self-efficacy was recognized as a consistent predictor of adherence to physical activity, medication and diet (30).

Self-efficacy play is a crucial factor in determining which activities a patient will perform or avoid. It is a strong predictor of health-related behaviour change (27) and should be considered as a key feature when planning a self-management education programme. To be effective, a self-management education programme has to promote the skills needed to carry out a specific medical regimen and to achieve behaviour change associated with a favourable health outcome. Through education based on self-management principles, we can provide guidance for patients to improve their ability to carry out daily activities and to adopt healthy behaviours such as physical activity. Patients who accept challenges and are able to persist

will not need as much support from the health professional as those who are not able to accept the necessity of change.

SELF-MANAGEMENT AND EXERCISE BEHAVIOUR MODIFICATION

Pulmonary rehabilitation, in which the physical training programme is often the primary focus, is one of the most effective treatments currently available to improve dyspnoea, exercise capacity limited by breathlessness and health-related quality of life in patients with COPD (1, 2). While the short-term benefits are well established, the challenge remains in understanding and promoting long-term exercise behaviour after the formal rehabilitation programme has ended.

There has been limited research in COPD regarding the interrelationship between self-management, self-efficacy and specific behaviour modification. Atkins et al. (31) have shown that cognitive and behavioural strategies as part of self-management are useful for motivating and maintaining participation in a regular walking programme among moderate to severe COPD patients. In other studies, the degree of self-efficacy has also been a significant factor in predicting the use of the treadmill, walking performance (32) and success in pulmonary rehabilitation (33). However, in these studies, assessment of physical activity behaviour was mostly during the adoption phase, i.e. from initiation to 6 months, and rarely during the maintenance phase, i.e. beyond 6 months. The maintenance phase includes the behaviour of exercise adherence, defined as an individual's free choice process of continuing an exercise programme initiated either alone or in collaboration with health care practitioners (34, 35). In the context of pulmonary rehabilitation, adherence is a measure of participation in exercise after completion of the formal programme.

Exercise behaviour research in chronic disease populations is beginning to emerge in the literature (36–39). In a cross-sectional survey of patients with mobility disorders from a variety of conditions (40), people with higher exercise self-efficacy and lower motivational barriers achieved better exercise maintenance at 6 months. In this study, demographic characteristics and disability-related and environmental barriers did not differentiate between patients who continued to exercise or not. To gain a better understanding of the factors contributing to exercise behaviour in chronic disease, it is also necessary to look at studies in the 65+ age group, as almost 90 per cent of these individuals have at least one chronic condition (41). In this group, exercise self-efficacy has been found to be the most consistent predictor of adherence to physical activity.

In longitudinal studies of the elderly with follow-up at or over 12 months (42, 43), exercise self-efficacy or changes in self-efficacy were predictors of exercise adherence. Outcome expectancies, defined as the estimate of expected benefits from regular exercise, were also associated with adherence (43). Confusion and depression were predictors of poor adherence to a home-based strength training programme in elderly people (44), but the role of affective factors is still unclear (30) and warrants further study.

In a review article of 27 cross-sectional and 14 longitudinal studies of individuals aged 65 years or more (45), it was shown that education level and past exercise behaviour correlate positively with the performance of regular exercise. Conversely, physical factors of perceived frailty and poor health were the greatest barriers to exercise adoption and maintenance. The finding of physical factors as a barrier to exercise behaviour change and maintenance is in agreement with a qualitative study conducted in COPD patients by Nault et al. (46). This qualitative study demonstrated that barriers to lifestyle changes frequently reported by patients were progression of COPD and associated co-morbid conditions.

In a recent study comparing enhanced follow-up with conventional follow-up, Brooks et al. (47) documented adherence to home exercises in COPD patients following completion of a pulmonary rehabilitation programme. Adherence was high shortly after completion of the rehabilitation programme, but dropped off in both groups (enhanced and conventional follow-up) over the next 6 months. The most consistently reported reasons for non-adherence were chest infection and disease exacerbation. Although not the primary focus of the study, the description of adherence to home exercise and reasons for non-adherence provide important insight into the pattern and predictors of physical activity behaviour modification following rehabilitation.

Adherence to exercise programmes is a crucial health behaviour in the management of a disease such as COPD and other chronic diseases. Self-management has potential use in interventions such as exercise training or a rehabilitation programme, where long-term adherence is dependent on self-efficacy and other behavioural variables as demonstrated in studies of elderly and chronic disease populations.

IMPLICATION FOR RESEARCH

Despite the progress made in recent years in the area of self-management, we are left with many unanswered questions. Studies are needed to examine which programme components are most effective in promoting lasting behavioural change, and which behaviours, apart from exercise training as part of a rehabilitation programme, contribute to improved health status. Finally, we need to know more about the determinants of lasting behaviour change, in order to plan intervention studies, and implement clinically effective and cost-effective strategies for the long-term therapeutic management of these patients.

Key points

- There is growing evidence of the effectiveness of self-management in improving patient well-being and reducing emergency room visits and hospitalizations; this is especially true for patients with reduced health status and exacerbation requiring health service use.

- For self-management to be successful it has to be implemented in the continuity of care, ensured by ongoing communication with a well trained health professional using standardized disease-specific teaching tools.
- A self-management programme with a multi-faceted approach is advocated, which implies not only teaching disease-specific information, but also designing and implementing therapeutic interventions that enhance self-efficacy and promote behaviour modification.
- Pulmonary rehabilitation should be part of the continuum of self-management, as self-management might be a powerful tool to help maintain long-term lifestyle skills and behaviour modification.

REFERENCES

◆1. Lacasse Y, Wong E, Guyatt GH et al. Meta-analysis of respiratory rehabilitation in chronic obstructive pulmonary disease. *Lancet* 1996; 348: 1115–19.

◆2. Lacasse Y, Brosseau L, Milne S et al. Pulmonary rehabilitation for chronic obstructive pulmonary disease. *Cochrane Library* 2003; 3: CD003793.

●3. Von Korff M, Gruman J, Schaefer J et al. Collaborative management of chronic illness. *Ann Intern Med* 1997; 127: 1097–102.

◆4. Monninkhof E, Van der Valk P, van Herwaarden C et al. Self-management education for patient with chronic obstructive pulmonary disease: a systematic review. *Thorax* 2003; 58: 394–8.

●5. Gallefoss F, Bakke PS. How does patient education and self-management among asthmatics and patients with chronic obstructive pulmonary disease affect medication? *Am J Respir Crit Care Med* 1999; 160: 2000–5.

●6. Littlejohns P, Baveystock CM, Parnell H, Jones PW. Randomised controlled trial of the effectiveness of a respiratory health worker in reducing impairment, disability, and handicap due to chronic airflow limitation. *Thorax* 1991; 46: 559–64.

●7. Watson PB, Town GI, Holbrook N et al. Evaluation of a self-management plan for chronic obstructive pulmonary disease. *Eur Respir J* 1997; 10: 1267–71.

◆8. Bourbeau J. Disease-specific self-management programs in patients with advanced chronic obstructive pulmonary disease. A comprehensive and critical evaluation. *Dis Manage Health* 2003; 11: 311–19.

●9. Bourbeau J, Julien M, Maltais F et al. Reduction of hospital utilization in patients with chronic obstructive pulmonary disease: a disease specific self-management intervention. *Arch Intern Med* 2003; 163: 585–91.

●10. Blake RL, Vandiver TA, Braun SR et al. A randomized controlled evaluation of a psychosocial intervention in adults with chronic lung disease. *Fam Med* 1990; 22: 365–70.

●11. Howland J, Nelson EC, Barlow PB et al. Chronic obstructive airway disease. Impact of health education. *Chest* 1986; 90: 233–8.

●12. Emery CF, Schein RL, Hauck ER, MacIntyre NR. Psychological and cognitive outcomes of a randomized trial of exercise among patients with chronic obstructive pulmonary disease. *Health Psychol* 1998; 17: 232–40.

13. Cockroft A, Bagnall P, Heslop A et al. Controlled trial of respiratory health worker visiting patients with chronic respiratory disability. Br Med J 1987; 294: 225–8.

14. Sassi-Dambron DE, Eakin EG, Ries AL, Kaplan RM. Treatment of dyspnea in COPD. A controlled clinical trial of dyspnea management strategies. Chest 1995; 107: 724–9.

15. Gourley GA, Portner TS, Gourley DR et al. Part 3. Humanistic outcomes in the hypertension and COPD arms of a multicenter outcomes study. J Am Pharm Assoc 1998; 38: 586–97.

16. Monninkhof E, Van der Valk P, Van der Palen J et al. Effects of a comprehensive self-management programme in patients with chronic obstructive pulmonary disease. Eur Res J 2003; 22: 815–20.

17. Hiss RG, Anderson RM, Hess GE, Stepien CJ, Davis WK. Community diabetes care. A 10 year perspective. Diabetes Care 1994; 17: 1124–34.

18. Rich MW, Beckhman V, Wittenberg C et al. A multidisciplinary intervention to prevent the re-admission of elderly patients with congestive heart failure. N Engl J Med 1995; 333: 1190–5.

19. Gibson PG, Coughlan J, Wilson AJ et al. Self-management education and regular practitioner review for adults with asthma (Cochrane Review), 2000.

20. Anthonisen NR, Manfreda J, Warren CP et al. Antibiotic therapy in exacerbations of chronic obstructive pulmonary disease. Ann Intern Med 1987; 106: 196–204.

21. Fletcher CM, Peto R, Anthonisen NR et al. The Lung Health Study: effects of smoking intervention and the use of an inhaled anticholinergic bronchodilator on the rate of decline of FEV1. J Am Med Assoc 1977; 272: 1497–507.

22. Parenteau S, Bourbeau J, Siok MA. Impact of an action plan that emphasizes the prompt use of oral prednisone and antibiotics in COPD exacerbation. Am J Resp Crit Care Med 2003; 167: A230.

23. Mazzuca SA. Does patient education in chronic disease have therapeutic value? J Chron Dis 1982; 35: 521–9.

24. Cockcroft DW, Murdock KY, Kirby J, Hargreave F. Prediction of airway responsiveness to allergen from skin sensitivity to allergen and airway responsiveness to histamine. Am Rev Respir Dis 1987; 135: 264–7.

25. Dang-Tan T. Efficacy of a Pulmonary Rehabilitation Program on Knowledge and Self-Efficacy for Elderly Chronic Obstructive Pulmonary Disease Patients. McGill, 2001.

26. Nault D, Pépin J, Renault V et al. Qualitative evaluation of a self-management program 'Living Well with COPD' offered to patients and their caregivers. Am J Respir Crit Care Med 2000; 161: A56.

27. Bandura A. Self-efficacy mechanism in human agency. Am Psychologist 1982; 33: 344–58.

28. Bandura A, Adams NE. Analysis of the self-efficacy theory of behavioral changes. Cogn Ther Res 1977; 1: 287–308.

29. Ferrini R, Edelstein S, Barrett-Corron E. The association between health beliefs and health behavior change in older adults. Prev Med 1994; 23: 1–5.

30. Culos-Reed SN, Rejeski WJ, McAuley E et al. Predictors of adherence to behavior change interventions in the elderly. Control Clin Trials 2000; 21: 200S–205S.

31. Atkins CJ, Kaplan RM, Timms RM et al. Behavioral exercise programs in the management of chronic obstructive pulmonary disease. J Consult Clin Psychol 1984; 52: 591–603.

32. Gormley J, Carrieri-Kohlman V, Douglas M, Stulbarg M. Treadmill self-efficacy and walking performance in patients with COPD. J Cardiopulm Rehabil 1993; 13: 424–31.

33. Kaplan RM, Ries AL, Prewitt LM, Eakin E. Self-efficacy expectations predict survival for patients with chronic obstructive pulmonary disease. Health Psychol 1994; 13: 366–8.

34. Meichenbaum D, Turk DC, Treatment Adherence: Terminology, Incidence and Conceptualization. Facilitating Treatment Adherence: a Practitioner's Guidebook. New York: Plenum Press, 1987.

35. Brawley LR, Culos-Reed S. Studying adherence to therapeutic regiments: overview, theories, recommendations. Contr Clin Trials 2000; 21(5 Suppl.): 156S–63.

36. Evangelista LS, Berg J, Dracup K. Relationship between psychosocial variables and compliance in patients with heart failure. Heart and lung. J Acute Crit Care 2001; 30: 294–301.

37. Hellman EA. Use of the stages of change in exercise adherence model among older adults with a cardiac diagnosis. J Cardiopulm Rehabil 1997; 17: 145–55.

38. Barlow JH. Understanding exercise in the context of chronic disease: an exploratory investigation of self-efficacy. Perp Motor Skills 1998; 29: 977–85.

39. Rejeski W, Brawley LR, Ettinger W et al. Compliance to exercise therapy in older participants with knee osteoarthritis: implications for treating disability. Med Sci Sports Exerc 1997; 29: 977–85.

40. Kinne S, Partrick DL, Maher EJ. Correlates of exercise maintenance among people with mobility impairments. Disabil Rehabil 1999; 21: 15–22.

41. Hoffman C, Rice D, Sung HY. Persons with chronic conditions. Their prevalence and costs. J Am Med Assoc 1996; 276: 1473–9.

42. McAuley E, Lox C, Duncan TE. Long-term maintenance of exercise, self-efficacy, and physiological change in older adults. J Gerontol Psych Sci 1993; 48: 218–24.

43. Brassington GS, Atienza AA, Perczek RE et al. Intervention-related cognitive versus social mediators of exercise adherence in the elderly. Am J Prev Med 2002; 23: 80–6.

44. Jette AM, Rooks D, Lachman M et al. Home-based resistance training: predictors of participation and adherence. The Gerontologist 1998; 38: 412–21.

45. Rhodes RE, Martin AD, Tawnton JE et al. Factors associated with exercise adherence among older adults. An individual perspective. Sport Med 1999; 28: 397–411.

46. Nault D, Dagenais J, Perreault V et al. Qualitative evaluation of a disease specific self-management program 'Living well with COPD©'. Eur Respir J 2000; 16: 317S.

47. Brooks D, Krip B, Mangovski-Alzamora S, Goldstein RS. The effect of postrehabilitation programmes among individuals with chronic obstructive pulmonary disease. Eur Res J 2002; 20: 20–9.

48. Solomon DK, Portner TS, Bass GE et al. Part 2. Clinical and economic outcomes in the hypertension and COPD arms of a multicenter outcomes study. J Am Pharm Assoc 1998; 38: 574–85.

49. Gallefoss F, Bakke PS, Rsgaard PK. Quality of life assessment after patient education in a randomized controlled study on asthma and chronic obstructive pulmonary disease. Am J Respir Crit Care Med 1999; 159: 812–17.

50. Gallefoss F, Bakke PS. Impact of patient education and self-management on morbidity in asthmatics and patients with chronic obstructive pulmonary disease. Respir Med 2000; 94: 279–87.

51. Bourbeau J, Nault D, Dang-Tan T. Self-management and behaviour modification in COPD. Patient Educ Couns 2004; 52: 271–7.

37

Exacerbations in chronic lung disease and rehabilitation

BARTOLOME R. CELLI, VICTOR PINTO-PLATA

INTRODUCTION

Chronic obstructive pulmonary disease (COPD) is the fourth leading cause of death in the United States for people over the age of 45 and the fourth cause of death in the world (1, 2). Its mortality rate continues to rise as death from other causes continues to decline. The recent Global Burden of Disease Study (2) predicted that COPD will be the third leading cause of death and the fifth cause of morbidity in the world by the year 2020. The cost of COPD is staggering, reaching $31.9 billion annually in the US alone. An important portion consists of direct expenditure due to recurrent exacerbations that lead to emergency visits and hospitalizations.

Unfortunately, there is currently no general agreement on the definition of an exacerbation of COPD. The most widely accepted is that proposed by Anthonisen *et al.* (3), who defined it as an increase in dyspnoea, cough and/or sputum purulence with or without symptoms of upper respiratory infection. The severity of the exacerbation is then graded according to the number of symptoms present. Other definitions have been developed for use in the field and pharmacotherapeutic trials and are based on worsening of symptoms requiring change in usual medications, or health care utilization patterns, such as number of hospitalizations.

EXACERBATIONS: EPIDEMIOLOGY AND CAUSATIVE FACTORS

Morbidity due to COPD increases with age and is greater in men than in women, although it is increasing faster in the latter (1). Large population studies have shown that the frequency of the exacerbations seems to be related to the severity of the disease (4–5) with low incidence (0–1 episodes/year) in mild to moderate disease (FEV_1 >50 per cent) and 1.3–1.5 episodes/year in more severe disease. Some studies have also reported a subgroup of patients with more frequent episodes (3 or more episodes/year), despite similar physiological characteristics. Because most patients enrolled in pulmonary rehabilitation programmes usually have more advanced disease, they are very prone to develop exacerbations.

The most important factors in the genesis of exacerbation of COPD are thought to be viral and/or bacterial infections and airway pollutants. Early studies identified a bacterial aetiology (*Haemophilus influenzae, Streptococcus pneumoniae, Moraxella catarrhalis* and *Chlamydia pneumoniae*) in 30–50 per cent of cases during the acute episode. However, a high percentage of the patients (25 per cent) had the same bacteria recovered during stable conditions (colonization vs. true infection). Using molecular biology typing, recent evidence suggests a higher probability of exacerbation with the same generic bacteria when the serotype of the organism changes (33 vs. 15 per cent) (6). Virus such as influenza and rhinoviruses seem to be involved in up to 30 per cent of exacerbations. Environmental studies have shown a temporal association between reduction of sulphur dioxide and ozone levels in the air with reduction in emergency room visits for COPD.

PATHOPHYSIOLOGICAL CHANGES DURING AN EXACERBATION

There is limited information regarding the pathophysiological events surrounding an exacerbation, because most studies have been conducted in the outpatient setting. This limits the capacity for close observation and better characterization of the physiological events occurring during an exacerbation.

Airflow worsening during exacerbation

During an exacerbation, there seems to be a component of airway inflammation that worsens the already compromised airways of these patients. Pulmonary function tests done in the first day after enrolment in a study evaluating the effect of corticosteroids on the clinical course of exacerbations (7) documented a worsening of FEV_1. Those patients treated with corticosteroids showed an improvement of approximately 0.2 L in FEV_1 during the first 3 days compared with patients not treated with this medication, whose FEV_1 improved by approximately 0.13 L. A smaller study by Thompson *et al.* (8) showed an 18 per cent improvement in FEV_1 on day 3 in 13 patients with exacerbation treated with corticosteroids compared with control group 1.6 per cent in patients not receiving this medication. Other studies have shown less important changes in spirometry during the acute episode (Table 37.1). However, they all show some worsening in the degree of obstruction. In a cohort of 101 outpatients, Seemungal *et al.* (9) reported a change of 0.024 L in FEV_1 and 0.008 L/min in peak expiratory flow rate (PEFR) on day 1 of an exacerbation. When patients manifested symptoms of dyspnoea or increased wheeze, they also found greater changes in PEFR with a correlation of 0.12 between symptoms and lung function change. Our group has also reported modest changes in FEV_1 in patients admitted and followed daily during an episode of acute exacerbation of chronic bronchitis (AECB) (10). The FEV_1 changed by 0.05 L while in the hospital (first 4 days) and by 0.29 L, or 6 per cent (relative change), after discharge (11).

Hyperinflation during the exacerbation

Dynamic hyperinflation (DH) is defined as the failure of the lungs to reach functional residual capacity (FRC) at the end of exhalation, also described as 'air trapping'. During an exacerbation, patients develop airway inflammation, bronchoconstriction, mucous secretion that generates higher airways resistance with expiratory airflow limitation, all leading to tachypnoea. The resulting increase in respiratory rate shortens the time of expiration and is likely to result in the development of DH (Fig. 37.1). Hyperinflation places the diaphragm in a disadvantageous position, decreasing its force-generating capacity. Elmaghraby *et al.* (10) performed daily measurements of pulmonary function test in patients admitted with the diagnosis of COPD exacerbation. The tests included inspiratory capacity (IC), an indirect measurement of DH, and the maximal inspiratory pressure (respiratory muscle strength measurement). Both tests showed larger improvement during the hospitalization and after recovery compared with those observed for the FEV_1 (Table 37.2). Likewise, there was a significant decrease in respiratory rate, which allowed longer time for exhalation and

Table 37.1 *Baseline pulmonary function values and changes during acute exacerbation (AE) of chronic obstructive pulmonary disease reported by different authors*

Reference	FEV_1 (L) ± SD	Change in FEV_1 (L) during AE
Niewoehner *et al.* (7)	0.76 ± 0.28	0.1
Thompson *et al.* (8)	1.04 ± 0.36	0.05
Seemungal *et al.* (9)	1.10 ± 0.50	0.024
Elmaghraby *et al.* (10)	0.79 ± 0.32	0.05

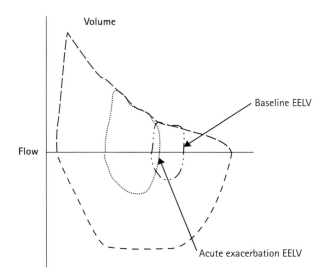

Figure 37.1 *Flow–volume envelope of a patient with severe COPD. The small dotted line shows the end-expiratory lung volume (EELV) at rest. As the respiratory rate increases and the expiratory time shortens during an acute exacerbation, there is a displacement of the tidal volume envelope to the left, signifying an increased in the EELV or air trapping. The increase in EELV has been associated with the degree of perceived dyspnoea.*

therefore improved the level of DH. All these changes, especially the reduction in respiratory rate, were associated with improvement in dyspnoea.

Alteration of gas exchange

The underlying abnormalities in gas exchange during the stable phase in patients with COPD worsen during an exacerbation. The non-uniform distribution of emphysematous lung causes areas with different ventilation/perfusion ratios. During an exacerbation, the increase in respiratory demand generates areas with more hyperinflation, particularly the more emphysematous portion of the lung which has higher compliance than that of the more normal lung. The systemic manifestations of exacerbation, including fever, increase cardiovascular demands, which in turn shorten the circulating time of blood through the pulmonary vasculature. This, coupled

Table 37.2 *Change over time in vital signs, dyspnoea visual analogue scale (VAS) and spirometric measurements in patients hospitalized with acute exacerbation of chronic obstructive pulmonary disease at the St Elizabeth's Medical Center*

Measurement	Day 1	Day 2	Day 3	Day 4	Recovery	P-value[a]
Respiratory rate (breaths/min)	28 ± 5	27 ± 4	23 ± 4	23 ± 3	20 ± 5	<0.001
Pulse (breaths/min)	98 ± 16	94 ± 13	90 ± 12	87 ± 11	82 ± 12	<0.001
VAS (cm)	7.1 ± 1.8	6.1 ± 1.9	4.8 ± 2.3	3.1 ± 1.7	2.2 ± 2.3	<0.001
FEV_1 (L)	0.79 ± 0.32	0.83 ± 0.34	0.80 ± 0.33	0.83 ± 0.33	1.08 ± 0.41	NS
FVC (L)	1.87 ± 0.64	1.89 ± 0.54	1.86 ± 0.52	1.90 ± 0.65	2.11 ± 0.61	<0.05
IC (L)	1.43 ± 0.54	1.36 ± 0.48	1.47 ± 0.47	1.66 ± 0.53	1.86 ± 0.59	<0.01
$P_{I,max}$ (cmH_2O)	43 ± 19	N.A.	53 ± 31	N.A.	63 ± 25	<0.02

FEV_1, forced expiratory volume in 1 s; FVC, forced vital capacity; IC, inspiratory capacity; $P_{I,max}$, maximum inspiratory pressure.
[a]P-value by ANOVA; NS, non-significant.

with the uneven hyperinflation, also creates changes in lung perfusion that affect the gas exchange process. According to the degree of the underlying lung disease, patients may only develop hypoxaemia, but if the abnormalities are more severe, patients may develop hypercapnia and ventilatory failure. Barbera *et al.* (12) studied 13 patients with severe disease ($FEV_1 = 0.91$ L), admitted with exacerbation and also followed them after discharge. The ventilation/perfusion ($\dot{V}/\dot{Q}$) relationship was assessed using the inert gas technique. They found an increased $\dot{V}/\dot{Q}$ inequality during exacerbation due to greater perfusion in poorly ventilated alveoli, amplified by the decrease in mixed oxygen tension that results from greater oxygen consumption. This alteration in ventilation/perfusion matching is the most important cause of the gas abnormalities during the exacerbation.

To correct these abnormalities, particularly in hypercapnic patients, invasive and non-invasive ventilation (NIPPV) have been used. NIPPV has gained popularity because it avoids the complications of endotracheal intubation, preserves airways' defence mechanisms and allows the patients to eat and speak. Compared with standard care, NIPPV decreases the need for invasive ventilation and reduces mortality, complication rates and hospital stay (13).

Intuitively, we would think that NIPPV improves gas exchange abnormalities by correcting abnormalities in $\dot{V}/\dot{Q}$. However, subsequent work by Diaz *et al.* (14) proved this to be wrong. They studied the effect of NIPPV on pulmonary gas exchange and haemodynamics during hypercapnic exacerbation of COPD. Using the same inert gas technique reported previously (12), patients were evaluated while breathing spontaneously, 15–30 min on NIPPV and 15 min after withdrawal. They found that the use of NIPPV significantly increased the P_aO_2 and decreased the P_aCO_2 and cardiac output, with no substantial changes in $\dot{V}/\dot{Q}$ mismatching. They concluded that the improvement in respiratory blood gases during NIPPV was due to improvement in alveolar ventilation and not to improvement in $\dot{V}/\dot{Q}$ relationships. These results suggest that respiratory muscle dysfunction and inadequate alveolar ventilation are more important factors in hypercapnic respiratory failure than ventilation/perfusion changes, and patients with severe disease are more likely to develop symptomatic exacerbation because they have minimal, if any, respiratory reserve.

EXACERBATION AND DISEASE PROGRESSION

The development of exacerbations, especially if they become recurrent, seems to have important effects on the natural course of the disease. In the outpatient studies conducted in London by Seemungal *et al.* frequent exacerbators (<2 episodes per year) scored better in the St George's Respiratory Questionnaire than patients who had more frequent episodes of exacerbations (15). In this and in a previous study (16), the best predictors of future exacerbations were the number of exacerbations on the previous year. Very importantly, two recent studies have shown that lung function declines faster in smokers with repeated exacerbations (17) and in frequent versus non-frequent exacerbators (18). In addition, the recovery from exacerbations is longer than once thought and in some patients neither lung function nor symptoms revert to the pre-exacerbation level (9). Therefore, the evidence recently accumulated is that exacerbations should be prevented and effectively treated, to avoid the dire consequences of those episodes.

GOALS OF TREATMENT

The goals in treating patients with acute exacerbation include relief of dyspnoea, correction of hypoxaemia and treatment of the precipitating events, such as respiratory infections. A possible algorithm detailing the approach to patients with exacerbations is shown in Fig. 37.2. However, as important as treating an exacerbation may be, it is also important to take measures to prevent recurrences. Hence the treatment has to include an acute outpatient or in-patient treatment phase and the implementation of preventive measures.

Outpatient therapy

The patients may be managed at home or in the hospital according to the severity of the exacerbation and the presence of co-morbid conditions. Patients managed at home usually require increasing dose of β_2-agonist and/or use of anticholinergic therapy until symptoms improve. Use of a spacer with metered

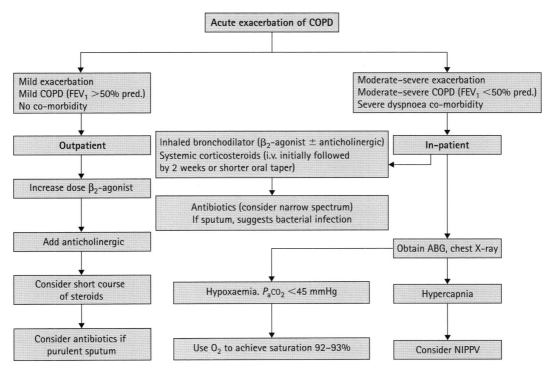

Figure 37.2 *Algorithm describing the approach to patients with an exacerbation of COPD. The decision to treat in an outpatient setting or in the in-patient setting depends on the severity of the exacerbation, the degree of co-morbidity and the available resources. ABG, arterial blood gases; FEV$_1$, forced expiratory volume in 1 s; NIPPV, non-invasive positive pressure ventilation; P$_a$CO$_2$, partial pressure of carbon dioxide.*

dose inhaler may improve drug airway penetration. In some patients with poor technical coordination the use of nebulized bronchodilator may prove more effective (19). In moderate to severe exacerbation, a short course of corticosteroid (less than 2 weeks) and antibiotics, especially in the presence of green purulent sputum, is indicated.

In-patient therapy

The decision to admit or treat patients at home may be difficult. Severe COPD (FEV$_1$ <1 L), very low peak flow (<100 L/min), hypoxaemia and hypercapnia are indications for hospital admission.

OXYGEN THERAPY

The aim of oxygen therapy is to maintain adequate oxygenation with near maximal haemoglobin saturation (P_aO_2 = 60–65 mmHg, or $O_{2,sat}$ >91–92 per cent) without worsening hypercapnia. Oxygen may be supplemented by nasal cannula or Venturi mask (less well tolerated but capable of providing a more even and steady oxygen concentration). Arterial blood gases on room air should be obtained. If the problem is hypoxaemia without hypercapnia, supplementation of low-flow oxygen as required to keep saturations at the desired level is usually sufficient. However, when the patient has hypercapnia and especially with compensated respiratory acidosis, monitoring with arterial blood gases is required.

BRONCHODILATOR THERAPY

Short-acting inhaled β_2-agonists are the preferred initial bronchodilator for the treatment of acute exacerbations of chronic bronchitis, although they have not been demonstrated to be superior to anticholinergic treatment. Usually given in nebulized form, despite evidence that, in very well selected groups of patients with intact sensorium and comprehension, administration via metered dose inhaler with spacer has equal efficacy. The nebulizer should be used with compressed air rather than oxygen while supplementing the oxygen via the nasal cannula. If the patient does not respond adequately, the dose of the medication can be increased to every 2–4 h or an anticholinergic agent may be added. There is no evidence that the combination of both drug agents is superior to either class alone, but there is clinical consensus that the combination may cause fewer side-effects than the progressive increase of each agent alone. The role of intravenous aminophylline is controversial, but if administered, the serum level should be not higher than 12–13 mg/dL and interactions with other medications should also be evaluated.

CORTICOSTEROIDS

Several randomized, placebo-controlled trials have shown that corticosteroids are effective in improving airflow, gas exchange and symptoms. One of these studies enrolled 271 hospitalized veterans and showed that patients treated with systemic corticosteroids had fewer treatment failures, better spirometry and shorter hospital stay (7). The duration of treatment should be limited to 2 weeks (similar outcome to 8-week course) to limit adverse side-effects. A recent study showed that the administration of a fixed dose of 10 mg/day of prednisone for a total of 10 days was significantly better than placebo in patients treated emergently and then sent home on that regimen (20). This should simplify the management of patients who until now were provided with relatively complex 'weaning' therapeutic schemas.

ANTIBIOTIC THERAPY

Bacterial infection may play a role in the development of an exacerbation either as a primary event or following an initial viral process. Two meta-analyses (one of them including 11 randomized, placebo-controlled studies) concluded that antibiotics are beneficial for the treatment of exacerbations, particularly those patients with more severe exacerbation (presence of three symptoms: increased dyspnoea, sputum volume and sputum production) (21). Patients with fewer symptoms, lower physician-assigned severity score or non-purulent sputum may not benefit from antibiotic treatment.

In most cases, sputum gram stain and cultures are not necessary because of the evidence of bacterial contamination in clinically stable patients. The selection of antibiotic depends on local bacterial flora and antibiotic policy. There is no definitive study to support the use of newer, more expensive antibiotics as first-line treatment. Amoxicillin may be used, except for those cases of known beta-lactamase-producing organism, severe exacerbation or failure to improve. In those cases, a second- or third-generation cephalosporin, a fluoroquinolone or a newer macrolide may be the treatment of choice. The duration of treatment has not been clearly defined, lasting between 3 and 14 days, with a common practice of 5–10 days.

RESPIRATORY FAILURE

Patients should be considered for ventilatory support if they have persistent hypoxaemia and/or hypercapnia with low pH (<7.35) despite maximal medical therapy. Several randomized controlled trials have shown that NIPPV is beneficial in selected patients with respiratory failure, decreasing the need for invasive mechanical ventilation and its complications, and possibly improving survival. Other benefits include lower in-hospital mortality rate, accelerated symptomatic and physiological improvement and shorter hospital stay (22). Certain conditions would make patients less likely to respond to NIPPV, including respiratory arrest, medical instability (shock, cardiac ischaemia), inability to protect the airway, excessive secretions, agitation or uncooperativeness, craniofacial trauma or deformity.

PREVENTION

Vaccinations

For patients enrolled in pulmonary rehabilitation, it is extremely important that the chances of decreasing recurrence

be maximized. The use of yearly influenza and pneumococcal vaccine every five years is recommended. Likewise, indoor protection during periods of high environmental pollution is salutatory (23). A healthy life style that includes regular exercise and nutrition are measures that may also improve overall well-being.

Medications

Because exacerbations are associated with increased airway inflammation, there has been much interest in the use of inhaled steroids to reduce exacerbation frequency. In the ISOLDE study, patients with moderate to severe COPD treated with the inhaled steroid fluticasone for a period of 3 years had a reduction in exacerbation frequency of around 25 per cent compared with placebo (4). This study also found that inhaled steroids significantly slowed the deterioration in quality of life scores that occurs over time in patients with the disease. However, the overall exacerbation frequency was relatively low in that study and this was probably due to a retrospective assessment of exacerbation. The effect of inhaled steroids was greater in patients with more impaired lung function, suggesting that this is the group most likely to benefit from long-term inhaled steroid therapy. In the Lung Health Study, the group treated with the inhaled steroid triamcinolone had significantly fewer visits to a physician due to respiratory illness (24). Another earlier study by Paggiaro et al. (5) suggested that the severity of exacerbations might be reduced with inhaled steroid therapy, although, once again, the exacerbation frequency in that study was relatively small. Interestingly, the number of exacerbations was increased following withdrawal of inhaled steroids during the run-in to the ISOLDE trial, although the inhaled steroid withdrawal was not placebo-controlled (25).

A number of recent studies have also shown that reductions in exacerbations can be achieved with bronchodilator therapy (26–29). Mahler et al. (26) found that the time to the first exacerbation was longer with therapy with the long-acting beta-agonist, salmeterol. In another study comparing salmeterol to ipratropium and placebo over a 12-week period, there was no difference in the effect of either treatment arm on exacerbation frequency (27). Van Noord et al. (28), in a similar study, suggested that the combination of salmeterol and ipratropium was most effective in reducing of exacerbation. Rossi et al. (29), over 12 months, compared two different dosages of the inhaled bronchodilator formoterol with placebo or theophylline in a randomized double-blind study. Formoterol reduced the number of hospitalizations, and thus severe exacerbations, compared with placebo and also significantly reduced the number of 'bad days' compared with placebo or treatment with theophylline (29). The new long-acting anticholinergic agent tiotropium has shown similar results. Over 1 year, treatment with tiotropium reduced exacerbations by 24 per cent, compared with ipratropium (30). There was also an increased time to the next exacerbation and increased time to first hospitalization. It is interesting that both long-acting

Library and Knowledge Service Derby Teaching Hospitals NHS Foundation Trust beta-agonists and long-acting anticholinergic agents have some effect on reducing exacerbation frequency and probably also reduce exacerbation severity. Calverley et al. (31) have recently reported a 12-month randomized study of the effect of inhaled fluticasone, salmeterol or the combination compared with placebo. All the active treatments reduced exacerbation frequency compared with placebo and the number of exacerbations that required therapy with oral corticosteroids. Patients with more severe COPD (i.e. FEV_1 <50 per cent of predicted) showed a greater effect of the active treatments on exacerbations than patients with an FEV_1 >50 per cent of predicted.

Pulmonary rehabilitation

Whether pulmonary rehabilitation can effectively help prevent the recurrence of exacerbations has not been formally tested. However, some indirect evidence seems to support this possibility. In 2000, Griffiths et al. (32) presented data on 200 patients with chronic lung disease who were randomized to either 6 weeks' multidisciplinary pulmonary rehabilitation or standard medical management. In addition to showing substantial improvements in exercise performance and health-related quality of life, the pulmonary rehabilitation intervention led to fewer days in the hospital and fewer primary care home visits in the 1-year follow-up period. Thus, this large randomized trial demonstrated a substantial reduction in health care utilization following pulmonary rehabilitation, confirming conclusions from non-controlled studies years earlier (33).

Thus the evidence suggests that during the rehabilitation programme, great care must be taken to optimize effective and complementary medication use to further enhance the value of the programme. Significant reductions in exacerbations can only help optimize patient outcomes.

CONCLUSION

Chronic obstructive pulmonary disease exacerbations are an important cause of morbidity, health-related quality of life and mortality in COPD. Exacerbations also have significant health economic consequences and affect disease progression and thus deserve attention. Inhaled bronchodilators, systemic corticosteroids for most patients, and antibiotics for those thought to have a bacterial infection causing the exacerbation are effective in hastening recovery from moderate to severe exacerbations. The judicious use of oxygen supplementation and non-invasive ventilation for the appropriate patients have improved our capacity to treat patients during an exacerbation. However, the overall aim of therapy is to reduce significantly the morbidity associated with COPD exacerbations and improve the quality of life of our patients with this disabling condition and this requires more effective prevention. There is a need to test whether pulmonary rehabilitation can have an impact on exacerbations and their frequency.

Key points

- Exacerbations of COPD are important causes of morbidity, decreased health status and mortality.
- The burden of exacerbation on the total cost of caring for patients with COPD is very large, and increasing.
- Viral or bacterial infections and environmental changes are all causative agents of exacerbation.
- In spite of significant recent advances, the pathophysiology of exacerbations remains poorly understood.
- Judicious use of bronchodilators, corticosteroids and oxygen help to ameliorate the acute course of exacerbations.
- Non-invasive ventilation has been shown to prevent morbidity and death in patients with exacerbation developing acute on chronic respiratory failure.
- Frequent exacerbations may be associated with more rapid decline of lung function.
- Prevention remains the best approach to prevent exacerbation.
- Smoking cessation in the smoker and vaccinations are logical preventive measures that may have an impact on exacerbation rate.
- Optimization of medical therapy and pulmonary rehabilitation are treatment modalities that have shown to reduce exacerbation rate.

REFERENCES

●1. National Heart, Lung and Blood Institute. *Morbidity & Mortality: 1998 Chart Book on Cardiovascular, Lung and Blood Diseases.* Bethesda, MD: NHLBI.

●2. Murray CJL, Lopez AD, eds. *The Global Burden of Disease: a Comprehensive Assessment of Mortality and Disability from Diseases, Injuries and Risk Factors in 1990 and Projected to 2020.* Cambridge, MA: Harvard University Press, 1996.

◆3. Anthonisen NR, Manfreda J, Warren CPW et al. Antibiotic therapy in exacerbations of chronic obstructive pulmonary disease. *Ann Intern Med* 1987; **106**: 196–204.

4. Burge PS, Calverley PMA, Jones PW et al. Randomized, double blind, placebo controlled study of fluticasone propionate in patients with moderate to severe chronic obstructive pulmonary disease: the ISOLDE trial. *Br Med J* 2000; **320**: 1297–303.

5. Paggiaro PL, Dahle R, Bakran I et al. Multicentre randomized placebo-controlled trial of inhaled fluticasone propionate in patients with chronic obstructive pulmonary disease. *Lancet* 1998; **351**: 773–80.

6. Sethi S, Evans N, Grant BJB, Murphy TF. New strains of bacteria and exacerbations of chronic obstructive pulmonary disease. *N Engl J Med* 2002; **347**: 465–71.

◆7. Niewoehner DE, Erbland ML, Deupree RH et al. Effect of systemic glucocorticoids on exacerbations of chronic obstructive pulmonary disease. *N Engl J Med* 1999; **340**: 1941–7.

8. Thompson WH, Nielson CP, Carvalho P et al. Controlled trial of oral prednisone in outpatients with acute COPD exacerbation. *Am J Respir Crit Care Med* 1996; **154**: 407–12.

9. Seemungal TAR, Donaldson GC, Bhowmik A *et al.* Time course and recovery of exacerbations in patients with chronic obstructive pulmonary disease. *Am J Respir Crit Care Med* 2000; **161**: 1608–13.

10. Elmaghraby Z, Hamada F, Pinto-Plata V *et al.* Dyspnea during acute exacerbation (AE) of COPD is best explained by dynamic hyperinflation (DH) [Abstract]. *Am J Respir Crit Care Med* 2001; **163**: A 812.

11. Livnat G, Pinto-Plata V, Girish M *et al.* Clinical and physiological correlates in acute excerbation (AE) of COPD. *Am J Respir Crit Care Med* 2001; **163**: A 769.

12. Barbera JA, Roca J, Ferrer A *et al.* Mechanisms of worsening gas exchange during acute exacerbations of chronic obstructive pulmonary disease. *Eur Respir J* 1997; **10**: 1285–91.

13. Brochard L, Mancebo J, Wysocki M. Noninvasive ventilation for acute exacerbations of chronic obstructive pulmonary disease. *N Engl J Med* 1995; **333**: 817–22.

14. Diaz O, Iglesia R, Ferrer M *et al.* Effects of noninvasive ventilation on pulmonary gas exchange and hemodynamics during acute hypercapnic exacerbations of chronic obstructive pulmonary disease. *Am J Respir Crit Care Med* 1997; **156**: 1840–5.

◆15. Seemungal T, Donaldson G, Paul E *et al.* Effect of exacerbation on quality of life in patients with chronic obstructive pulmonary disease. *Am J Respir Crit Care Med* 1998; **157**: 1418–22.

16. Ball P, Harris J, Lowson D *et al.* Acute infective exacerbations of chronic bronchitis. *Q J Med* 1995; **88**: 61–8.

17. Kanner RA, Anthonisen N, Connett J *et al.* Lower respiratory illnesses promote FEV_1 decline in current smokers but not ex-smokers with mild chronic obstructive pulmonary disease. *Am J Respir Crit Care Med* 2001; **164**: 358–64.

18. Donaldson G, Seemungal T, Bhowmik A *et al.* Relationship between exacerbation frequency and lung function decline in chronic obstructive pulmonary disease. *Thorax* 2002; **57**: 847–85.

19. Turner MO, Patel A, Ginsberg S *et al.* Bronchodilator delivery in acute airflow obstruction. A meta-analysis. *Arch Inter Med* 1997; **157**: 1736–44.

◆20. Aaron S, Vandenheur K, Hebert P *et al.* Outpatient oral prednisone after emergency treatment of chronic obstructive pulmonary disease. *N Engl J Med* 2003; **348**: 2618–25.

●21. McCrory DC, Brown C, Gelfand SE, Bach PB. Management of acute exacerbation of COPD. A summary and appraisal of published evidence. *Chest* 2001; **119**: 1190–209.

●22. Stoller JK. Acute exacerbations of chronic obstructive pulmonary disease. *N Engl J Med* 2002; **346**: 988–94.

23. Pawels RA, Buist AS, Calverly P *et al.* Global strategy for the diagnosis, management and prevention of chronic obstructive pulmonary disease. *Am J Respir Crit Care Med* 2002; **163**: 1256–76.

◆24. The Lung Health Study research Group. Effect of inhaled triamcinolone on the decline in pulmonary function in chronic obstructive pulmonary disease. *N Eng J Med* 2000; **343**: 1902–9.

25. Jarad N, Wedzicha JA, Burge PS, Calverley PMA. An observational study of inhaled corticosteroid withdrawal in patients with stable chronic obstructive pulmonary disease. *Respir Med* 1999; **93**: 161–6.

◆26. Mahler DA, Donohue JF, Barbee RA *et al.* Efficacy of salmeterol xinafoate in the treatment of COPD. *Chest* 1999; **115**: 957–65.

◆27. Rennard S, Anderson W, Zuwallack R *et al.* Use of a long-acting inhaled beta2 adrenergic agonis salmeterol xinafoate in patients with COPD. *Am J Respir Crit Care Med* 2001; **163**: 163–9.

◆28. Van Noord JA, de Munck DRAJ, Bantje ThA *et al.* Long-term treatment of chronic obstructive pulmonary disease with salmeterol and the additive effect of ipratropium. *Eur Resp J* 2000; **15**: 878–85.

◆29. Rossi A, Kristufek P, Levine B *et al.* Comparison of the efficacy, tolerability and safety of formoterol dry powder and oral slow-release theophylline in treatment of COPD. *Chest* 2002; **121**: 1058–69.

30. Vincken W, van Noord JA, Greefhorst APM. Improved health outcomes in patients with COPD during 1 year's treatment with tiotropium. *Eur Respir J* 2002; **19**: 209–16.

◆31. Calverley P, Pauwels R, Vestbo J *et al.* Combined salmeterol and fluticasone in the treatment of chronic obstructive pulmonary disease: a randomised controlled trial. *Lancet* 2003; **361**: 449–56.

32. Griffiths TL, Burr ML, Campbell IA *et al.* Results at 1 year of outpatient multidisciplinary pulmonary rehabilitation: a randomised controlled trial. *Lancet* 2000; **355**: 362–8.

33. Griffiths TL, Phillips CJ, Davies S *et al.* Cost effectiveness of an outpatient multidisciplinary pulmonary rehabilitation programme. *Thorax* 2001; **56**: 779–84.

38

Long-term compliance after chronic obstructive pulmonary disease rehabilitation

ROGER S. GOLDSTEIN, RICHARD ZUWALLACK

INTRODUCTION

Patient compliance is the extent to which patients adhere to recommendations by health care providers. Non-compliance with medical management occurs commonly, and there is often a wide gap between the regimen recommended by the health care provider and that followed by the patient (1). In a study of asthmatics aged 18–70 years, 37 of the 72 patients who participated took less than 70 per cent of the prescribed dose of medications over the study period (2). Kribbs *et al.* (3) reported that patients with obstructive sleep apnoea provided poor estimates of actual continuous positive airway pressure (CPAP) use and that objective recordings reflected a discrepancy of $69 \pm 110 \, \text{min}$ between patient reports and actual usage. Outpatient medical management of chronic obstructive pulmonary disease (COPD) remains suboptimal despite the publication of several practice guidelines (4).

The operational definitions of compliance vary depending on the specific management recommendation that is being monitored. Approaches to monitoring compliance include subjective self-reports or impressions of health care providers and objective assessments such as pill counting, canister weighing and covert microprocessors to measure activation of delivery devices or usage of machines. Subjective reports are less reliable than objective measures.

Non-compliance with medical advice influences patient outcomes in many conditions such as diabetes, epilepsy, renal transplantation, asthma and tuberculosis (Box 38.1). Lack of compliance not only negates the gains associated with treatment, but results in unnecessary diagnostic tests and

---

Box 38.1 Consequences of reduced compliance with medical advice[a]

- Diabetes – an increased rate of hospital admission
- Epilepsy – increased seizure activity
- Post-renal transplant – the third commonest cause of renal allograft failure
- Asthmatics – fewer symptom-free periods and increased exacerbations
- Tuberculosis – treatment failure and multi-drug resistance

[a]Lack of compliance not only negates gains associated with treatment, but results in unnecessary diagnostic tests and procedures.

---

procedures, invariably increasing health care resource utilization. Patients with chronic conditions often fail to recall elements of potentially important medical advice and often do not adhere to the advice that is recalled (5).

WHY ARE SOME PATIENTS POORLY COMPLIANT?

The explanation as to why some patients do not adhere to medical advice includes many contributing variables (6, 7):

- *Patient factors* include knowledge, health beliefs and attitude to their condition. The interaction with the

Box 38.2 Approaches that might influence compliance

- Combined strategies – more effective than a single intervention
- Family education reinforced by health care professionals
- Verbal and written instructions
- Simplified schedule with fewer demands
- Realistic routines with frequent supervision
- Positive feedback and encouragement

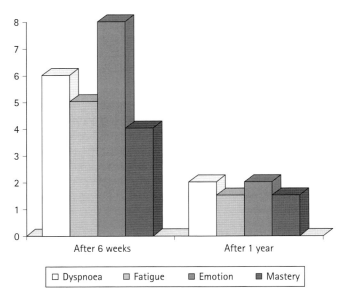

Figure 38.1 *Randomized controlled trial of outpatient rehabilitation. Between-group differences in health-related quality of life (dyspnoea, fatigue, emotional function and mastery) are shown after 6 weeks (at the end of the rehabilitation programme) and after 1 year. Note that although between-group differences persist, there has been a diminution of benefits at 1 year. Reproduced with permission from Goldstein et al. (6).*

health care provider will probably influence the patient's adherence, as will the presence of anxiety or depression. A previous history of non-adherence is often predictive of future behaviour.

- *Practitioner factors* include the quality of the explanation and the amount of individual attention given to the patient.
- *Regimen factors* are important in determining the commitment of the patient, e.g. the number and frequency of medications prescribed or the complexity and duration of an exercise programme.
- *External factors*, such as the presence of a stable social support network, family cohesiveness, positive environmental attitudes and interpersonal resources, may all have a bearing on compliance with medical advice.

Approaches that might increase compliance are summarized in Box 38.2. Although the determinants of poor compliance are often complex, with many of the sociodemographic variables still to be defined, an improved understanding of this issue will assist health care providers in identifying those individuals at high risk.

DIMINUTION OF BENEFITS

Pulmonary rehabilitation is an accepted therapeutic intervention which has been shown in a variety of well designed randomized controlled trials, in which valid, reproducible and interpretable outcome measures were used, to improve functional exercise capacity and health-related quality of life (8–12). It also reduces health resource utilization (6, 12). However, the benefits of rehabilitation diminish with time (Fig. 38.1). Reis *et al.* (10) noted that the initial improvements in exercise gained during rehabilitation diminished over the subsequent 18 months. Wedzicha *et al.* (13) reported that, at 1 year, no significant improvements in health status or exercise tolerance remained. Foglio *et al.* (14) noted (in asthmatics and patients with COPD) that at 12 months post-rehabilitation only 52 per cent of subjects had clinically relevant improvements in health status. Griffiths *et al.* (6) attributed the loss of effect following rehabilitation to poor self-management practices and a lack of adherence to treatment protocols after discharge.

REHABILITATION AND SURVIVAL

To date we do not have convincing evidence that rehabilitation influences survival in patients with COPD. However, we do know (15) that after adjustments for other physiological variables such as forced expiratory volume in 1 s (FEV_1), health status is an independent predictor of mortality (Fig. 38.2). In this study by Domingo-Salvany *et al.* (15), 321 male patients with COPD were followed for 6 years. Those who died (106) were older (69.8 vs. 62.5 years, $P < 0.05$), had a lower body mass index (25.4 vs. 27.1, $P < 0.05$), were more impaired (FEV_1 = 34 vs. 51 per cent of predicted, $P < 0.05$) and had reduced health status, compared with survivors. A reduction of 1 standard deviation (SD) in the FEV_1 was associated with a 60 per cent increase in mortality, confirming the important influence of pulmonary mechanics on survival. However a reduction of 1 SD in the St George's Respiratory Questionnaire (16) was associated with a 30 per cent increase in total mortality. This study noted that health status was an important, independent marker of survival in patients with COPD.

Gerardi *et al.* (17) evaluated the predictors of mortality among 158 patients with COPD, who completed rehabilitation. During the study period of 40 ± 17 months, 43 patients (27 per cent) died, representing a 3-year survival of 80 per cent. The most significant variable associated with survival was the post-rehabilitation walking distance (12-min walking test). This applied to both respiratory deaths and all-cause mortality. Subsequently, Bowen *et al.* (18) reported on the survival characteristics of patients who had been enrolled in

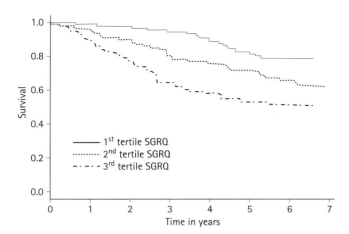

Figure 38.2 *Survival against time for patients with COPD showing various tertiles of the St George's Respiratory Questionnaire, a disease-specific quality of life measure. Note that those with the poorest quality of life have the lowest survival. Reproduced with permission from Domingo-Salvany et al. (15).*

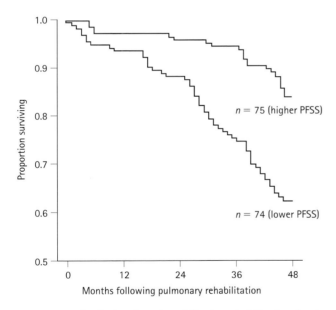

Figure 38.3 *Survival against time, following rehabilitation, for the post-rehabilitation pulmonary function status scale (PFSS). Note that the worst survival is among those with the greatest impairment. Reproduced with permission from Bowen et al. (18).*

10 rehabilitation programmes in Connecticut, between 1993 and 1994. Survival data were recorded from 149 subjects (91 per cent) over a period of 44 ± 12 months. Survival post-rehabilitation was 95 per cent (1 year), 92 per cent (2 years), 85 per cent (3 years) and 73 per cent (4 years). In their analysis of factors relating to increased survival following rehabilitation, functional activities as measured by the pulmonary function status scale (19) and exercise (6-min walking test) (Figs 38.3 and 38.4) were both better predictors of survival than pulmonary mechanics. One might therefore speculate

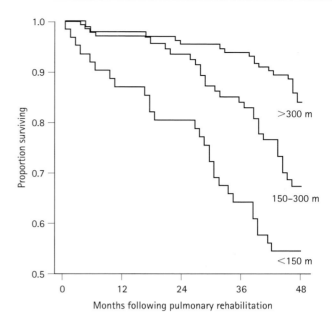

Figure 38.4 *Survival against time, following rehabilitation, for the 6-min walk test. Note that the worst survival is among those with the greatest impairment. Reproduced with permission from Bowen et al. (18).*

that the maintenance of improved functional activities and health status following rehabilitation could have an important influence on patient survival.

PATIENT FACTORS

Not everyone improves in a similar way following rehabilitation. Ketelaars *et al.* (20) used hierarchical cluster analysis to define patients in whom long-term benefits of rehabilitation were sustained 9 months after completion of an in-patient programme. Complete data sets were obtained from 77 patients with similar pulmonary function characteristics. In one group ($n = 44$), health status was moderate on admission, improved with rehabilitation and subsequently deteriorated at follow-up. In the second group ($n = 33$) health status reflected severe impairment on admission with little improvement after rehabilitation and no further change at follow-up. The second group would be unlikely to improve further even if additional resources were allocated for maintenance. This information is important in developing strategies for aftercare at home that aim to maintain the benefits of rehabilitation (Fig. 38.5).

PROGRAMME LOCATION

The immediate benefits of rehabilitation are not site-specific. Excellent improvements have been reported among in-patient (8), outpatient (6, 21) and community-based programmes

(11). However, programme location may influence the longer term patient adherence. Strijbos *et al.* (22) described 41 subjects who completed an 18-month study in which they were randomized to enrol in a hospital outpatient pulmonary rehabilitation programme or a home-based programme. Each programme offered supervision twice a week for 12 weeks. Similar improvements in both groups were noted at 3 and 6 months. However, only those who underwent the home-based programme experienced a sustained improvement at 18 months (Fig. 38.6). A possible explanation is that an initial

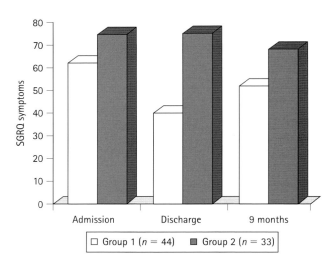

Figure 38.5 *Hierarchical cluster analysis, showing two groups of patients with COPD following rehabilitation. In group 1, improvements with rehabilitation are followed by a diminution of benefit. In group 2 the initial impairment is greater. There is minimal change with rehabilitation and no further change 9 months later. Reproduced with permission from Ketelaars et al. (20).*

familiarity with exercising at home might enable subjects to more readily continue their exercises at home and therefore extend its duration of benefit. This conclusion was supported by the patient's diary cards, which reflected greater participation during the unsupervised home period.

PROGRAMME DURATION

In their meta-analysis of rehabilitation, Lacasse *et al.* (9) noted consistent modest improvements in nearly all of the programmes evaluated. In a post hoc analysis, the magnitude of the improvement appeared to be influenced by the programme duration. This hypothesis was tested prospectively by Troosters *et al.* (23) and Guell *et al.* (24). Troosters *et al.* (23) reported on 100 patients randomized to 6 months of outpatient rehabilitation versus control. Sixty-two were evaluated at 6 months and 49 at 18 months. The between-group differences in 6-min walk (52 m, confidence interval [CI] 15–89) and health status (CRDQ 14 points, CI 6–21) noted at 6 months were sustained at 18 months, at which time they still remained above the minimal clinically important difference (Fig. 38.7). In a subsequent study by Guell *et al.* (24), 60 subjects received 12 months of outpatient rehabilitation versus usual care (Fig. 38.8). Between-group differences in dyspnoea, health status and functional exercise were evident by the third month and continued with somewhat diminished magnitude into the second year of follow-up (24-month between-group exercise difference: 81 m, 95 per cent CI, 38–125 m, $P < 0.001$). In this study the number needed to treat to achieve a significant benefit in health status for a 2-year period was approximately three. In support of the importance of programme duration in contributing to the effects of rehabilitation, Green *et al.* (25) noted lesser improvements following rehabilitation

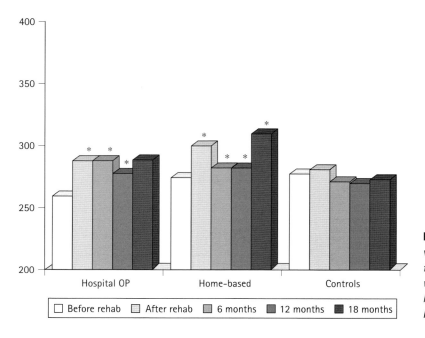

Figure 38.6 *Hospital outpatient (op) rehabilitation versus home-based rehabilitation. The results shown are for the 6-min walk test. Both groups improved compared with control subjects. However, only those treated at home maintained their improvement at 18 months. Reproduced with permission from Strijbos et al. (22).*

among 23 subjects randomized to 4 weeks of rehabilitation versus 21 subjects randomized to a 7-week programme.

EXERCISE MAINTENANCE

In a retrospective report of 51 patients who completed outpatient pulmonary rehabilitation, Vale *et al.* (26) noted that 19 individuals had participated in a structured weekly, post-rehabilitation exercise maintenance programme, whereas 32 had not. In both groups, functional exercise capacity (12-min walk) and health-related quality of life (CRQ) decreased at the time of follow-up (11.0 ± 6.1 months) although these measures remained above the baseline. There were no between-group differences attributable to the post-rehabilitation exercise maintenance programme (Fig. 38.9).

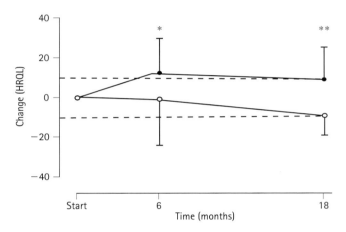

Figure 38.7 *Change in health status following 6 months of outpatient rehabilitation versus control. Note the between-group differences at 6 months were sustained at 18 months. HRQL, health-related quality of life. Reproduced with permission from Troosters et al. (23).*

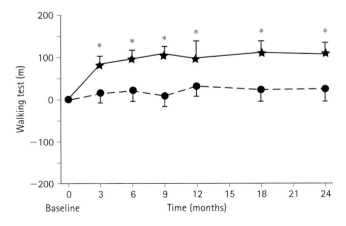

Figure 38.8 *Change in 6-min walking test (from baseline) following 12 months of rehabilitation. Note the study group (upper tracing) maintained improved function at 24 months. Reproduced with permission from Güell et al. (24).*

PROGRAMME REPEAT

Foglio *et al.* (27) reported a pilot study in which 61 stable patients (26 COPD, 35 asthma) who completed rehabilitation were randomized to receive a repeat programme 12 months later and again at 24 months, or just to receive a 24-month repeat. Only 36 subjects completed this study. Although subsequent yearly interventions resulted in comparable short-term gains in exercise capacity and health status, there were no additive long-term benefits from a standard annual programme repeat.

ENHANCED FOLLOW-UP

Brooks *et al.* (7) reported on a randomized controlled trial of enhanced aftercare versus usual aftercare among 109 individuals with COPD who completed pulmonary rehabilitation. The enhanced follow-up group were enrolled in monthly hospital group sessions and also received telephone contact 2 weeks after each visit to the centre. All subjects were seen in follow-up every 3 months. At 6 months, the distance walked in 6 min was slightly greater in the enhanced follow-up group compared with control subjects. At 1 year, this difference had disappeared (Fig. 38.10). Health-related quality of life did not differ between groups. When asked (self-reported compliance), 'Are you doing any regular exercises at home?', the percentage of subjects who continued to exercise declined in both groups with no between-group difference (Fig. 38.11). Brooks *et al.* noted that individuals complied differently with different exercises. Good compliance was noted with breathing exercises and with aerobic exercise, but compliance with interval training and muscle strengthening was poor in both

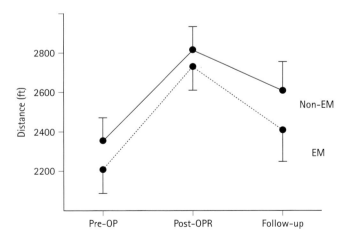

Figure 38.9 *Twelve-minute walk distance before outpatient rehabilitation (OPR), immediately after outpatient rehabilitation and at follow-up after 12 months. Note that there were no differences between subjects participating in an enhanced maintenance programme (EM) and those who did not (non-EM). Reproduced with permission from Vale et al. (26).*

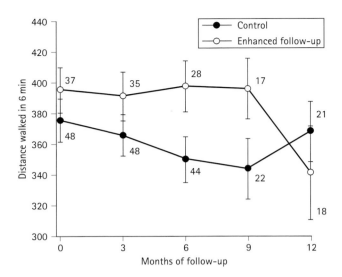

Figure 38.10 *Six-minute walk distance among control subjects and those receiving enhanced follow-up. Between-group differences have disappeared at 1 year. Reproduced with permission from Brooks et al. (7).*

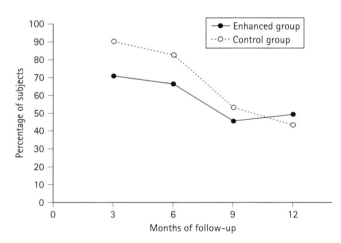

Figure 38.11 *Percentage of subjects who reported participating in a home exercise programme plotted against time. Note that there were no differences between those who received enhanced follow-up and control subjects. Reproduced with permission from Brooks et al. (7).*

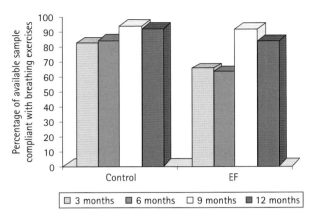

Figure 38.12 *Compliance with breathing exercises among control subjects and those involved in enhanced follow-up (EF), both groups shown for 3, 6, 9 and 12 months. Note the high compliance in both groups with no between-group differences. Reproduced with permission from Brooks et al. (7).*

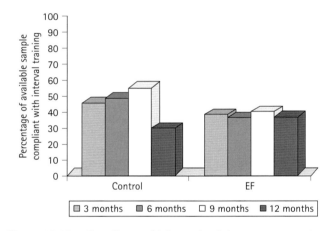

Figure 38.13 *Compliance with interval training among control subjects and those involved in enhanced follow-up (EF), both groups shown for 3, 6, 9 and 12 months. Note the low compliance in both groups with no between-group differences. Reproduced with permission from Brooks et al. (7).*

groups (Figs 38.12 and 38.13). This raises important issues regarding the best content for a maintenance programme, an area in which little information is available. When asked why they discontinued exercise, many individuals identified a respiratory exacerbation as the trigger after which they dropped out of the programme. Conceivably, an effective strategy to maintain function following rehabilitation might be to apply additional resources soon after an exacerbation.

Ries *et al.* (21) reported on 172 individuals randomized to 1 year of maintenance treatment or usual care following 8 weeks of pulmonary rehabilitation. During the maintenance programme, patients received weekly telephone calls in addition to their monthly visits to the centre. Subjects adhered well to the trial, with 138 subjects completing their 12-month assessments and 131 subjects completing their 24-month assessments. However, when compared with the control group, there were only minimal improvements in maximal treadmill exercise, 6-min walk test and health status during the 12-month maintenance period, and by 24 months these differences had disappeared (Fig. 38.14).

COMMENTS

Although there is good evidence that rehabilitation improves health-related quality of life and functional exercise capacity, these improvements diminish with time almost certainly because of reduced patient compliance. Although longer programmes will extend the clinical benefits of rehabilitation, programme enhancements with regular facility visits and

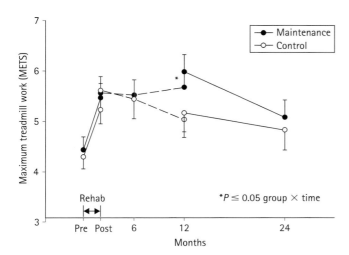

Figure 38.14 *Maximal treadmill work against time. Subjects involved in a 12-month enhanced maintenance programme versus control. Note that, pre- to post-rehabilitation, both groups improved. Randomization occurred post-rehabilitation. The intervention was completed at 12 months. At 24 months, there were no between-group differences. Reproduced with permission from Ries et al. (21).*

phone calls have resulted in only minimal gains. Conceivably, rehabilitation applied following a respiratory exacerbation may be of more value in improving compliance and extending the duration of benefits.

The observation that behavioural interventions rarely produce long-term effects is not unique to pulmonary rehabilitation but has been reported in trials of smoking cessation, weight loss and exercise adherence (28–30). Variables responsible for a short-term behavioural change might well differ from those responsible for a long-term change (31). The best suited to improve health status and functional exercise capacity among patients with COPD remain to be established.

Key points

- Adherence (compliance) with medical advice is a widespread challenge in all branches of health care.
- Non-adherence results in increased morbidity, mortality and health care resource utilization.
- Rehabilitation is effective in improving health status and functional exercise capacity.
- Post-rehabilitation improvements diminish with time, probably because of poor adherence with recommendations from health care providers.
- Various approaches to maintain benefit include longer programmes, repeat programmes and enhanced follow-up.
- Patients will adhere differently to different components of health care, depending on the complexity, frequency and constitution of the activities recommended.

- Therapeutic interventions aimed at maintenance following the intensive phase of rehabilitation, might best be positioned following an acute exacerbation, as many subjects indicate that this is the precipitating event that results in non-adherence to the programme.

REFERENCES

◆1. Haynes RB, Taylor DW, Sackett DL. *Compliance in Healthcare.* Baltimore: Johns Hopkins University Press, 1979.

2. Bosley CM, Fosbury JA, Cochrane GM. The psychological factors associated with poor compliance with treatment in asthma. *Eur Respir J* 1995; **8**: 899–904.

3. Kribbs NB, Pack AI, Kline LR et al. Objective measurement of patterns of nasal CPAP use by patients with obstructive sleep apnea. *Am Rev Respir Dis* 1993; **147**: 887–95.

4. Ramsey SD. Suboptimal medical therapy in COPD. exploring the causes and consequences. *Chest* 2000; **117**: 33S–7S.

5. Kravitz RL, Hays RD, Sherbourne CD et al. Recall of recommendations and adherence to advice among patients with chronic medical conditions. *Arch Intern Med* 1993; **153**: 1869–78.

●6. Griffiths TL, Burr ML, Campbell IA et al. Results at 1 year of outpatient multidisciplinary pulmonary rehabilitation: a randomised controlled trial. *Lancet* 2000; **355**: 362–8.

7. Brooks D, Krip B, Mangovski-Alzamora S, Goldstein RS. The effect of postrehabilitation programmes among individuals with chronic obstructive pulmonary disease. *Eur Respir J* 2002; **20**: 20–9.

●8. Goldstein RS, Gort EH, Stubbing D et al. Randomised controlled trial of respiratory rehabilitation. *Lancet* 1994; **344**: 1394–7.

◆9. Lacasse Y, Wong E, Guyatt GH et al. Meta-analysis of respiratory rehabilitation in chronic obstructive pulmonary disease. *Lancet* 1996; **348**: 1115–19.

●10. Ries AL, Kaplan RM, Limberg TM, Prewitt LM. Effects of pulmonary rehabilitation on physiologic and psychosocial outcomes in patients with chronic obstructive pulmonary disease. *Ann Intern Med* 1995; **122**: 823–32.

●11. Wijkstra PJ, Ten Vergert EM, van Altena R et al. Long term benefits of rehabilitation at home on quality of life and exercise tolerance in patients with chronic obstructive pulmonary disease. *Thorax* 1995; **50**: 824–8.

●12. Bourbeau J, Julien M, Maltais F et al. Reduction of hospital utilization in patients with chronic obstructive pulmonary disease: a disease-specific self-management intervention. *Arch Intern Med* 2003; **163**: 585–91.

●13. Wedzicha JA, Bestall JC, Garrod R et al. Randomized controlled trial of pulmonary rehabilitation in severe chronic obstructive pulmonary disease patients, stratified with the MRC dyspnoea scale. *Eur Respir J* 1998; **12**: 363–9.

14. Foglio K, Bianchi L, Bruletti G et al. Long-term effectiveness of pulmonary rehabilitation in patients with chronic airway obstruction. *Eur Respir J* 1999; **13**: 125–32.

15. Domingo-Salvany A, Lamarca R, Ferrer M et al. Health-related quality of life and mortality in male patients with chronic obstructive pulmonary disease. *Am J Respir Crit Care Med* 2002; **166**: 680–5.

◆16. Jones PW, Quirk FH, Baveystock CM, Littlejohns P. A self-complete measure of health status for chronic airflow limitation. The St

George's Respiratory Questionnaire. *Am Rev Respir Dis* 1992; **145**: 1321–7.

17. Gerardi DA, Lovett L, Benoit-Connors ML *et al*. Variables related to increased mortality following out-patient pulmonary rehabilitation. *Eur Respir J* 1996; **9**: 431–5.

18. Bowen JB, Votto JJ, Thrall RS *et al*. Functional status and survival following pulmonary rehabilitation. *Chest* 2000; **118**: 697–703.

19. Weaver TE, Narsavage GL. Physiological and psychological variables related to functional status in chronic obstructive pulmonary disease. *Nurs Res* 1992; **41**: 286–91.

20. Ketelaars CA, Abu-Saad HH, Schlosser MA *et al*. Long-term outcome of pulmonary rehabilitation in patients with COPD. *Chest* 1997; **112**: 363–9.

21. Ries AL, Kaplan RM, Myers R, Prewitt LM. Maintenance after pulmonary rehabilitation in chronic lung disease: a randomized trial. *Am J Respir Crit Care Med* 2003; **167**: 880–8.

22. Strijbos JH, Postma DS, van Altena R *et al*. A comparison between an outpatient hospital-based pulmonary rehabilitation program and a home-care pulmonary rehabilitation program in patients with COPD. A follow-up of 18 months. *Chest* 1996; **109**: 366–72.

23. Troosters T, Gosselink R, Decramer M. Short- and long-term effects of outpatient rehabilitation in patients with chronic obstructive pulmonary disease: a randomized trial. *Am J Med* 2000; **109**: 207–12.

24. Guell R, Casan P, Belda J *et al*. Long-term effects of outpatient rehabilitation of COPD. A randomized trial. *Chest* 2000; **117**: 976–83.

25. Green RH, Singh SJ, Williams J, Morgan MD. A randomised controlled trial of four weeks versus seven weeks of pulmonary rehabilitation in chronic obstructive pulmonary disease. *Thorax* 2001; **56**: 143–5.

26. Vale F, Reardon JZ, Zuwallack RL. The long-term benefits of outpatient pulmonary rehabilitation on exercise endurance and quality of life. *Chest* 1993; **103**: 42–5.

27. Foglio K, Bianchi L, Ambrosino N. Is it really useful to repeat outpatient pulmonary rehabilitation programs in patients with chronic airway obstruction? A 2-year controlled study. *Chest* 2001; **119**: 1696–704.

28. Pomerlau OAD, Pertschuck M. Predictors of outcome and recidivism in smoking cessation treatment. *Addict Behav* 1978; **3**: 65–70.

29. Foreyt JP, Goodrick GK, Gotto AM. Limitations of behavioral treatment of obesity: review and analysis. *J Behav Med* 1981; **4**: 159–74.

30. Martin JE, Dubbert PM. Exercise applications and promotion in behavioral medicine: current status and future directions. *J Consult Clin Psychol* 1982; **50**: 1004–17.

31. Epstein LH. Role of behavior theory in behavioral medicine. *J Consult Clin Psychol* 1992; **60**: 493–8.

39

Ethical/regulatory issues concerning long-term mechanical ventilation

ALLEN I. GOLDBERG

The purpose of this chapter is to enhance understanding about ethical and regulatory issues concerning long-term mechanical ventilation (LTMV). Based on US experience and international observations (1–3), it provides global insights for:

- health care consumers – patients, families, employers, other purchasers of health care
- health care, educational, social service professionals; all service providers participating within the community
- health public policy experts/agencies; funding organizations involved with managed care and global budgets.

This chapter will provide readers means to:

- *Learn from the past* – understand the background of issues resulting from the creation of the initial and subsequent populations of patients who required LTMV
- *Consider for the present* – analyse the complexity of concerns of families, professionals and organizations seeking services to meet health care, psychosocial, developmental, educational and vocational patient needs
- *Apply for the future* – plan strategies to develop and manage comprehensive and integrated approaches for patients and families who require LTMV that will consider ethical choices and operate within the framework of global health and managed care.

INTRODUCTION/BACKGROUND

Long-term mechanical ventilation may represent a life-sustaining alternative for selected persons with chronic respiratory insufficiency. All participants must understand the perspectives of rehabilitation team members, patients and their families, and others involved. We all face global issues of health care systems challenged by many similar realities.

Every nation in the world faces escalating health care expenditures competing with restricted resources needed for social, economic and other priorities. This was anticipated in developing countries and in former communist nations undergoing economic transformation. However, industrial nations, especially during reduced economic productivity and dramatic societal change, also face this challenge. A prominent reason for the escalation of health care costs is exploding development and application of life-sustaining technologies (4–6).

This challenge creates an opportunity to adapt existing health systems to evolving needs making greater demands on traditional health care delivery. Growing numbers of elderly persons, people with disabilities, and patients facing newer health issues (AIDS, technology-dependent persons) require care for chronic conditions from health systems that were established based on an industrial era model focused on acute care. These patients' long-term care needs are outcomes of progress that result from successes of modern medical science and advanced medical technology. Current systems are not prepared for their new demands.

A global search has begun for new and 'non-traditional' approaches to health systems as a result of these concerns. In November 1990, the Max-Planck-Institut held a health care summit to analyse alternative delivery models suitable for the elderly and people with chronic conditions (7). Participants reviewed the evolution of different community-based models in countries with national health systems (England/Italy), national health insurance (France/Germany), and evolving market/regulatory approaches (USA, Canada). In addition to analysis of finance systems, trans-national analysis was undertaken to evaluate differences between nations' health care delivery models based on the same financial approach.

Among the concerns raised were:

- What are suitable models for persons with long-term requirements for health care and medical technology?
- What can other nations' experiences tell us about optimal economic/finance systems to avoid limited access to care?

Conclusions reached were fundamental to understanding future global health system reform. No matter what organizational model was described (traditional hospital, home care, community centres, nursing homes, other long-term care alternatives), what happens in each nation is based on two factors:

- Funding – the finance system does not matter; what matters is that funding is provided as an incentive to develop an organizational system
- Culture – variations between nations with the same health care finance system are best understood in the context of cultural differences between nations and within regional and local levels. National policy makes a major difference. However, in the community, people can work together to design a variety of innovative local solutions accomplished, encouraged by or despite national health care policy.

The home care matrix: the scope of home care practice

Home care is one appealing organizational model that will compete with others for restricted financial resources in global health care reform. Home care growth is driven by the increasing number of disabled and elderly persons as a percentage of the total population, although children with chronic disease/ disability comprise the fastest growing segment (8).

Home care means the provision by one or more organizations of physician-prescribed nursing care, social work, therapies (physical, occupational, nutritional, speech), vocational and social services, homemaker, home health aide and/or personal assistance services, to disabled, sick or convalescent persons in their home. This regulatory (US Medicare) home care definition requires that the patient be home-bound. LTMV patients with portable devices may be mobile and denied services until statutory/regulatory changes recognize this reality.

Home care can be best classified considering dimensions of three needs:

- duration of time – acute (<7 days), subacute (1–6 weeks) or long-term (>6 weeks)
- level of professional/personal support – none (self, family member); intermittent skilled professional visits; or continuous (private duty nursing/personal attendant)
- involvement of technology – none; low technology (aids for daily living, communication, mobility); or high technology (life-sustaining devices).

People needing prolonged high-technology home care (HTHC) will face changing public policy and marketplace dynamics early in the 21st century (9). Patients requiring LTMV are at greatest risk for service denial (10, 11).

The home care culture: how it differs from the 'medical model' (12)

THE MEDICAL MODEL

All service providers involved with home care must accept a different 'mind set' from the institutional way of thinking and relating to patients. Home care is not an extension of the medical model into the home.

In the medical model, the physician is in charge with the patient/family dependent upon professional authority for decisions and actions. When care is being given in a hospital or ambulatory care setting, patients and family members have a power disadvantage and are not in control. They are more likely to accept medical decisions based on scientific authority and technical information which may take less account of their wishes and desires. In these settings, the physician and other health professionals control decisions and implementation of the plan subject to patient/family compliance. The goals are illness reversal and, when possible, cure.

THE HOME CARE MODEL

In contrast to the medical model, home care represents a culture with attitudes, beliefs, values, and norms of behaviour that differ from those of the more traditional 'medical model'. Home care demonstrates a person-centred social concept typified by the independent living model of persons with disabilities. In this model, physicians are collaborators of care and invited care partners, with the patient/family unit active in making decisions, running the plan and providing feedback for evaluation and improvement. In family-centred care, the patient/family is central and in charge; properly prepared patients/families consider multiple options since they have been empowered and are aware decision-makers. Families rely on information that comes from self-help and mutual aid groups. Their focus is wellness and desire to improve their health status and life situation rather than expect total cure. They are active participants taking responsibility for their own health. Patients/families have important management insights and can make decisions enhancing safety, reducing risk, improving quality and reducing costs. They become essential participants in health self-management.

UNDERSTANDING THE PAST

Long-term mechanical ventilation has evolved globally with local variations. The following provides insights into how it began and developed.

The polio era: creation of the first population of LTMV patients (13)

TECHNOLOGICAL ADVANCES

Countless infants, children and young adults were stricken with paralytic respiratory polio during the poliomyelitis pandemic of the 1950s. Universal fear among the population and the medical community resulted from this plague-like crisis of catastrophic proportions. The polio crisis stimulated advances in upper airway management (tracheostomy) and mechanical ventilation (14). Use of such technology reduced bulbar polio mortality from 90 to 20 per cent (15).

ORGANIZATIONAL ADVANCES

The response to the pandemic included the creation of designated respiratory polio centres (16). Centres were established by voluntary organizations worldwide.

In the US, Americans gave millions of dollars to the March of Dimes of The National Foundation for Infantile Paralysis (16). Polio centres were unique since they featured interdisciplinary teams of health care professionals, including physicians, nurses, social workers and therapists – all working together. Among the 'new' professions were rehabilitation (physical) medicine and respiratory (inhalation) therapy which were 'born' during World War II. The focus was not only on acute survival but on long-term rehabilitation and education. Hence, the team included the active participation of multiple disciplines of therapy: physical, occupational, speech, vocational as well as social support and educational professionals.

COMMUNITY-BASED SOLUTIONS

Most people are aware of the scientific breakthrough to prevent poliomyelitis. After a quarter of a century of leadership by Franklin D. Roosevelt and research efforts of Jonas Salk and others at The National Foundation, the payoff was population-based immunization in the US in 1956.

A less well known development at this time was a significant community-based accomplishment: high-technology home care (HTHC). Portable home respirators were designed in response to the thousands of poliomyelitis victims with respiratory insufficiency who chose to live in the community with families as an alternative to long-term institutions. Consumers working with their doctors and manufacturers helped design technology and the home care programmes (17).

Gini Laurie, noted historian of the poliomyelitis era stated (16):

> The centers and home care resulted in tremendous financial savings and greater degree of independence and self-sufficiency than was ever dreamed possible for people so severely disabled....The average hospital time was cut from more than a year to seven months; the home care costs were one-tenth to one-fourth hospital costs.

Home care was not a new concept in America. The home was the traditional site of health care from the colonial times (18). Furthermore, the idea of 'home visiting' to support the health, social, educational and other needs of children was also well established (19). However, with HTHC, life could be sustained on a prolonged basis at home by augmenting or replacing a breathing ability with a machine. HTHC programmes were developed in partnerships with patients/families, physicians and other health care professionals, and organizational leaders

all working together on a local basis. HTHC had similar evolution at this time in other nations (1–3). Creative cost-saving solutions were found to make HTHC less expensive and more desirable than institutional care (e.g. the use of personal care attendants/alternative care providers) (16).

The critical care era

ADVANCES IN CRITICAL CARE AND REHABILITATION MEDICINE (20)

The technological and organizational advances from the polio era laid the foundation for the development of critical care and rehabilitation medicine. Physician leaders around the world began to apply new knowledge and skills to other challenges. Many pioneers of intensive care units were those with polio experience (20). Units 'housing' LTMV poliomyelitis survivors evolved into ICUs. Other units developed due to medical/surgical advances and the need to concentrate technology and interdisciplinary teams. In these ICUs, critically ill patients could recover from life-threatening acute illness with dramatically improved survival rates and recovery with rehabilitation.

In the US, nearly all of the 'respiratory polio centres' of the National Foundation were 'disassembled' in the late 1950s as it redefined its focus to birth defects (16). The exceptions were centres supported with public financing: Goldwater, Texas Institute for Rehabilitation Research, Rancho los Amigos (21). There, long-term mechanical ventilation for chronic respiratory insufficiency, 'lost' to acute care physicians, was applied by rehabilitation teams to patients with a spinal cord injuries and neuromusculoskeletal disorders. Technology support was provided and adapted for home use.

INITIAL HOSPITAL-BASED SOLUTIONS

The 'price to pay' for ICU miracles was survival of a small number of patients who required LTMV. For all concerned, ventilator-dependent patients were considered 'treatment failures'. With changes in reimbursement to prospective payment, they became expensive failures. When removed too early from technology, they became medically unstable after discharge at home where they died or required hospital readmission.

Initial hospital-based efforts to address LTMV focused on creation of 'step-down' units. Solutions required an integrated team approach involving patients and families in self-care. 'Optimal support' (optimal ventilation, pharmacology, nutrition and psychosocial stimulation) changed the outcome and proved that patients on LTMV could 'thrive'. The initial specially designated units featured a patient-centred team approach led by a primary-care nurse and fostered team interaction. Families became involved in learning skills, adapting procedures, providing care, making management decisions and, if they chose, planning for transitional care. It was in these units that the family members could be thoroughly prepared for care-giver roles and responsibilities for care at home.

Over time, it became clear that additional solutions were needed. This led to other transitional care settings. Several centres considered LTMV a challenge for the extension of their mission. In these centres, the focus was on chronic care and the family as a social unit; professionals were available to deal with long-term developmental, social and educational needs. For adults, special 'weaning units' were developed to attempt to stabilize and withdraw mechanical ventilation over longer periods of time by weaning protocols (22–23).

INITIAL HOME CARE EXPERIENCES

Initial home care initiatives for LTMV were undertaken with encouragement from patients and families as the preferred option. By the mid-1980s, the paediatric literature reported several home care discharge experiences (24–27). Initial reports came from the earliest developed units responsible for major advances in neonatology and critical care. Each described organizational and funding concerns. However, initial demonstrations determined that resources could be found and financing arranged with 'creative solutions' by establishing collegial relationships among health care providers, administrators and funders. This was also the approach of European models for adults established in the 1960s and 1970s (28, 29).

The recent past: making change happen

The following account documents how change has been made to respond to the needs of patients who require LTMV.

BRINGING PUBLIC ATTENTION TO THE POPULATION REQUIRING LTMV

US Surgeon General C. Everett Koop MD (1981–1989) believed in care for life-supported children at home. Moreover, he shared the vision that meeting the needs of technology-dependent children and their families led to solutions for all children with special needs due to disabilities and/or chronic illness. To facilitate system change, he designed the Surgeon General's Workshop (30).

Dr Koop invited all categories of stakeholders needed to understand the issues as participants in planning and implementing change. His interactive format had 'at the table': national leaders of relevant programmes/policies, health care professionals, organizational leaders and informed consumers (ventilator users).

PUBLIC POLICY RESPONSES TO MEET THE NEEDS OF LTMV

By the early 1980s, ventilator-dependent patients were not rare. Julie Beckett had learned that home care for children like her daughter Katie was possible in Illinois. With the support of her health care team, funding was sought in Iowa but blocked by Medicaid 'bureaucratic red-tape'. With resourcefulness, determination and conviction, she contacted the right political people who brought the plight of these children and barriers created by government policy to the attention of Vice-President Bush. President Reagan highlighted Katie Beckett at a 1981 press conference; Katie was sent home as 'an exception to policy' (31).

When the US president makes an exception to policy, legislation/regulation must deal with anticipated future cases. US Health and Human Services (HHS) Secretary Schweiker charged Dr Koop to chair an ad-hoc task force and Congressman Waxman charged his health care subcommittee to design a public policy response. Community-based 'waivers' were proposed to existing policy. They were determined by strict criteria with financial risk limited to a defined number of beneficiaries. Since 1982, public funding for LTMV children has been obtained as a waiver from Medicaid (Title XIX) policy. The waiver provided a mechanism to utilize public funds without requiring co-payment by families that would reduce financial assets to poverty level. However, not all states applied for waivers; waiver benefits depended upon insights and understanding of authors who submitted them. Waivers limited the number of beneficiaries and took an excessive amount of time for approval. Waivers' restrictive policies and procedures replaced what had been innovative 'creative financing' by negotiations and flexible public funding arrangements for individual cases. The ultimate result from Dr Koop's efforts was the public policy (Title V) designation of children with disabilities and chronic disease as 'children with special needs'. This permitted development of funding and programmes for this segment of the population.

PRIVATE REIMBURSEMENT PRACTICES

Not all patients on LTMV required public funding. Some had some private indemnity benefits, often with major medical insurance. Although these policies did not cover this new category of patient, insurance company administrators (medical directors) and employers who determined benefit programmes were open to direct dialogue for creative solutions to best utilize the remaining funds obligated to spend. Less restricted by rules and regulations, they permitted more innovative ways to meet the individual needs of their employees' families. Many consulted public agencies knowledgeable about community-based resources and had public funds to supplement private benefits.

SERVICE DELIVERY DEVELOPMENT

Initial discharge efforts found durable medical equipment vendors and home health agencies hesitant to provide devices and personnel in the home due to potential medical liability risk and lack of funding. But as insurance companies and 'waiver cases' began to provide potentially limitless funding streams, home care organizations began to develop programmes. Families could obtain equipment, supplies and support but they faced fragmented services in the community. LTMV at home, previously delivered at significant cost-savings compared with hospitalization, started to equal or exceed costs of care in an institutional alternative. This was due to inadequate coordination of service delivery and to funding approaches lacking cost management mechanisms. A new 'industry' developed which resulted in exploding costs/utilization (32, 33).

Excessive growth became a major public policy concern (8). Subsequent regulations required that home care must cost less than alternatives.

ANALYSING THE PRESENT

In some countries, systems have been established for LTMV (34, 35). In the US, patients and families face disorganized and fragmented sources of funding and services for health care, social, educational and rehabilitation needs. The cost of lack of integration is high. With a 'non-system', LTMV needs may not be met or, if met, actual expenditures may be excessive. Patients and families are victims of cost and operational inefficiencies which may put at risk their home care option since costs might exceed institutional alternatives. This becomes critical with managed care and global health budgets.

Current reimbursement policies and programmes for LTMV

PUBLIC SECTOR

Not all patients at home require public funding assistance. However, over time, those with finite private indemnity insurance or managed care restrictive policies will become dependent on public funding. Over a lifetime, insurance policy limits are commonly exceeded and home care benefits will be determined by public policy with or without 'waiver' exceptions. For the elderly eligible for Medicare (social/health insurance), LTMV patients face more restrictive payment policies to physicians, home health agencies and durable medical equipment suppliers. Most recently, they face an enormous burden of regulatory-mandated co-payments and deductibles they must pay and the limitation of services due to competitive bidding for government contracts (10).

In the US, each state varies in its Medicaid (Title XIX) policy and available funding. Additionally, for children, each state also has a designated programme for 'children with special needs' (Title V). These funds have defined categorical criteria with/without supplementation by social security benefits. Compared with Medicaid funding, Title V funding is much more limited. Title V programmes provide involvement by concerned professionals who want to meet the comprehensive needs of these special children. In Illinois, Title V has been a valuable resource for information about community-based services and as a case-manager of Medicaid 'waiver' funds.

Other public funds have been identified and applied for LTMV children. For example, under-utilized budgeted state funds identified by resourceful parents were the basis of a state-wide case-management programme for ventilator-dependent children in Pennsylvania. This was accomplished by one resourceful parent who had chosen LTMV at home for her developmentally delayed child as a preferable situation to prolonged institutionalization.

PRIVATE SECTOR

Private sector funding from traditional indemnity insurance previously paid health care costs retrospectively 'at cost'. 'Cost shifting' by health care providers placed an added burden upon private insurers to compensate for under-funded public payment. For private insurers, LTMV represents 'catastrophic cost'. In 1983, private insurers (Aetna; Blue Cross-Blue Shield) responded with 'case management' strategies that required a health care professional (nurse/physician) to review and approve costs for such exceptional cases. Despite 'policy restrictions', case managers were approachable as colleagues to develop flexible, individualized programmes. Utilizing case management for exceptional cases has been a similar strategy by those employers who have developed self-insurance programmes with/without third party administrators.

During the 1990s, the penetration of managed care organizations (MCOs) into regional health care markets was dramatic. By 1995, 56 million Americans were enrolled, up 10 per cent/year, a fivefold increase since 1992. MCOs assume full financial risk for enrolled members by accepting premiums for total comprehensive care. MCOs then attempt to locate hospitals and health care providers who agree to financial contracts which transfer part/all of the financial risk to them for providing medically necessary services. The line between funder and provider can become fuzzy depending upon the contract. Arrangements vary with each contract's formulas for exceptional cost situations. No funding is designed for health, social support and rehabilitation needs of LTMV.

Exceptional programmes and people can be found in managed care organizations. MCOs have also incorporated 'case management' as a strategy to limit financial exposure that might exceed anticipated expenditures. In some cases, 'benefit management' is interpreted very narrowly, limiting/rejecting payment for services needed for LTMV. However, innovative programmes can result in significant cost saving and quality programmes for LTMV (36).

ALTERNATIVE FUNDING SOURCES

Managed care expansion

A recent US regulatory initiative has encouraged managed care Medicaid and the federal government now provides a managed care Medicare option. Presently, all MCOs attempt to manage care by managing costs. Up to now, this has been done with volume discount contracts with providers or by establishing limited provider networks. In some cases, MCOs transfer all financial risk to providers by capitation: 'per patient per month' payment for all health care needs. Although this is meant to provide incentives for health promotion/prevention, it encourages limited expenditures since cost overruns are provider liabilities. LTMV costs may not be considered 'medically necessary'.

MCOs attempt to control costs by determining 'medical necessity' by requiring approval of all benefits by a 'gatekeeper' who is often a primary care physician (family physician/generalist). Since LTMV potentially represents catastrophic costs, MCOs also utilize case managers. Both 'gatekeepers' and case managers may or may not agree to medical necessity that would improve the well-being and health of their beneficiaries. However, they are educable and will work with families and professional advocates collegially.

Family contributions

Families are exposed to both direct and indirect costs for LTMV. More public/private programmes now consider or require annual deductibles and co-payments for covered benefits which may also have upper major medical limits. Furthermore, there are many uncovered health-related expenses the family must face. Families may need to expand or modify their home, which may result in increased energy costs and taxes when they face loss of earnings due to time required for providing direct care. They may require new means of transportation and mobility and face payments for technical aids for education and rehabilitation purposes. Although these may not seem 'medically necessary', they are all justified since they promote health and indirectly affect direct health care expenditures. They permit continuity of home care which, properly designed and managed, can limit health care costs and extend benefits.

Voluntary and community agencies

Non-profit voluntary/community agencies exist which could potentially provide funding for 'categorical' needs. For example, organizations designated 'by diagnosis or condition' raise funds for research/services directly or via United Way (e.g. Muscular Dystrophy Association, United Cerebral Palsy, Easter Seals). Such agencies will not fund catastrophic health costs; rather, they may provide supplementary funding for designated purposes, e.g. purchase of devices.

Community agencies have been more helpful responding to rehabilitation (health-affecting) needs. Some charitable organizations (Rotary International) have carried out fundraising for individual children/special populations.

Creative financing (combining funding from private, public, community sources), designed by concerned professionals, organizations and parents working together, has done much to fund extraordinary costs for LTMV on an individual case basis.

Current service provision

Services for complex chronic conditions are provided without a coordinated, integrated management approach. Fragmentation frustrates patients/families, professionals and payers. Operational inefficiencies, gaps and duplications result in cost overruns or payment denials.

HEALTH CARE

Long-term mechanical ventilation at home requires a variety of services for medical, psychosocial and rehabilitation needs that all promote health. Few designated programmes or resources target LTMV or can provide 'one-stop shopping' including case management.

PSYCHOSOCIAL AND REHABILITATION

Psychosocial/rehabilitation needs of LTMV patients affect health directly. Services to meet these needs are at times available from home health agencies, but they may also be found in other community agencies designated for other purposes. Many of these have 'home visiting' as part of their programmes

(19). However, they are not integrated with services provided by home health agencies.

Families have often found that they can get more support for health and related needs by turning to other families and concerned persons who join together as self-help and mutual aid groups (38). Self-help groups such as IVUN (International Ventilator Users Network) are a major source of support for families which supplement information and provide needed help not within the realm of professionals (39). Other consumer-directed groups (Family Voices, CoACH) provide care coordination skills, advocacy and serve as social change catalysts (40, 41).

EDUCATION

As LTMV has become more prevalent, community educational systems have faced major challenges beyond special educational programming. In some school districts, developmental therapies (physical, occupational, speech therapy) are available to prepare children for school; these services do not depend upon health insurance. Federal laws mandate that states develop early intervention programmes. Families, health and funding agencies have joined together in local area councils to facilitate case finding, system design and coordination of services to prepare children for school. Unfortunately, recent regulatory changes limit innovative approaches intended by the law.

APPROACHING THE FUTURE

The future of LTMV is intricately tied into the future of HTHC. Due to unconstrained growth of the home care industry and costs, the future of HTHC has been questioned on ethical grounds (32, 33).

Ethical conflicts result when multiple ethical principles reflecting different perspectives are considered. What judgment principles relate to HTHC?

Beneficence-based judgment: If a treatment has merit and meets the individual's health needs, it ought to be instituted and continued. Only harmful interventions ought to be stopped; there is no obligation to continue non-beneficial intervention. Minimal benefit interventions may be continued or stopped, but intervention ought to be instituted and/or continued only if clinical judgment determines that it is more than minimally beneficial.

This is the ethical principle used by professionals concerning treatment options they offer to patients, considering each individual at times without enough concern for the needs of society or primarily what the patient wants.

Autonomy-based judgment: Interventions are only justified when they are based on informed opinion of the patient/family unit. These decisions are made in their best interest and reflect their perspective. Home care differs from traditional care since patients' and families' wants are valued, person/family-centred care is a core belief, and decisions involving the patient/family unit are the norm of behaviour.

This is the ethical principle used by persons/families that require and want to be supported by life-sustaining technology at home.

Justice-based judgment: Only interventions that result in social utility are justified since finite resources must be distributed equitably for the most good for society.

Given that freedom-based, merit-based and needs-based interests all generate justice-based obligations, there is no uncontended theory of justice that prevails.

Clearly, there is conflict regarding what the professional wants to do, what the patient/person/family wants to have done, and what society can afford to do. Since one option demands trade-off with another, LTMV/HTHC raises an ethical debate which is a part of the more difficult, larger issue of allocation of limited resources especially in a managed care environment. This is exacerbated by the universal growth in populations with chronic disease/disability served by 'systems' designed for acute interventions.

What will the future of LTMV reimbursement look like?

Health care cost expansion exceeding the general rate of inflation cannot continue unabated forever. For over a decade, various strategies have been attempted and failed to control cost (case-mix average prospective payment for diagnostic-related groups [DRGs], volume discount contracting with preferred providers, catastrophic complex care case management, regulation of physician fees by resource-based relative value scales [RBRVS]). These strategies have tried to limit expenditures and have affected quantity, and potentially quality, of care. These 'managed care' tactics have focused more on managing costs than on maintaining or improving quality.

Global health care reform will return. Recent efforts have been incremental, focusing more on financial reform than on system delivery; instead of federal reform, states have failed experiments with managed care Medicaid; MCOs no longer want to participate in Medicare. Market-driven health care reform has intensified. Many players are publicly traded (investor-financed). To realize expected return on investments, rigorous cost management will be put in place. Ultimately, all payers – and the public – will realize that global health management is inevitable. LTMV cases represent complex expensive care, 'outliers' to any managed care approach; and payment for their health care costs may be at risk without special considerations and arrangements which will limit the options for LTMV.

LTMV needs also include family social support and rehabilitation services. The constraints on health care revenues extend to social and educational budgets as well. Politicians seek to reduce government expenditures. Although not specific, budgets for all federal, state and local social programmes are at risk. State/local governments have responded to public referenda to limit debt and tax financing and have already put in cost controls (balanced/neutral budget requirements) that demand fiscal responsibility. Public sector funding for all services will be constricted and growth-limited. All this will intensify during economic cycle downturns and increasing budgetary deficits.

What organizational strategies may make sense in this future funding environment?

Market/political health care reform, proposed or real, has already resulted in market-driven experiments that may predict future realities. Health care providers may consolidate into integrated delivery systems (IDSs). All facility- (acute, subacute, long-term care) and non-facility-based components (home care) will have to operate within finite cost constraints that encourage cost-saving mechanisms: replacement of professionals with trained non-professionals and volunteers; and replacement of 'people' with advanced medical information and communication technologies. IDSs employ components of managed care: primary-care focus with generalist gatekeepers to restrict access to specialists and case management. Cost management will limit approval of services not considered 'medically necessary.'

Health care is not the only need of LTMV patients and families. Other community-based services (social support, rehabilitation, educational, vocational), which are also under funding/budgetary constraints, must consider integration and cost-limiting strategies as well. Public, voluntary and self-help organizations should realize the value of coalition-building and resource-sharing. They can achieve synergy by creating community health networks that foster organizational interdependency. Social service organizations also provide home visits and case management. Many community-based service organizations will coordinate similar services meeting multiple needs simultaneously. In the future, they will find that integration of services from multiple sources enhances client benefit and maximize resource utilization. Public funders providing oversight will contract with social agency preferred providers that implement such strategies (public sector integration of social agency funding). Visionary philanthropy may encourage coalitions and community-driven and focused solutions that feature such collaboration.

What organizational planning approaches (processes) will make them happen?

Organizations serving LTMV patients and their families in the future will require systems thinking. The complexity of changes in the political, market and public policy environment will require that they respond as learning organizations utilizing systems approaches. Meeting the multiple needs of LTMV patients with fragmented, isolated and competing services will no longer be possible. Today LTMV is a 'non-system'; tomorrow, a systems approach will be mandatory. Organizations will entertain considerations of strategic alliances in a variety of forms, including joint ventures on a programme/organizational basis, staged mergers or provider/payer/patient system development. Complementary services can be better coordinated and managed; home visiting can serve multiple purposes, including medical/social service delivery, technical support and case management.

Future action planning should consider a process whereby systems development identifies and invites all stakeholders, including consumers, into the process of system planning, implementation and evaluation; outcome analysis will be used as feedback for further system development. These systems will be in the form of stakeholder partnerships, each representing unique perspectives essential for successful operation of the system: patient/provider/payer partnerships.

CONCLUSION

In conclusion, it is worth considering three questions: what then will the future for LTMV patients look like; will they survive in a managed care world; and what can be established; how will it be established (42)?

- *An integrated family-directed community health system will operate within finite predetermined financial constraints.* The financial risk to manage available resources and respond to the multiple needs of all beneficiaries will be the burden of the system. Community-based alternatives (e.g. LTMV) cannot survive if costs exceed institutional-based alternatives.

- *The system must be operated by an integrated management approach which involves and links all stakeholders in system development.* Stakeholders include health care, social service, rehabilitation and educational professionals; patients/families; community-based providers/agencies, and funders. Ethical/management conflicts can be resolved by a process of planning, implementing, evaluating and modifying the system which respects multiple viewpoints and perspectives. In this way, the evolution of the system will be flexible and adaptable, meeting the needs of each individual participant and group while maximizing the utilization of resources. The system will not survive if it is fragmented, inflexible and unable to change nor innovate.

- *The system must be designed 'smartly', utilizing available technologies of management information systems and advanced communications which can extend the impact of each player.* The central role must be given to the person/family at home who has valuable insight and skills in self-management and management of their own programme needs.

- *The system must integrate a variety of services targeted to meet multiple needs.* The system must present a total service package which will offer options depending upon the needs of each individual situation. Such an integrated system must be designed and operated locally, since its success will be based on dedicated collaborative efforts of professionals and parents, providers and payers who will all benefit if given the opportunity to work together within the constraints of managed care/global health budgets.

- *The system must responsibly accomplish multiple goals: universal access, medical necessity as determined by system criteria, quality improvement and cost containment.* It must prove itself by pre-setting desirable outcomes and acceptable quality indicators for continuous improvement. Only by achieving desired results as determined by rigorous evaluation (outcomes) research will the system justify required resources for growth and survival.

Key points

- In the middle of the twentieth century, patients, families, physicians, concerned health care professionals and organizations formed voluntary organizations to create community-based solutions. This occurred worldwide in many nations in response to the long-term needs of poliomyelitis survivors.
- In the more recent past, changes occurred by a process that featured involvement of all potential beneficiaries, including 'consumers'. Change designed at the national/global level required local implementation.
- In the US, current funding and services are fragmented. Unlimited cost escalation and lack of chronic care models can no longer be tolerated. International models of coordinated and integrated systems of care exist (43–46).
- The future of LTMV, facing global limitations of resources, will require a systems approach to change that is community-focused and driven.

REFERENCES

●1. Goldberg AI. Home health for the chronically ill in the United States: the market oriented system. In: Hollingsworth JR, Hollingsworth EJ, eds. *Care for the Chronically and Severely Ill: Comparative Social Policies.* New York: Aldine de Gruyter, 1994.
2. Goldberg AI. *Home Care and Alternatives to Hospitalization in France for Medical Technology Dependent Children and Adults with Severe Chronic Respiratory Insufficiency: the Associative System.* World Health Organization, Fellowship Report. Geneva, Switzerland: WHO, 1986.
3. Goldberg AI. Home care services for severely physically disabled people in England and France. Case-example: the ventilator-dependent person. *International Exchange of Experts and Information in Rehabilitation Fellowship Report.* New York: World Rehabilitation Fund: 1983.
4. Institute of Medicine. *Assessing Medical Technology.* Washington, DC: National Academy Press, 1985.
5. US Congress Office of Technology Assessment. *Life-sustaining Technologies and the Elderly.* (OTA-BA-306). Washington, DC: US Government Printing Office, 1987.
6. Weisbrod BA. The health care quadrilemma: an essay on technology change, insurance, quality of care, and cost containment. *J Econ Lit* 1991; **29**: 523–52.
7. Hollingsworth JR, Hollingsworth EJ, eds. *Care of the Chronically and Severely Ill. Comparative Social Policies.* New York: Aldine de Gruyter, 1994.
8. Vladek BC. *Home-Based Care for a New Century.* Keynote Address at Arden House (Harriman, New York). New York: Milbank Fund and Visiting Nurse Services of New York, 1993.

●9. Goldberg AI. Can high-technology home care survive in a world in search of health care reform? In: Robert D, ed. *Home Mechanical Ventilation*. Paris: Arnette-Blackwell, 1995.

10. Robinson JC. Renewed emphasis on consumer cost sharing in health insurance benefit design. *Health Affairs* 2002. Online (http://www.healthaffairs.org/WebExclusives/Robinson_Web_Escl_030202.htm).

11. Anonymous. Reimbursement for ventilatory equipment: how it works. *IVUN News* 2003; **17**: 9.

12. Brooks D, King AJ, Tonak M *et al*. Ventilator user's perspectives on important elements of health-related quality of life. A Canadian qualitative study. Online (http://www.post-polio.org/ivun). St Louis, MO: Post-Polio Health International – International Ventilator Users Network, 2002.

13. Goldberg AI, Faure EAM, eds. *Whatever Happened to the Polio Patient? Proceedings of an International Symposium*. Chicago: Northwestern University Press, 1981.

14. Engstrom CG. Treatment of severe cases of respiratory paralysis by the Engstrom Universal Respirator. *Br J Med* 1952; **2**: 666.

15. Kristensen HS, Neukirch F. Very long-term artificial ventilation (twenty-eight years). In: Rattenborg CC, Via-Reque E, eds. *Clinical Use of Mechanical Ventilation*. Chicago: Yearbook, 1981.

16. Laurie G. Introductory remarks. In: Goldberg A, Faure EAM, eds. *What Ever Happened to the Polio Patient? Proceedings of an International Symposium*. Chicago: Northwestern University Press, 1981.

17. National Foundation for Infantile Paralysis. *Roundtable Conference on Poliomyelitis Equipment (May 28–29, 1953)*. New York: National Foundation for Infantile Paralysis, 1953.

18. Ginsberg E *et al*. *Home Care: Its Role in a Changing Health Services Market*. Totawa, NJ: Roman and Allanhead, 1984; 6.

19. Gomby DS, Larson CS, eds. *The Future of Children: Home Visiting*, vol. 3 no. 3. Los Altos, CA: The David and Lucile Packard Foundation, 1993.

●20. Goldberg AI. Pediatric high-technology home care. In: Rothkopf MN, Askanazi J, eds. *Intensive Home Care*. Baltimore: Williams & Wilkins, 1992; 199–214.

21. Goldberg AI. Home care for a better life for ventilator-dependent people. *Chest* 1983; **84**: 365–6.

22. Gracey DR, Naessens JM, Viggiano RW *et al*. Outcomes of patients cared for in a ventilator-dependent unit in a general hospital. *Chest* 1995; **107**: 494–9.

23. Dasgupta A, Rice R, Mascha E *et al*. Four-year experience with a unit for long-term mechanical ventilation (Respiratory Special Care Unit) at the Cleveland Clinic Foundation. *Chest* 1999; **116**: 447–55.

24. Burr BH, Guyer B, Todres ID *et al*. Home care for children on respirators. *N Engl J Med* 1983; **309**: 1319–23.

25. Goldberg AI, Faure EAM, Vaughn C *et al*. Home care for life supported persons: an approach to program development. *J Pediatrics* 1984; **104**: 785–95.

26. Kettrick RG, Donar M. The ventilator-dependent child: medical and social care. In: *Critical Care, State of the Art*. Fullerton, CA: Society of Critical Care Medicine 1985; **4**: 1–38.

27. Frates RC, Splaingard M *et al*. Outcomes of home mechanical ventilation in children. *J Pediatrics* 1985; **106**: 850–6.

28. Goldberg AI. The regional approach to home care for life-supported persons. *Chest* 1984; **86**: 345–6.

●29. Goldberg AI. Home care for life-supported persons. Is a national approach the answer? *Chest* 1986, 1983; **90**: 744–8.

◆30. Report on the Surgeon General's Workshop. *Children with Handicaps and Their Families: Case Example – the Ventilator-Dependent Child* (PHS-83–50194). Washington, DC: US Department of Health and Human Services.

31. New York Times. *Girl Cited by Reagan Received Medicaid Under a Special Rule* (11 November 1981) New York: New York Times.

32. Arras JD. *Bringing the Hospital Home: Ethical and Social Implications of High-Technology Home Care*. Baltimore, MD: The Johns Hopkins University Press 1995.

33. Caring for an aging world- allocating scarce resources. The technology tether: an introduction to ethical and social issues. In: *An Introduction to Ethical and Social Issues in High Technology Home Care*. Hastings Cent Rep 1994; (Sep–Oct); S1–28.

●34. Goldberg AI. Home care for life-supported persons: the French system of quality control, technology assessment, and cost containment. *Public Health Report* 1989; **104**: 329–35.

●35. Goldberg AI. Technology assessment and support of life-sustaining devices in home care: The home care physician's perspective. *Chest* 1994; **105**: 1448–53.

36. Goldberg AI, Trubitt MJ. An integrated approach to home health care. *Physician Executive* 1994; **20**: 45–6.

37. Gomby DS, Larson CS, Lewit EM, Berhman RE. Home visiting: analysis and recommendations. *Future Child* 1993; **3**: 6–22.

38. Katz AH, Hedrich HL, Isenberg H *et al*. *Self-Help: Concepts and Applications*. Philadelphia: The Charles Press, 1992.

39. International Ventilator Users Network. Online (http://www.post-polio.org/ivun/). St Louis, MO: Post Polio Health International.

40. Family Voices. Online (www.familyvoices.org).

41. Coordinating Action for Children's Health (coACh). Online (http://www.coachcarecenter.org).

●42. Goldberg AI. Health care networks for long term mechanical ventilation. In: Hill NS, ed. *Long-Term Mechanical Ventilation*. New York: Marcel Dekker, 2001.

●43. Goldberg AI, Faure EAM. Home care for life-supported persons in England: the Responaut Program. *Chest* 1984; **86**: 910–14.

●44. Goldberg AI, Faure EAM. Home care for life-supported persons in France: the regional association. *Rehabil Lit* 1986; **47**: 60–4.

45. Goldberg AI. Mechanical ventilation and respiratory care in the home for the 1990s. Some personal observations. *Respir Care* 1990; **35**: 247–59.

46. Goldberg AI. Outcomes of home care for life-supported persons. Long-term oxygen and prolonged mechan ventilation. *Chest* 1996; **109**: 595–6.

40

End-of-life issues in advanced chronic obstructive pulmonary disease

GRAEME ROCKER, PAUL HERNANDEZ

INTRODUCTION

The purpose of this chapter is to raise awareness of the key end-of-life issues facing chronic obstructive pulmonary disease (COPD) patients and their care-givers. The potential benefits of pulmonary rehabilitation as a setting conducive to addressing these issues are also addressed. End-of-life issues in COPD are explored from the perspective of the patient and the health care professional. This chapter is of particular interest to health care professionals who provide care for COPD patients with advanced disease. An edited version of this chapter has been adapted by the Canadian Thoracic Society COPD Guidelines Committee for inclusion in a supplement published in the *Canadian Respiratory Journal* in early 2004.

BACKGROUND

Chronic obstructive pulmonary disease is a chronic, slowly progressive and disabling condition that typically leads to increasingly severe dyspnoea and compromised quality of life for many years prior to death. It is the fourth leading cause of death in North America; currently, it is the only major cause of adult mortality to increase over the past 35 years. Globally it is predicted to be the third major cause of death by 2020 (1). In the advanced stages of COPD, acute exacerbations lead to frequent hospitalizations, including admissions to the intensive care unit (ICU) for treatment of respiratory failure. Few published guidelines exist to assist patients with COPD or their care-givers in dealing with end-of-life issues (2), despite the importance of this chronic disease in terms of its prevalence,

negative impact on health-related quality of life and ultimately on the manner of patients' death.

People in the Western, developed world live in a 'death denying' culture that often fails to serve the needs of individuals facing imminent death. Most individuals with advanced COPD have not taken the opportunity to clearly articulate the level of care they wish to receive as COPD progresses, including decisions about advanced life support (3–5). Until recently, descriptions of experiences of COPD patients as they approached the end of their lives have been limited (6). Recent survey data and studies using qualitative approaches have led to improved understanding of these experiences that should assist patients, their families and health care providers in exploring concerns and planning for issues that they will face at the end of life.

In the current climate of shared decision-making, accurate data are needed to better inform patients of their prognoses and treatment options (7, 8). Unfortunately, in COPD, accurate predictions for individual patients usually cannot be made for several critical aspects of management (e.g. rates of short- and long-term survival during acute exacerbation). However, data from recent significant studies of outcome of hospital admissions for COPD acute exacerbation and predictors of long-term survival in stable COPD should provide insights to both care-givers and patients involved in the decision-making process (9–13).

COPD PATIENTS' PERSPECTIVES

What do our COPD patients tell us?

A desire to improve the care of patients with COPD implies a commitment to listening to patients and taking subsequent action based upon this information. Singer *et al.* (14) described five domains of quality end-of-life care reported by patients suffering from chronic health conditions (Box 40.1) (14). COPD patients have indicated specific qualities and skills that they expect of their physicians in order for them to be able to provide high-quality end-of-life care (Box 40.2) (15).

In contrast to these ideals, major sources of dissatisfaction described by patients with 'end stage' COPD in a UK study included perceptions of inadequate provision of information about their illness, treatment options and availability of social supports (16); 78 per cent of patients felt that they did not have enough information about their prognosis and issues related to future management, while 30 per cent of patients felt that diagnostic information was lacking or provided insensitively. Of particular concern, 26 per cent of patients didn't know that COPD was potentially fatal. In addition, much patient information was derived at the time of hospital admission and often from conversations with other non-physician health care professionals (16).

Our understanding of the experiences of patients living with severe COPD has been enhanced by research conducted using qualitative methodology. Guthrie *et al.* (17) conducted in-depth, semi-structured interviews in the UK with 37 patients living with severe COPD. The interviewer focused on psychosocial issues, including patients' thoughts about death. The authors concluded that patients were preoccupied with personal and interpersonal matters rather than with physical distress or medical issues. Patients spoke of fear of isolation and the manner in which they might die. Several subjects raised the option of suicide. The authors called for an extension of palliative care services to cover a wider spectrum of advanced chronic diseases like COPD (17). In another qualitative research study, entitled 'Death stories: acute exacerbations of chronic obstructive pulmonary disease', Bailey (6) described patients as living in the 'shadow of fear and uncertainty cast by their near-death experiences'.

Functional status and quality of life in advanced COPD

There are numerous determinants of functional status in COPD, including severity of airflow obstruction, blood gas abnormalities, frequency and severity of acute exacerbations, age, presence of co-morbidities (e.g. anxiety and depression, malnutrition, peripheral muscle dysfunction) and level of social support (18). Health-related quality of life scores were worse for the patients with COPD in the Study to Understand Prognoses and Preferences for Outcomes and Risks of Treatment (SUPPORT) than for patients who had survived cardiopulmonary resuscitation (19). In addition, 80 per cent of the patients interviewed at 6 months after admission considered their quality of life to be no better than fair or poor (9). In a study of 321 men with COPD of varying severity, health-related quality of life (HRQL) worsened as severity increased and was impaired, relative to the general population, even when FEV_1 exceeded 50 per cent of predicted (20). More recently Fan *et al.* (21) reported that lower quality of life and particularly low scores in the physical domain were powerful predictors of hospital admission – odds ratio (OR) 6.0, 95 per cent CI, 3.1–11.5 – and subsequent death (OR 6.8, 95 per cent CI, 3.3–13.8).

In a study comparing patients with non-small-cell lung cancer and COPD, those with COPD reported lower scores ($P < 0.05$) for activities of daily living, social and physical functioning, more depression (90 vs. 52 per cent) and lack of access to palliative care services (0 vs. 30 per cent) (16). This underscores the general lack of effective end-of-life care for many patients dying of diseases other than cancer. In the SUPPORT study, cancer patients tended to die away from critical care settings with good symptom control (22). However, for patients with COPD, death often came in the ICU setting, with technically assisted support being provided (e.g. mechanical ventilator, feeding tubes) and surrogates reporting poor symptom control (22).

HEALTH CARE PROVIDERS' PERSPECTIVE

What do physicians discuss with their COPD patients?

A recent survey of Canadian respirologists focused on questions such as where, when, and how physicians discussed end-of-life

---

Box 40.1 Determinants of quality end-of-life care: patients' perspective. Adapted from Singer *et al.* (14).

- Receiving adequate pain and symptom management
- Avoiding inappropriate prolongation of dying
- Achieving a sense of control
- Relieving burden placed upon loved ones
- Strengthening relationships with loved ones

Box 40.2 Qualities physicians need to provide high-quality end-of-life care to COPD patients. Adapted from Curtis *et al.* (15).

- Ability to provide emotional support
- Ability to communicate effectively
- Accessibility
- Provision of continuity of care
- Provision to patients with information in five content areas:
  - diagnosis and disease progression
  - treatment options
  - prognosis
  - expectations of death from COPD
  - advance care planning

issues with COPD patients (4). When discussing mechanical ventilation for 'end-stage COPD', 41 per cent of respondents stated that these discussions take place in the ICU, and only 23 per cent in the clinic or office (4). The degree of dyspnoea influenced timing of these discussions; 84 per cent of respondents wait until dyspnoea is severe, while 75 per cent of respondents wait until the FEV_1 is <30 per cent of predicted. When discussing mechanical ventilation, almost all physicians spontaneously mention intubation (96.8 per cent) but most (70 per cent) wait until asked by the patient to discuss weaning or extubation. Certain biases creep into these conversations. For example, mechanical ventilation is discouraged by physicians in a setting of alcohol abuse, severe depression and smoking >2.5 packs per day by 16, 17 and 26 per cent of respondents, respectively (4). The authors wrote: 'At the very least, this observation suggests that physicians should question their beliefs and biases when making end-of-life recommendations' (4). Physicians need to be aware of the influence on patients' choices relating to the way in which they frame end-of-life discussions (23).

How could physicians improve end-of-life discussions with their COPD patients?

Curtis (24) described three critical phases to end-of-life care discussions: making preparations, conducting and closing discussions. In making preparations, physicians should review their knowledge of patients' illness, their attitudes and knowledge of their own disease. An appropriate setting, time and decision about who will be present should be arranged prior to the meeting. In conducting the discussions, following introductions, physicians should find out how much patients know and want to know. Discussions should be frank and honest without removing all hope. Physicians should acknowledge strong emotions, tolerate silence and encourage patients and families to express their feelings. In closing these discussions, an understanding of what to expect for the disease course and treatment options should be restated. Patients often need reminding that withholding resuscitation measures does not equate to withdrawing care. Patients and families should leave knowing how to reach the physician after the meeting closes to reinforce that they are not being abandoned.

Physicians should encourage specific discussions about patients' fears, support systems, including whether to involve palliative care services, preferences for where patients want to die and for use of mechanical ventilation versus comfort measures in the setting of respiratory failure. The importance of kindness in these discussions cannot be overemphasized (25).

Who should be involved in end-of-life discussions?

Many physicians leave end-of-life discussions about COPD until the time of the ICU admission (4). There is little about the typical ICU environment that lends itself to the optimal conduct of end-of-life discussions. Discussions in the primary

care setting might be one potential answer (26). In a survey, most (72.5 per cent) of the 214 responding GPs thought that discussions of prognosis were necessary or essential, and 82 per cent felt they had an important role (26). In contrast, only 41 per cent of GPs reported often or always discussing prognosis with their COPD patients. Of the 33 GPs who reported they rarely or never discussed prognosis with their patients, most felt ill-prepared for this task (26). The authors concluded that 'the palliative care approach of open communication, whilst seen to be relevant to severe COPD, is not applied routinely in managing the disease in primary care'(26).

The shift in emphasis of goals of care (Fig. 40.1) that occurs as COPD advances fits well with the principles of palliative care medicine. Palliative care has been defined as a holistic approach to the alleviation of symptoms and suffering (physical, emotional and spiritual) when finding a cure or reversing the underlying disease process is no longer possible (27). One goal of palliative care is to provide the best possible quality of life for patients and their families. Control of symptoms is of paramount importance. This approach is applicable to the care of all COPD patients, independent of stage of disease, but is especially relevant for those with advanced disease at the end-of-life. To narrow the gap between patients' needs and what health care professionals provide, more formal links with palliative care programmes might help. However, where access to formal palliative care services is unavailable, respirologists and GPs (who currently report being ill-prepared for the task) will continue to provide the bulk of care to dying COPD patients.

What is the role of pulmonary rehabilitation programmes in end-of-life discussions?

A pulmonary rehabilitation programme seems an ideal venue for end-of-life discussions to take place. The multidisciplinary team has frequent contact with patients and family members during exercise and education sessions to develop a trusting relationship. Pulmonary rehabilitation programmes emphasize patient and family education which enables them to make

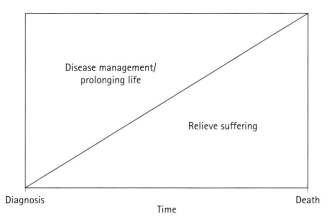

Figure 40.1 *Palliative care: a shift in emphasis in goals of chronic obstructive pulmonary disease care.*

decisions to improve their health and quality of life. When questioned, nearly all patients attending one pulmonary rehabilitation programme reported a desire for a patient–physician discussion about both advance directives and life support. Despite this, however, these discussions had actually taken place for only 19 and 15 per cent of patients, respectively (5). Only 14 per cent of patients thought that physicians involved in the programme understood their wishes in regard to end-of-life care (5).

Seventy-eight per cent of 214 pulmonary rehabilitation programmes surveyed in the USA considered their programme an appropriate site for education about advance directives, and 86 per cent were willing to add this to their educational programmes (28). However, two-thirds indicated that they did not provide education regarding advance directives, and 48 per cent of programmes failed to provide any educational material. Most programmes 'had no knowledge of their patients' advance directives' (3). Although only a minority of COPD patients is able to attend pulmonary rehabilitation, we should ensure that at least these patients are given the opportunity to discuss end-of-life issues with their health care providers.

Other data suggest that when patients are provided educational materials and an opportunity to document their wishes, the rate of writing advance directives improves (28). However, a recent multicentre international observational study reported that advance directives had been established within 24 h of an ICU admission for only 11 per cent of close to 3000 patients (29).

COPD OUTCOME DATA TO INFORM END-OF-LIFE DISCUSSIONS

Acute exacerbations of COPD requiring hospitalization

In 1998, COPD accounted for over 5000 deaths, or 4 per cent of all deaths in Canada. Mortality rates were highest among the elderly, especially those over 70 years of age. Mortality rates were markedly higher in men than in women (31). As the population ages, mortality rates due to COPD are expected to climb, especially among women.

Two recent studies have reported outcomes of more than 1000 admissions due to acute exacerbations of COPD (AECOPD) (9, 11). The SUPPORT study published outcomes of 1016 patients admitted to five US hospitals with hypercapnia complicating AECOPD (9). Patients had an average age of 70 years, were 51.5 per cent male, and 78.1 per cent had more than two significant co-morbid illnesses. The mortality rate for the index admission was 11 per cent. Mortality was progressively higher at 60 days, 180 days, 1 year and 2 years (20, 33, 43 and 49 per cent, respectively). Six-month mortality increased from 21 per cent for patients not readmitted, to 36 per cent for those readmitted two or more times.

The SUPPORT study data were collated between 1989 and 1994 from only five US centres before widespread use of non-invasive mechanical ventilation (NIV) for AECOPD complicated by hypercapnia (32). This limits some of the inferences that can be made. Other limitations apply to a UK data set from a British Thoracic Society (BTS) clinical audit (11). In the BTS study, data were collated from 1400 admissions from 1997 to 2001, but 'only 13 per cent of potentially eligible patients' received some form of ventilatory support. These limitations not withstanding, both studies reported factors that independently increased risk of mortality at 6 months (9) and 3 months (11), respectively, that clinicians should factor into their discussions about prognosis and end-of-life decisions with their COPD patients.

Other recent substantial studies of more than 100 patients hospitalized for AECOPD reported similar index admission mortality rates from 11 to 24 per cent (12, 13, 33, 34). Studies that have focused on specific population subsets suggest increased mortality in patients using long-term oxygen (50 per cent index admission mortality in a Spanish Study) (35) and patients who could not be weaned after 21 days of mechanical ventilation (68 per cent 2-year mortality) (36).

Age is the most consistent predictor of death in patients admitted for AECOPD. In the BTS study, relative to patients <65 years old, the odds ratios (95 per cent CI) of death at 3 months for those aged 75–79 years and >80 years, were 2.2 (1.3–1.7) and 3.0 (1.8–4.9), respectively (11). Meanwhile survival subsequent to successful discharge varies. In two studies of 270 and 362 patients, median survivals were reported as 3.1 years and 224 days, respectively (10, 34). Age and presence of co-morbidities again proved to be predictors of death (10, 34).

Other predictive factors include the degree of acidosis on presentation and pre-existing functional status. A bed-bound functional status prior to hospital admission increased the risk of death by a factor of 20 (11). Whilst the BTS study showed that a presenting pH <7.26 increased the relative risk of mortality at 3 months (relative to pH >7.35) to 3.8 (CI 2.7–5.4), this was not confirmed in SUPPORT study. Finally, in the BTS study, a presenting haemoglobin oxygen saturation of S_aO_2 <86 per cent increased the mortality risk by a factor of 2.3 (95 per cent CI 1.6–3.2) relative to a S_aO_2 >92 per cent (11).

Predictors of survival in stable COPD

In 985 COPD patients followed for 3 years, initial FEV_1 and age were the most important predictors of survival (37). In a Dutch retrospective study of 400 patients with COPD, low body mass index (BMI), age and low P_aO_2 were significant independent predictors of increased mortality (37). In a prospective study of 203 COPD patients, weight gain through nutritional therapy with or without anabolic steroids had a positive impact on survival (38). A low BMI was also associated with increased mortality in the Copenhagen City Heart Study, in which 2132 subjects with airflow obstruction were followed for 17 years (relative risk 7.11, 95 per cent CI 2.97–17.05) (39), and in a recent UK prospective cohort study of 137 elderly patients with COPD (40).

Readmission rates

Among the 1400 BTS study patients, there was a 34 per cent readmission rate within 3 months of the index hospitalization (11). Of the 900 SUPPORT study patients who survived to index discharge, 446 (50 per cent) were readmitted 754 times over the next 6 months: 254 patients (28 per cent) once, 116 (13 per cent) twice and 76 (9 per cent) three times or more. In a review of the last 6 months of life of the 416 patients who died with COPD, these patients spent 15–25 per cent of their remaining time in hospital (19). Data from Ontario, Canada, also demonstrated that the majority of patients with COPD die in hospital (41).

In the BTS study, the following factors were the major independent predictors (OR, 95 per cent CI) of hospital readmission: previous admission (2.5, 2.0–3.2); lower percentage of predicted FEV_1 (1.8, 1.4–2.3) and more than five medications at the time of readmission (2.7, 2.0–3.7) (11).

SYMPTOM MANAGEMENT

Dyspnoea is a disturbing and complex symptom that can be described as the subjective awareness of the uncomfortable sensation of one's own breathing (42). The vast majority of patients with advanced COPD report moderate to severe dyspnoea as the overriding complaint affecting their quality of life (19). Clinical assessment of 'respiratory difficulty' often fails to match patients' perception of their level of dyspnoea. However, validated measurement tools exist that allow researchers to quantify dyspnoea in COPD (43, 44). It is possible (but unproven) that these tools may also have a role in helping clinicians and family care-givers to quantify dyspnoea severity in COPD patients in order to establish the effectiveness of treatment interventions.

Whether or not specific treatment for COPD is effective in alleviating dyspnoea, all patients with advanced disease should receive non-specific palliative measures. A variety of pharmacological and non-pharmacological interventions can help. Simple measures such as directing cool air onto the face with a fan, a change in body position and teaching patients to conserve energy and pace themselves can effectively reduce dyspnoea (45, 46).

Psychological factors such as anxiety, fear and panic frequently play a role in heightening dyspnoea in COPD, especially at the end of life (47). The concerns of patients and family care-givers need to be addressed in a supportive and empathetic manner. Anxiety can often be partially alleviated by simply clarifying the aetiology of dyspnoea and treatment options available to the patient. Relaxation and breathing techniques (e.g. pursed-lip breathing) may be of help to patients during panic attacks. Other forms of psychological support (e.g. stress management, coping skills training and cognitive restructuring) have been less well-studied in severe COPD (47). Despite conflicting results in studies, anxiolytic medication may also be helpful when non-pharmacological measures have failed (46, 47).

Oxygen administration can reduce ventilation by decreasing hypoxic drive mediated by peripheral chemoreceptors, one mechanism postulated to account for the reduction of dyspnoea (42). Individual responses vary. There is some evidence that acute administration of oxygen can reduce dyspnoea in patients with terminal cancer (48, 49). The benefit in terms of survival, haemodynamics and neurocognitive function of long-term oxygen in appropriately chosen, stable COPD patients has been recognized for two decades (50–52). However, palliation of dyspnoea through supplemental oxygen administration in mildly hypoxaemic patients with COPD has not yet been adequately investigated to recommend its routine use at this time.

Opioids reduce dyspnoea and ventilation in COPD in response to a variety of stimuli (42). The mode of action by which opioids relieve dyspnoea is poorly understood. Clinically, respiratory depression is an uncommon problem if patients are initiated on a low dose and titrated slowly according to response and side-effects. Tolerance to the respiratory depressant effect develops quickly (53). Risk of respiratory depression increases with dose, rate of administration, prior opioid use, combined use with any other respiratory depressants, and advanced age (54). In a review of the use of opioids in dyspnoea management, adverse effects were reported more often in the studies using multiple doses in opioid naive patients (55). These potential problems notwithstanding, physicians have a duty to relieve the burden of distress experienced by dyspnoeic patients with advanced COPD. Opioid medications should be considered for palliation of severe dyspnoea in the terminal stages of COPD.

Comfort care may also include medications to reduce cough and retained respiratory secretions (56). Opioids and inhaled local anaesthetic agents may be helpful in alleviating cough. Retained respiratory secretions may be dried temporarily with the use of anticholinergic agents. Alternatively, adequate patient hydration may reduce viscosity of respiratory secretions, making them easier to expectorate either spontaneously or with chest physiotherapy.

Emotional consequences of severe COPD

Depression is frequently reported to reduce the quality of life of individuals with severe COPD, with prevalence rates ranging from 7 to 42 per cent (57). Lacasse et al. (58) demonstrated that in a group of severe, oxygen-dependent COPD patients, 57 per cent reported depressive symptoms and 18 per cent were found to be severe. Depression can heighten patients' awareness of physical symptoms while diminishing their capacity to cope with the struggles of living with a chronic, debilitating illness such as COPD. Effective management of depression in COPD can be complicated by under-diagnosis, under-treatment due to fear of side-effects and lack of timely referral to appropriate resources (47).

Is there a role for palliative non-invasive mechanical ventilation?

The long-term prognosis for patients who are hospitalized with AECOPD is poor. However, the likelihood of short-term survival to hospital discharge is high, approximately 90 per cent. For COPD patients with acute respiratory failure complicating an episode of AECOPD, survival rates fall to between 75 and 90 per cent (34, 59). This still suggests that acute respiratory failure complicating AECOPD has a more favourable short-term prognosis than acute respiratory failure from other causes. A more favourable prognosis has accrued with more widespread use of NIV for AECOPD (32). Many patients with AECOPD are able to avoid intubation.

At the end of life, the rationale for providing technically assisted support (e.g. NIV) should be grounded firmly in the need to provide comfort care. Two uncontrolled trials reported that NIV can reduce dyspnoea and preserve patient autonomy in appropriately selected patients (60, 61). There are no controlled trials demonstrating that NIV provides more comfort than medical management alone. This does not preclude the use of NIV for patients who would otherwise choose not to be intubated, with the understanding that if it cannot achieve its aims within an accepted time-frame, it can and should be withdrawn. Patients may benefit from the extra time it allows them to complete important tasks. If the patient, care-givers and health care team feel that benefits outweigh the risks, then there may be a time-limited role for palliative NIV (62).

CARE–GIVER BURDEN

The current trend in health care is to shift patient care delivery to the outpatient setting. This adds to the substantial burden that care-givers already experience in supporting a family member with advanced COPD. The impacts on family care-givers can be divided broadly into three categories (56):

- physical demands of providing care
- emotional demands of supporting a loved one with a chronic or terminal illness
- financial expense.

A number of instruments have been developed as tools to measure care-giver burden. Unfortunately, many lack adequate reliability, validity or content specificity for application in research (63). Few COPD studies have reported measures of care-giver burden. A recent Veterans Affairs study from the US reported the effectiveness of team-managed, home-based primary care on patient outcomes, care-giver burden and care-giver HRQL (64). This randomized, controlled, multicentre trial involved 1966 patients suffering from a terminal illness, congestive heart failure or COPD. Compared with usual care, the team-managed, home-based primary care model significantly reduced care-giver burden and improved care-giver HRQL.

DECISION AIDS AND ADVANCE DIRECTIVES

Dales *et al.* (65) have described a decision aid for COPD patients considering mechanical ventilation. In a preliminary report, 10 out of 10 women and two out of 10 men declined mechanical ventilation after considering the descriptions of their disease, mechanical ventilation and a hypothetical scenario. Decision aids may be helpful, but their value needs to be further assessed in more substantial studies.

Formalizing plans following end-of-life discussions in an advance directive should improve the likelihood that patients receive the level of care they desire (66). There are many barriers to both the creation and adoption of advance directives, but none is insurmountable (2). Plans need to be subject to ongoing review and include an understanding of the flexibility or rigidity of such directives in specific circumstances (2). Martin *et al.* (67) have provided a useful overview of advance care planning in general, including the goals of care, and types and utility of advance directives.

Quill (68) reminds us that: 'When physicians provide their patients with the honesty, expertise, compassion and commitment they would want for themselves and their families, they provide the highest quality medical care possible.' He concludes: 'There is little or nothing to lose in initiating palliative care discussions earlier and more systematically in a patient's final trajectory, and so much is lost when these discussions are avoided.' If these discussions take place, our COPD patients will be better informed and more confident that their health care providers will not abandon them at the end of life.

Key points

- COPD is a common, progressive, disabling condition that negatively impacts on quality of life and ultimately ends in respiratory failure and death.
- Mortality during admission for treatment of an AECOPD ranges from 10 to 20 per cent. Age, presence of gas exchange abnormalities, body mass index and functional status are important predictors of death. Unfortunately, it remains difficult to accurately predict short- and long-term survival of individual COPD patients.
- Pharmacological and non-pharmacological treatments are available to alleviate distressing respiratory symptoms, such as dyspnoea, cough and retained respiratory secretions.
- Emotional consequences of living with advanced COPD include anxiety, fear, panic and depression. These psychological factors can impose a barrier to effective symptom control, reduce quality of life and require multidimensional management strategies.
- Care-giver burden is likely to be substantial but is largely unmeasured in COPD patients and their families.
- There is a considerable disparity between patients' expectations for information about their disease and its prognosis and what physicians provide. Discussions about end-of-life issues are often held too late and in

inappropriate settings. Lack of access to formal palliative care services means that family physicians provide the majority of end-of-life care to COPD patients, a task they feel ill-prepared to face.

● Informed discussions among patients, families and physicians regarding advance directives should improve the likelihood that patients receive the levels of care that they would choose. Decision aids may assist patients when considering intubation and mechanical ventilation.

REFERENCES

1. Murray CJ, Lopez AD. Alternative projections of mortality and disability by cause 1990–2020: Global Burden of Disease Study. *Lancet* 1997; **349**: 1498–504.

2. Heffner JE. Chronic obstructive pulmonary disease: ethical considerations of care. *Clini Pulmon Med* 1996; **3**: 1–8.

3. Heffner JE, Fahy B, Barbieri C. Advance directive education during pulmonary rehabilitation. *Chest* 1996; **109**: 373–9.

4. McNeely PD, Hebert PC, Dales RE *et al.* Deciding about mechanical ventilation in end-stage chronic obstructive pulmonary disease: how respirologists perceive their role. *Can Med Assoc J* 1997; **156**: 177–83.

●5. Heffner JE, Fahy B, Hilling L, Barbieri C. Attitudes regarding advance directives among patients in pulmonary rehabilitation. *Am J Respir Crit Care Med* 1996; **154** (6 Pt 1): 1735–40.

6. Bailey PH. Death stories: acute exacerbations of chronic obstructive pulmonary disease. *Qual Health Res* 2001; **11**: 322–38.

7. Emanuel EJ, Emanuel LL. Four models of the physician-patient relationship. *J Am Med Assoc* 1992; **267**: 2221–6.

8. Heyland DK, Rocker GM, Dodek P *et al.* Decision-making in the ICU. Perspectives of the substitute decision-maker. *Am J Respir Crit Care Med* 2002; **165**: A254.

●9. Connors AF, Jr, Dawson NV, Thomas C *et al.* Outcomes following acute exacerbation of severe chronic obstructive lung disease. The SUPPORT investigators (Study to Understand Prognoses and Preferences for Outcomes and Risks of Treatments). *Am J Respir Crit Care Med* 1996; **154** (4 Pt 1): 959–67.

10. Antonelli Incalzi R, Fuso L, De Rosa M *et al.* Co-morbidity contributes to predict mortality of patients with chronic obstructive pulmonary disease. *Eur Respir J* 1997; **10**: 2794–800.

●11. Roberts CM, Lowe D, Bucknall CE *et al.* Clinical audit indicators of outcome following admission to hospital with acute exacerbation of chronic obstructive pulmonary disease. *Thorax* 2002; **57**: 137–41.

12. Moran JL, Green JV, Homan SD *et al.* Acute exacerbations of chronic obstructive pulmonary disease and mechanical ventilation: a reevaluation. *Crit Care Med* 1998; **26**: 71–8.

13. Nevins ML, Epstein SK. Predictors of outcome for patients with COPD requiring invasive mechanical ventilation. *Chest* 2001; **119**: 1840–9.

●14. Singer PA, Martin DK, Kelner M. Quality end-of-life care. Patients' perspectives. *J Am Med Assoc* 1999; **281**: 163–8.

15. Curtis JR, Wenrich MD, Carline JD *et al.* Patients' perspectives on physician skill in end-of-life care: differences between patients with COPD, cancer, and AIDS. *Chest* 2002; **122**: 356–62.

16. Gore JM, Brophy CJ, Greenstone MA. How well do we care for patients with end stage chronic obstructive pulmonary disease (COPD)? A comparison of palliative care and quality of life in COPD and lung cancer. *Thorax* 2000; **55**: 1000–6.

17. Guthrie SJ, Hill KM, Muers ME. Living with severe COPD. A qualitative exploration of the experience of patients in Leeds. *Respir Med* 2001; **95**: 196–204.

18. Curtis JR, Deyo RA, Hudson LD. Pulmonary rehabilitation in chronic respiratory insufficiency. 7. Health-related quality of life among patients with chronic obstructive pulmonary disease. *Thorax* 1994; **49**: 162–70.

19. Lynn J, Ely EW, Zhong Z *et al.* Living and dying with chronic obstructive pulmonary disease. *J Am Geriatr Soc* 2000; **48** (5 Suppl.): S91–100.

20. Ferrer M, Alonso J, Morera J *et al.* Chronic obstructive pulmonary disease stage and health-related quality of life. The Quality of Life of Chronic Obstructive Pulmonary Disease Study Group. *Ann Intern Med* 1997; **127**: 1072–9.

21. Fan VS, Curtis JR, Tu SP *et al.* Using quality of life to predict hospitalization and mortality in patients with obstructive lung diseases. *Chest* 2002; **122**: 429–36.

22. Claessens MT, Lynn J, Zhong Z *et al.* Dying with lung cancer or chronic obstructive pulmonary disease: insights from SUPPORT. Study to Understand Prognoses and Preferences for Outcomes and Risks of Treatments. *J Am Geriatr Soc* 2000; **48** (5 Suppl.): S146–53.

●23. Sullivan KE, Hebert PC, Logan J *et al.* What do physicians tell patients with end-stage COPD about intubation and mechanical ventilation? *Chest* 1996; **109**: 258–64.

●24. Curtis JR. Communicating with patients and their families about advance care planning and end-of-life care. *Respir Care* 2000; **45**: 1385–94 (discussion 1394–8).

25. Rousseau P. Kindness and the end of life. *West J Med* 2001; **174**: 292.

●26. Elkington H, White P, Higgs R, Pettinari CJ. GPs' views of discussions of prognosis in severe COPD. *Fam Pract* 2001; **18**: 440–4.

27. Heffner JE, Fahy B, Hilling L, Barbieri C. Outcomes of advance directive education of pulmonary rehabilitation patients. *Am J Respir Crit Care Med* 1997; **155**: 1055–9.

28. MacDonald N. *Palliative Medicine, Pain Control and Symptom Assessment. In: Caring for the Dying – Identification and Promotion of Physician Competency.* Philadelphia: American Board of Internal Medicine, 1999; 11–26.

29. Cook DJ, Guyatt G, Rocker G *et al.* Cardiopulmonary resuscitation directives on admission to intensive-care unit: an international observational study. *Lancet* 2001; **358**: 1941–5.

30. Roy D. The times and places of palliative care. *J Palliat Care* 2000; **16** (Suppl.): S3–4.

31. McFarlane A, Goldstein, R. COPD. In: *Respiratory Disease in Canada.* Ottawa, Canada: Health Canada, 2001; 45–55.

32. Plant PK, Owen JL, Elliott MW. Non-invasive ventilation in acute exacerbations of chronic obstructive pulmonary disease: long term survival and predictors of in-hospital outcome. *Thorax* 2001; **56**: 708–12.

33. Esteban A, Anzueto A, Frutos F *et al.* Characteristics and outcomes in adult patients receiving mechanical ventilation: a 28-day international study. *J Am Med Assoc* 2002; **287**: 345–55.

34. Seneff MG, Wagner DP, Wagner RP *et al.* Hospital and 1-year survival of patients admitted to intensive care units with acute exacerbation of chronic obstructive pulmonary disease. *J Am Med Assoc* 1995; **274**: 1852–7.

35. Anon JM, Garcia de Lorenzo A, Zarazaga A *et al.* Mechanical ventilation of patients on long-term oxygen therapy with acute exacerbations of chronic obstructive pulmonary disease: prognosis and cost-utility analysis. *Intensive Care Med* 1999; **25**: 452–7.

36. Nava S, Rubini F, Zanotti E *et al.* Survival and prediction of successful ventilator weaning in COPD patients requiring mechanical ventilation for more than 21 days. *Eur Respir J* 1994; **7**: 1645–52.

37. Anthonisen NR, Wright EC, Hodgkin JE. Prognosis in chronic obstructive pulmonary disease. *Am Rev Respir Dis* 1986; **133**: 14–20.

38. Schols AM, Slangen J, Volovics L, Wouters EF. Weight loss is a reversible factor in the prognosis of chronic obstructive pulmonary disease. *Am J Respir Crit Care Med* 1998; **157** (6 Pt 1): 1791–7.

39. Landbo C, Prescott E, Lange P *et al.* Prognostic value of nutritional status in chronic obstructive pulmonary disease. *Am J Respir Crit Care Med* 1999; **160**: 1856–61.

40. Yohannes AM, Baldwin RC, Connolly M. Mortality predictors in disabling chronic obstructive pulmonary disease in old age. *Age Ageing* 2002; **31**: 137–40.

41. Heyland DK, Lavery JV, Tranmer JE, Shortt SED. The final days: an analysis of the dying experience in Ontario. *Annals RCPSC* 2000; **33**: 365–1.

42. American Thoracic Society. Dyspnea. Mechanisms, assessment, and management: a consensus statement. *Am J Respir Crit Care Med* 1999; **159**: 321–40.

43. Borg GA. Psychophysical bases of perceived exertion. *Med Sci Sports Exerc* 1982; **14**: 377–81.

44. Mahler DA, Rosiello RA, Harver A *et al.* Comparison of clinical dyspnea ratings and psychophysical measurements of respiratory sensation in obstructive airway disease. *Am Rev Respir Dis* 1987; **135**: 1229–33.

45. Schwartzstein RM, Lahive K, Pope A *et al.* Cold facial stimulation reduces breathlessness induced in normal subjects. *Am Rev Respir Dis* 1987; **136**: 58–61.

46. Hernandez P. Dyspnea in palliative care. *Can J CME* 2000; **13**: 57–72.

47. Nault D, Siok MA, Borycki E *et al.* Psychological considerations in COPD. In: Boubeau J, Naul D, Borycki E, eds. *Comprehensive Management of COPD.* Hamilton: BC Decker, 2002; 215–44.

48. Bruera E, de Stoutz N, Velasco-Leiva A *et al.* Effects of oxygen on dyspnoea in hypoxaemic terminal-cancer patients. *Lancet* 1993; **342**: 13–14.

49. Booth S, Kelly MJ, Cox NP *et al.* Does oxygen help dyspnea in patients with cancer? *Am J Respir Crit Care Med* 1996; **153**: 1515–18.

50. Nocturnal Oxygen Therapy Trial Group. Continuous or nocturnal oxygen therapy in hypoxemic chronic obstructive lung disease: a clinical trial. *Ann Intern Med* 1980; **93**: 391–8.

51. Medical Research Council Working Party. Long term domiciliary oxygen therapy in chronic hypoxic cor pulmonale complicating chronic bronchitis and emphysema. *Lancet* 1981; **1**: 681–6.

52. Anthonisen NR. Long-term oxygen therapy. *Ann Intern Med* 1983; **99**: 519–27.

53. Bruera E, Macmillan K, Pither J, MacDonald RN. Effects of morphine on the dyspnea of terminal cancer patients. *J Pain Symptom Manage* 1990; **5**: 341–4.

◆54. Davis CL. ABC of palliative care. Breathlessness, cough, and other respiratory problems. *Br Med J* 1997; **315**: 931–4.

55. Jennings AL, Davies AN, Higgins JP *et al.* A systematic review of the use of opioids in the management of dyspnoea. *Thorax* 2002; **57**: 939–44.

56. Heffner J. Chronic obstructive pulmonary disease. In: Curtis J, Rubenfield G, eds. *Managing Death in the ICU: The Transition from Cure to Comfort.* New York: Oxford University Press, 2000; 319–28.

57. van Ede L, Yzermans CJ, Brouwer HJ. Prevalence of depression in patients with chronic obstructive pulmonary disease: a systematic review. *Thorax* 1999; **54**: 688–92.

58. Lacasse Y, Rousseau L, Maltais F. Prevalence of depressive symptoms and depression in patients with severe oxygen-dependent chronic obstructive pulmonary disease. *J Cardiopulm Rehabil* 2001; **21**: 80–6.

59. Plant PK, Owen JL, Elliott MW. Early use of non-invasive ventilation for acute exacerbations of chronic obstructive pulmonary disease on general respiratory wards: a multicentre randomised controlled trial. *Lancet* 2000; **355**: 1931–5.

60. Benhamou D, Girault C, Faure C *et al.* Nasal mask ventilation in acute respiratory failure. Experience in elderly patients. *Chest* 1992; **102**: 912–17.

61. Meduri GU, Fox RC, Abou-Shala N *et al.* Noninvasive mechanical ventilation via face mask in patients with acute respiratory failure who refused endotracheal intubation. *Crit Care Med* 1994; **22**: 1584–90.

62. Benditt JO. Noninvasive ventilation at the end of life. *Respir Care* 2000; **45**: 1376–81 (discussion 1381–4).

◆63. Kinsella G. A review of the measurement of caregiver and family burden in palliative care. *J Palliat Care* 1998; **14**: 37–45.

64. Hughes SL, Weaver FM, Giobbie-Hurder A *et al.* Effectiveness of team-managed home-based primary care: a randomized multicenter trial. *J Am Med Assoc* 2000; **284**: 2877–85.

●65. Dales RE, O'Connor A, Hebert P *et al.* Intubation and mechanical ventilation for COPD: development of an instrument to elicit patient preferences. *Chest* 1999; **116**: 792–800.

66. Lynn J, Goldstein NE. Advance care planning for fatal chronic illness: avoiding commonplace errors and unwarranted suffering. *Ann Intern Med* 2003; **138**: 812–18.

67. Martin DK, Emanuel LL, Singer PA. Planning for the end of life. *Lancet* 2000; **356**: 1672–6.

68. Quill TE. Perspectives on care at the close of life. Initiating end-of-life discussions with seriously ill patients: addressing the 'elephant in the room'. *J Am Med Assoc* 2000; **284**: 2502–7.

Index

Page numbers in **bold type** refer to figures; those in *italics* to tables and boxes.

Derby Hospitals NHS Foundation
Trust
Library and Knowledge Service